Nutrition and Health

Adrianne Bendich, Ph.D., FACN, FASN, Series Editor

More information about this series at http://www.springer.com/series/7659

Rajkumar Rajendram
Victor R. Preedy • Vinood B. Patel
Editors

Glutamine in Clinical Nutrition

Humana Press

Editors
Rajkumar Rajendram
Department of Intensive Care
Barnet and Chase Farm Hospitals
Royal Free London NHS
Foundation Trust
London, UK

Victor R. Preedy
Department of Nutrition and Dietetics
Diabetes and Nutritional Sciences
School of Medicine
King's College London
London, UK

Vinood B. Patel
Department of Biomedical Sciences
University of Westminster
London, UK

ISBN 978-1-4939-1931-4 ISBN 978-1-4939-1932-1 (eBook)
DOI 10.1007/978-1-4939-1932-1
Springer New York Heidelberg Dordrecht London

Library of Congress Control Number: 2014957307

Printed on acid-free paper

Humana Press is a brand of Springer
Springer is part of Springer Science+Business Media (www.springer.com)

Preface

Glutamine was originally considered a nonessential amino acid due the fact that it can be synthesized from glutamate. Glutamine is also the most abundant amino acid and a major contributor to whole body nitrogen metabolism in man. However, over several decades, evidence has supported the notion that glutamine is "conditionally essential" and thus important in human health. For example, glutamine protects the intestinal tract, skeletal muscle, and neuronal tissue against metabolic stress. Some of the earlier studies showed that reduced intracellular glutamine in muscle was associated with loss of lean tissue or wasting. This led to the development of nutritional support regimens in which glutamine was administered by enteral or parental routes. However, this is rather a simplistic notion of glutamine's role and potential in disease. It is now known that glutamine has an almost ubiquitous function and is important in maintaining the cellular milieu of virtually every organ in the human body. Thus, its supplementation not only modulates skeletal muscle mass in postsurgical stress but also improves lymphocyte count, enhances outcome scores, and ameliorates the peroxidation of lipids as just a few examples. However, more recent studies have suggested that the administration of glutamine conjugated, or co-administered, with substrates provides greater efficacy that glutamine alone. Furthermore the efficacy of conjugated glutamine is enhanced when administered in complex cocktails that may contain other nutraceuticals. The science of glutamine is thus complex, and finding all the relevant information in a single source has hitherto been problematic. This is however addressed in *Glutamine in Clinical Nutrition*.

It has five major sections:

Section 1: Basic Processes at the Cellular Level and in Animal Models
Section 2: Glutamine Use in Critically Ill Patients and Their Diagnosis
Section 3: Glutamine in Normal Metabolism and Under Surgical Stress
Section 4: Clinical Aspects of Glutamine in the Intestine
Section 5: Clinical Aspects of Glutamine in Certain Patient Populations

Coverage includes glutamine structure and function, amino acid transporters, glutamine transaminases, one-carbon metabolism, uptake and immunomodulation, the pituitary gland, thyroid-stimulating hormone release, the TCA cycle, *mammary tissue*, cancer cells, metabolic imaging, endotoxemia, metabolic stress, major surgery, intensive care, *multiple trauma*, sepsis, dipeptides, insulin sensitivity, critically ill children, liver cirrhosis, *ammonia*, *encephalopathy*, the glutamine-glutamate-alpha-ketoglutarate axis, glutamine cycling, metabolic syndrome, glucagon-like peptide-1, presurgery, malnutrition, diabetic foot ulcers, epithelial tight junction, colitis, *Helicobacter pylori* infection, intestinal hypoxic injury, dipeptides, intestinal microcirculation, manganese toxicity, epilepsy, glutamine synthetase deficiency, plasma antioxidants, HIV, ischemia reperfusion injury, cancer immunosuppression, exercise, cancer cachexia, skeletal muscle, myostatin, and many other areas. Finally there is a chapter on "Web-Based Resources and Suggested Readings."

Contributors are authors of international and national standing, leaders in the field, and trendsetters. Emerging fields of science and important discoveries are also incorporated in *Glutamine in Clinical Nutrition*.

This book is designed for nutritionists and dietitians, public health scientists, doctors, epidemiologists, health care professionals of various disciplines, policy makers, and marketing and economic strategists. It is designed for teachers and lecturers, undergraduates and graduates, researchers and professors.

The Editors

London, UK

Rajkumar Rajendram
Victor R. Preedy
Vinood B. Patel

Series Editor Page

The great success of the Nutrition and Health Series is the result of the consistent overriding mission of providing health professionals with texts that are essential because each includes (1) a synthesis of the state of the science; (2) timely, in-depth reviews by the leading researchers and clinicians in their respective fields; (3) extensive, up-to-date fully annotated reference lists; (4) a detailed index; (5) relevant tables and figures; (6) identification of paradigm shifts and the consequences; (7) virtually no overlap of information between chapters, but targeted, interchapter referrals; (8) suggestions of areas for future research; and (9) balanced, data-driven answers to patient as well as health professionals questions that are based upon the totality of evidence rather than the findings of any single study.

The series volumes are not the outcome of a symposium. Rather, each editor has the potential to examine a chosen area with a broad perspective, both in subject matter and in the choice of chapter authors. The international perspective, especially with regard to public health initiatives, is emphasized where appropriate. The editors, whose trainings are both research and practice oriented, have the opportunity to develop a primary objective for their book; define the scope and focus; and then invite the leading authorities from around the world to be part of their initiative. The authors are encouraged to provide an overview of the field, discuss their own research, and relate the research findings to potential human health consequences. Because each book is developed de novo, the chapters are coordinated so that the resulting volume imparts greater knowledge than the sum of the information contained in the individual chapters.

Glutamine in Clinical Nutrition, edited by Rajkumar Rajendram, Victor Preedy, and Vinood Patel, is a very welcome addition to the Nutrition and Health Series and fully exemplifies the series' goals. Although glutamine is not an essential amino acid and can be synthesized de novo, it is the most abundant amino acid in the human body. Glutamine has numerous valuable metabolic functions: nitrogen transport, maintenance of the cellular redox state, serves as a metabolic intermediate and can be used as a source of energy, and is a required component of glutathione, the major intracellular antioxidant. Its central role in human physiology and metabolism in healthy individuals and its critical importance during the stresses of injury, inflammation, chronic diseases, and fetal development make it sufficiently important to warrant this 40 chapter, comprehensive volume. This book is designed as a resource for nutritionists and dietitians, public health scientists, physicians, epidemiologists, and health care professionals of various disciplines who interact with clients, patients, and/or family members. This important volume provides objective, relevant information for teachers and lecturers, advanced undergraduates and graduates, researchers and professors who require extensive, up-to-date literature reviews, instructive tables and figures, and excellent references on major aspects of glutamine related to human health and disease.

The volume contains in-depth chapters that review the cellular and genetic aspects of glutamine's actions. Relevant animal models are described that help us to better understand the tissue and organs that are most affected by glutamine metabolism; both healthy and clinically relevant models are reviewed. The majority of the volume examines the importance of glutamine in patients as glutamine is considered a conditionally essential amino acid when the body is under the severe stress of sepsis, cancer, premature birth, and immunosuppression, as examples. It must be noted that this is the first volume to be published for health professionals and advanced students that examines the biochemistry, clinical nutrition, and therapeutic aspects of glutamine.

The editors of this volume are experts in their respective fields and represent the medical profession as well as the academic research community. Dr. Rajkumar Rajendram is an intensive care physician, anesthetist, and perioperative physician. He was trained in general medicine and intensive care in Oxford, and he attained membership in the Royal College of Physicians (MRCP) in 2004. Dr. Rajendram then trained in anesthesia and intensive care in the Central School of Anesthesia, London Deanery and became a Fellow of the Royal College of Anaesthetists (FRCA) in 2009. He is one of the first intensivists to become a Fellow of the Faculty of Intensive Care Medicine (FFICM). Dr. Rajendram recognized that nutritional support was a fundamental aspect of critical care and, as a visiting research Fellow in the Nutritional Sciences Research Division of King's College London, he has published over 50 textbook chapters, review articles, peer-reviewed papers, and abstracts. Professor Victor Preedy is a senior member of King's College London where he is a Professor of Nutritional Biochemistry and Professor of Clinical Biochemistry at King's College Hospital. He is also Director of the Genomics Centre and a member of the School of Medicine. He is a member of the Royal College of Pathologists, a Fellow of the Society of Biology, the Royal College of Pathologists, the Royal Society for the Promotion of Health, the Royal Institute of Public Health, the Royal Society for Public Health, and in 2012 a Fellow of the Royal Society of Chemistry. Dr. Patel is a Senior Lecturer in Clinical Biochemistry at the University of Westminster and honorary Fellow at King's College London. Dr. Patel obtained his degree in Pharmacology from the University of Portsmouth, his Ph.D. in protein metabolism from King's College London, and completed postdoctoral research at Wake Forest University School of Medicine. Dr. Patel is a recognized leader in alcohol research and was involved in several NIH-funded biomedical grants related to alcoholic liver disease. Dr. Patel has edited biomedical books in the area of nutrition and health and disease prevention and has published over 160 articles.

The volume is organized into five major sections. *Section One*, containing ten related chapters, discusses the basic biochemical processes that involve glutamine at the cellular level and the physiological functions as well as certain pathophysiological functions that have been identified using animal models. The first chapter provides a broad-based perspective on the functions of glutamine and its importance in serving as a major source of molecules used in the synthesis of other amino acids, proteins, and other complex molecules within the human body. Glutamine is a critical nutrient for all rapidly proliferating cells and growing tissues, including cancerous tissues. In addition to providing building blocks for immune and other proliferating cells, glutamine contributes to the maintenance of redox balance by providing reducing equivalents that are also necessary for the synthesis of fatty acids. The chapter also explores the potential uses of glutamine supplementation in cases where its synthesis is insufficient to maintain muscle mass. Tables and figures included describe major metabolic cycles and the importance of glutamine as a source of nitrogen. The second chapter describes the molecules, at the cellular level, that are involved in the transport of glutamine in and out of cells. The authors focus mainly on the description of the functional properties of the physiologically important and Na+-dependent glutamine transporters belonging to the solute carrier 1 and SLC38 families. The chapter includes excellent figures and detailed descriptions of the regulation and the functional properties of the Sodium-Coupled Neutral Amino Acid Transporters (SNATs) of the SLC38 gene family that control influx and efflux of glutamine from cells.

Another important function of glutamine is to serve as a precursor for the neurotransmitter glutamate in the glutamate-glutamine cycle in the mammalian brain. This cycle is illustrated in the included figures that describe the brain cells and enzymes involved in this cycle. Chapter 3 examines the glutamine-glutamate cycle in depth. In the central nervous system, glutamate is locally converted from glutamine, which is absorbed into the neurons and acts as a neurotransmitter. Glutamate is an important excitatory amino acid neurotransmitter in the brain. The authors of Chap. 3 describe the recent laboratory animal studies on the function of glutamine and glutamate as extracellular signal mediators in the autocrine and/or paracrine system of the endocrine tissues. Glutamine and glutamate have been shown to play a dual role as excitatory neurotransmitters in the central nervous system as well as extracellular signaling molecules in endocrine tissues such as the adrenal gland, pancreas, and testis and in the pituitary gland. Specific models of in vitro and in vivo signaling of thyroid-stimulating hormone release from the pituitary gland provide a new avenue for exploring the role of glutamine in pituitary gland functions. Chapter 4 describes the central role of glutamine in the metabolism of cells of the immune system. Glutamine, in addition to glucose, is used as an energy source by immune cells especially when stimulated by antigens that trigger cellular proliferation. The cell culture studies that are reviewed clearly indicate the important roles of glutamine as an energy source as well as a precursor of the antioxidant, glutathione, to protect immune and surrounding cells from oxidative damage.

The fifth chapter examines the roles of the glutamine transaminases. The authors describe and include important figures to help the reader to visualize several glutaminase pathways and suggest that the glutaminase II pathway can provide metabolically critical molecules to epithelial cells in several tissues, including the brain (choroid plexus), prostate, bladder, and pancreas. Recent interest has focused on the glutaminase II pathway as it is found in a number of human cancer tissues; the presence of the glutaminase II pathway may be of fundamental importance in cancer biology. Given all of the metabolic pathways that involve glutamine, it is not surprising that the importance of glutamine for cancer cells is an area of intense research. Chapter 6 examines a glucose-independent, glutamine-driven tricarboxylic acid cycle that serves as an alternative energy-generating pathway for the survival and growth of tumor cells despite hypoxic and nutrient-deprived microenvironments. Cell culture studies have documented that glutamine is a viable alternative source of energy for glucose-deprived cancer cells. New studies are looking at drug candidates that can disrupt cancer cell use of glutamine as an energy source. Chapter 7 describes the role of glutamine in the multiple metabolic pathways of breast tumor cells. Glutamine metabolism differs significantly in basal compared to luminal breast cancer cells in that basal breast cancer cells require exogenous glutamine while luminal breast cancer cells are independent of exogenous glutamine. The chapter describes the metabolic differences between these two tumor cell types and suggests that these differences present therapeutic opportunities. Chapter 8 provides an historic perspective of the research to find cancer drug candidates. Because glutamine is so central to normal cell function, there has been limited success in finding a drug candidate that provides an acceptable risk:benefit ratio; however, research continues. Chapter 9 expands upon the role of glutamine in cancer cells by exploring the diagnostic potential of this activity to find active sites of cancer cell metabolism. The authors indicate that since the 1950s, glutamine has been recognized as an important tumor nutrient that contributes to key metabolic processes in proliferating cancer cells. Glutamine participates in bioenergetics, supports cell defenses against oxidative stress, complements glucose metabolism, and is an obligate nitrogen donor for nucleotide and amino acid synthesis. Glutamine also influences a number of signaling pathways that contribute to tumor growth. The chapter reviews the mechanisms involved in using glutamine plus positron emission tomography (PET) imaging to describe the metabolic activities of cancer cells.

The final chapter in the first section reviews the alterations in glutamine metabolisms that occur during sepsis and septic shock that are seen in patients and can be best studied using animal models and cell cultures. Chapter 10 describes the cellular responses to bacterial infections in animal models exposed to endotoxins that can lead to sepsis, septic shock, and to multiple organ dysfunction syndrome. We learn that endotoxemia markedly modifies glutamine metabolism in tissues with a decrease of intestinal glutamine uptake and metabolism, and a decrease in oxygen consumption. In skeletal muscle, endotoxemia increases endogenous glutamine synthesis and release resulting in a decrease in the muscle glutamine content. In lungs, endotoxemia results in a decrease of glutamine uptake with increased endogenous glutamine synthesis and release. Supplementation with glutamine in its free form or in its dipeptide form resulted in a decrease in intestinal permeability and bacterial translocation and decreased intestinal inflammation. In the lung, glutamine supplementation attenuated pulmonary inflammation and injury. The results of these studies have led to preliminary studies in patients with septic shock that are reviewed in the next section.

Section Two contains eight chapters that review the use of glutamine in critically ill patients and in the diagnosis of the status of certain critically ill patients. The first chapter in this section, Chap. 11, examines the normal rate of glutamine turnover and the effects of critical illness on the turnover of glutamine. The total pool of free glutamine in the human body turns over every 24 h. The extracellular glutamine pool is approximately 2 g and it has a rapid turnover; the intracellular glutamine pool contains more than 50 g and turns over more slowly. The author stresses the need for monitoring serum glutamine levels in critically ill patients especially when glutamine is provided either via the enteral or parenteral routes. Chapter 12 describes in detailed tables and figures the clinical studies using glutamine in the intensive care setting in surgical and critically ill patients. Although the laboratory animal data appear promising, current clinical data are not consistent and this may be due to the heterogeneity of the patient populations and their disease states, the lack of studies using pretreatment as used in laboratory animal studies, and differing doses and duration of treatments. Related to this chapter is the analysis of the use of glutamine in critically ill and less critically ill patients in intensive care units. Chapter 13 reviews the clinical studies that have examined the potential for glutamine supplementation to improve the outcomes of patients with multiple traumas. As with other chapters, these authors recommend the initiation of more well-controlled studies that can help to clarify the levels of benefit.

Chapter 14 reviews the immune responses to sepsis and the use of glutamine containing enteral and parenteral preparations. The authors note that glutamine is of value to immune responses to infections, yet the patient intervention data are inconsistent.

Chapter 15 examines the potential roll of glutamine in preserving insulin sensitivity in critically ill patients. The authors explain that hyperglycemia is a key metabolic feature associated with the stress response in critically ill patients. The stress response causes an exaggerated production of catecholamines and cortisol that combined with the presence of inflammatory cytokines results in insulin resistance. Stress hyperglycemia has been linked to poor outcomes, and the authors review the clinical studies that control high glucose levels using supplemental glutamine in the form of a dipeptide. They review the positive clinical data on the use of glutamine-enriched total parenteral nutrition in critically ill adult patients. Chapter 16 focuses on an in-depth review of the clinical data on the use of glutamine supplementation in critically ill adult patients in order to develop a rationale for glutamine use in critically ill children. In critically ill adults, plasma glutamine levels decrease quickly and significantly, remaining low for up to 21 days, and are associated with increased morbidity and mortality. Data have consistently shown benefits of glutamine supplementation in this patient population, and these studies have resulted in the American Society of Parenteral and Enteral Nutrition (ASPEN) and the European Society of Enteral and Parenteral Nutrition (ESPEN) recommending that 0.3–0.5 g of glutamine/kg bw be added to parenteral nutrition in critically ill adults. The authors review the limited studies with preterm and very low birth weight infants who have been given glutamine and the studies in limited numbers of children with severe infections and illnesses and indicate that the findings are inconsistent. Differing routes of administration, dose, degree of illness, and cause of childhood illnesses may be some of the reasons for the inconsistent findings. Further clinical studies that are randomized and double blind, of sufficiently long duration, and with a physiologically efficacious dose of glutamine for preterm infants are recommended as a first step in developing criteria for use in this patient population that is known to be at significant risk for sepsis and septic shock.

As mentioned above, in critically ill patients, glutamine is often given enterally and it is metabolized mainly in the liver as a source of energy. Glutamine is also metabolized to glutamate and ammonia by the liver type of the mitochondrial enzyme glutaminase. It is critical to determine the level of liver function especially in patients with liver cirrhosis. Chapter 17 describes a diagnostic test, the oral glutamine challenge, which is used to monitor liver function. The high protein meal that is used in this test induces an increase in blood ammonia in patients with cirrhosis but not in healthy controls or liver transplant patients. When the blood ammonia levels increase, it is transported to the central nervous system where ammonia may promote toxic effects including hepatic encephalopathy. Of interest, the oral glutamine test is also used in drug development to assess the effect of new drugs on liver function. The final chapter in this section, Chap. 18, discusses the biochemical reactions that result in ammonia formation in patients with hepatic encephalopathy, the effects on brain and other tissues, and the potential for glutamine supplementation to reduce certain of the adverse effects in these critically ill patients.

Section Three contains six chapters that examine the interactions between glutamine and insulin. The first chapter in this section, Chap. 19, provides an overview of the molecular interactions required to affect insulin secretion. The chapter describes how the glutamine-glutamate-α-ketoglutarate axis regulates amino acid and glucose-stimulated insulin secretion based on studies of mouse models of congenital hyperinsulinism and studies of human islet cells. The importance of glutamine-stimulated insulin secretion is examined using several knock-out mouse models and cell culture studies that are explained in detail in the excellent figures in this chapter. Chapter 20 reviews the multifactorial nature of the metabolic syndrome and the role of glutamine and glutamate in its development and adverse health effects, especially cardiovascular disease. The authors indicate that the metabolic syndrome is a complex disorder that can include highly related diseases such as type 2 diabetes, dyslipidemias, central obesity, arterial hypertension, nonalcoholic fatty liver disease (NAFLD), prothrombotic and proinflammatory states, and polycystic ovarian syndrome. The pathogenesis of the metabolic syndrome is linked to insulin resistance. The first link between the metabolic syndrome and glutamine/glutamate is the finding of significantly higher concentrations of serum glutamate in obese patients compared to normal weight, age and sex-matched individuals. Newer data linking genetic mutations resulting in enzyme changes has shown that an enzyme, glutamate decarboxylase 1, acts as an autoantigen in insulin-dependent diabetes. Excellent tables and figures help to illustrate the candidate genes and their interactions in the development and progression of the metabolic syndrome. The next chapter (Chap. 21) examines the functions of glutamine that are related to insulin and glucose responses to food intake. Low serum glutamine concentrations have been documented in individuals with impaired fasting glucose and impaired glucose tolerance and in type 2 diabetes patients. Large cohort studies have reported that low circulating glutamine levels predict type 2 diabetes incidence. The chapter reviews the clinical studies that found a beneficial reduction in gastric emptying when glutamine was given as a supplement with a meal.

The next three chapters examine the potential for glutamine to improve the overall metabolic status of patients undergoing surgery. Chapter 22 describes the unique circumstances of repair of the congenital defect, cleft lip, and the surgery's effects on glycemic control. The authors describe their blinded clinical study in age and defect-matched boys who were given glutamine parenterally prior to and during surgery or placebo and the supplemented group was found to have significantly better glycemic control and less stress responses following surgery. The authors of Chap. 23 also report on the results of their blinded intervention study in a cohort of moderately malnourished adults who are scheduled for gastric surgery. Three groups were identified prospectively. One group got parenteral glutamine in the postoperative period; another got parenteral glutamine both preoperatively and postoperatively. The third group got no additional glutamine. The authors report that the group that had both doses of glutamine had a trend of fewer admissions to intensive care and reduced duration of parenteral nutrition following surgery. The incidence of hyperglycemia was lowest in this supplemented group. Chapter 24 describes the serious adverse effects of diabetes that can result in diabetic foot ulcers. Ulcers affecting the lower limbs of diabetics are among the most frequent and costly clinical complications of the disease. The authors describe recent studies using a glutamine-containing supplement in diabetic patients with foot ulcer wounds and found enhanced healing and greater collagen formation. These preliminary studies add to the need for further data on glutamine use in patients undergoing surgical procedures and wound healing.

Section Four includes five chapters that provide the reader with basic information on the role of glutamine in maintaining the integrity of the intestinal wall, a review of the models used to examine the effects of a breach in the intestinal wall, and the importance of glutamine. We learn that enterocytes prefer glutamine as a source of energy, but these cells lack the capacity to synthesize glutamine. Glutamine is essential in maintaining gastrointestinal structure and barrier function. In vitro studies using cell monolayers demonstrated a direct influence of glutamine on tight junction integrity in the intestinal epithelium. Chapter 25 includes useful figures that describe cellular and laboratory studies that show the importance of glutamine in the intestine. The next, related chapter (Chap. 26) examines the importance of glutamine in animal models of colitis. The author explains that inflammatory bowel disease (IBD) is an idiopathic chronic condition of the gastrointestinal tract characterized by intermittent periods of inflammation and remission. The pathogenesis of IBD includes interactions between genetic, enteric microbiota, environmental, and immunological factors. The anti-inflammatory and immunoenhancing functions of glutamine have led to its use in animal models of this complex disease. Although benefits have been seen in animal models, there have not been consistent improvements in clinical trials.

There is a unique chapter that explores the effects of *Helicobacter pylori* infection in the GI tract and the potential for adverse effects in infected patients if they are treated with glutamine. Chapter 27 examines the interplay between the effects of *H. pylori* on the GI tract's metabolism, the finding that *H. pylori* can use glutamine as an energy source and that glutamine supplementation in *H. pylori* models actually enhanced inflammation, most likely by enhancing the production of ammonia. Obviously, in vitro and laboratory animal models were of great value in determining the potential for harm in supplementing patients with glutamine as a therapy for *H. pylori* infection.

As indicated above, preterm infants are at risk for glutamine and other amino acid deficiencies as the placenta is no longer supplying amino acids and the stressed preterm infant may not be able to synthesize sufficient glutamine and/or arginine. The next chapter examines the serious effects of intestinal dysfunction and the role of glutamine and arginine in the preterm infant and term infant. Chapter 28 reviews the laboratory animal studies that suggest a potential use of arginine, glutamine, and arginyl-glutamine (Arg-Gln) dipeptide to prevent and treat small intestinal hypoxic injury in pediatric patients especially in neonates. The final chapter (Chap. 29) reviews the effects of sepsis on glutamine metabolism and the use of glutamine by intestinal cells as a source of energy. Intestinal microcirculatory dysfunction is a key factor in the development of sepsis. Proposed mechanisms by which glutamine beneficially affects intestinal microcirculation include maintenance of functional capillary density, microvascular integrity, enhancement of leukocyte rolling, and adherence to intestinal microcirculation. Glutamine also influences the expression of adhesion molecules, and production of cytokines, the reduction of oxidation stress and nitric oxide-related mechanisms, heat shock proteins, and other effectors. The authors agree with other chapter authors that glutamine should be examined as a therapeutic strategy for patients with sepsis under controlled conditions.

The last section in the volume, *Section Five*, includes 11 chapters that examine a number of clinical conditions, most of which either have been shown to benefit from glutamine supplementation or are a consequence of disruption in glutamine metabolism. The first three chapters examine the importance of glutamine in the human brain and the adverse consequences to disruption in normal glutamine levels. The first chapter (Chap. 30) describes the interactions between glutamine and manganese. Manganese is an essential mineral and is found in the active site of several metalloenzymes including glutamine synthetase. However, chronic exposure to high levels of manganese can be toxic and result in a neurological disorder, referred to as manganism. The authors explain that exposure to high levels may be from consumption of well water containing high levels of the metal, exposure to a fuel additive used in some unleaded gasolines, exposure to organic manganese-containing pesticides, occupational exposure of miners, battery manufacturers, automotive repair technicians, and others.

Manganism is characterized by neuropsychiatric symptoms resembling those observed in idiopathic Parkinson's disease including hypokinesia, rigidity and tremor, postural instability, dystonia and bradykinesia, micrographia, mask-like facial expression, and speech disturbances. Manganese competes with glutamine for entry into brain cells. Manganese toxicity is associated with the disruption of glutamine and glutamate transport in astrocytes and can result in glutamine-mediated neurotoxicity. Chapter 31 reviews the importance of glutamine in the glutamine-glutamate-GABA cycle in the brain, which controls the balance between the excitatory and inhibitory nerve transmission. This chapter focuses on the association between the disruption of the cycle and resultant seizures or epilepsy. Epileptic seizures result from abnormal, excessive neuronal activity in the brain that may be due to the imbalance between excitability and inhibition in neurotransmission. There are data that suggest that in the epileptic brain, there is a lower than normal concentration of glutamine that appears to be linked to decreased functioning of glutamine synthetase. It is not clear at present whether glutamine supplementation would be of help in epilepsy. Chapter 32 describes the consequences of a unique congenital genetic defect that results in the lack of the enzyme glutamine synthetase that is often associated with fetal and early neonatal death. One case is described in an infant who suffered from neonatal onset severe epileptic encephalopathy and was entered into a clinical case study. Fortunately, when glutamine supplementation was provided, it resulted in relatively beneficial effects on patient alertness and reduced several but not all of the adverse brain effects.

Chapter 33 describes the oxidative damage associated with HIV infection and their current drug treatments. The link with glutamine is through glutamate as this amino acid is required for glutathione synthesis. Glutathione is a major antioxidant and treated HIV patients have significantly lower glutathione levels than non-HIV infected individuals. Glutathione (L-y-glutamyl-l-cysteinyl-glycine) is the major intracellular water-soluble antioxidant involved in metabolic processes and cell viability. Glutamine supplementation significantly increased glutathione concentrations in a clinical study with treated HIV patients, and the authors found that glutamine supplementation not only increased glutamate levels but also contributed to increasing cysteine and glycine through alterations in their metabolism.

Two chapters examine the impact of glutamine status on the oxidative tissue damage that is a consequence of ischemia/reperfusion injury. Chapter 34 reviews the model systems that strongly suggest that end-stage renal disease patients who are candidates for kidney transplant should be given glutamine supplementation prior to surgery. The models predict that supplementation results in an increase in glutathione levels that would be of value during the expected ischemia/reperfusion associated with kidney transplant. Also, as it is well accepted that the kidney that is to be transplanted is exposed to ischemia when removed from the donor, followed by reperfusion when it is transplanted. Thus, the kidney may also benefit by being bathed with a solution containing glutamine. Chapter 35 expands upon the data discussed in the previous chapter and describes the effects of ischemia/reperfusion (I/R) injury and its consequences in other tissues and organs. Intestinal I/R injury occurs in a variety of clinical settings. Intestinal ischemia/reperfusion can result from many causes including major trauma, hemorrhage, small bowel transplantation, superior mesenteric artery and vein thrombosis, acute pancreatitis, sepsis, cardiopulmonary bypass, and burn injuries. The injury leads to the generation of inflammatory factors, release of cytotoxic substances, activation of pathologic enzymes, and activation of immune cells in the intestine. These changes can result in intestinal mucosal injury, enhanced intestinal permeability, and inflammation, leading to gut dysfunction or even multiple organ dysfunction syndrome. The chapter includes discussions of injury to the liver, heart, brain, and kidney. Animal model research is critical to achieving the maximum beneficial effect of glutamine as the delivery route, dose, and timing need to be optimized for each organ system and each patient population.

As reviewed in earlier chapters, cancer cells utilize glutamine as an energy source and for the synthesis of molecules that have adverse effects on many tissues and organs within the body. The next two chapters look at some of these adverse effects to determine the potential for balancing the risk/benefits of glutamine supplementation for cancer patients. Chapter 36 describes in detail the mechanisms by which tumor cells downregulate immune cells through the synthesis of cytokines and altering receptors so that immune cells that would kill tumor cells can no longer function. In cell culture and laboratory animal studies, depletion of glutamine from culture media benefits immune cells and reduces the function of tumor cells. Yet, the potential to reduce systemic glutamine levels has not proven to be efficacious, and the more favorable targeting of intracellular glutamine is considered a more viable research focus. Chapter 37, in contrast, reviews the potential for glutamine supplementation to improve the muscle functions of patients with cancer cachexia so that they can benefit physically and emotionally from an exercise program. We learn that cachexia is characterized by involuntary body weight loss due to the cancer's production of cytokines that result in deep lean body mass loss and decreased fat stores and accounts for over 20 % of all cancer deaths. In the hypercatabolic state seen in cancer patients, where a negative nitrogen balance and increased muscle breakdown occur, glutamine demand increases, resulting in a significant reduction in plasma levels. The authors review the biochemical changes associated with cancer cachexia and conclude that in the cancer catabolic state, glutamine nutritional supplementation and exercise as adjuvant therapy can improve patient response, quality of life, and survival.

Two chapters continue the examination of the role of glutamine in muscle under varying physiological and pathological conditions. Chapter 38 reviews the effects of exercise as well as certain disease states on muscle use of glutamine. Muscle glutamine metabolism can be altered in a number of catabolic conditions, including cancer, sepsis, diabetes, and/or prolonged or exhausting physical exercise. Serious muscle damage and catabolism lead to the activation of local and acute inflammatory response. These processes increase the cell consumption of glutamine, promoting the imbalance of the synthesis and degradation of this amino acid. The reduction of glutamine and the increased inflammatory response increase protein breakdown, which can reduce the cell antioxidant concentrations and promote immunosuppression. The authors note that in athletes, glutamine supplementation may not prevent the inflammatory response and muscle damage or enhance performance, but may help the recovery of cells, including skeletal muscle. Chapter 39 discusses the substance that causes muscle wasting and how glutamine can affect this process. Myostatin is the negative regulator of muscle mass and its overexpression results in muscle atrophy. The authors explain that high myostatin circulating levels have been associated with weight loss in patients with AIDS, in the sarcopenia of aging, in atrophy due to muscle denervation or disuse, as well as in cancer patients as discussed above. Cell culture and laboratory animal studies suggest that glutamine supplementation can reduce levels of myostatin in a number of model systems. As with many of the clinically relevant outcomes discussed throughout this important volume, the preclinical findings consistently point to the potential for glutamine supplementation to either reduce the adverse effect or, in some instances, improve clinical outcomes. The final chapter in this comprehensive, clinically relevant volume provides a wealth of information on web-based resources and suggested readings for the health provider interested in the myriad of data concerning glutamine's role in human physiology and pathology.

The above description of the contents of the 40 chapters in this volume attest to the depth of information currently available concerning the central role of glutamine in maintaining the health of the individual as well as providing benefits as a supplement for certain patient populations. Each chapter includes Key Points, Keywords, and complete definitions of terms with the abbreviations fully defined for the reader and consistent use of terms between chapters. Key features of this comprehensive volume includes over 200 detailed tables and informative figures, an extensive, detailed index, and more than 1,800 up-to-date references that provide the reader with excellent sources of worthwhile information.

In conclusion, *Glutamine in Clinical Nutrition*, edited by Rajkumar Rajendram, Victor R. Preedy, and Vinood B. Patel, provides health professionals in many areas of research and practice with the most up-to-date, well-referenced volume on the importance of glutamine in maintaining the overall health of the individual as well as serving as a critical source of energy and precursor of other amino acids and glutathione that are especially critical in the disease conditions discussed in the chapters. This unique volume will serve the reader as the benchmark in this complex area of interrelationships between nonessential and conditionally essential amino acid functions and the unique role of glutamine specifically in the synthesis of brain neurotransmitters, collagen formation, insulin and glucose modulation, and the functioning of all organ systems that are involved in the maintenance of the body's metabolic integrity. Moreover, the physiological, genetic, and pathological interactions between plasma levels of glutamine, glutamate, and related nonessential amino acids that are synthesized through glutamine metabolism are clearly delineated in clear and useful tables and figures so that students as well as practitioners can better understand the complexities of these interactions. Unique chapters examine the effects of glutamine status that can be significantly altered by the effects of genetic mutations. Chapters review the consequences of these mutations from prepregnancy, during fetal development, in the neonate and infancy. The editors are applauded for their efforts to develop the most authoritative and unique resource on the role of glutamine in health and disease to date, and this excellent text is a very welcome addition to the Nutrition and Health Series.

Adrianne Bendich, Ph.D., F.A.C.N., F.A.S.N.
Series Editor

About the Series Editor

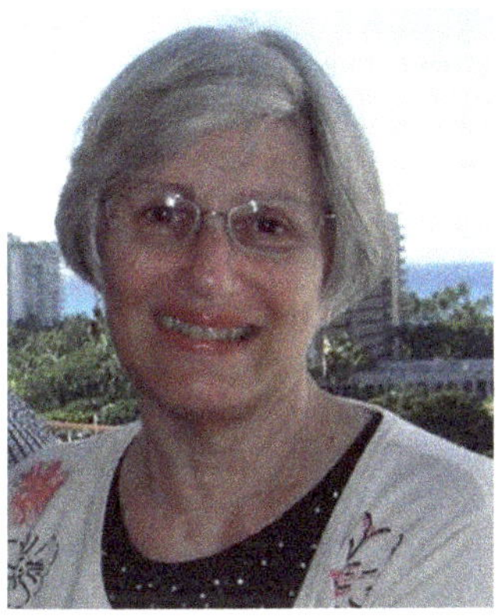

Dr. Adrianne Bendich Ph.D., F.A.S.N., F.A.C.N. has served as the "Nutrition and Health" Series Editor for over 15 years and has provided leadership and guidance to more than 120 volume editors that have developed the 60+ well-respected and highly recommended volumes in the Series.

In addition to "**Glutamine in Clinical Nutrition,**" **edited by Rajkumar Rajendram M.D., Victor Preedy Ph.D., and Vinood Patel Ph.D., major new editions** in 2012–2014 include:

1. **Handbook of Clinical Nutrition and Aging, Third Edition**, edited by Connie W. Bales Ph.D., R.D., Julie L. Locher Ph.D., M.S.P.H., and Edward Saltzman, M.D., 2014
2. **Nutrition and Oral Medicine, Second Edition**, edited by Dr. Riva Touger-Decker, Dr. Connie C. Mobley, and Dr. Joel B. Epstein, 2014
3. **Fructose, High Fructose Corn Syrup, Sucrose and Health**, edited by Dr. James M. Rippe, 2014
4. **Nutrition in Kidney Disease, Second Edition**, edited by Dr. Laura D. Byham-Gray, Dr. Jerrilynn D. Burrowes, and Dr. Glenn M. Chertow, 2014
5. **Handbook of Food Fortification and Health, volume I** edited by Dr. Victor R. Preedy, Dr. Rajaventhan Srirajaskanthan, and Dr. Vinood B. Patel, 2013
6. **Handbook of Food Fortification and Health, volume II** edited by Dr. Victor R. Preedy, Dr. Rajaventhan Srirajaskanthan, and Dr. Vinood B. Patel, 2013
7. **Diet Quality: An Evidence-Based Approach, volume I** edited by Dr. Victor R. Preedy, Dr. Lan-Ahn Hunter, and Dr. Vinood B. Patel, 2013
8. **Diet Quality: An Evidence-Based Approach, volume II** edited by Dr. Victor R. Preedy, Dr. Lan-Ahn Hunter, and Dr. Vinood B. Patel, 2013

9. **The Handbook of Clinical Nutrition and Stroke**, edited by Mandy L. Corrigan, MPH, RD, Arlene A. Escuro, MS, RD, and Donald F. Kirby, M.D., FACP, FACN, FACG, 2013
10. **Nutrition in Infancy**, **volume I** edited by Dr. Ronald Ross Watson, Dr. George Grimble, Dr. Victor Preedy, and Dr. Sherma Zibadi, 2013
11. **Nutrition in Infancy**, **volume II** edited by Dr. Ronald Ross Watson, Dr. George Grimble, Dr. Victor Preedy, and Dr. Sherma Zibadi, 2013
12. **Carotenoids and Human Health**, edited by Dr. Sherry A. Tanumihardjo, 2013
13. **Bioactive Dietary Factors and Plant Extracts in Dermatology**, edited by Dr. Ronald Ross Watson and Dr. Sherma Zibadi, 2013
14. **Omega 6/3 Fatty Acids**, edited by Dr. Fabien De Meester, Dr. Ronald Ross Watson, and Dr. Sherma Zibadi, 2013
15. **Nutrition in Pediatric Pulmonary Disease**, edited by Dr. Robert Dumont and Dr. Youngran Chung, 2013
16. **Magnesium and Health**, edited by Dr. Ronald Ross Watson and Dr. Victor R. Preedy, 2012.
17. **Alcohol, Nutrition and Health Consequences**, edited by Dr. Ronald Ross Watson, Dr. Victor R. Preedy, and Dr. Sherma Zibadi, 2012
18. **Nutritional Health, Strategies for Disease Prevention, Third Edition**, edited by Norman J. Temple, Ted Wilson, and David R. Jacobs, Jr., 2012
19. **Chocolate in Health and Nutrition**, edited by Dr. Ronald Ross Watson, Dr. Victor R. Preedy, and Dr. Sherma Zibadi, 2012
20. **Iron Physiology and Pathophysiology in Humans**, edited by Dr. Gregory J. Anderson and Dr. Gordon D. McLaren, 2012

Earlier books included **Vitamin D, Second Edition** edited by Dr. Michael Holick; "**Dietary Components and Immune Function**" edited by Dr. Ronald Ross Watson, Dr. Sherma Zibadi, and Dr. Victor R. Preedy; "**Bioactive Compounds and Cancer**" edited by Dr. John A. Milner and Dr. Donato F. Romagnolo; "**Modern Dietary Fat Intakes in Disease Promotion**" edited by Dr. Fabien De Meester, Dr. Sherma Zibadi, and Dr. Ronald Ross Watson; "**Iron Deficiency and Overload**" edited by Dr. Shlomo Yehuda and Dr. David Mostofsky; "**Nutrition Guide for Physician**s" edited by Dr. Edward Wilson, Dr. George A. Bray, Dr. Norman Temple, and Dr. Mary Struble; "**Nutrition and Metabolism**" edited by Dr. Christos Mantzoros; and "**Fluid and Electrolytes in Pediatrics**" edited by Leonard Feld and Dr. Frederick Kaskel. Recent volumes include "**Handbook of Drug-Nutrient Interactions**" edited by Dr. Joseph Boullata and Dr. Vincent Armenti; "**Probiotics in Pediatric Medicine**" edited by Dr. Sonia Michail and Dr. Philip Sherman; "**Handbook of Nutrition and Pregnancy**" edited by Dr. Carol Lammi-Keefe, Dr. Sarah Couch, and Dr. Elliot Philipson; "**Nutrition and Rheumatic Disease**" edited by Dr. Laura Coleman; "**Nutrition and Kidney Disease**" edited by Dr. Laura Byham-Grey, Dr. Jerrilynn Burrowes, and Dr. Glenn Chertow; "**Nutrition and Health in Developing Countries**" edited by Dr. Richard Semba and Dr. Martin Bloem; "**Calcium in Human Health**" edited by Dr. Robert Heaney and Dr. Connie Weaver; and "**Nutrition and Bone Health**" edited by Dr. Michael Holick and Dr. Bess Dawson-Hughes.

Dr. Bendich is President of Consultants in Consumer Healthcare LLC and is the editor of ten books including "**Preventive Nutrition: The Comprehensive Guide for Health Professionals, Fourth Edition**" coedited with Dr. Richard Deckelbaum (www.springer.com/series/7659). Dr. Bendich serves on the Editorial Boards of the *Journal of Nutrition in Gerontology and Geriatrics*, and *Antioxidants*, and has served as Associate Editor for *Nutrition* the International Journal; served on the Editorial Board of the *Journal of Women's Health and Gender-based Medicine* and served on the Board of Directors of the American College of Nutrition.

Dr. Bendich was Director of Medical Affairs at GlaxoSmithKline (GSK) Consumer Healthcare and provided medical leadership for many well-known brands including TUMS and Os-Cal. Dr. Bendich had primary responsibility for GSK's support for the Women's Health Initiative (WHI) intervention study. Prior to joining GSK, Dr. Bendich was at Roche Vitamins Inc. and was involved with the groundbreaking clinical studies showing that folic acid-containing multivitamins significantly reduced major classes of birth defects. Dr. Bendich has coauthored over 100 major clinical research studies in the area of preventive nutrition. She is recognized as a leading authority on antioxidants, nutrition and immunity and pregnancy outcomes, vitamin safety, and the cost-effectiveness of vitamin/mineral supplementation.

Dr. Bendich received the Roche Research Award, is a *Tribute to Women and Industry* Awardee, and was a recipient of the Burroughs Wellcome Visiting Professorship in Basic Medical Sciences. Dr. Bendich was given the Council for Responsible Nutrition (CRN) Apple Award in recognition of her many contributions to the scientific understanding of dietary supplements. In 2012, she was recognized for her contributions to the field of clinical nutrition by the American Society for Nutrition and was elected a Fellow of ASN. Dr. Bendich is an Adjunct Professor at Rutgers University. She is listed in Who's Who in American Women.

About the Volume Editors

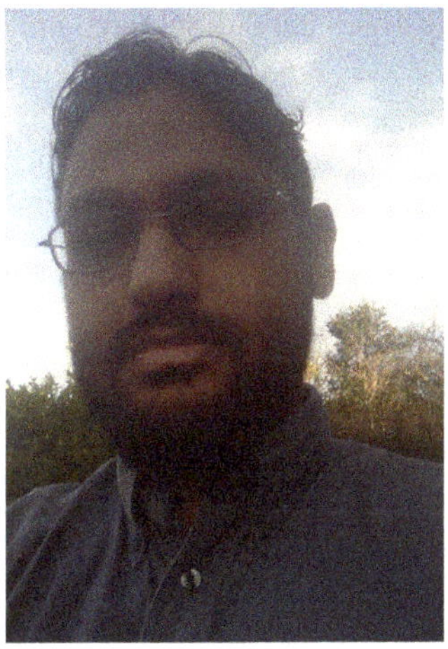

Dr. Rajkumar Rajendram is an intensivist, anesthetist, and perioperative physician. He graduated in 2001 with a distinction from Guy's, King's and St. Thomas Medical School, in London. As an undergraduate he was awarded several prizes, merits, and distinctions in preclinical and clinical subjects. This was followed by training in general medicine and intensive care in Oxford, during which period he attained membership of the Royal College of Physicians (MRCP) in 2004. Dr. Rajendram went on to train in anesthesia and intensive care in the Central School of Anaesthesia, London Deanery and became a fellow of the Royal College of Anaesthetists (FRCA) in 2009. He has completed advanced training in intensive care in Oxford and was one of the first intensivists to become a fellow of the faculty of intensive care medicine (FFICM) by examination. He coauthored the Oxford Case Histories in Cardiology which was published by the Oxford University Press in 2011. He is currently preparing the text for the Oxford Case Histories in Intensive Care. His unique training and experience has been tailored for a career in intensive care with a subspecialty interest in perioperative medicine.

Dr. Rajendram recognizes that nutritional support is a fundamental aspect of critical care. He has therefore devoted significant time and effort into nutritional science research. As a visiting research fellow in the Nutritional Sciences Research Division of King's College London, he has published over 50 textbook chapters, review articles, peer-reviewed papers, and abstracts from his work.

Victor R. Preedy B.Sc., Ph.D., D.Sc., F.S.B., F.R.S.H., F.R.I.P.H.H., F.R.S.P.H., F.R.C.Path., F.R.S.C. is a senior member of King's College London (Professor of Nutritional Biochemistry) and King's College Hospital (Professor of Clinical Biochemistry; Hon.). He is attached to both the Diabetes and Nutritional Sciences Division and the Department of Nutrition and Dietetics. He is also Director of the Genomics Centre and a member of the School of Medicine. Professor Preedy graduated in 1974 with an Honours Degree in Biology and Physiology with Pharmacology. He gained his University of London Ph.D. in 1981. In 1992, he received his Membership of the Royal College of Pathologists and in 1993 he gained his second doctoral degree, for his contribution to the science of protein metabolism in health and disease. Professor Preedy was elected as a Fellow of the Institute of Biology in 1995 and to the Royal College of Pathologists in 2000. Since then he has been elected as a Fellow to the Royal Society for the Promotion of Health (2004) and the Royal Institute of Public Health and Hygiene (2004). In 2009, Professor Preedy became a Fellow of the Royal Society for Public Health and in 2012 a Fellow of the Royal Society of Chemistry. In his career Professor Preedy worked at the National Heart Hospital (part of Imperial College London) and the MRC Centre at Northwick Park Hospital. He has collaborated with research groups in Finland, Japan, Australia, the USA, and Germany. He is a leading expert on biomedical sciences and has a longstanding interest in how nutrition and diet affects well-being and health. He has lectured nationally and internationally. To his credit, Professor Preedy has published over 500 articles, which include peer-reviewed manuscripts based on original research, reviews, and numerous books and volumes.

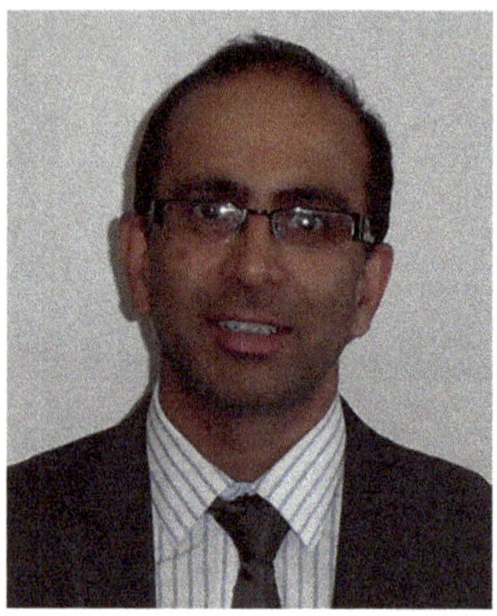

Dr. Vinood B. Patel is currently a Senior Lecturer in Clinical Biochemistry at the University of Westminster and honorary fellow at King's College London. He presently directs studies on metabolic pathways involved in liver disease, particularly related to mitochondrial energy regulation and cell death. In addition, research is being undertaken to study the role of nutrients, phytochemicals, and fatty acids in the development of fatty liver disease and iron homeostatic regulation. Another area includes identifying new biomarkers that can be used for diagnosis and prognosis of liver disease. Dr. Patel graduated from the University of Portsmouth with a degree in Pharmacology and completed his Ph.D. in protein metabolism from King's College London in 1997. His postdoctoral work was carried out at Wake Forest University Baptist Medical School studying structural-functional alterations to mitochondrial ribosomes, where he developed novel techniques to characterize their biophysical properties. Dr. Patel is a nationally and internationally recognized alcohol researcher and was involved in several NIH-funded biomedical grants related to alcoholic liver disease. Dr. Patel has edited biomedical books in the area of nutrition and health prevention, autism, and biomarkers and has published over 160 articles.

Acknowledgments

The development of this book is built upon the foundation of the excellent work provided by the staff of Humana, and we are very thankful to them. In particular we wish to acknowledge the outstanding support, advice, and patience of the Series Editor, Dr. Adrianne Bendich; the Developmental Editor, Michael Griffin; and the Associate Editor, Amanda Quinn.

The Editors

Contents

Contributors

Iman Afif, B.A. Division of Gastrointestinal and Liver Pathology, Department of Pathology, Johns Hopkins University School of Medicine, Baltimore, MD, USA

Sayaka Aizawa, Ph.D. Area of Regulatory Biology, Division of Life Science, Graduate School of Science and Engineering, Saitama University, Saitama, Japan

Ruqaiya M. Al Balushi, B.Sc., M.Sc., Ph.D. Health and Nutrition Department, College of Food and Agriculture, United Arab Emirates University, Al Ain United Arab Emirates

Nadia A. Al-Banna, Ph.D. Department of Pharmacology, Dalhousie University, Halifax, NS, Canada

Thomas Albers, Ph.D. Department of Chemistry, Binghamton University, Binghamton, NY, USA

Javier Ampuero, M.D. Unit for Clinical Management of Digestive Diseases, Valme University Hospital, Sevilla, Spain

Mireille Andriamihaja, Ph.D. Dr. INRA/AgroParisTech, UMR 914 Nutrition Physiology and Ingestive Behavior, Paris, France

Michael Aschner, Ph.D. Department of Molecular Pharmacology, Albert Einstein College of Medicine, Bronx, NY, USA

Francesco M. Baccino, M.D. Department of Clinical and Biological Sciences, University of Turin, Torino, Italy

Lasse K. Bak Department of Drug Design and Pharmacology, Faculty of Health and Medical Sciences, University of Copenhagen, Copenhagen, Denmark

Kechen Ban, Ph.D. Department of Surgery, University of Texas Medical School at Houston, Houston, TX, USA

Merrilyn Banks, B.Sc., M. Hlth. Sc., Ph.D. Department of Nutrition and Dietetics, Royal Brisbane & Women's Hospital, Brisbane, QLD, Australia

Annabel E. Barber, M.D. Department of Surgery, University of Nevada School of Medicine, Las Vegas, NV, USA

François Blachier, Ph.D. Dr. INRA/AgroParisTech, UMR 914 Nutrition Physiology and Ingestive Behavior, Paris, France

Andrea Bonetto, Ph.D. Indiana University School of Medicine - IUPUI, Indianapolis, IN, USA

Maria Dorotéia Borges-Santos Centre for Nutritional and Physical Exercise Metabolism, Department of Public Health, Botucatu Medical School, Sao Paulo State University – UNESP, Botucatu, SP, Brazil

Marco Braga, M.D. Department of Surgery, San Raffaele Hospital, Milan, Italy

Efrossini Briassouli, M.D. 1st Department of Internal Medicine–Propaedeutic, "Laiko" Hospital, University of Athens, Athens, Greece

George Briassoulis, M.D., Ph.D. Paediatric Intensive Care Unit, Department of Paediatric Intensive Care, School of Medicine, University of Crete, Heraklion, Crete, Greece

Roberto Carlos Burini, Ph.D. Centre for Nutritional and Physical Exercise Metabolism, Department of Public Health, Botucatu Medical School, Sao Paulo State University – UNESP, Botucatu, SP, Brazil

Cervantes Caporossi, Ph.D. Clinical Surgery Department of Julio Muller Hospital, UFMT Brazil (Federal University of Mato Grosso), Mato Grosso, Brazil

Carol Lorencio Cárdenas, M.D. Intensive Care Department, Hospital Josep Trueta, Girona, Spain

Ana Augusta Monteiro Cavalcante, M.Sc., Ph.D. Dr. R&D, Nutrimed Industrial Ltda., Fortaleza, Ceará, Brazil

Kamaljit Chaudhry, Ph.D. Department of Physiology, University of Tennessee Health Science Center, Memphis, TN, USA

Zhong Chen, Ph.D. Department of Pharmacology, Key Laboratory of Medical Neurobiology of the Ministry of Health of China, Zhejiang Province Key Laboratory of Neurobiology, College of Pharmaceutical Sciences, Zhejiang University, Hangzhou, China

Jen-Tsan Chi, M.D., Ph.D. Department of Molecular Genetics & Microbiology, Center for Genomics and Computational Biology, Duke Medical Center, Durham, NC, USA

Seok Rye Choi, Ph.D. Department of Radiology, University of Pennsylvania School of Medicine, Philadelphia, PA, USA

Maria Rosa Ciriolo, Ph.D. Department of Biology, University of Rome "Tor Vergata", Rome, Italy

Jeremy Cohen, M.R.C.P, F.R.C.A., Ph.D. Department of Intensive Care Medicine, Royal Brisbane & Women's Hospital, Brisbane, QLD, Australia

Burns, Trauma & Critical Care Research Centre, School of Medicine, The University of Queensland, Brisbane, QLD, Australia

Arthur J.L. Cooper, Ph.D., D.Sc. Department of Biochemistry and Molecular Biology, New York Medical College, Valhalla, NY, USA

Sara Coppola, M.D. Department of Surgery, University of Milano-Bicocca-San Gerardo Hospital, Monza, Italy

Paola Costelli, Ph.D. Department of Clinical and Biological Sciences, University of Turin, Torino, Italy

Vinicius Fernandes Cruzat Department of Food Science and Experimental Nutrition, Faculty of Pharmaceutical Sciences, University of São Paulo, São Paulo, SP, Brazil

Sherry Dadsetan Department of Drug Design and Pharmacology, Faculty of Health and Medical Sciences, University of Copenhagen, Copenhagen, Denmark

Enrico Desideri, Ph.D. Department of Biology, University of Rome “Tor Vergata”, Rome, Italy

Thambi Dorai, Ph.D. Department of Urology, New York Medical College, Valhalla, NY, USA

Bhuvaneswari Dorai, M.D. Department of Pathology, Nyack Hospital, Nyack, NY, USA

José Ferreira da Cunha Filho Bairro: Dionísio Torres, Fortaleza-CE, Brasil

Department of Surgery, Federal University of Ceará, School of Medicine, Bairro: Rodolfo Teófilo, Fortaleza, Ceará, Brazil

Kenneth Frauwirth, Ph.D. Department of Cell Biology and Molecular Genetics, University of Maryland, College Park, MD, USA

Luca Gianotti, M.D., Ph.D. Department of Surgery, University of Milano-Bicocca-San Gerardo Hospital, Monza, Italy

Maria Cristina Cintra Gomes-Marcondes, Ph.D. Department of Structural and Functional Biology, Biology Institute, State University of Campinas – UNICAMP, Campinas, São Paulo, Brazil

Valter Torezan Gouvêa Junior, Ph.D. Clinical Surgery Department of Julio Muller Hospital, UFMT Brazil (Federal University of Mato Grosso), Mato Grosso, Brazil

Teodoro Grau-Carmona M.D., Ph.D. Intensive Care Department, Hospital Universitario Doce de Octubre, Madrid, Spain

Jerry R. Greenfield, M.B.B.S (Hons 1), Ph.D., F.R.A.C.P. Diabetes and Obesity Program, Garvan Institute of Medical Research, Faculty of Medicine, University of New South Wales, Sydney, NSW, Australia

Department of Endocrinology, St Vincent’s Hospital, Sydney, NSW, Australia

Christof Grewer, Ph.D. Department of Chemistry, Binghamton University, Binghamton, NY, USA

Johannes Häberle, M.D. Division of Metabolism, University Children’s Hospital Zurich, Zürich, Switzerland

Susan J. Hagen, Ph.D. Roberta and Stephen R. Weiner Department of Surgery, Beth Israel Deaconess Medical Center, Harvard Medical School, Boston, MA, USA

André Hallen, B.Sc. Department of Chemistry and Biomolecular Sciences, Macquarie University, North Ryde, NSW, Australia

Ines Hammami, B.Eng., M.Sc.A., Ph.D. Department of Chemical Engineering, Ecole Polytechnique de Montréal, Montreal, QC, Canada

Weiwei Hu, Ph.D. Department of Pharmacology, Key Laboratory of Medical Neurobiology of the Ministry of Health of China, Zhejiang Province Key Laboratory of Neurobiology, School of Basic Medical Sciences, Zhejiang University, Hangzhou, Zhejiang, P. R. China

Benjamin Jung Hwang, B.A. Division of Gastrointestinal and Liver Pathology, Department of Pathology, Johns Hopkins University School of Medicine, Baltimore, MD, USA

Mario Jolicoeur, B.Eng., M.Sc.A., Ph.D. Department of Chemical Engineering, Ecole Polytechnique de Montréal, Montreal, QC, Canada

Maris S. Jones, M.D. Department of Surgery, University of Nevada School of Medicine, Las Vegas, NV, USA

Xiangfeng Kong, Ph.D. Key Laboratory of Agro-ecological Processes in Subtropical Region, Institute of Subtropical Agriculture, Chinese Academy of Sciences, Changsha, Hunan, China

Rosemary A. Kozar, M.D., Ph.D. Department of Surgery, University of Texas Medical School at Houston, Houston, TX, USA

Boris F. Krasnikov, Ph.D. Department of Biochemistry and Molecular Biology, New York Medical College, Valhalla, NY, USA

Hank F. Kung, Ph.D. Department of Radiology, University of Pennsylvania School of Medicine, Philadelphia, PA, USA

Hsiu-Ni Kung, Ph.D. Department of Anatomy and Cell Biology, School of Medicine, National Taiwan University, Taipei, Taiwan

Antonio Lancha, Jr., Ph.D. Laboratory of Applied Nutrition and Metabolism, School of Physical Education and Sports, University of Sao Paulo, Brazil, Sao Paulo, Brazil

Anne Le, M.D. Division of Gastrointestinal and Liver Pathology, Department of Pathology, Johns Hopkins University School of Medicine, Baltimore, MD, USA

Josep Manel Llop Talaverón, Pharm. D. Hospitalet de Llobregat, Department of Pharmacy, Hospital Universitari Bellvitge/Universitat de Barcelona, Barcelona, Spain

Christian Lehmann M.D., Ph.D., F.R.C.P.C. Department of Anesthesia, Pain Management and Perioperative Medicine, QE II Health Sciences Centre, Dalhousie University, Halifax, NS, Canada

Department of Pharmacology & Microbiology and Immunology, Dalhousie University, Halifax, NS, Canada

Department of Anesthesiology and Operative Intensive Care Medicine, Charité – Universitätsmedizin, Berlin, Germany

Changhong Li, M.D., Ph.D. Division of Endocrinology, The Children's Hospital of Philadelphia, Perelman School of Medicine, University of Pennsylvania, Philadelphia, PA, USA

Jianyong Li, D.V.M., Ph.D. Department of Biochemistry, Virginia Tech, Blacksburg, VA, USA

Nan Li, M.D. Department of Pediatrics, University of Florida, Gainesville, FL, USA

Brian P. Lieberman Department of Radiology, University of Pennsylvania School of Medicine, Philadelphia, PA, USA

Liya Ma, M.D. Shenzhen Baoan Maternity and Child Health Hospital, Shenzhen, China

Luise Victoria Marino, B.Sc. (Hons.), Ph.D. Department of Paediatrics, Imperial College London, London, UK

Carlos Augusto Fernandes Molina, Ph.D. Department of Surgery and Anatomy of São Paulo University, USP, São Paulo, Brazil

Fernando Moreto, Ph.D. Centre for Nutritional and Physical Exercise Metabolism, Department of Public Health, Botucatu Medical School, Sao Paulo State University – UNESP, Botucatu, SP, Brazil

Luca Nespoli, M.D. Department of Surgery, University of Milano-Bicocca-San Gerardo Hospital, Monza, Italy

Josef Neu, M.D. Department of Pediatrics, University of Florida, Gainesville, FL, USA

Massimo Oldani, M.D. Department of Surgery, University of Milano-Bicocca-San Gerardo Hospital, Monza, Italy

Gabriel Mercadal-Orfila, Pharm. D. Mateu Orfila/Department of Pharmacy, Maó-Menorca, Spain

Jennifer D. Paratz, M.Phty, Ph.D., F.A.C.P. Department of Intensive Care Medicine, Royal Brisbane & Women's Hospital, Brisbane, QLD, Australia

Burns, Trauma & Critical Care Research Centre, School of Medicine, The University of Queensland, Brisbane, QLD, Australia

Joshua K. Park, B.S. Division of Gastrointestinal and Liver Pathology, Department of Pathology, Johns Hopkins University School of Medicine, Baltimore, MD, USA

Vinood B. Patel, B.Sc., Ph.D. Department of Biomedical Sciences, Faculty of Science & Technology, University of Westminster, London, UK

Fabio Penna, Ph.D. Department of Clinical and Biological Sciences, University of Turin, Torino, Italy

John Thomas Pinto, Ph.D. Department of Biochemistry and Molecular Biology, New York Medical College, Valhalla, NY, USA

Carlos J. Pirola, M.D., Ph.D. Department of Molecular Genetics and Biology of Complex Diseases, Institute of Medical Research A Lanari-IDIM, University of Buenos Aires-National Scientific and Technical Research Council, Ciudad Autónoma de Buenos Aires, Argentina

Karl Ploessl, Ph.D. Department of Radiology, University of Pennsylvania School of Medicine, Philadelphia, PA, USA

Brad Poore, B.S. Division of Gastrointestinal and Liver Pathology, Department of Pathology, Johns Hopkins University School of Medicine, Baltimore, MD, USA

Victor R. Preedy, B.Sc., Ph.D., D.Sc. Nutritional Sciences Division, Department of Nutrition and Dietetics, School of Biomedical and Health Sciences, King's College London, London, UK

Rajkumar Rajendram, M.R.C.P., F.R.C.A., F.F.I.C.M. Department of Intensive Care, Barnet and Chase Farm Hospitals, Royal Free London NHS Foundation Trust, London, UK

RadhaKrishna Rao, Ph.D., A.G.A.F. Department of Physiology, University of Tennessee Health Science Center, Memphis, TN, USA

Manuel Romero-Gómez, M.D., Ph.D. Unit for Clinical Management of Digestive Diseases, Valme University Hospital, Sevilla, Spain

Takafumi Sakai, Ph.D. Area of Regulatory Biology, Division of Life Science, Graduate School of Science and Engineering, Saitama University, Saitama, Japan

Ichiro Sakata, Ph.D. Area of Regulatory Biology, Division of Life Science, Graduate School of Science and Engineering, Saitama University, Saitama, Japan

Emilianne Miguel Salomão, Ph.D. Department of Structural and Functional Biology, Biology Institute, State University of Campinas – UNICAMP, Campinas, São Paulo, Brazil

Dorit Samocha-Bonet, Ph.D., M.Sc., B.Sc. Diabetes & Obesity Program, Garvan Institute of Medical Research, Faculty of Medicine, University of New South Wales, Sydney, NSW, Australia

Arne Schousboe Department of Drug Design and Pharmacology, Faculty of Health and Medical Sciences, University of Copenhagen, Copenhagen, Denmark

Nicholas Siegel, B.S. Division of Gastrointestinal and Liver Pathology, Department of Pathology, Johns Hopkins University School of Medicine, Baltimore, MD, USA

Marta Sidoryk-Wegrzynowicz, Ph.D. Department of Pediatrics, Vanderbilt University School of Medicine, Nashville, TN, USA

Peter B. Soeters, M.D., Ph.D. Emeritus Professor of Surgery, Maastricht University Medical Center, Lanaken, Belgium

Silvia Sookoian, M.D., Ph.D. Department of Clinical and Molecular Hepatology, Institute of Medical Research A Lanari-IDIM, University of Buenos Aires-National Scientific and Technical Research Council, Ciudad Autónoma de Buenos Aires, Argentina

Patrizio Tatti Department of Endocrinology and Diabetes, ASL RMH, Marino (Roma), Italy

Julio Tirapegui, Ph.D. Department of Food Science and Experimental Nutrition, Faculty of Pharmaceutical Sciences, University of São Paulo, São Paulo, SP, Brazil

Daniel Tomé, Ph.D. INRA/AgroParisTech, UMR 914 Nutrition Physiology and Ingestive Behavior, Paris, France

Paulo Roberto Leitão de Vasconcelos, D.Phil Department of Surgery, School of Medicine, Federal University of Ceará, Fortaleza, Ceará, Brazil

Helle S. Waagepetersen Department of Drug Design and Pharmacology, Faculty of Health and Medical Sciences, University of Copenhagen, Copenhagen, Denmark

Jan Wernerman, M.D., Ph.D. Karolinska University Hospital Huddinge, Karolinska Institutet, Stockholm, Sweden

Guoyao Wu, Ph.D. Department of Animal Science, Texas A&M University, College Station, TX, USA

Hongyu Xue, M.D., Ph.D. Department of Anesthesiology, University of Colorado Denver, Aurora, CO, USA

Yulong Yin, Ph.D. Key Laboratory of Agro-ecological Processes in Subtropical Region, Institute of Subtropical Agriculture, Chinese Academy of Sciences, Changsha, Hunan, China

Yong-Ming Yu, Ph.D. Department of Surgery, Shriners Burns Hospital, Massachusetts General Hospital, Harvard Medical School, Boston, MA, USA

Catherine Zander Department of Chemistry, Binghamton University, Binghamton, NY, USA

Marco Zanello, M.D. IRCCS Istituto di Science Neurologiche, University Alma Mater of Bologna, Bologna, Italy

Zhou Zhang, Ph.D. School of Life Science and Biopharmaceutics, Shenyang Pharmaceutical University, Shenyang, Liao Ning Province, China

Lin Zhu, Ph.D. Department of Radiology, University of Pennsylvania School of Medicine, Philadelphia, PA, USA

College of Chemistry, Beijing Normal University, Beijing, China

Part I
Basic Processes at the Cellular Level and in Animal Models

Chapter 1
Glutamine Structure and Function: A Starter Pack

Peter B. Soeters

Key Points

- The main function of glutamine is to support cell proliferation in all situations where proliferation is enhanced (inflammatory states, growth). Another important function is to produce NADPH in the first steps of glutamine breakdown, which serves to maintain the redox state.
- Glutamine is an anaplerotic substrate. Its breakdown yields glutamic acid and subsequently α-oxoglutarate, which replenishes intermediates of the Krebs-cycle that can branch off at several sites and deliver building stones for cells and matrix.
- In addition to the utilization of the carbon skeleton, the two nitrogen atoms are also utilized for the synthesis of purines and pyrimidines. Other important products are proline, aspartic acid and other nonessential amino acids.
- When cell proliferation and wound healing are required, glutamine is furnished by increased synthesis in peripheral tissues (mainly muscle). Precursors are glucose and glutamic acid, derived from carbon skeletons and amino groups of amino acids and synthesized in the liver. Branched chain amino acids in peripheral tissues supply amino groups for glutamine synthesis.
- The net release of glutamine from peripheral tissues is in principle the best indicator of an adequate supply of glutamine, but has not consistently been measured and related to outcome.
- In severe liver failure peripheral release of glutamine fails to be metabolized by these organs, leading to pathologically elevated levels.
- Especially parenterally administered glutamine(peptide) enriched amino acid mixtures have beneficial effects on infections and bowel integrity in inflammatory states of long duration. In view of the maximal production rate of approximately 30 g/24 h in sepsis, dosages administered above this level are pharmacological and may be deleterious in patients with primary or secondary liver failure.

Keywords Glutamine metabolism • Anaplerosis • Cataplerosis • Redox status • Cell proliferation • Glutamine production • Inflammatory activity • Glutamine administration • Glutamine status

P.B. Soeters, M.D., Ph.D. (✉)
Maastricht University Medical Center, Lanaken, Belgium
e-mail: pb.soeters@maastrichtuniversity.nl

R. Rajendram et al. (eds.), *Glutamine in Clinical Nutrition*, Nutrition and Health,
DOI 10.1007/978-1-4939-1932-1_1, © Springer Science+Business Media New York 2015

Abbreviations

ICW	Intracellular water
AIDS	Acquired immunodeficiency syndrome
NIDDM	Non-insulin-dependent diabetes mellitus
Rd	Rate of disposal
Ra	Rate of disappearance
NADPH	Reduced nicotinamide adenine diphosphate
NH_3	Ammonia

Introduction

The important role of glutamine in metabolism has been appreciated since more than 40 years [1–4]. In the early seventies the focus was mainly on glutamine utilization in the intestine (in cell cultures, in vivo and in the isolated vascularly perfused rat intestine), showing that glutamine is taken up by the intestine in far higher quantities than other amino acids. Its carbon is partly incorporated in tissue insoluble material, CO_2, citrulline, proline, and organic acids (lactic acid and citric acid). The nitrogen appeared largely in citrulline, alanine, ammonia, and proline. Nitrogen appearing in cell components (tissue insoluble material, e.g., protein, nucleotides) was not specified. The proximal small intestine accounted for most of the glutamine uptake and consequently for most of the ammonia release. Decades earlier, ammonia was proposed to cause hepatic encephalopathy, and systemic hyperammonemia was mainly ascribed to ammonia generated in the colon by bacterial degradation of urea and amino acids. This ammonia could escape hepatic detoxification by shunting of portal blood around the liver through collaterals (varices) formed as a consequence of portal hypertension due to liver cirrhosis or presinusoidal inhibition of portal flow. Consequently patients with hepatic failure and encephalopathy were treated with antibiotics and protein restriction. In the eighties, it became clear that ammonia formation largely occurs in the jejunum due to glutamine breakdown, which is not directly influenced by antibiotics. At the same time also immunocytes were found to metabolize substantial amounts of glutamine in vitro [4]. To acquire maximal proliferation rates in culture all cell types require, apart from other components in the medium in lower concentrations, glutamine and glucose, which in the absence of other oxidizable substrate were found to be partly oxidized but also to deliver the components earlier described.

In other studies incubations with whole muscle led to a catabolic state delivering amino acids into the medium but especially glutamine and alanine in larger quantities than their presence in muscle protein [5]. This implies that these two amino acids must have been newly produced. Later experiments in vivo demonstrated that glutamine and alanine production in muscle was greatly enhanced after any stressful event (trauma, endotoxin challenge, cecal ligation and puncture, burns) and this was found even earlier in vivo when measuring net arteriovenous release of amino acids across extremities in septic patients [6]. These findings led to the hypothesis that in stressful or/and malnourished states glutamine is lacking and that supplementation of glutamine improves the response to stress/trauma, etc. [7, 8] Benefit was considered to be especially achievable in the intestine.

The hypothesis was supported by low plasma and tissue levels of glutamine, found in critically ill patients and considered to indicate glutamine deficiency [9]. Basic research and clinical application of modulated nutritional formulas have simultaneously been undertaken before metabolism had been clearly defined and shortages confirmed. Still today modulated feeds are administered without full knowledge of their metabolism. In several publications, the benefit of the supplementation of glutamine has been postulated to result from different mechanisms without apparent

Table 1.1 Proposed roles of glutamine in stressed states (infection, trauma, inflammation, growth)

Proposed roles of glutamine in stress/trauma/infection
Adapted from Wischmeyer [10]
Tissue protection
Enhanced heat shock protein expression
Antiapoptotic effect
Fuel source for epithelial cells
Anti-inflammatory
Attenuation of NF-κB/stress kinase activation
Enhanced peroxisome proliferator-activated receptor-γ activation
Attenuation of cytokine expression
Preservation of tissue metabolic function in stress states
Preservation of ATP levels following sepsis and ischemia/reperfusion
Preservation of mitochondrial function
Antioxidant/attenuation of inducible nitric oxide synthase expression
Enhanced glutathione levels following stress
Attenuation of iNOS synthase activation in sepsis and ischemia/reperfusion
Reduction of oxidant stress

connection and without trying to outline the central role of glutamine in intermediate metabolism (Table 1.1) [10]. In this chapter we describe the role of glutamine in intermediary metabolism in health and disease, the likelihood that its production may be deficient and how to assess this, and situations in which supplementation with glutamine may be beneficial, how much should be supplemented, and in what manner.

Glutamine as a Universal Precursor in Intermediary Metabolism

In this section we describe the central role, played by glutamine, in intermediary metabolism, delivering carbon skeletons and nitrogen containing molecules to support the synthesis of cells and matrix in trauma and disease.

Glutamine (Fig. 1.1) is readily transported into cells and deamidated in several tissues (intestine, spleen, immune cells, kidney) to yield glutamate and NH_3. Glutamate in turn is either transformed to α-ketoglutarate by means of its dehydrogenase or transaminated to equally yield α-ketoglutarate, which serves as an intermediate in the Krebs cycle. In this way, glutamine and glutamic acid (together with glucose) serve as anaplerotic substrates, replenishing Krebs-cycle intermediates in proliferating tissues (Fig. 1.2). In these tissues, the intermediates are only partly regenerated as would happen when the Krebs cycle would exclusively operate to oxidize acetyl-coA, because intermediates branch off at several sites to provide substances supporting cell proliferation in the immune response, wound repair, and growth, and to maintain redox balance. This is called cataplerosis (Fig. 1.3).

In starvation combined with stress (disease, trauma, infection) peripheral tissues (predominantly muscle) become catabolic, implying that protein synthesis is lower than degradation (Fig. 1.4). The resulting amino acids are released in the circulation. A large proportion of these amino acids is taken up by the liver, producing substantial amounts of glucose, glutamic acid, acute phase proteins, and other products in lower quantities (Figs. 1.5 and 1.6). Glucose and glutamic acid are in turn released into the circulation, and are, besides fatty acids, which largely function as fuel, the only substances taken up in peripheral tissues, (skin, adipose tissue, bone but predominantly muscle) in stressed conditions. There they donate their carbon skeletons and amino groups to form glutamine, glycine, alanine,

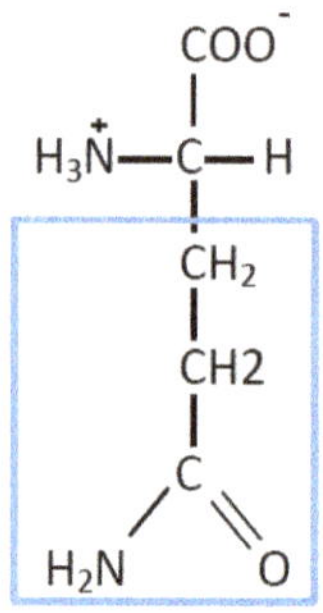

Fig. 1.1 Structure formula of glutamine. The formula shows the ionization at neutral pH (7.0). The part of the molecule inside the *blue box* shows the "R-group" responsible for the specific properties of the amino acid. The part outside the box is common to all amino acids (adapted from Lehninger. Principles of Biochemistry. D.L. Nelson, M.M.Cox. Publisher W.H. Freeman and Company. New York, USA, 2005)

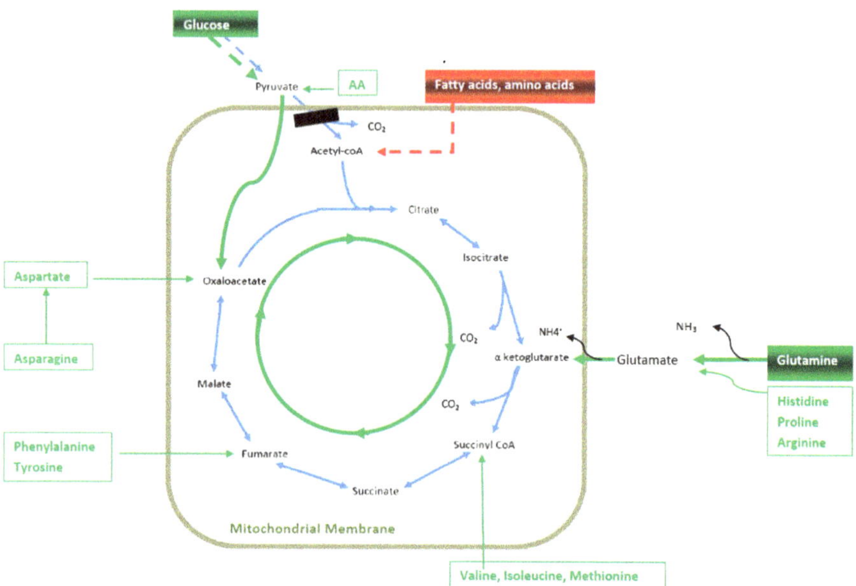

Fig. 1.2 Proliferating cells/growing tissues. *Anaplerosis*. Anaplerosis in activated immune cells and cells in growing tissues. Glutamine, glutamate, and glucose are the main anaplerotic substrates in activated/proliferating cells. Other amino acids probably have a minor role in anaplerosis and are preferentially used in protein synthesis. Complete oxidation of glucose and glutamine is inhibited. Acetyl-coA introduced in the TCA cycle is largely derived from fatty acids and ketone bodies and little from amino acids. Glutamine and glucose furnish little acetyl-coA (see block at pyruvate dehydrogenase step)

and proline in far higher amounts than the quantities present in muscle protein and released after net protein degradation [11]. Which carbon skeleton and which nitrogen ends up where is not exactly specified in vivo in humans but may be estimated on a stoichiometric basis. The amino group of glutamate and branched chain amino acids supplies most of the amino-nitrogen of glycine, alanine, and proline. Glutamine is produced partly from amidation of glutamic acid by ammonia derived from purine metabolism or/and taken up from the circulation, partly from transamination and subsequent amidation of glucose derived α-oxoglutarate. Alanine, produced in muscle after transamination of glucose derived pyruvate and the amino group of glutamic acid, is the major gluconeogenic amino

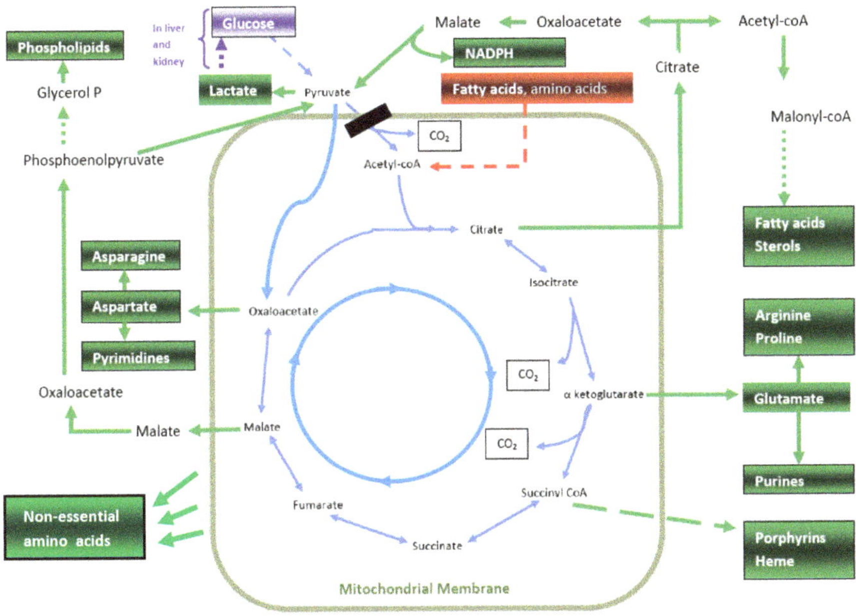

Fig. 1.3 Proliferating cells/growing tissues. *Cataplerosis.* Cataplerosis in activated immune cells and cells in growing tissues. Cataplerosis furnishes acetyl-coA for FA and sterol synthesis, NADPH in the malate-pyruvate cycle, glutamate for the synthesis of purines, aspartate for pyrimidines. Pyruvate is partly transaminated with glutamic acid to yield alanine (not shown). It is not exactly known how many and which intermediates are cataplerotically transaminated with glutamic acid to yield other non-essential amino acids. Glycolysis furnishes lactate. Lactate and alanine are exported and can serve as precursors of gluconeogenesis in liver and kidney

Fig. 1.4 Multicatheterized pig model of sepsis (after 24-h endotoxin infusion) [11]. *Upper panel*: Disposal (protein synthesis) and production (protein degradation) of phenylalanine in muscle of pigs 24 h after an endotoxin challenge. *Lower panel*: Disposal (protein synthesis) and production (protein degradation) of phenylalanine, corrected for oxidation in liver of pigs 24 h after an endotoxin challenge. The net balance represents the release of amino acids in the hindquarter and uptake in the liver. (Figure adapted from data in Bruins MJ et al, Clin Sci (Lond). 2003 Feb;104(2):127–41. PubMed PMID: 12546635 with permission [11])

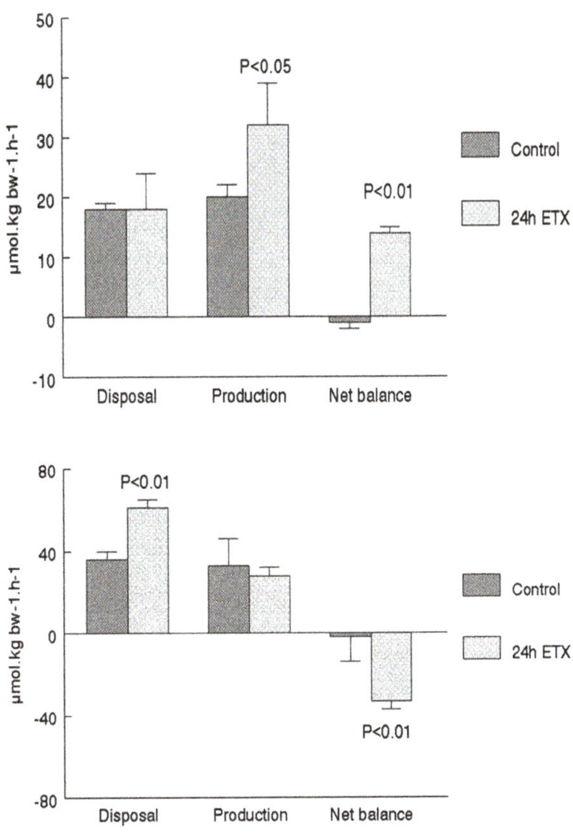

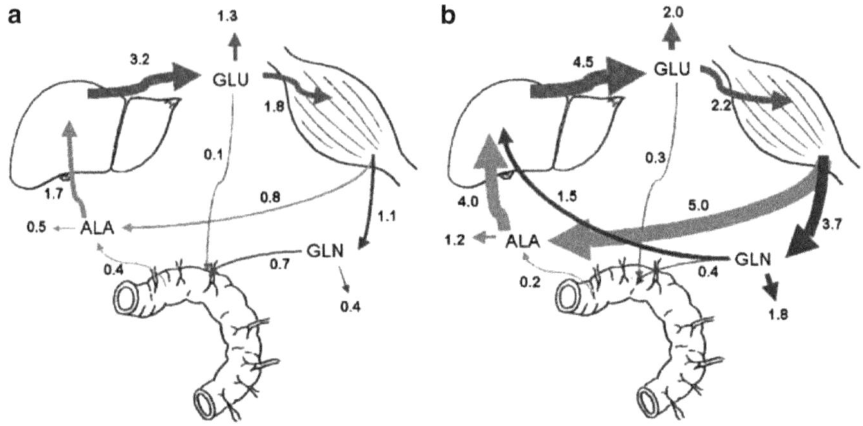

Fig. 1.5 Fluxes of glutamic acid, glutamine, and alanine between liver, muscle, and intestine [11]. Fluxes of glutamate (GLU), glutamine (GLN), and alanine (ALA) between liver, muscle, and portal-drained viscera after a 24-h infusion of (**a**) saline or (**b**) endotoxin. Release of other amino acids by muscle and intestine and uptake by liver are not shown. The release of glutamic acid by the liver should be emphasized, because it is utilized in peripheral tissues to furnish building blocks for rapidly proliferating cells (figures reproduced from Bruins MJ et al. Clin Sci (Lond). 2003 Feb;104(2): 127–41. PubMed PMID: 12546635 with permission [11])

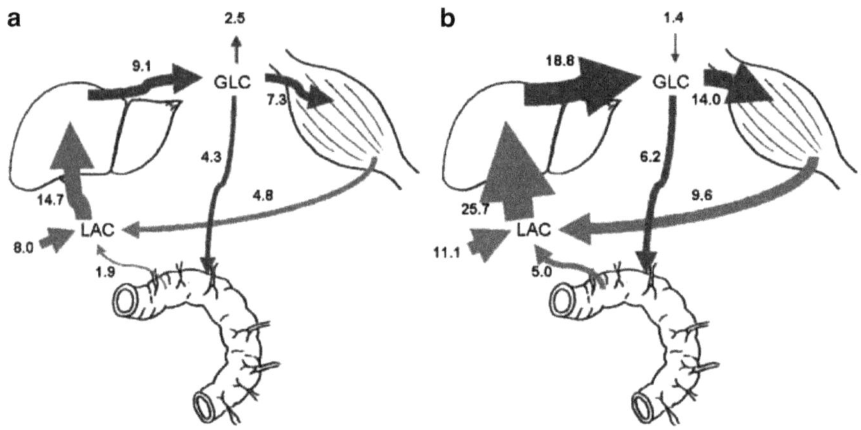

Fig. 1.6 Fluxes of glucose and lactate between liver, muscle and intestine [11]. Fluxes of glucose (GLC) and lactate (LAC) between liver, muscle and portal-drained viscera after a 24-h infusion of (A) saline or (B) endotoxin. Fluxes are given as μmol/minute/kg bodyweight (figures reproduced from Bruins MJ et al, Clin Sci (Lond). 2003 Feb;104(2): 127–41. PubMed PMID: 12546635 with permission [11])

acid in the liver, in addition producing urea or donating its amino group to α-oxoglutarate, forming glutamic acid. Another major substrate for hepatic glucose formation is lactate, accounting for less than 50 % of the products of glucose breakdown in peripheral tissues and in a variable rate in rapidly proliferating cells in the stress response (Cori cycling) (Fig. 1.6). The complex cycling of glucose and amino acids across several organs is an example of many of the metabolic processes in the body. It ensures continuous availability of necessary substrates and allows instantaneous regulation. Glucose and ammonia formation in the kidney with glutamine as substrate is part of this cycling and probably serves in the kidney to excrete superfluous nitrogen, to preserve anaplerotic substrate and to maintain acid base balance. Accelerated gluconeogenesis in liver and kidney is necessarily accompanied by increased urea and ammonia production, respectively. Not only peripheral tissues are catabolic, but the anabolic synthesis of immune cells, wound cells, matrix, etc. does not match peripheral nitrogen losses, so that in stress situations there is net nitrogen loss in the whole body. Hepatic glutamic acid production in (stress-) starvation can be considered to be a nitrogen sparing mechanism, but hepatic amino acid induced gluconeogenesis inevitably is accompanied to some degree by urea formation, although this is very low in pure starvation, when, in contradistinction with stress starvation, gluconeogenesis largely occurs in the kidney, utilizing mainly glutamine and producing ammonia, which is partly excreted in the urine.

Altogether in stress situations muscle in collaboration with the liver releases high quantities of glutamine, glycine, proline, alanine, and lower quantities of the remaining 16 amino acids present in muscle protein [11]. These processes increase quantitatively when the inflammatory response or growth rates are stronger. Muscle catabolism therefore plays a useful adaptive role in host response and inhibiting this response may be deleterious but cannot or only modestly be accomplished by nutritional means. Supplementation with glutamine-enriched parenteral nutrition increases the total appearance in plasma although endogenous glutamine (and alanine) production in peripheral tissues continues [12]. Metabolism in the liver is complex because, in addition to its role in intermediary metabolism, the liver has an important immune function, producing immune cells and proteins, active in host response.

It is noteworthy that matrix (collagen), comprising at least a quart of the solids in peripheral tissues, contains high amounts of alanine, glycine, and proline and that it is synthesized during tissue formation and wound healing. The degree with which its catabolism in peripheral tissues contributes to the amino acid mix that is released in the circulation is probably modest, because turnover of collagen is low, possibly with the exception of a small more rapidly turning over pool [13].

In the tissues responsible for host response and growth, besides glucose (via pyruvate carboxylase), glutamine (via glutamic acid), and to a lesser degree other glucogenic amino acids are taken up as anaplerotic substrate (Fig. 1.2), furnishing the carbon for purines, pyrimidines, sterols, and fatty acid synthesis (Fig. 1.3). In addition both nitrogens of glutamine are built into pyrimidines (via aspartic acid) and purines. Furthermore glutamine yields substantial amounts of proline used in collagen synthesis especially in growing states and in (wound) healing. Glycine is produced in high quantities via 3-phosphoglycerate (branching off from glycolysis) via serine formation and also provides nitrogen for pyrimidine synthesis. Another role of the high production rate of glycine in peripheral tissues consists of, together with alanine-, glutamine-, and glutamine-derived proline, the synthesizing collagen, because these amino acids are present in collagen in far higher amounts than in myofibrillar protein.

In addition to the production of nucleic acids, rapidly proliferating cells take up a normal amino acid mix for protein synthesis and cover their energy requirements to a limited degree by glycolysis, partial oxidation of glucose (6- to 5-carbon) in the pentose phosphate pathway and of glutamine in the step from α-oxoglutarate to succinyl-coA (5- to 4- carbon). Contrary to general belief more recent literature supports fatty acid oxidation as a main source of energy in rapidly proliferating cells (especially reported in cancer [14] and pregnancy [15]) whereas glucose oxidation via pyruvate - dehydrogenase and the formation of acetyl-coA oxidized in the Krebs cycle is substantially inhibited [16]. This is supported by a simple calculation that in stress starvation or in starving cancer patients a net loss of 14 g of nitrogen/24 hours, excreted in the urine, reflects a protein loss of approximately 87 g, yielding 45 g of glucose (nitrogen should be subtracted and not all amino acids are glucogenic), assuming that this nitrogen is largely derived from amino acids. Forty-five grams of glucose together with maximally 10 g of glycerol derived glucose would cover less than half of energy requirements of the brain, if fully oxidized, but even this is unlikely because of the role of glucose in proliferative pathways. These changes in metabolism constitute the hallmark of insulin resistance, inhibiting glucose oxidation and promoting Cori-cycling (glucose-pyruvate/lactate-glucose) and pentose phosphate pathway flux [17]. Therefore fatty acid oxidation must provide most of the energy (90 %) in stress starvation.

Importantly in the breakdown of glutamine NADPH is produced. Outside the mitochondrion, glucose yields NADPH in the first two steps of the pentose phosphate pathway and inside the mitochondrion in several pathways, the most important ones probably being the isocitrate-dehydrogenase pathway and the conversion of glutamine via glutamic acid to α-oxoglutarate. NADPH is crucial in maintaining redox balance (e.g., reducing oxidized glutathione and proteins), supporting fatty acid synthesis, cholesterol and other components and allowing an oxidative burst of macrophages in dealing with debris and microorganisms.

Why are even in vitro specifically glucose and glutamine necessary to allow rapid cell proliferation? [4, 18]

In vivo small bowel enterocytes rely to a substantial degree on glucose and glutamine to maintain their integrity [19]. Newsholme suggested that the specific need for glutamine and glucose in immune cells (probably all rapidly proliferating cells; see above) arises from the need to produce NADPH [20]. In addition, glutamine is very suitable for cell proliferation because it is abundantly present in the body and can function as an anaplerotic substrate for the Krebs cycle, delivering α-oxoglutarate. All subsequent intermediates can branch off and deliver other substrates for further processing to produce for instance nonessential amino acids. Glutamine is therefore a universal precursor of the carbon of many cell elements, and contains two nitrogen atoms, both of which can be utilized for the synthesis of the bases of nucleic acids and the amino nitrogen also playing an important role in transamination reactions.

The described trafficking of glutamine between organs plays another role. In the first step of the degradation of glutamine NH_3 is generated, which has toxic effects on the brain if it reaches the circulation in large amounts. The glutamine that is metabolized in tissues for other purposes (e.g., cycling) than its incorporation in protein, predominantly yields NH_3 in the first degradation step. These tissues are anatomically located in such a way that the NH_3 that is released is immediately scavenged. This applies to the intestine, producing substantial amounts of ammonia in the jejunum and via bacterial action in the colon, which is metabolized by the liver. The kidney also produces ammonia which is partly excreted in the urine and partly released in the systemic circulation, where it may reach the brain but to an even higher degree peripheral tissues (muscle, adipose tissue) where it may provide some of the amide-nitrogen for the synthesis of glutamine, binding toxic NH_3. After synthesis glutamine can be released in the systemic circulation, where glutamine serves as a non-toxic nitrogen carrier despite present in far higher concentrations than any other amino acid.

It has been suggested that supplementation with glutamine may increase glutathione synthesis (via glutamic acid). The evidence put forward is not very convincing. Even more, cysteine availability is more likely to be limiting than glutamic acid. It is more likely that its connection with glutathione consists of the important role of glutamine to produce NADPH in its breakdown which in turn promotes reduction of oxidized glutathione maintaining redox balance.

A fourth more specific role of glutamine may be as one of the osmolytes regulating cell homeostasis in hyper- and hypo-osmolar conditions. Cell swelling or shrinkage have been claimed to play a role in the regulation of protein synthesis [21]. The original correlation found between intracellular glutamine concentrations and protein synthesis has not consistently been confirmed in later research [22].

It may be concluded that in traumatized/diseased/growth conditions, glutamine has more specific roles as nontoxic nitrogen carrier, as anaplerotic substrate required for cell proliferation, as driver of NADPH production required for fatty acid synthesis and maintenance of redox balance, countering oxidative stress, and as an osmolyte. In view of its central place in intermediary metabolism, a shortage in glutamine availability would imply that flux in biosynthetic processes would be compromised. This will specifically be harmful in situations where rapid cell proliferation is required. The functions ascribed to glutamine (Table 1.1) are all resulting from this central role of glutamine in metabolism and not from separate unrelated metabolic pathways.

The Significance of Amino Acid Concentrations and Fluxes

Glutamine is by far the most abundant free amino acid in plasma and tissues in humans and varies in plasma in healthy man between 450 and 650 μmol/L. Plasma concentrations drop to 75 % of preoperative values after surgical trauma in non-depleted colorectal cancer patients to around 450 μmol/L and generally decrease in inflammatory states [23]. Plasma levels have been found to correlate more closely with disease severity than with malnutrition [24]. In tissues levels vary between 2 and 4 mmol/L intracellular water (ICW) in intestinal mucosa [23] and between 12 and 20 mmol/L intracellular water in muscle and liver (ICW) [9, 21, 25], whereas in pancreatitis patients with multiple organ failure, levels may drop as low as 5 mmol/L [26]. An exception exists in acute fulminant liver failure where very high levels have been found amounting to 1,000–3,000 μmol/L in plasma, which may be aggravated by renal failure [27, 28]. Apart from true liver failure, secondary liver failure may arise (shock, acute pulmonary hypertension and right heart failure) and eventual renal failure that may lead to failure to metabolize glutamine and other amino acids released by peripheral tissues in catabolic states. The liver and the kidney both metabolize glutamine and detoxify (liver) or excrete ammonia (kidney). Failure therefore leads to hyperaminoacidemia including high glutamine levels and hyperammonemia. In cerebral spinal fluid very high levels have been found in acute hepatic failure [27]. Recent data confirm the association between hyperglutaminemia and ICU mortality [29]. In this study low glutamine levels did not correlate with APACHE II score at admittance, but scrutiny of the detailed patient data is required to explain the discrepancy with an earlier study [24].

The steep concentration difference between plasma and tissue levels most likely is maintained by active Na^+/K^+-ATPase driven ion pump transport. This provides the drive for secondary transporters like the Na^+- glutamine co-transporter and other transporters and is partly responsible for the strong uphill gradient for many substances including amino acids and specifically glutamine. Intracellular glutamine concentrations may however also be influenced by glutamine delivery, intracellular production (from de novo synthesis or protein degradation), uptake (glutamine degradation and protein synthesis), and transport from inside to outside the cell. The fivefold difference between mucosal and muscle intracellular glutamine concentration shows that tissue-specific factors must also play a role. Different metabolic situations may exert specific effects on tissue amino acid concentrations via the mechanisms mentioned. Examples are sepsis [26], surgical trauma [30] or mono-organ failure [31].

A glutamine shortage can in principle be demonstrated by decreased release of glutamine and other amino acids (A–V concentration x leg or arm plasma flow x a factor extrapolating from this limb flow to total peripheral flow) from peripheral tissues (muscle, skin, bone) to tissues, requiring these amino acids and playing a crucial role in the response to trauma and disease (splanchnic tissues, immune system, wound) (Table 1.2). Clowes et al. reasoned that stable plasma amino acid concentrations prove that peripheral production balances central uptake [6]. He demonstrated in 1983 that septic cirrhotic patients with a low peripheral release of glutamine and other amino acids and thus metabolizing low quantities in their splanchnic tissues died of sepsis, while those with a high peripheral release survived [6].

Modern technology has allowed measuring the rate of appearance (Ra) in and disposal (Rd) from plasma of a certain substrate by the organism and it has been proposed that these measures might be an adequate measure for the supply of the substrate to the splanchnic and healing tissues. This is questionable because the relevant measure is the <u>net</u> release by peripheral tissues to the central tissues. Net release and uptake by organs are determined by the difference between Ra and Rd across an organ. Because both components can change in individual organs and total body Ra and Rd is determined by the sum of Ra's and Rd's of all organs, total Ra and Rd do not necessarily need to increase to nevertheless induce increased release from peripheral tissues and uptake by central tissues (Fig. 1.8). This means that the whole body Ra and the Rd of glutamine is not an adequate measure of the net release of glutamine from peripheral tissues to central tissues, active in host response.

Table 1.2 Net production (Arterio-Venous difference times flow) of amino acids, glutamine and alanine from peripheral tissues, considered to represent predominantly muscle in human studies in different clinical conditions [6, 55–59]

First authors	Unit of measurement	Control	Trauma	Sepsis	Septic Survivers	Septic non-survivers
Net peripheral release of AMINO ACIDS (g/m^2/24 h or g/1.7 $m^2$24 h) or (g/100 ml muscle and skin mass/24 or g/40 L of assumed total muscle and skin volume/24 h)						
Clowes (Ann. Surgery) ICU	g/m^2/24 h g/1.7 m^2/24 h	23.9 40.6			76.7 130.4	49.5 84.1
Vesali (Clin Nutr) ICU				0.056 23.3		
Gore (JPEN) Burns				0.14 56.7		
Carli (Clin Sci Lnd)	g /100 ml leg volume/24 h or total g/24 h (extrapolated to 40 L of assumed peripheral tissue)	0.051 20.4		0.11 44		
Mjaaland (Ann Surgery)		0.12 46.7		0.15 61.5		
Net peripheral release of GLUTAMINE (g/m^2/24 h or g/1.7 $m^2$24 h) or (g/100 ml muscle and skin mass/24 or g/40 L of assumed total muscle and skin volume/24 h)						
Clowes (Ann. Surg.) ICU	g/m^2/24 h g/1.7 m'/24 h				13.8 23.6	12.2 (NS) 20.8
Fong (Surgery)		0.056 22.3		0.065 25.8		
Vesali (Clin Nutr)				0.020 8.2		
Gore (JPEN)				0.014 5.4		
Carli (Clin Sci Lnd)	g /100 ml leg volume/24 h or total g/24 h (extrapolated to 40 L of assumed peripheral tissue)	0.048 19.1		0.083 33.0		
Mjaaland (Ann Surgery)		0.012 4.9		0.029 11.5		
Net peripheral release of ALANINE (g/m^2/24 h or g/1.7 $m^2$24 h) or (g/100 ml muscle and skin mass/24 or g/40 L of assumed total muscle and skin volume/24 h)						
Clowes (Ann. Surgery	g/m^2/24 h g/1.7 m/24 h				10.3 17.5	6.5 11.1
Vesali (Clin Nutr)				0.019 7.5		
Gore (JPEN)		0.014 5.4				
Carli (Clin Sci Lnd)	g/100 ml/24 h or total g/24 h (extrapolated to 40 L of assumed peripheral tissue)	0.051 12.1	0.068 27.0			
Mjaaland (Ann Surgery)		0.017 6.9	0.027 10.8			

Is There a Shortage in Disease and Trauma?

In the clinical literature decreases in plasma glutamine have generally been interpreted as a shortage and an indication to supplement glutamine in these presumed deficiency states.

Sources of Glutamine in plasma

Glutamine is a normal constituent of muscle protein. Breakdown of muscle protein therefore yields free glutamine which will appear in the cytosol and can be exported from the cell into the plasma compartment. Another source of glutamine consists of *de novo synthesis*, which is increased after trauma and other inflammatory conditions (Table 1.2). A third source of glutamine consists of the free pool, which shrinks in diseased states and therefore releases glutamine in the systemic circulation. The amount appearing in this manner would cover only the amount metabolized in half a day after trauma and during severe illness. This amount is therefore negligible in longer disease processes. An additional source of glutamine consists of exogenous supply as free amino acid, as dipeptide or as protein.

What Do Depressed Glutamine Concentrations in Plasma and Tissues Mean?

We discussed in the previous sections that several factors influence plasma amino acids levels, which makes it difficult to pinpoint one of them as the causative factor. This includes glutamine shortage. The decrease in plasma glutamine and most other amino acids [26, 31] has been found to correlate more significantly with the severity of disease than with nutritional state [24, 26] In patients with gastrointestinal diseases plasma and tissue glutamine levels did not correlate with percentage weight loss or percentage ideal body weight, but rather with the sedimentation rate and with leucocyte counts in blood as measures reflecting inflammatory activity [23]. The postoperative drop of plasma glutamine levels in cancer patients on the second day after operation, also indicates that these levels reflect the inflammatory influence of trauma and resuscitation rather than glutamine shortage [25].

An important factor, potentially influencing the generalized hypoaminoacidemia in most (sub-) acute inflammatory states, consists of the increased endo- and extravascular extracellular distribution spaces. The intravascular volume increases due to vasodilatation in most patients, if they are well resuscitated. Inflammation due to any non-infectious or infectious causes leads to increased capillary permeability, which in turn increases the escape rate of albumin, electrolytes, amino acids, fluid, and other components from the circulation to the extravascular extracellular space and increases extravascular extracellular volume. These effects of inflammatory activity may be connected with membrane permeability and decreases in membrane potential. Solute concentrations drop as a consequence of dilution in this increased volume. These distribution abnormalities develop within hours after the onset of illness and correlate with its severity. This explains in part why plasma glutamine levels correspond better with disease severity and poor survival than with the state of undernutrition. As mentioned before, additional factors may also contribute to hypoaminoacidemia, but it is impossible to define the contribution of each single factor. We conclude that it is unlikely that low plasma levels of glutamine can be reliably interpreted as reflecting a shortage.

Tissue concentrations of glutamine are much higher than plasma levels. In patients considered to require parenteral nutrition because of intestinal disease, mucosal glutamine levels were significantly lower (and intestinal permeability higher) in the group exhibiting inflammatory activity, whereas percentage weight loss in the absence of inflammatory activity was not significantly paralleled by a decrease in mucosal glutamine levels [23]. Similar as plasma concentrations, the tissue concentration drop results from alterations in transmembrane transport and permeability. TNF- α, produced in inflammatory states or after an endotoxin challenge, has been shown to inhibit the activity of the Na^+/K^+-ATPase pump in the kidney and Caco-2 cells of the rat (effects partially reversed by Indomethacin) [32, 33]. These changes lead to altered activity of secondary active transporters, passive transport, and, importantly, tight junction proteins [34]. Consequently steep uphill gradients of solutes cannot be maintained in critical illness and after trauma, explaining the decrease of several intracellular solutes, including glutamine. In conclusion low tissue concentrations of glutamine reflect inflammatory activity and not always glutamine shortage. However, long-standing inflammatory activity induces catabolism leading to malnutrition. In that situation malnutrition may possibly contribute to decreased glutamine production and delivery.

Do Glutamine Fluxes Represent a Shortage?

The results of studies regarding the release of glutamine (and other amino acids) from peripheral tissues, considered to represent predominantly muscle tissue) are expressed either as g/m^2/min [6] or as g/100 ml leg volume/minute. We extrapolated these data to g/1.7 m^2/24 h and to g/40 L of total muscle and skin volume/24 h to compare the amount of glutamine peripherally released per day in adults (Table 1.2). When plasma amino acid levels are stable, the peripheral release of amino acids is assumed to be taken up in "central tissues" including the liver, immune system, kidney, and healing tissues. Accordingly, the amount of glutamine released in non-stressed postabsorptive states ranges from 5 to 20 g per 24 h. All papers except one [35] express the release of glutamine as nmol/100 ml leg or arm volume/minute but the methods used to measure total leg or arm volume and the extrapolation to whole body release is not always precisely described, which may explain the variability. In sepsis or after operative trauma the release increased 15–135 % compared with healthy postabsorptive individuals. The highest value (33 g/24 h) was found in sepsis. (Table 1.2)

In a pig model of operative trauma, we confirmed the hypothesized net efflux from peripheral tissues and the increased uptake by liver and spleen, whereas uptake of glutamine by the intestine decreased (Fig. 1.7) [36]. This finding shows that immune cells (as represented by the spleen)

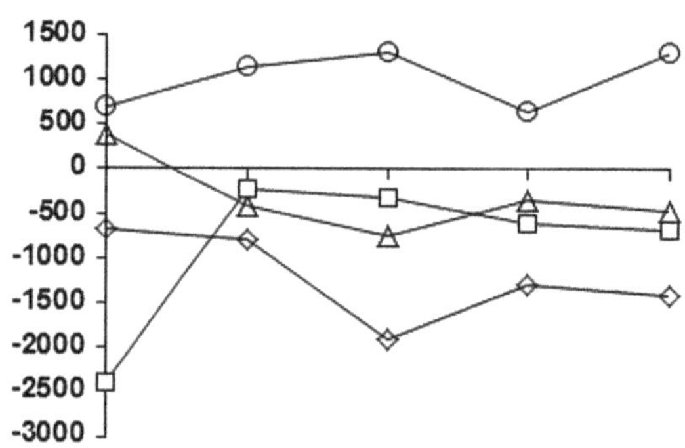

Fig. 1.7 Net fluxes (A-V differences times flow) of glutamine across liver, intestine, spleen, and muscle. Fluxes of glutamine across liver (*open triangle*) intestine (*open diamond*), hindquarter (muscle) (*open square*) and spleen (*open circle*) in nmol/kg/min measured 1,2,3 and 4 days after operative trauma in pigs. Control values were obtained 12 days after operation (figure adapted from Deutz NE et al, Clin Sci (Lond). 1992 Nov;83(5):607–14. PubMed PMID: 1335399. Epub 1992/11/01. Eng with permission [35])

preferentially take up glutamine (along with glucose) in vivo, as well as other amino acids in lower quantities, and modest amounts of fatty acids.

In conclusion, release of amino acids and specifically glutamine by peripheral tissues may be viewed as a measure of the adequacy of the metabolic response to trauma and all other situations where rapid cell and matrix deposition is required or taking place. This applies to a long list of situations including for instance pregnancy, during host defence and in cancerous states [37]. In view of the global interest in cancer, much basic research in this area has been performed in tumour models. The general conclusions, that can be derived from this large body of research, are that glucose and glutamine predominantly serve as building blocks for proliferation of cancer cells and stroma cells, supporting tumour cell proliferation, and producing reducing equivalents [37–41]. In these situations glucose and glutamine are oxidized only to a very limited degree and probably only as far as necessary to furnish the crucial products for synthesis of biomass. The body largely relies on fatty acid oxidation to cover energy requirements (see earlier) [16]. Unfortunately, no consistent data exist regarding the efflux of glutamine in severely undernourished patients. Although this measure might throw light on whether the body furnishes sufficient quantities of amino acids (specifically glutamine) to central tissues, such studies were not continued.

Does (Diminished) Appearance of Glutamine Indicate a Shortage?

It is possible that net glutamine release by muscle was not further investigated, because three decades ago stable isotope technology was introduced, which promised to furnish more in depth knowledge without necessitating unpopular invasive techniques in patients. As indicated previously, glutamine labelled with stable or radioactive isotopes was used to measure appearance rates (Ra) of glutamine in plasma. Amounts appearing in plasma ranged between 60 and 100 g/24 h depending on the label used. Appearance rates where highest when the amino-nitrogen at the 2 position of glutamine was labelled implying that transamination reactions with glutamine derived glutamic acid must be very active. This amount exceeds the amount that is released from peripheral tissues into the circulation (see previous section). A difficulty with the glutamine tracer methodology is firstly that even after 11 h tracer enrichment in glutamine has still not plateaued [42]. This implies that the turnover rates obtained early during the tracer infusion are an overestimation compared to the rates found with later measurements. Secondly as mentioned earlier the tracer methodology used in principle measures rates of appearance of <u>all</u> glutamine released in plasma and not the net release from peripheral tissues to the "central" tissues active in host response (arteriovenous concentration differences x flow) (Fig. 1.8).

With the amino nitrogen label the different laboratories found rather similar turnover rates despite different clinical conditions. The uncertain value of the Ra of glutamine into plasma as an indicator of glutamine adequacy is highlighted by data in the literature. While there is a significant increase in the Ra of weight losing patients with GI disease compared to volunteers [43] and wasting AIDS patients [44], the Ra was unaltered in NIDDM [45], in critical illness [46], before and after operation [25], and decreased in patients that were weight stable with short bowel syndrome [47] and in burn patients compared to volunteers receiving endotoxin [48]. In view of the finding that in traumatized or septic patients the net release of glutamine from muscle increases (Table 1.2), we can explain our finding that glutamine turnover does not increase after operation by assuming that an increased net release from muscle to central tissues is generated by decreasing the uptake component (Rd) in muscle and concomitantly decreasing the production component (Ra) in central tissues (Fig. 1.8).

These findings support our views expressed in a previous section, based on theoretical grounds, that Ra and Rd of glutamine do not furnish reliable information regarding glutamine availability. The multiple roles of glutamine in a multitude of reactions central in intermediary metabolism and the

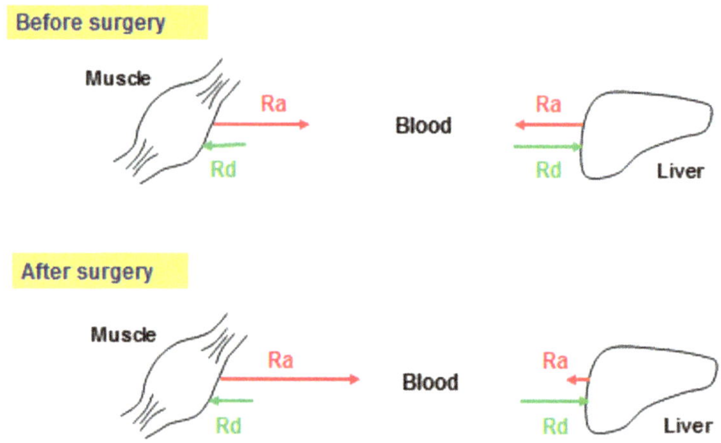

Fig. 1.8 Proposed kinetics of glutamine before and after surgery. Potential kinetics of glutamine after surgical trauma. In view of the fact that turnover did not increase and net release from muscle must have increased, the figure proposes that flux is generated by increasing the rate of appearance (Ra) in muscle and simultaneously decreasing the Ra in the other organs. In this way, flux can be generated without increasing whole body turnover

slow mixing with the large intracellular nitrogen pool may explain the absence of stable enrichment values of the tracer, which casts doubt on the validity of the Ra's found [42].

We conclude that the highest dosages of glutamine, administered till recently in clinical practice (approximately 30 g) approximates the maximal amount that has been found to be released in septic or traumatized states, approximating half of the values found for the total flux. These dosages should therefore be considered to be physiological rather than a pharmacological dose.

When Is Extra Glutamine Necessary and What For?

In view of the role of glutamine in intermediary metabolism a theoretical rationale may be proposed for its supplementation, but ultimately beneficial effects of the supplementation of glutamine should provide proof for the presence of glutamine deficiency.

Theoretical Reasons for Increased Glutamine Requirements

The inflammatory state is present in acute trauma/infection but many inflammatory elements also play a role for instance in cancer and pregnancy [37]. In host response efficient operation of the immune system is required to repair damaged tissues and to synthesize biomass. For that purpose especially substantial amounts of glutamine as well as glucose are utilized, which are acquired from the host. In trauma/infection this may require supplementation if endogenous supply is deficient. In theory, glutamine production by peripheral tissues may be compromised in the severely malnourished state, in which diminished muscle mass may preclude sufficient release of amino acids for the production of glucose and subsequently glutamine, as well as a mix of other amino acids to synthesize protein and other cell components in proliferating cells operative in host response. Along similar lines, inflammation may require large quantities of glutamine, which may fail to be produced when severe inflammation is prolonged. These theoretical considerations may be supported in practice by studies showing a better effect of glutamine when supplemented to patients who are critically ill for a long period of critical illness and for as long as the patient stays in that critical condition. Vice versa, well-nourished patients that are not critically ill or only for a very short period may not benefit from glutamine supplementation.

Practical Facts Supporting a Shortage of Glutamine

There is some support for the claim that enteral glutamine supplementation is beneficial in patients with burns or trauma, while studies looking at other categories of critically ill patients failed to prove benefit. This might be due to relatively well preserved enteral tolerance in patients with trauma and burns, while in patients with severe sepsis or septic shock, intolerance to enteral nutrition is a common finding. An additional explanation for lack of benefit of enterally administered glutamine may be the strong first pass uptake of glutamine in the intestine. Consequently, much less glutamine reaches the systemic circulation when enterally administered compared to parenteral administration. This may explain why more evidence is available showing a decrease in infections but no effect on mortality, supporting parenteral supplementation of glutamine in critically ill patients, i.e., patients with substantial and long-standing inflammatory activity [49–51]. However, in a recent observational study it was shown that 55–60 g of glutamine supplementation increased mortality [52]. This amount is twice the maximal amount that has been shown to be produced (and thus metabolized) in adult critically ill patients (see earlier). Since long it is known that patients with acute fulminant liver failure or secondary liver failure due to acute pulmonary hypertension cannot metabolize the amino acids derived from peripheral protein breakdown, which results in strongly elevated amino acid levels [27, 28]. This was the case in some patients in the study [52], which nevertheless received the enriched formula. It should be emphasized that any single amino acid administered in abundance can cause toxic symptoms. This may interfere among others with neurotransmitter metabolism and it has been proposed that high glutamine levels in the astrocytes cause brain edema and encephalopathy [53]. "Enrichment" of the nutrition formula with a single amino acid should therefore be within levels, not higher than the maximal fluxes of the amino acid found in humans in vivo and against a background of a normal composition of essential and nonessential amino acids. In practice this means that glutamine should be supplemented to a normal amino acid mixture in amounts between 12 and approximately 30 g in adults with normal built and normal liver and kidney function.

No unequivocal benefit is obtained while studying the effect of glutamine supplementation on bowel integrity. These results may be skewed by the fact that only a proportion of patients receiving glutamine supplementation did suffer from severe inflammatory activity [54].

Interestingly, in some of the studies referred to, insulin sensitivity appears to be improved in critically ill patients receiving supplemental alanyl-glutamine in their parenteral nutrition mixture [50, 51].

In summary, the results of glutamine supplementation suggest that benefit is only achieved in the presence of overt and long-standing inflammation, a situation in which clinical research has shown that more glutamine is utilized by the immune system, as well as healing and growing tissues. This beneficial effect supports the claim that, in these conditions, the organism may suffer from glutamine shortage. The amounts of glutamine supplemented represent between 33 and 100 % of maximal amounts released by peripheral tissues in sepsis, reported in the literature (Table 1.2). This implies that glutamine effects do not result from the administration of pharmacological dosages. In host response other amino acids are also produced in excess of their composition in muscle protein. This applies to glycine, alanine, and proline. Hypothetically, supplementation of the normal mix of amino acids in food or formulas with these amino acids may have additional beneficial effects.

Conclusions

Solid scientific data supporting an absolute shortage of glutamine in patients are lacking. Decreased plasma concentrations are determined by many factors, including acute inflammatory activity and the resulting distribution abnormalities, changes in synthesis and breakdown, and other factors, and therefore are not a reliable indicator of glutamine shortage. Release of glutamine by muscle in disease states and especially in the depleted state might be a good indicator, but has not been thoroughly studied. Tracer data regarding the turnover of glutamine in plasma (Ra and Rd) in well- or undernourished individuals in inflammatory and control conditions do not provide reliable information regarding glutamine status.

Sufficient data exist showing that glutamine is an essential nutrient in all rapidly proliferating cells and growing tissues, including cancer. It provides many different building blocks for these cells and their stroma and simultaneously contributes to maintenance of redox balance by providing reducing equivalents, which are also necessary to synthesize fatty acids and to allow the immune system to repair tissue damage. Theoretically therefore, glutamine supplementation may be beneficial in patients with long standing inflammatory activity, that are not producing sufficient quantities of glutamine either due to malnutrition or because they cannot meet the demands of the extremely severe inflammatory illnesses of patients in our present day intensive care units. In line with this, clinical data show that benefit of parenteral glutamine supplementation is especially achieved in critically ill patients, i.e., patients with substantial inflammation or sepsis. Benefit may possibly be also achieved in traumatized or burn patients, receiving extra glutamine enterally. Although controversial results exist, in some large multicenter studies in critically ill patients, infectious complications have been shown to be decreased and interestingly, insulin sensitivity to be improved. On the basis of these beneficial effects, one may assume that these patients suffer from glutamine shortage. This is supported by the fact that the amounts supplemented are not larger than the amounts newly produced by the body itself and therefore are not in the pharmacological range. When pharmacological dosages are administered, patients with marginal liver and (metabolic) kidney function have to deal with excess glutamine and may fail to metabolize these amounts, leading to adverse events. Consequently, it is recommended to supplement single amino acids always in (patho)physiological dosages together with an amino acid mix in normal composition.

References

1. Windmueller HG, Spaeth AE. Uptake and metabolism of plasma glutamine by the small intestine. J Biol Chem. 1974;249(16):5070–9.
2. Watford M, Lund P, Krebs HA. Isolation and metabolic characteristics of rat and chicken enterocytes. Biochem J. 1979;178(3):589–96.
3. Ardawi MS. Skeletal muscle glutamine production in thermally injured rats. Clin Sci. 1988;74(2):165–72.
4. Ardawi MS, Newsholme EA. Glutamine metabolism in lymphocytes of the rat. Biochem J. 1983;212(3):835–42.
5. Garber AJ, Karl IE, Kipnis DM. Alanine and glutamine synthesis and release from skeletal muscle. II The precursor role of amino acids in alanine and glutamine synthesis. J Biol Chem. 1976;251(3):836–43.
6. Clowes Jr GH, Hirsch E, George BC, Bigatello LM, Mazuski JE, Villee Jr CA. Survival from sepsis. The significance of altered protein metabolism regulated by proteolysis inducing factor, the circulating cleavage product of interleukin-1. Ann Surg. 1985;202(4):446–58.
7. Souba WW, Wilmore DW. Postoperative alteration of arteriovenous exchange of amino acids across the gastrointestinal tract. Surgery. 1983;94(2):342–50.
8. Wilmore DW, Smith RJ, O'Dwyer ST, Jacobs DO, Ziegler TR, Wang XD. The gut: a central organ after surgical stress. Surgery. 1988;104(5):917–23.
9. Vinnars E, Bergstom J, Furst P. Influence of the postoperative state on the intracellular free amino acids in human muscle tissue. Ann Surg. 1975;182(6):665–71.

10. Wischmeyer PE. Glutamine: mode of action in critical illness. Crit Care Med. 2007;35(9 Suppl):S541–4.
11. Bruins MJ, Deutz NE, Soeters PB. Aspects of organ protein, amino acid and glucose metabolism in a porcine model of hypermetabolic sepsis. Clin Sci (Lond). 2003;104(2):127–41.
12. van Acker BA, Hulsewe KW, Wagenmakers AJ, von Meyenfeldt MF, Soeters PB. Response of glutamine metabolism to glutamine-supplemented parenteral nutrition. Am J Clin Nutr. 2000;72(3):790–5.
13. Rennie MJ. Teasing out the truth about collagen. J Physiol. 1999;521:Pt 1:1.
14. Bayley J-P, Devilee P. The Warburg effect in 2012. Curr Opin Oncol. 2012;24(1):62–7. doi:10.1097/CCO.1090b1013e32834deb32839e.
15. Oey NA, den Boer ME, Wijburg FA, et al. Long-chain fatty acid oxidation during early human development. Pediatr Res. 2005;57(6):755–9.
16. Pike LS, Smift AL, Croteau NJ, Ferrick DA, Wu M. Inhibition of fatty acid oxidation by etomoxir impairs NADPH production and increases reactive oxygen species resulting in ATP depletion and cell death in human glioblastoma cells. Biochim Biophys Acta. 2011;1807(6):726–34.
17. Soeters MR, Soeters PB. The evolutionary benefit of insulin resistance. Clin Nutr. 2012;31(6):1002–7.
18. Ardawi MS. Glutamine and glucose metabolism in human peripheral lymphocytes. Metabolism. 1988;37(1):99–103.
19. Souba WW, Smith RJ, Wilmore DW. Glutamine metabolism by the intestinal tract. JPEN J Parenter Enteral Nutr. 1985;9(5):608–17.
20. Newsholme P. Why Is L-Glutamine Metabolism Important to Cells of the Immune System in Health, Postinjury, Surgery or Infection? J Nutr. 2001;131(9):2515S–22.
21. Haussinger D, Soboll S, Meijer AJ, Gerok W, Tager JM, Sies H. Role of plasma membrane transport in hepatic glutamine metabolism. Eur J Biochem. 1985;152(3):597–603.
22. Olde Damink SW, de Blaauw I, Deutz NE, Soeters PB. Effects in vivo of decreased plasma and intracellular muscle glutamine concentration on whole-body and hindquarter protein kinetics in rats. Clin Sci (Lond). 1999;96(6):639–46.
23. Hulsewe KW, van der Hulst RW, van Acker BA, von Meyenfeldt MF, Soeters PB. Inflammation rather than nutritional depletion determines glutamine concentrations and intestinal permeability. Clin Nutr. 2004;23(5):1209–16.
24. Oudemans-van Straaten HM, Bosman RJ, Treskes M, van der Spoel HJ, Zandstra DF. Plasma glutamine depletion and patient outcome in acute ICU admissions. Intensive Care Med. 2001;27(1):84–90.
25. van Acker BA, Hulsewe KW, Wagenmakers AJ, Soeters PB, von Meyenfeldt MF. Glutamine appearance rate in plasma is not increased after gastrointestinal surgery in humans. J Nutr. 2000;130(6):1566–71.
26. Roth E, Zoch G, Schulz F, et al. Amino acid concentrations in plasma and skeletal muscle of patients with acute hemorrhagic necrotizing pancreatitis. Clin Chem. 1985;31:1305–9.
27. Record CO, Buxton B, Chase RA, Curzon G, Murray-Lyon IM, Williams R. Plasma and Brain Amino Acids in Fulminant Hepatic Failure and their Relationship to Hepatic Encephalopathy. Eur J Clin Investig. 1976;6(1):387–94.
28. Iber FLRH, Levenson SH, Chalmers TC. The plasma amino acids in patients with liver failure. J Lab Clin Met. 1957;50(3):417–25.
29. Rodas PC, Rooyackers O, Hebert C, Norberg A, Wernerman J. Glutamine and glutathione at ICU admission in relation to outcome. Clin Sci (Lond). 2012;122(12):591–7.
30. Petersson B, Vinnars E, Waller SO, Wernerman J. Long-term changes in muscle free amino acid levels after elective abdominal surgery. Br J Surg. 1992;79(3):212–6.
31. Suliman ME, Qureshi AR, Stenvinkel P, et al. Inflammation contributes to low plasma amino acid concentrations in patients with chronic kidney disease. Am J Clin Nutr. 2005;82(2):342–9.
32. Schmidt C, Hocherl K, Schweda F, Kurtz A, Bucher M. Regulation of renal sodium transporters during severe inflammation. J Am Soc Nephrol. 2007;18(4):1072–83.
33. Markossian S, Kreydiyyeh SI. TNF-alpha down-regulates the Na+-K+ATPase and the Na+-K+-2Cl-cotransporter in the rat colon via PGE2. Cytokine. 2005;30(6):319–27.
34. Fink MP, Delude RL. Epithelial barrier dysfunction: a unifying theme to explain the pathogenesis of multiple organ dysfunction at the cellular level. Crit Care Clin. 2005;21(2):177–96.
35. Clowes Jr GH, Randall HT, Cha CJ. Amino acid and energy metabolism in septic and traumatized patients. JPEN J Parenter Enteral Nutr. 1980;4(2):195–205.
36. Deutz NE, Reijven PL, Athanasas G, Soeters PB. Post-operative changes in hepatic, intestinal, splenic and muscle fluxes of amino acids and ammonia in pigs. Clin Sci (Lond). 1992;83(5):607–14.
37. Soeters PB, Grimble RF. The conditional role of inflammation in pregnancy and cancer. Clin Nutr. 2013;32(3):460–5.
38. Munoz-Pinedo C, El Mjiyad N, Ricci JE. Cancer metabolism: current perspectives and future directions. Cell Death Dis. 2012;3:e248.
39. Liu W, Le A, Hancock C, et al. Reprogramming of proline and glutamine metabolism contributes to the proliferative and metabolic responses regulated by oncogenic transcription factor c-MYC. Proc Natl Acad Sci. 2012;109(23):8983–8.

40. Son J, Lyssiotis CA, Ying H, et al. Glutamine supports pancreatic cancer growth through a KRAS-regulated metabolic pathway. Nature. 2013;496(7443):101–5.
41. Daye D, Wellen KE. Metabolic reprogramming in cancer: unraveling the role of glutamine in tumorigenesis. Semin Cell Dev Biol. 2012;23(4):362–9.
42. Van Acker BA, Hulsewe KW, Wagenmakers AJ, et al. Absence of glutamine isotopic steady state: implications for the assessment of whole-body glutamine production rate. Clin Sci (Lond). 1998;95(3):339–46.
43. Carbonnel F, Messing B, Darmaun D, et al. Energy and protein metabolism in malnutrition due to nonneoplastic gastrointestinal diseases. Metabolism. 1995;44(9):1110–5.
44. Yarasheski KE, Zachwieja JJ, Gischler J, Crowley J, Horgan MM, Powderly WG. Increased plasma gln and Leu Ra and inappropriately low muscle protein synthesis rate in AIDS wasting. Am J Physiol. 1998;275(4 Pt 1):E577–83.
45. Stumvoll M, Perriello G, Nurjhan N, et al. Glutamine and alanine metabolism in NIDDM. Diabetes. 1996;45(7): 863–8.
46. Jackson NC, Carroll PV, Russell-Jones DL, Sonksen PH, Treacher DF, Umpleby AM. The metabolic consequences of critical illness: acute effects on glutamine and protein metabolism. Am J Physiol. 1999;276(1 Pt 1):E163–70.
47. Darmaun D, Messing B, Just B, Rongier M, Desjeux JF. Glutamine metabolism after small intestinal resection in humans. Metabolism. 1991;40(1):42–4.
48. Gore DC, Jahoor F. Glutamine kinetics in burn patients. Comparison with hormonally induced stress in volunteers. Arch Surg. 1994;129(12):1318–23.
49. Goeters C, Wenn A, Mertes N, et al. Parenteral L-alanyl-L-glutamine improves 6-month outcome in critically ill patients. Crit Care Med. 2002;30(9):2032–7.
50. Dechelotte P, Hasselmann M, Cynober L, et al. L-alanyl-L-glutamine dipeptide-supplemented total parenteral nutrition reduces infectious complications and glucose intolerance in critically ill patients: the French controlled, randomized, double-blind, multicenter study. Crit Care Med. 2006;34(3):598–604.
51. Grau T, Bonet A, Minambres E, et al. The effect of L-alanyl-L-glutamine dipeptide supplemented total parenteral nutrition on infectious morbidity and insulin sensitivity in critically ill patients. Crit Care Med. 2011;39(6): 1263–8.
52. Heyland D, Muscedere J, Wischmeyer PE, et al. A randomized trial of glutamine and antioxidants in critically ill patients. N Engl J Med. 2013;368(16):1489–97.
53. Brusilow SW, Cooper AJ. Encephalopathy in acute liver failure resulting from acetaminophen intoxication: new observations with potential therapy. Crit Care Med. 2011;39(11):2550–3.
54. Hulsewe KW, van Acker BA, Hameeteman W, et al. Does glutamine-enriched parenteral nutrition really affect intestinal morphology and gut permeability? Clin Nutr. 2004;23(5):1217–25.
55. Fong YM, Tracey KJ, Hesse DG, Albert JD, Barie PS, Lowry SF. Influence of enterectomy on peripheral tissue glutamine efflux in critically ill patients. Surgery. 1990;107(3):321–6.
56. Vesali RF, Klaude M, Rooyackers OE, TJader I, Barle H, Wernerman J. Longitudinal pattern of glutamine/glutamate balance across the leg in long-stay intensive care unit patients. Clin Nutr. 2002;21(6):505–14.
57. Gore D, Wolf S, Herndon D, Wolfe R. Relative influence of glucose and insulin on peripheral amino acid metabolism in severely burned patients. J Parenter Enter Nutr. 2002;26(5):271–7.
58. Carli F, Webster J, Ramachandra V, et al. Aspects of protein metabolism after elective surgery in patients receiving constant nutritional support. Clin Sci (Lond). 1990;78(6):621–8.
59. Mjaaland M, Unneberg K, Larsson J, Nilsson L, Revhaug A. Growth hormone after abdominal surgery attenuated forearm glutamine, alanine, 3-methylhistidine, and total amino acid efflux in patients receiving total parenteral nutrition. Ann Surg. 1993;217(4):413–22.

Chapter 2
Amino Acid Transporters and Glutamine

Catherine Zander, Zhou Zhang, Thomas Albers, and Christof Grewer

Key Points

- Glutamine, a nonessential but physiologically important amino acid, is transported across cell membranes by a variety of amino acid transport systems.
- Cloned glutamine transporters have been assigned to classically characterized transport systems by their substrate and inhibitor specificity, as well as cation dependence and mechanistic properties.
- The molecular identification of the relevant genes has allowed the determination of physical transport mechanisms, as well as the identification of tissue distribution and regulatory pathways that affect expression levels and transport rates.
- This review focuses on the current knowledge of glutamine transport by the Na^+-dependent transport systems ASC (ASCT2), N (SNATs 3, 5, and 7), and A (SNATs 1, 2, and 4).
- Mechanistic properties and regulatory pathways are described, as well as the involvement of glutamine transporters in the glutamate-glutamine cycle in the brain.
- These transport systems are targets of ongoing research that will further our understanding of glutamine transfer between organs and cells.

Keywords Amino acid transport • Glutamine transport • ASCT2 • SNAT • System A • System N • System ASC • Glutamate-glutamine cycle

Abbreviations

APC	Amino acid polyamine and organocation transporter
ASC/ASCT	Alanine serine cysteine transporter
ATB^{0+}	Sodium- and chloride-dependent neutral and basic amino acid transporter
BetP	Sodium betaine symporter

C. Zander • T. Albers, Ph.D. • C. Grewer, Ph.D. (✉)
Department of Chemistry, Binghamton University, 4400 Vestal Pkwy East, Binghamton, NY 13902, USA
e-mail: czander1@binghamton.edu; talbers@binghamton.edu; cgrewer@binghamton.edu; cgrewer@stny.rr.com

Z. Zhang, Ph.D.
School of Life Science and Biopharmaceutics, Shenyang Pharmaceutical University, 103-22#, Wenhua Rd, Shenhe District, Shenyang, Liaoning Province, China
e-mail: zhouzhang@hotmail.com

R. Rajendram et al. (eds.), *Glutamine in Clinical Nutrition*, Nutrition and Health,
DOI 10.1007/978-1-4939-1932-1_2,

Cl^-	Chloride
EAAT	Excitatory amino acid transporters
EGF	Epidermal growth factor
GABA	γ-Aminobutyric acid
GltPh	Archaeal aspartate transporter
K_i	Dissociation constant
K_m	Michaelis–Menten constant
LAT	Large-neutral amino acid transporter
LeuT	Bacterial leucine transporter
MAPK	Mitogen-activated protein kinases
MeAIB	2-(Methylamino)-isobutyrate
Mhp1	Sodium-hydantoin transporter
mTOR	Mammalian target of rapamycin
Nedd4-2	E3 ubiquitin-protein ligase
NMDA	*N*-methyl-D-aspartate
PI3-kinase	Phosphatidylinositide 3-kinase
PKA/PKB	Protein kinase A/B
PMA	Phorbol-12-myristate 13-acetate
RVI	Regulatory volume increase
SGK	Serum- and glucocorticoid-induced protein kinase
SLC	Solute carrier
SNAT	Sodium-coupled neutral amino acid transporter
TM	Transmembrane domain
TOR	Serine threonine kinase/target of rapamycin
VGLUT	Vesicular glutamate transporter
vSGLT	Sodium-galactose symporter

Introduction

Glutamine transporters play important roles in metabolism and amino acid homeostasis of cells in most tissues [1]. While glutamine has been classified to be a nonessential amino acid, it has been shown that glutamine supply may become limiting for metabolism under conditions of stress and illness [2]. Furthermore, glutamine is a critical nutrient for rapidly proliferating cells, such as dividing cancer cells [3, 4]. On a cellular level, glutamine is imported into cells, or exported from cells, by plasma membrane glutamine transporters (see [1] for a review). Many glutamine transporters have been characterized traditionally by their specificity profile for substrates and inhibitors, their cation dependence, and mechanistic properties. Most of these transport systems have now been cloned, enabling the detailed investigation of their functional properties, tissue distribution, regulation, and pharmacology. In this review, we focus mainly on the description of the functional properties of the physiologically important and Na^+-dependent glutamine transporters belonging to the solute carrier 1 (SLC1, [5]) and SLC38 families [6]. These transporters were assigned to the classically-identified transport systems ASC (neutral amino acid transporters from the SLC1 family [5]), and systems A and N (SLC38 members [6]), summarized in Table 2.1. $ATB^{0,+}$ is another Na^+-dependent amino acid transporter with broad specificity and below mM affinity for glutamine. It belongs to the SLC6 family of transporters and is also Cl^- dependent [7]. Due to the low activity of this transport system in most non-proliferating cells, it will not be discussed in this review. One of the major Na^+-independent transport systems is system L, which exchanges glutamine for other amino acids and may use the

Table 2.1 Basic characteristics of the transporters of the SLC1 and SLC38 families

Human gene name	Protein name	Alias	Predominant substrate	Transporter type/coupling ions	Tissue distribution	Sequence accession ID	Human gene locus
SLC1A4	ASCT1, SATT	System ASC	A, S, C, T	C/Na^+, E/amino acids	Widespread	Q76GL9	2p15-p13
SLC1A5	ASCT2, AAAT	System ASC	A, S, C, T, Q, N	C/Na^+, E/amino acids	Lung, skeletal muscle, large intestine, kidney, testis, adipose tissue	Q15758	19q13.3
SLC38A1	SNAT1	ATA1,NAT2,SAT1	Q,A,N,C,H,S	C/Na^+	Brain, retina, heart, placenta, adrenal gland	Q9H2H9.1	12q13.11
SLC38A2	SNAT2	ATA2,SAT2	A,N,C,Q,G,H,M,P,S	C/Na^+	Ubiquitous	CAG33548.1	12q13.11
SLC38A3	SNAT3	SN1	Q,H,A,N	C/Na^+, E/H^+	Liver, skeletal muscle, kidney, pancreas	CAG33251.1	3p21.31
SLC38A4	SNAT4	ATA3,NAT3,PAAT	A,N,C,G,S,T	C/Na^+	Brain, retina, liver, kidney, adipose tissue	Q969I6.1	12q13.11
SLC38A5	SNAT5	SN2	Q,N,H,S	C/Na^+, E/H^+	Stomach, brain, liver, lung, small intestine, spleen, colon, kidney	Q8WUX1.1	Xp11.23
SLC38A6	SNAT6	–	–	–	Brain, eye, heart, liver, kidney	Q8IZM9.2	14q23.1
SLC38A7	SNAT7	–	Q,H,S,A,N	?/Na^+	Brain, liver, skeletal muscle, uterus, pituitary	Q9NVC3.1	16q21

For detailed information about the SLC gene tables, please visit: http://www.bioparadigms.org. SNAT8–11 are omitted from the table
Abbreviations for transport type: *C* cotransporter, *E* exchanger

transmembrane [glutamine] gradient as a driving force for the import of leucine [8]. System L has been described classically through leucine transport [9], as well its preference of amino acids with bulky, hydrophobic side chains. This system will not be described in this review in detail.

System ASC Transporters of the SLC1 Family

System ASC has traditionally been characterized by its preference for short-chain amino acids, such as *a*lanine, *s*erine, and *c*ysteine, from which its name was derived [10]. However, system ASC also transports glutamine with an affinity that is comparable to that for the prototypical substrate alanine [5], although glutamine is transported with a lower v_{max}. System ASC was distinguished from other glutamine transport systems by its insensitivity to N-methylated amino acids, such as MeAIB ((2-(methylamino) isobutyric acid)).

cDNA cloning resulted in the identification of two sequences that are now accepted to code for system ASC transporters, namely ASCT1 and ASCT2 [5] (ASCT=alanine serine cysteine transporter). Both transporters belong to the SLC1 family of amino acid transporters. The cloning of the transporters revealed an interesting transmembrane topology with 6 N-terminal transmembrane domains followed by a C-terminal domain, which has a difficulty to interpret hydrophobicity profile. The crystal structure of the homologous bacterial glutamate transporter GltPh revealed that the C-terminal transport domain consists of a repeat of a reentrant-loop-helix motif, which is inserted into the membrane in opposing orientation [11]. Although the crystal structure of ASCTs is not known, homology models predict that this C-terminal domain harbors the binding site for the amino acid [12].

Substrate Selectivity and Pharmacology

While ASCT1 showed no measurable transport activity for glutamine, ASCT2 is able to transport glutamine with reasonably high affinity (K_m in the range of 20–70 μM, [5, 13, 14]). This affinity is in the same range as that of the other preferred substrates, alanine, serine, and cysteine. Because this review focuses on glutamine transporters, we will only discuss ASCT2. Asparagine is also transported by ASCT2, as are methionine, glycine, leucine, and valine, to some extent, although with low affinities [5]. Glutamate is a transported substrate only at acidic pH, in contrast to transport of neutral amino acids, which is pH independent [13], indicating that glutamate is protonated at the γ-carboxylate when interacting with ASCT2.

The pharmacology of ASCT2 is not well established. Inhibitors were developed on the basis of structural homology with glutamate transporter inhibitors [12, 14] (Fig. 2.1a). Benzylserine (Fig. 2.1b (1)), which is structurally related to a glutamate transporter inhibitor blocks ASCT2 function, although with low apparent affinity (K_i=0.8 mM). Inhibitory potency was increased by adding hydrophobic bulk to the benzyl group. The resulting inhibitor serine biphenyl-4-carboxylate blocked ASCT2 activity with a K_i of 30 μM [12]. Interestingly, it was found that the amount of hydrophobic bulk of the substituent not only correlated with affinity, but also with the ability of compounds to be transported [12] (Fig. 2.1b (2) shows a potent inhibitor with large hydrophobic bulk). In another report, compounds were identified based on *N*-γ-substituted glutamine [15] (Fig. 2.1b (3)). Several aromatic substituents were used, leading to the characterization of an amide that inhibits with an apparent K_i in the 250 μM range (at 100 μM glutamine). Based on the analysis of electron-withdrawing properties of the substituent, the authors predict the existence of an important hydrogen bond formed between the transporter-binding site and the amide hydrogen [15].

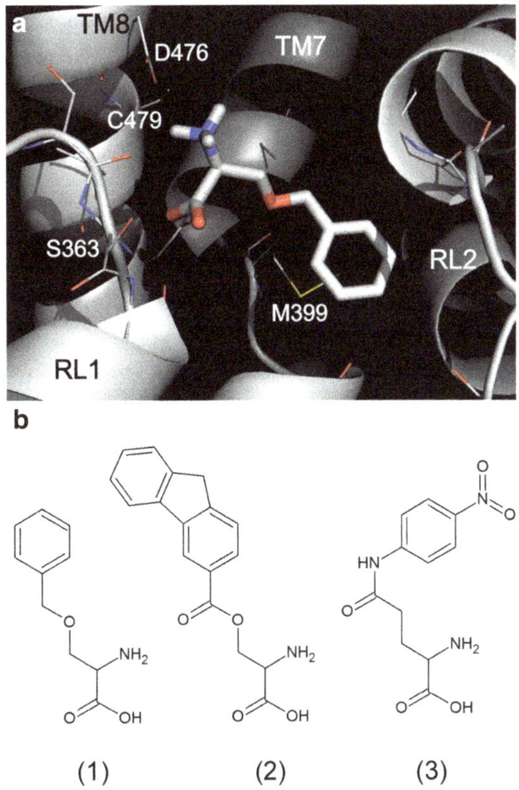

Fig. 2.1 (**a**) Proposed binding pose of the inhibitor benzylserine in the ASCT2 substrate-binding site (adapted from [12]). (**b**) Structures of selected ASCT2 blockers

Tissue Distribution and Subcellular Expression

Northern blot analysis detected mRNA coding for rat ASCT2 in most tissues, except for brain, liver, and heart tissue [5]. However, it was later found that ASCT2 is expressed in the brain as well [13]. In the intestine and kidney, ASCT2 is expressed mainly in epithelial cells [4].

In the brain, ASCT2 expression was found in dendrites of neurons, whereas the cell bodies showed little detectable ASCT2 expression [16]. Functional evidence for ASCT2 presence in nerve terminals was obtained by measuring D-serine uptake [16]. The functional significance of ASCT2 expression in neurons is not clear, although it has been implicated in the uptake of glutamine and D-serine, which is an endogenous NMDA (*N*-methyl-D-aspartate) receptor ligand. A connection to regulation of oxidative stress may also be possible, since L-cysteine, as a regulator of glutathione levels, is a transported ASCT2 substrate [5].

Expression of ASCT2 in astrocytes is more controversial. While several reports have detected mRNA and protein expression in neonatal glial cell cultures [17], no immunostaining was found in adult brain astrocytes [16]. The reasons behind this discrepancy are not clear. It is possible that ASCT2 is only expressed in developing astrocytes, or that results from cell culture expression cannot be transferred to native tissue.

ASCT2 has been found to be highly overexpressed in many cancer cells [3, 4], as well as rapidly growing cell lines, and has been particularly studied in hepatoma cells [18]. While ASCT2 is not expressed in the normal liver, it is expressed in rapidly growing and aggressive human hepatomas [18]. Glutamine uptake in these cells can be enhanced up to 20-fold compared to normal cells.

Glutamine uptake by ASCT2 appears to be essential for the survival of this rapidly-growing tissue, due to its high nitrogen demand. In fact, ASCT2 antisense RNA expression resulted in apoptotic cell death, a response that is similar to that of glutamine deprivation [3]. These findings indicate that ASCT2 may be a useful target for pharmacological intervention to prevent rapid growth of cancerous cells.

Functional and Predicted Structural Properties

The transport mechanism of natively expressed system ASC and ASCT2 has been analyzed using radiotracer flux studies and electrophysiology [5, 13, 14, 19]. Most importantly, it was observed that ASCT2 is unable to support inward transport of amino acids in the absence of cytosolic amino acids. However, transport activity was found when internal amino acid was present [19]. This has led to the conclusion that ASCT2 catalyzes obligate amino acid exchange across the cell membrane (Fig. 2.2a). Native system ASC as well as ASCT1 and ASCT2 are electroneutral transporters [19, 20], consistent with the obligate exchange hypothesis. Consistently, no steady-state transport currents can be detected in ASCT2 upon substrate application [14].

ASCT2 is, however, not fully electrically silent. Upon substitution of chloride with more hydrophobic anions, such as NO_3^- or SCN^-, amino acid-induced currents were observed that were dependent on the electrochemical gradient of the anion across the membrane [14, 19] (Fig. 2.2a). Interestingly, the anion current was dependent on the extracellular Na^+ concentration [14, 19], similar to observations made previously for the related glutamate transporters. It was concluded that the substrate-induced anion conductance is conserved between the acidic and neutral amino acid transporters of the SLC1 family.

Amino acid transport by ASCT2 is strongly dependent on the Na^+ concentration [19] (Fig. 2.2a), on the extracellular and intracellular sides of the membrane, indicating that Na^+ must be bound to the transporter for amino acid translocation. However, ASCT2 is independent of K^+ [14]. Furthermore, proton cotransport is not required for ASCT2 function.

The effect of Na^+ has been incorporated into proposed transport mechanisms. Here, Na^+ binds to the transporter after amino acid association is complete, resulting in a Na^+-amino acid-bound transporter [19]. Recent evidence, however, points to association of Na^+ with the empty transporter before amino acid binds [14]. The "fully loaded" transporter then undergoes conformational change resulting in amino acid translocation. In this model, Na^+ binding has a regulatory effect, as it has been found that the affinity for Na^+ is high (low mM range). Thus, Na^+ would never dissociate from the transporter, unless its concentrations became unphysiologically low [21].

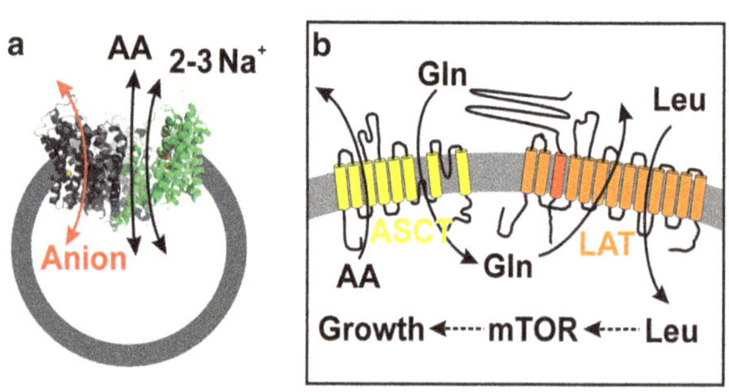

Fig. 2.2 ASCT2 coupling stoichiometry and anion fluxes (**a**) and importance for cell growth in rapidly growing cells (**b**, adapted from [8])

Regulation

Mechanisms for regulation of ASCT2 expression have been identified. First, ASCT2 expression levels in tumor cell lines were proposed to be stimulated by glutamine and inhibited by glutamine deprivation [4]. A transcriptional mechanism was identified as the cause for this stimulation. Second, regulation of membrane expression occurs through growth factors, such as epidermal growth factor (EGF), as well as insulin and insulin growth factor (IGF) [22]. Signaling pathways involve mitogen-activated kinase (MAPK), protein kinase C (PKC), as well as PI3 kinase [22]. The downstream targets in the latter signaling pathway are serum and glucocorticoid inducible kinase (SGK) isoforms. Consistently, expression of constitutively active SGK1 and SGK3, as well as protein kinase B (PKB), increased ASCT2 transport activity in *Xenopus* oocytes [22].

The function of ASCT2 as a glutamine importer was proposed to be connected to mammalian target of rapamycin (mTOR) [3]. TOR is a serine/threonine kinase, which is involved in signaling related to energy status and nutrient supply. ASCT2 activates the mTOR pathway by importing glutamine into the cell, which in turn leads to leucine influx through transporters of the LAT family, in exchange with intracellular glutamine [8] (illustrated in Fig. 2.2b). Glutamine and leucine then activate mTOR by mechanisms that are currently not well understood.

System N Transporters of the SLC38 Gene Family

According to regulation and the functional properties, the *S*odium-*C*oupled *N*eutral *A*mino acid *T*ransporters (SNATs) of the SLC38 gene family are classically described as system A and system N transport activities [6, 23]. Unlike system A subtypes (described in the next section), which transport small, aliphatic amino acids and are rheogenic and pH sensitive, the system N subtypes (SNAT3, SNAT5, and SNAT7) counter transport H^+, which may be a key property to allow their operation in reverse and catalyze glutamine efflux from cells [24] (Fig. 2.3a). The system N subtypes have narrower substrate profiles than do the system A subtypes [6]. The system A transporters show substrate selectivity for the amino acid analog MeAIB, as well as a broad range of amino acids such as glycine, L-alanine, L-cysteine, and L-glutamine, whereas, as its name suggests, system N preferentially

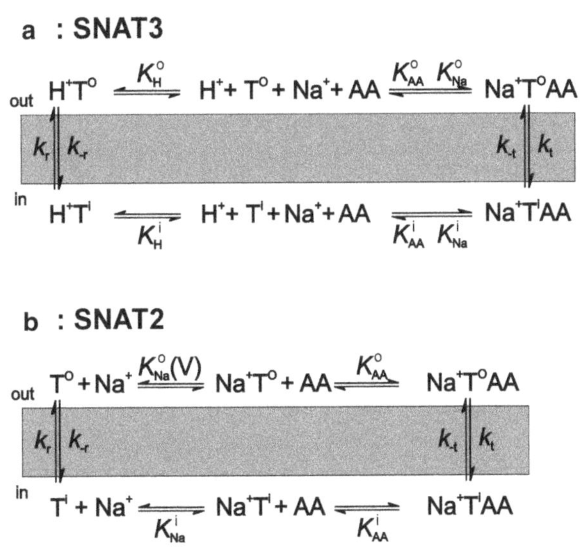

Fig. 2.3 Proposed mechanism of amino acid transport by SNAT3 (**a**, adapted from [48]) and SNAT1/2 (**b**, adapted from [24])

transports amino acids containing nitrogen in the side chain, such as L-glutamine, L-histidine, and L-asparagine [6].

So far, three isoforms of system N transporters have been identified, namely, SNAT3, SNAT5, and SNAT7 [6, 25]. Amino acid transport is coupled to the cotransport of Na^+. Activities classified as system N-like have been studied in neurons. Since L-glutamine is preferred as a substrate, the system N glutamine transporters of the SLC38 family have been suggested to be part of the synthesis of the neurotransmitter glutamate, and are therefore likely involved in altering both γ-aminobutyric acid (GABA) and glutamate levels as well as the cycling of glutamate [26] (detailed below).

SNAT7 is a recently cloned system N amino acid transporter [25]. SLC38A7 bears the hallmarks of system N, with preference for L-glutamine, L-histidine, and L-asparagine, and is insensitive to MeAIB. However, the preferred substrate profile of SLC38A7 is unusually broad compared with other known system N transporters, SNAT3 and SNAT5. Therefore, it was suggested that SLC38A7 is a new system N amino acid transporter on the basis of the expression profile, showing high expression in liver, and substrate selectivity [25].

Tissue Distribution and Subcellular Expression

Most of the system N SLC38 family members have relatively broad expression profiles. In contrast to SNAT1 and SNAT2, which are present in neurons, SNAT3 (also referred to as SN1 or NAT) expression in the brain is largely confined to astrocytes. Abundant expression of the SNAT3 protein is detected in astrocytes throughout the brain and the retina, but SNAT3 is absent from neurons and oligodendrocytes. SNAT3 mRNA is also abundant in liver, kidney, heart, skeletal muscle, and adipose tissue [27]. SNAT5 mRNA transcript was detected in multiple brain regions, lung, colon, small intestine, and spleen, whereas three other transcripts are observed in other tissues, including a 2.6-kb transcript in liver and kidney and a 1.4-kb transcript that is dramatically expressed in stomach [26].

Functional data showed that system N transporters are expressed in retinal Müller cells and that system N is the principal mediator of glutamine transport in these cells. SNAT3 and SNAT5 are also expressed robustly in retinal ganglion cells.

Functional and Predicted Structural Properties

SNAT3 (SLC38A3) cotransports glutamine together with one Na^+ ion into the cell, in exchange for H^+ (Fig. 2.3a). H^+ countertransport was identified by the ability of SNAT3 to make the cell interior more alkaline upon extracellular glutamine application, a principal feature distinguishing system N subtypes from the system A subfamily [24]. Due to the coupling stoichiometry, glutamine transport by SNAT3 is unaffected by changes of the membrane potential and is, therefore, thought to be electroneutral [24]. Despite the proposed eletroneutral nature, currents could be measured in response to application of glutamine to SNAT3-expressing *Xenopus* oocytes [28]. It is not clear whether these currents are caused purely by uncoupled, glutamine induced ion fluxes across the membrane, or if there is also electrogenic function associated with SNAT3. It should be noted that in another study the coupling stoichiometry was found to be 1 glutamine to 2 Na^+ ions, suggesting electrogenic nature of transport [27].

The three-dimensional structure of the system N transporters is not known. However, the SLC38 family is distantly related to the amino acid/polyamine/organocation transporter family APC [29]. Crystal structures of members of the APC family have been determined and the SNAT3 structure was modeled by using the Mhp1 transporter structure as a template [28]. According to this homology model, predicted transmembrane segment 1 contributes to a conserved Na^+ binding site. Interestingly, asparagine 76 of SNAT3, which is a conserved residue in transmembrane domain 1 (TM1), is critical for the substrate-induced ion conductance of SNAT3 and mutations to N76 affect binding of the cosubstrate Na^+. Therefore, it was hypothesized that this residue is likely to be localized in the translocation pore in the center of the membrane [28].

SNAT5 mediates Na^+/amino acid cotransport and counter transport of H^+, but differs from SNAT3 in its substrate profile. Human SNAT5 favors serine along with the classic system N substrates glutamine, asparagine and histidine. Assigning SNAT5 to the system N subfamily is therefore based on its countertransport of H^+ and its 61 % sequence identity to SNAT3, and not on its substrate profile [6]. Amino acid transport activity of SNAT5 exhibited marked pH sensitivity, with influx of substrate increasing with pH in the range of 7.0–8.0 [30].

It has been demonstrated that SNAT5 is capable of mediating bidirectional fluxes of amino acid substrate. The ability of SNAT5 to mediate both accumulation of glutamine from an external supply and efflux of glutamine into amino acid-free medium demonstrates the important capability of system N to facilitate net movement of amino acid across the plasma membrane both into and out of cells, a property that is shared between SNAT3 and SNAT5 [23].

Regulation

The primary sequence of SNAT3 contains a number of putative phosphorylation sites [31]. PKC isoforms are activated by a variety of pathways that are involved in cell growth, migration, and differentiation. It has been shown that SNAT3 is rapidly downregulated by activating PKC through the treatment of *Xenopus laevis* oocytes with phorbol-12-myristate-13-acetate (PMA). This downregulation occurs in a caveolin-dependent, dynamin-independent manner and was suggested to be independent of the direct phosphorylation of the transporter [32], although phosphorylation at a particular serine residue has later been shown [31]. SNAT3 is also regulated by pathways involving serum and glucocorticoid inducible kinase SGK and PKB [33], by protein degradation through the ubiquitin ligase Nedd4-2, an effect which is reversed by coexpression of SGK1 [33]. Regulation of SNAT3 expression by insulin and serum starvation was found in the liver [34]. Dietary restriction increased plasma membrane expression, whereas chronic insulin application resulted in downregulation [34], likely involving PI3 kinase.

In the kidney, it has been demonstrated that diets and conditions that stimulate renal ammoniagenesis and urinary ammonium excretion, such as potassium restriction, high protein intake, and metabolic acidosis, lead to higher expression of the SNAT3 transporter. This correlation and the localization of SNAT3 to the basolateral membrane of the late proximal tubule strongly suggest that SNAT3 plays a pivotal role in supplying the proximal tubule with glutamine for ammoniagenesis. Some of these proposed regulatory processes are illustrated in Fig. 2.4.

Not much is known regarding the regulatory processes affecting SNAT5 function. It has been proposed that the C-terminal histidine residue (H471) of SNAT5 is a pH-sensing residue which regulates substrate (Na^+ plus amino acid) transport activity, at least partly by allosteric effects on Na^+ binding and which may, therefore, be important for physiological functioning of the transporters [30].

System A Transporters of the SLC38 Family

Within the SLC38 family, three distinct isoforms with hallmarks of system A activity were identified through cDNA cloning: SNAT1, SNAT2, and SNAT4 [35, 36]. Although no crystal structure is available, useful information of the fold is provided by distantly related transporter families.

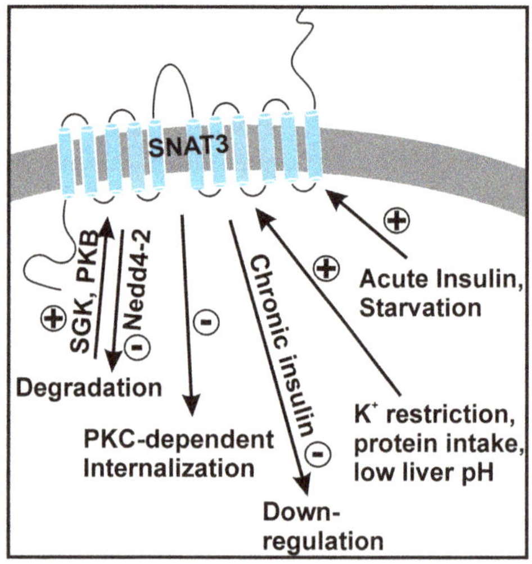

Fig. 2.4 Potential regulatory mechanisms that control SNAT3 expression

At present, sequence homology has been established with transporters of the mammalian SLC32 and SLC36 families, as well as with the more distantly related plant auxin carriers and the bacterial APC family [29]. Considering the established structural relationship between the APC-family transporters and those of the SLC6 family, it is reasonable to assume that the system A transporters adopt a fold that is similar to LeuT(Aa) and Mhp1, for which crystal structures are known (see for example [37]). LeuT(Aa) has been one of the most useful templates for SNAT2 structural homology modeling [38]. The inverted repeat topology is proposed to be shared with many different families of transporters despite low sequence homology.

Based on hydropathy analysis, SNAT1 and SNAT2 are predicted to have 11 transmembrane domains; with an intracellular N terminus and an extracellular C terminus and a large glycosylated loop between TM5 and TM6 [6]. The intracellular location of the N-terminus is consistent with the absence of an N-terminal signaling sequence for membrane insertion.

Substrate Selectivity and Pharmacology

All three system A isoforms are secondary active transporters, which cotransport one aliphatic, zwitterionic amino acid with one Na^+ ion down the Na^+ concentration gradient [39]. The preference for amino acid substrates between isoforms varies. SNAT1 and 2 have similar substrate specificity, transporting most hydrophilic or small neutral amino acids. System A is so named because of its affinity for alanine. SNAT1 has a much higher affinity for glutamine than SNAT2, $K_m = 230$ μM and $K_m = 1.65$ mM, respectively. The reverse is found for alanine; SNAT1's K_m for alanine is 520 ± 80 μM, and SNAT2's 200 ± 17 μM [38, 39]. SNAT4's K_m for alanine however, is significantly lower, 3.52 ± 0.62 mM.

MeAIB, a non-metabolizable amino acid analogue, is thought to be a specific transportable substrate for system A transporters. It has long been considered the paradigm system A substrate, used to differentiate system A activity in native cells from that of other amino acid transporters [9]. Although MeAIB is specific to system A transporters, it originally caused mistaken family assignment of SNAT4. At low concentrations, MeAIB works poorly as an inhibitor. It has been strongly recommended to use caution when using MeAIB as an inhibitor to characterize system A transporters [6, 41].

Tissue Distribution and Subcellular Expression

SNAT2 is ubiquitously expressed within mammalian and avian cells [6]. SNAT2 mRNA has been found in every tissue analyzed by using Northern blotting. SNAT2's mRNA and protein levels are increased by amino acid deprivation in many different cell types [42, 43]. Hypertonic stress also increases the abundance of SNAT2 mRNA in most studied cell types. In the brain, SNAT2 is expressed in excitatory neurons in the hippocampus [44], but is not found in astrocyte-enriched cultures. In the pancreas, SNAT2 is responsible for the majority of glutamine uptake within α-cells of the islets of Langerhans [45].

The placenta requires expression of SNAT4 for proper mammalian fetal development and healthy birth weight. SNAT4 is also found in large concentrations within the liver. The full function of SNAT4 within the liver is not yet fully understood. When liver cells are incubated in alanine and glutamine they have a higher gluconeogenesis activity [46]; insulin, which up regulates SNAT4 mRNA inhibits gluconeogenesis [9].

In the brain, SNAT1 is expressed mainly in GABAergic and glutamatergic neurons [6]. It contributes to the plasticity of inhibitory synapses. SNAT1 transports glutamine as a precursor of synaptic GABA within hippocampal cells and synaptosomes. SNAT1 is expressed within the larger microvessels within the cortex [47]. The cortical expression aids in shuffling glutamine from the astrocytes into the neurons [6]. SNAT1 is also expressed in the heart, placenta and the adrenal gland.

Functional and Predicted Structural Properties

For SNAT1, it was proposed that binding of Na^+ and the substrate is sequential: Sodium binding occurs before amino acid binding (Fig. 2.3b). Once both Na^+ and the amino acid are bound, the complex is translocated across the membrane in the same step [40] (Fig. 2.3b). In both SNAT1 and 2, when alanine was rapidly applied in the presence of Na^+, an "instantaneous," rapidly decaying inward transient current was observed [40]. If the alanine binding step is electroneutral, because at neutral pH alanine has no net charge, then either movement of Na^+ and/or movement of charges of the binding sites cause this rapid charge movement. The bimolecular rate constant of alanine binding to SNAT1 and 2 was estimated as $>2\times10^7\ M^{-1}\ s^{-1}$ [40], indicating close to diffusion-controlled substrate binding.

SNAT2 has a large anion leak that is not stoichiometrically coupled to the transport current. The presence of extracellular Na^+ increases the size of the leak current [48]. The binding of amino acid in SNAT2 inhibits this anion leak [48]. The SNATs function poorly at low pH. They have the largest activity at a pH of 7.4 for SNAT1, pH 8.0 for SNAT2, and 8.5 for SNAT4 [35, 49]. Protons regulate the transporters by raising the K_m for Na^+ through allosteric changes. System A transporters are electrogenic, and display voltage-dependent inward substrate transport currents, which increase in size at more negative voltage [35, 39, 41].

Like other transporters related to the APC family, SNAT2 was proposed to adopt a fold based on an inverted repeat topology [38], likely resulting from gene-duplication and fusion events, with 11 transmembrane domains (topology illustrated in Fig. 2.5a). TM1-5 and TM 6-10 are placed in the membrane mirrored with opposite vertical orientations. These two TM sections have similar structural characteristics although they do not have high sequence homology. The inverted topology motif was proposed to be instrumental for the cotransport of the substrates through a slight tilting of the 5-TM bundle motifs, or a "rocking" bundle mechanism, as hypothesized for the SLC6 transporters [50].

Analysis of the SNAT2 Na^+-binding site through site-directed mutagenesis experimentally supports the hypothesis that the LeuT(Aa) fold is shared with the SLC38 system A family. Threonine 384 on TM8 was identified as being part of the Na^+ binding site. Asparagine 82, located on TM1, was also hypothesized to be involved in the Na^+ binding site [38], in analogy to studies of the homologous N76

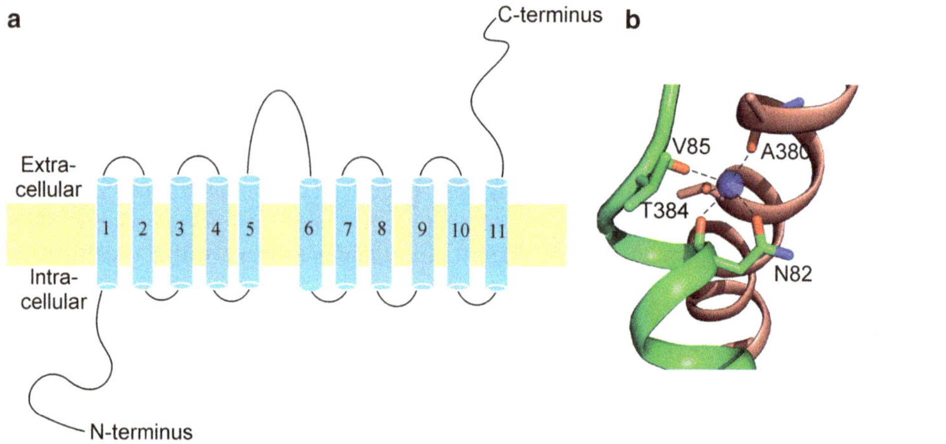

Fig. 2.5 Structural features of SNATs. (**a**) Transmembrane topology (SNAT1/2). (**b**) Predicted SNAT2 Na⁺-binding site (adapted from [38])

residue in SNAT3 [28] (Fig. 2.5b). The Na^+ binding site for SNAT2 is situated in the region where predicted TM1 and 8 intersect one another, creating a v-motif similar to that of LeuT(Aa), BetP, vSGLT and Mhp1, as predicted by X-ray crystallography (see for example [37]).

The deletion of TM11 in SNAT2 produced an inactive transporter. This is hypothesized to be due to poor cell surface expression and not a change in transport ability. The C-terminus in SNAT2 is important for voltage regulation and necessary for transport at physiological potentials. The pH dependence was only partially retained with the truncation of the C-terminus. A mutation of histidine 504 to alanine in the c-terminus of SNAT2 reduces pH sensitivity without changing the K_m for Na^+ [30].

Regulation

Because SNAT2 is assumed to be the prototypical, ubiquitously-expressed system A transporter, much of what is known about the regulation of system A transporters is thought to be related to regulation of SNAT2 function/expression levels. Several reviews have summarized regulatory pathways in more detail (see for example [6]). Therefore, we present here only a brief summary.

When cells are amino acid starved or in hypertonic conditions they undergo a regulatory volume increase (RVI). SNAT2 is upregulated in response to these situations of deprivation and is responsible for short term RVI. The upregulation of SNAT2 is both short term through the redistribution of SNAT2 proteins from intracellular stores into the membrane, and long term by increased transcription. SNAT2 is also upregulated in response to insulin [51]. In some cell types, such as oligodendrocytes, where SNAT2 expression is not seen under basal conditions, SNAT2 is upregulated under systemic hypertonic conditions. When any system A substrate is available, SNAT2's mRNA is downregulated, and if the hypertonic conditions are corrected, the speed of downregulation is increased through a reduction in mRNA stability and changes in gene expression [52].

SNAT1 and 4 likely play very specific roles in specialized cell types to maintain pools of glutamine as metabolic precursors. SNAT1 is regulated intrinsically within inhibitory hippocampal cells through transporter activity and not substrate availability, via depolarization and developmental cues, in order to maintain a supply of glutamine to serve as a GABA precursor. Within these cells, SNAT2 is upregulated with age, while SNAT1 is downregulated [53]. SNAT4 is upregulated within mouse liver, specifically within the basolateral layers of hepatocyte-like cells, by insulin through a PI3-kinase-dependent pathway.

Amino Acid Transporters and the Glutamate Glutamine Cycle

A physiologically important function of glutamine is to serve as a precursor for the neurotransmitter glutamate in the glutamate-glutamine cycle in the mammalian brain. In this cycle (Fig. 2.6), glutamate, released into the synapse during neurotransmission, is taken up into adjacent glia cells. Within glia cells, glutamate is converted to glutamine by glutamine synthase. Glutamine is then shuttled back into neurons, in which glutamate is regenerated by glutaminase. Shuttling of glutamine from glia cells to neurons requires release through transporters in the glia cell membrane, followed by neuronal glutamine uptake (see for example [54, 55]).

Amino acid transporters are critically involved in many of these steps. Uptake of glutamate into glia cells is performed by high-capacity glutamate transporters of the excitatory amino acid transporter (EAAT) family. Subtype EAAT2 is mainly responsible for this uptake. Glutamine release from glia cells requires a transporter that can catalyze efflux. Although the exact nature of the transport systems involved in efflux is still discussed, SNAT3 is a potential candidate that has the functional pre-requisites to serve as an efflux system [56]. Most importantly, glutamine transport by SNAT3 is thought to be electroneutral, rendering efflux possible even at negative transmembrane potentials [24]. However, another report suggests electrogenic glutamine transport by SNAT3 [27], caused by the cotransport of two Na^+ ions. If this was the case, glutamine efflux would be hindered at negative voltage. In addition to system N, ASCT2 and the system L transporter LAT2 may contribute to glutamine release, in particular in cultured astrocytes [57], in exchange for other extracellular amino acids. However, the lack of ASCT2 expression in mature brain astrocytes makes its physiological importance for glutamine efflux less clear [16]. Furthermore, an unidentified transporter has been implicated in the efflux mechanism [57].

Once glutamine is released from glia cells, it is taken up into neurons by amino acid transporters. The identity of the transport systems involved is also not well established, although evidence points to SNAT2 and SNAT1 (system A) as a major contributor to neuronal uptake. SNAT2 is strongly expressed in neurons and the inhibition of SNAT2 by the specific transported substrate MeAIB results in an elevation of extracellular glutamine.

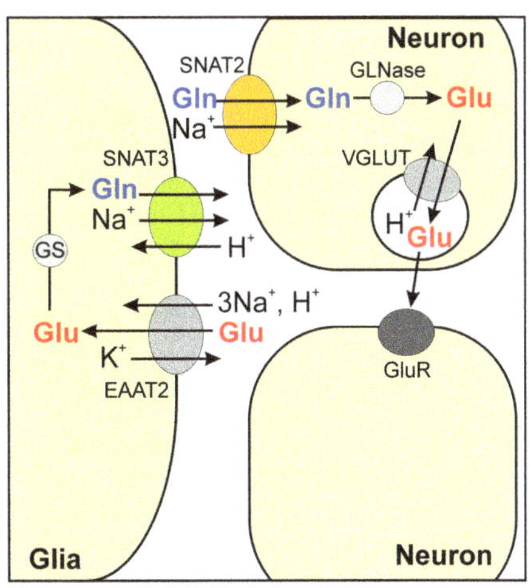

Fig. 2.6 Proposed involvement of several amino acid transporters in the glutamate-glutamine cycle

After entering the presynaptic terminal, glutamine is converted to glutamate by glutaminase, and subsequently repackaged into synaptic vesicles. Transport into the vesicles is accomplished by the vesicular glutamate transporters (VGLUTs) [58].

Conclusions

The preceding sections have highlighted the function of glutamine transporters in many physiological processes, as well as the molecular properties and regulatory processes that determine transporter activity. Understanding of the biophysical transport mechanism, structure function relationships, as well as development of specific pharmacological tools for manipulation of glutamine transporter function remain challenges that require future investigation. These issues are particularly important with respect to recent reports that implicate glutamine transporters in the growth of rapidly dividing cells, such as tumor cells. Our ability to manipulate glutamine uptake by these cells, either through pharmacological intervention, or through modulation of transporter expression or activity by targeting regulatory pathways, at either the transcriptional or trafficking level, will be paramount to the identification of new avenues to inhibit cell growth.

Acknowledgements This work was supported by the National Institutes of Health Grant 2R01NS049335-06A1 awarded to C.G.

References

1. Bode BP. Recent molecular advances in mammalian glutamine transport. J Nutr. 2001;131:2475S–85.
2. Neu J, Shenoy V, Chakrabarti R. Glutamine nutrition and metabolism: where do we go from here? FASEB J. 1996;10:829–37.
3. Fuchs BC, Bode BP. Amino acid transporters ASCT2 and LAT1 in cancer: partners in crime? Semin Cancer Biol. 2005;15:254–66.
4. McGivan JD, Bungard CI. The transport of glutamine into mammalian cells. Front Biosci. 2007;12:874–82.
5. Utsunomiya-Tate N, Endou H, Kanai Y. Cloning and functional characterization of a system ASC-like Na+-dependent neutral amino acid transporter. J Biol Chem. 1996;271:14883–90.
6. Mackenzie B, Erickson JD. Sodium-coupled neutral amino acid (System N/A) transporters of the SLC38 gene family. Pflugers Arch. 2004;447:784–95.
7. Sloan JL, Mager S. Cloning and functional expression of a human Na(+) and Cl(-)-dependent neutral and cationic amino acid transporter B(0+). J Biol Chem. 1999;274:23740–5.
8. Nicklin P, Bergman P, Zhang B, et al. Bidirectional transport of amino acids regulates mTOR and autophagy. Cell. 2009;136:521–34.
9. Oxender DL, Christensen HN. Distinct mediating systems for the transport of neutral amino acids by the Ehrlich cell. J Biol Chem. 1963;238:3686–99.
10. Christensen HN, Liang M, Archer EG. A distinct Na+-requiring transport system for alanine, serine, cysteine, and similar amino acids. J Biol Chem. 1967;242:5237–46.
11. Yernool D, Boudker O, Jin Y, Gouaux E. Structure of a glutamate transporter homologue from Pyrococcus horikoshii. Nature. 2004;431:811–8.
12. Albers T, Marsiglia W, Thomas T, Gameiro A, Grewer C. Defining substrate and blocker activity of alanine serine cysteine transporter 2 (ASCT2) ligands with novel serine analogs. Mol Pharmacol. 2011;81:356–65.
13. Broer A, Brookes N, Ganapathy V, et al. The astroglial ASCT2 amino acid transporter as a mediator of glutamine efflux. J Neurochem. 1999;73:2184–94.
14. Grewer C, Grabsch E. New inhibitors for the neutral amino acid transporter ASCT2 reveal its Na+-dependent anion leak. J Physiol. 2004;557:747–59.
15. Esslinger CS, Cybulski KA, Rhoderick JF. Ngamma-aryl glutamine analogues as probes of the ASCT2 neutral amino acid transporter binding site. Bioorg Med Chem. 2005;13:1111–8.
16. Gliddon CM, Shao Z, LeMaistre JL, Anderson CM. Cellular distribution of the neutral amino acid transporter subtype ASCT2 in mouse brain. J Neurochem. 2009;108:372–83.

17. Dolinska M, Zablocka B, Sonnewald U, Albrecht J. Glutamine uptake and expression of mRNA's of glutamine transporting proteins in mouse cerebellar and cerebral cortical astrocytes and neurons. Neurochem Int. 2004;44:75–81.
18. Fuchs BC, Perez JC, Suetterlin JE, Chaudhry SB, Bode BP. Inducible antisense RNA targeting amino acid transporter ATB0/ASCT2 elicits apoptosis in human hepatoma cells. Am J Physiol Gastrointest Liver Physiol. 2004;286:G467–78.
19. Broer A, Wagner C, Lang F, Broer S. Neutral amino acid transporter ASCT2 displays substrate-induced Na+ exchange and a substrate-gated anion conductance. Biochem J. 2000;346:705–10.
20. Zerangue N, Kavanaugh MP. ASCT-1 is a neutral amino acid exchanger with chloride channel activity. J Biol Chem. 1996;271:27991–4.
21. Zander CB, Albers T, Grewer C. Voltage-dependent processes in the electroneutral amino acid exchanger ASCT2. J Gen Physiol. 2013;141(6):659–72. doi:10.1085/jgp.201210948.
22. Palmada M, Speil A, Jeyaraj S, Bohmer C, Lang F. The serine/threonine kinases SGK1, 3 and PKB stimulate the amino acid transporter ASCT2. Biochem Biophys Res Commun. 2005;331:272–7.
23. Baird FE, Beattie KJ, Hyde AR, Ganapathy V, Rennie MJ, Taylor PM. Bidirectional substrate fluxes through the system N (SNAT5) glutamine transporter may determine net glutamine flux in rat liver. J Physiol. 2004;559: 367–81.
24. Chaudhry FA, Krizaj D, Larsson P, et al. Coupled and uncoupled proton movement by amino acid transport system N. EMBO J. 2001;20:7041–51.
25. Hagglund MG, Sreedharan S, Nilsson VC, et al. Identification of SLC38A7 (SNAT7) protein as a glutamine transporter expressed in neurons. J Biol Chem. 2011;286:20500–11.
26. Umapathy NS, Dun Y, Martin PM, et al. Expression and function of system N glutamine transporters (SN1/SN2 or SNAT3/SNAT5) in retinal ganglion cells. Invest Ophthalmol Vis Sci. 2008;49:5151–60.
27. Fei YJ, Sugawara M, Nakanishi T, et al. Primary structure, genomic organization, and functional and electrogenic characteristics of human system N 1, a Na+- and H+-coupled glutamine transporter. J Biol Chem. 2000;275: 23707–17.
28. Broer S, Schneider HP, Broer A, Deitmer JW. Mutation of asparagine 76 in the center of glutamine transporter SNAT3 modulates substrate-induced conductances and Na+ binding. J Biol Chem. 2009;284:25823–31.
29. Jack DL, Paulsen IT, Saier MH. The amino acid/polyamine/organocation (APC) superfamily of transporters specific for amino acids, polyamines and organocations. Microbiology. 2000;146(Pt 8):1797–814.
30. Baird FE, Pinilla-Tenas JJ, Ogilvie WL, Ganapathy V, Hundal HS, Taylor PM. Evidence for allosteric regulation of pH-sensitive System A (SNAT2) and System N (SNAT5) amino acid transporter activity involving a conserved histidine residue. Biochem J. 2006;397:369–75.
31. Nissen-Meyer LS, Popescu MC, el Hamdani H, Chaudhry FA. Protein kinase C-mediated phosphorylation of a single serine residue on the rat glial glutamine transporter SN1 governs its membrane trafficking. J Neurosci. 2011;31:6565–75.
32. Balkrishna S, Broer A, Kingsland A, Broer S. Rapid downregulation of the rat glutamine transporter SNAT3 by a caveolin-dependent trafficking mechanism in Xenopus laevis oocytes. Am J Physiol Cell Physiol. 2010;299: C1047–57.
33. Boehmer C, Okur F, Setiawan I, Broer S, Lang F. Properties and regulation of glutamine transporter SN1 by protein kinases SGK and PKB. Biochem Biophys Res Commun. 2003;306:156–62.
34. Gu S, Villegas CJ, Jiang JX. Differential regulation of amino acid transporter SNAT3 by insulin in hepatocytes. J Biol Chem. 2005;280:26055–62.
35. Sugawara M, Nakanishi T, Fei YJ, et al. Structure and function of ATA3, a new subtype of amino acid transport system A, primarily expressed in the liver and skeletal muscle. Biochim Biophys Acta. 2000;1509:7–13.
36. Varoqui H, Zhu H, Yao D, Ming H, Erickson JD. Cloning and functional identification of a neuronal glutamine transporter. J Biol Chem. 2000;275:4049–54.
37. Boudker O, Verdon G. Structural perspectives on secondary active transporters. Trends Pharmacol Sci. 2010;31:418–26.
38. Zhang Z, Albers T, Fiumera HL, Gameiro A, Grewer C. A conserved Na(+) binding site of the sodium-coupled neutral amino acid transporter 2 (SNAT2). J Biol Chem. 2009;284:25314–23.
39. Yao D, Mackenzie B, Ming H, et al. A novel system A isoform mediating Na+/neutral amino acid cotransport. J Biol Chem. 2000;275:22790–7.
40. Zhang Z, Papageorgiou G, Corrie JE, Grewer C. Pre-steady-state currents in neutral amino acid transporters induced by photolysis of a new caged alanine derivative. Biochemistry. 2007;46:3872–80.
41. Mackenzie B, Schafer MK, Erickson JD, Hediger MA, Weihe E, Varoqui H. Functional properties and cellular distribution of the system A glutamine transporter SNAT1 support specialized roles in central neurons. J Biol Chem. 2003;278:23720–30.
42. Hyde R, Cwiklinski EL, MacAulay K, Taylor PM, Hundal HS. Distinct sensor pathways in the hierarchical control of SNAT2, a putative amino acid transceptor, by amino acid availability. J Biol Chem. 2007;282:19788–98.

43. Ling R, Bridges CC, Sugawara M, et al. Involvement of transporter recruitment as well as gene expression in the substrate-induced adaptive regulation of amino acid transport system A. Biochim Biophys Acta. 2001; 1512:15–21.
44. Gonzalez-Gonzalez IM, Cubelos B, Gimenez C, Zafra F. Immunohistochemical localization of the amino acid transporter SNAT2 in the rat brain. Neuroscience. 2005;130:61–73.
45. Gammelsaeter R, Jenstad M, Bredahl MK, Gundersen V, Chaudhry FA. Complementary expression of SN1 and SAT2 in the islets of Langerhans suggests concerted action of glutamine transport in the regulation of insulin secretion. Biochem Biophys Res Commun. 2009;381:378–82.
46. Desy F, Burelle Y, Belanger P, Gascon-Barre M, Lavoie JM. Effects of acute exercise on the gluconeogenic capacity of periportal and perivenous hepatocytes. J Appl Physiol. 2001;91:1099–104.
47. Ruderisch N, Virgintino D, Makrides V, Verrey F. Differential axial localization along the mouse brain vascular tree of luminal sodium-dependent glutamine transporters Snat1 and Snat3. J Cereb Blood Flow Metab. 2011;31:1637–47.
48. Zhang Z, Grewer C. The sodium-coupled neutral amino acid transporter SNAT2 mediates an anion leak conductance that is differentially inhibited by transported substrates. Biophys J. 2007;92:2621–32.
49. Zhang Z, Zander CB, Grewer C. The C-terminal domain of the neutral amino acid transporter SNAT2 regulates transport activity through voltage-dependent processes. Biochem J. 2011;434:287–96.
50. Forrest LR, Rudnick G. The rocking bundle: a mechanism for ion-coupled solute flux by symmetrical transporters. Physiology (Bethesda). 2009;24:377–86.
51. Kashiwagi H, Yamazaki K, Takekuma Y, Ganapathy V, Sugawara M. Regulatory mechanisms of SNAT2, an amino acid transporter, in L6 rat skeletal muscle cells by insulin, osmotic shock and amino acid deprivation. Amino Acids. 2009;36:219–30.
52. Gazzola RF, Sala R, Bussolati O, et al. The adaptive regulation of amino acid transport system A is associated to changes in ATA2 expression. FEBS Lett. 2001;490:11–4.
53. Brown MN, Mathews GC. Activity- and age-dependent modulation of GABAergic neurotransmission by system A-mediated glutamine uptake. J Neurochem. 2010;114:909–20.
54. Broer S, Brookes N. Transfer of glutamine between astrocytes and neurons. J Neurochem. 2001;77:705–19.
55. Conti F, Melone M. The glutamine commute: lost in the tube? Neurochem Int. 2006;48:459–64.
56. Chaudhry FA, Reimer RJ, Krizaj D, et al. Molecular analysis of system N suggests novel physiological roles in nitrogen metabolism and synaptic transmission. Cell. 1999;99:769–80.
57. Deitmer JW, Broer A, Broer S. Glutamine efflux from astrocytes is mediated by multiple pathways. J Neurochem. 2003;87:127–35.
58. Fremeau Jr RT, Burman J, Qureshi T, et al. The identification of vesicular glutamate transporter 3 suggests novel modes of signaling by glutamate. Proc Natl Acad Sci U S A. 2002;99:14488–93.

Chapter 3
Role of Glutamine Transaminases in Nitrogen, Sulfur, Selenium, and 1-Carbon Metabolism

Arthur J.L. Cooper, Thambi Dorai, Bhuvaneswari Dorai, Boris F. Krasnikov, Jianyong Li, André Hallen, and John Thomas Pinto

Key Points

- Glutamine transaminases (GTK and GTL) and possibly other aminotransferases catalyze the transamination of glutamine with a suitable α-keto acid, generating α-ketoglutaramate (KGM) and the corresponding L-amino acid.
- KGM is hydrolyzed by ω-amidase to α-ketoglutarate and ammonia.
- Glutamine transaminase plus ω-amidase constitute the glutaminase II pathway for the anaplerotic conversion of glutamine to α-ketoglutarate and ammonia, a process that may be important in regulation of growth of cancer cells.
- The glutaminase II pathway is responsible for the salvage of α-keto acids arising through non-specific transamination reactions.
- The glutaminase II pathway closes the methionine salvage pathway in mammals and many other organisms.
- The glutaminase II pathway is prominent in epithelial cells and may be important for the uptake and metabolism of circulating α-keto acids.
- Glutamine transaminases catalyze non-physiological β-elimination reactions leading to the bioactivation of certain xenobiotics.
- GTK catalyzes transamination of sulfur-containing amino acids giving rise to cyclic ketimines, some of which may be neuroactive.

A.J.L. Cooper, Ph.D., D.Sc. (✉) • B.F. Krasnikov, Ph.D. • J.T. Pinto, Ph.D.
Department of Biochemistry and Molecular Biology, New York Medical College, Valhalla, NY, USA
e-mail: arthur_cooper@nymc.edu; ajlc@bestweb.net

T. Dorai, Ph.D.
Department of Urology, New York Medical College, Valhalla, NY, USA

B. Dorai, M.D.
Department of Pathology, Nyack Hospital, Nyack, NY, USA

J. Li, D.V.M., Ph.D.
Department of Biochemistry, Virginia Tech, Blacksburg, VA, USA

A. Hallen, B.Sc.
Department of Chemistry and Biomolecular Sciences, Macquarie University, Balaclava Road, North Ryde, Australia

R. Rajendram et al. (eds.), *Glutamine in Clinical Nutrition*, Nutrition and Health,
DOI 10.1007/978-1-4939-1932-1_3, © Springer Science+Business Media New York 2015

- L-Selenomethionine is a good transaminase substrate of GTL, whereas *Se*-methyl-L-selenocysteine is a good transaminase/β-lyase substrate of GTK—the corresponding α-keto acids are good inhibitors of histone deacetylases.
- The chemoprotective action of selenium may be due to the action of glutamine transaminases on selenium-containing amino acids.

Keywords ω-Amidase • Glutamine transaminase K • Glutamine transaminase L • α-Keto acid transport • α-Ketoglutaramate • α-Keto-γ-methiolbutyrate • Methionine salvage pathway • Seleno amino acids • Seleno keto acids

Abbreviations

AECK	Aminoethylcysteine ketimine
CK	Cystine ketimine
CRYM	μ-Crystallin
CysK	Cystathionine ketimine
DAB	3,3′-Diaminobenzidine
DCVC	*S*-(1,2-Dichlorovinyl)-L-cysteine
GTK	Glutamine transaminase K
GTL	Glutamine transaminase L
HDAC	Histone deacetylase
KAT	Kynurenine aminotransferase
KGM	α-Ketoglutaramate
KMB	α-Keto-γ-methiolbutyrate [2-oxo-4-(methylthio)butyrate]
KMSB	α-Keto-γ-methylselenobutyrate
LK	Lanthionine ketimine
MSC	*Se*-Methyl-L-selenocysteine
MSP	β-Methylselenopyruvate
MTA	5′-Methylthioadenosine
PLP	Pyridoxal 5′-phosphate
SM	L-Selenomethionine
TCA	Tricarboxylic acid
TFEC	*S*-(1,1,2,2-Tetrafluoroethyl)-L-cysteine

Introduction: Historical

Work in the 1940s showed that rat tissues contain phosphate-activated glutaminase (Eq 3.1) (glutaminase I; now simply referred to as glutaminase) and an apparent pyruvate-activated glutaminase (glutaminase II). Glutaminase is now known to consist of a liver type glutaminase isozyme (LGA; GLS1), a kidney type glutaminase isozyme (KGA; GLS2), and a shortened form (glutaminase C, GAC).

$$\text{L-Glutamine} + H_2O \rightarrow \text{L-glutamate} + NH_3 \tag{3.1}$$

In the 1950s Meister and colleagues showed that the glutaminase II of rat liver consists of a glutamine transaminase (EC 2.6.1.-; (Eq. 3.2)) coupled to an ω-amidase (ω-amidodicarboxylate amidohydrolase, EC 3.5.1.3; (Eq. 3.3)) [1]. [Note that the word aminotransferase is now more generally used than the word transaminase, but the former word has been retained for enzymes catalyzing transfer of the amino group of glutamine.] The net (glutaminase II) reaction is shown in (Eq. 3.4). The partially purified rat liver glutamine transaminase was shown to have a broad α-keto acid specificity [1].

$$\text{L-Glutamine} + \alpha\text{-keto acid} \rightleftarrows \alpha\text{-ketoglutaramate}\left(\text{KGM}\right) + \text{L-amino acid} \tag{3.2}$$

$$\text{KGM} + \text{H}_2\text{O} \rightarrow \alpha - \text{ketoglutarate} + \text{NH}_3 \tag{3.3}$$

$$\text{Net: L-Glutamine} + \alpha\text{-keto acid} + \text{H}_2\text{O} \rightarrow \alpha\text{-ketoglutarate} + \text{L-amino acid} + \text{NH}_3 \tag{3.4}$$

Mammalian Tissues Contain at Least Three Aminotransferases that Can Utilize Glutamine as an Amino Donor

In the 1970s, Cooper and Meister showed that rat tissues contain a kidney type (glutamine transaminase K, GTK) and a liver type (glutamine transaminase L, GTL) [2]. Other workers studying the degradation of tryptophan in the production of NAD^+ identified the kynurenine pathway and characterized kynurenine aminotransferase I (KAT I) as an important enzyme that catalyzes the transamination of kynurenine to kynurenate. Subsequent studies demonstrated that this enzyme is identical to GTK, and investigations by Han et al. using a recombinant human enzyme (hKAT I) reported on the K_{cat}/K_m values for glutamine and five other "best" substrate amino acids using α-ketobutyrate as α-keto acid co-substrate [3]. Han et al. reported K_{cat}/K_m values for glutamine, phenylalanine, leucine, kynurenine, tryptophan and methionine of 157, 54, 45, 43, 36, and 34 min^{-1} mM^{-1}, respectively [3]. In another study, Han et al. investigated the amino acid specificity of another kynurenine aminotransferase, namely mouse kynurenine aminotransferase III (mKAT III) [4]. These authors showed that glutamine was also the most favorable amino acid substrate of this enzyme with a K_{cat}/K_m value of 194 min^{-1} mM^{-1}. K_{cat}/K_m values for the next six "best" amino acid substrates, namely histidine, methionine, phenylalanine, asparagine, cysteine, and kynurenine, were reported to be 171, 162, 147, 126, 114, and 92 min^{-1} mM^{-1}, respectively. We have shown that KAT III is identical to GTL [5]. Inasmuch as (a) GTK and GTL were described prior to the identification of KAT I and KAT III as distinct kynurenine aminotransferases, (b) glutamine is a better substrate than is kynurenine, (c) mammalian tissues contain far more glutamine than kynurenine, and (d) the present chapter focuses on glutamine, we have assumed the nomenclature GTK and GTL throughout the present chapter, except where it is necessary to indicate the KAT nomenclature often presented in basic scientific literature. Finally, Han et al. have investigated the substrate specificity of yet another KAT, namely hKAT II [6]. Historically, KAT II was first described as an aminoadipate aminotransferase. As determined for GTK/KAT I and GTL/KAT III, the amino acid (and α-keto acid) specificity of KAT II is also broad. Thus, K_{cat}/K_m values for aminoadipate, kynurenine, methionine, and glutamate were reported to be 196, 126, 124, and 119 min^{-1} mM^{-1}, respectively [6]. The K_{cat}/K_m value for glutamine was lower, but still appreciable (11.8 min^{-1} mM^{-1}) [6]. All three enzymes are discussed later in this chapter with reference to their ability to transaminate seleno amino acids.

Glutamine transaminases and ω-amidase activities are widespread in rat tissues, and are especially active in rat liver and kidney [7]. In rat liver and kidney, both activities are present in cytosol and mitochondria [7]. Both GTK and GTL generally "prefer" amino acids [$RCH(NH_3^+)CO_2^-$] and co-substrate keto acids [$RC(O)CO_2^-$] in which R is a hydrophobic group or a polar but uncharged group. An exception is glyoxylate [$HC(O)CO_2^-$], which is a good substrate of both GTL and GTK. [Glyoxylate is an α-aldehydic acid, rather than an α-keto acid, and as such is much more hydrated (>90 %) to the corresponding gem diol [$HC(OH)_2CO_2^-$] under physiological conditions than are typical α-keto acids [5–10 % present as $RC(OH)_2CO_2^-$], and transamination of glyoxylate is greatly favored over transamination of glycine.]

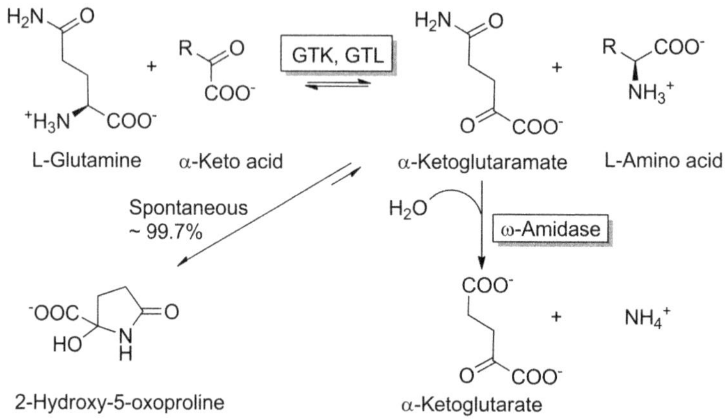

Fig. 3.1 The glutamine transaminase—ω-amidase (glutaminase II) pathway for the metabolism of L-glutamine. Note that the glutamine transaminase reaction is freely reversible, but due to (**a**) the cyclization of product α-ketoglutaramate (KGM) to lactam (2-hydroxy-5-oxoproline) (99.7 % lactam; 0.3 % open-chain form at pH 7.4) and (**b**) conversion of the open-chain form to α-ketoglutarate by ω-amidase, the glutamine transaminase reaction is drawn toward glutamine utilization and amination of α-keto acid substrate [$RC(O)CO_2^-$]. GTK, glutamine transaminase K; GTL, glutamine transaminase L. Modified from ref. [12]

Although aminotransferase reactions are generally freely reversible, those involving glutamine (Eq. 3.2) are drawn in the direction of glutamine utilization because KGM cyclizes to a lactam [8] and is also removed by the action of ω-amidase (Fig. 3.1). Under physiological conditions, 99.7 % of KGM is in the lactam form (2-hydroxy-5-oxoproline) and only about 0.3 % is in the open-chain form (substrate of ω-amidase) (Fig. 3.1) [8]. The interconversion between open and closed forms of KGM is specific base (OH^-)-catalyzed [8]. At physiological pH values the interconversion is slow enough that despite the high affinity of ω-amidase for the open-chain form [8–12], KGM is present in rat tissues at steady state levels in the μM range [12].

The glutaminase and glutaminase II pathways constitute the main mechanisms by which glutamine is metabolized. Most work in the area of glutamine metabolism has been devoted to the glutaminase pathway. However, compelling data suggest that the glutaminase II pathway is quantitatively important in humans. Thus, turnover of glutamine through the glutaminase II pathway has been demonstrated by Darmaun et al. to occur in human volunteers administered L-[N^{15}]glutamate, L-[2-^{15}N] glutamine and L-[5-^{15}N]glutamine [13]. The authors noted that their data strongly suggest that the nitrogen flux from the amine moiety is greater than that from the amide of glutamine. Thus, the data appear to show that the transamination pathway (Eq. 3.2) is quantitatively more important than the glutaminase pathway (Eq. 3.1) for the metabolism of glutamine in humans. On the other hand, the authors raised the caveat that because aminotransferases are reversible their findings do not mean that nitrogen fluxes from the amine are necessarily greater than those from the amide nitrogen or even result in a net amine turnover [13]. However, as noted above, unlike most aminotransferase reactions, those involving glutamine are largely irreversible. Thus, the work of Darmaun et al. [13] is crucial in understanding whole body glutamine metabolism and suggests that in humans the glutaminase II pathway (Eq. 3.4) may be physiologically as critical as the glutaminase pathway (Eq. 3.1) and possibly even more so. In this chapter we summarize the biological roles of the glutaminase II pathway (i.e., glutamine transaminase plus ω-amidase) and suggest that this pathway is much more important than hitherto realized both in terms of the magnitude of the overall metabolic flux of nitrogen and the possible contribution of the individual enzymes to cancer prevention and control.

Salvage of α-Keto Acids

Enzymes occasionally "make mistakes" and convert an inappropriate/non-physiological substrate to a potentially toxic or a metabolically wasteful product. Thus, repair/salvage enzymes are essential. For example, the cytosolic and mitochondrial isozymes of aspartate aminotransferase can catalyze transamination to some extent of amino acids other than the "usual" substrates, aspartate and glutamate. Such "unscheduled" amino acid substrates of mitochondrial aspartate aminotransferase include, for example, cysteine, methionine, isoleucine and the aromatic amino acids [14]. The α-keto acid products of these transamination reactions are good substrates of the glutamine transaminases. Because of the irreversible nature of the glutaminase II pathway, losses of sulfur and "essential" carbon and the accumulation of potentially neurotoxic α-keto acids (e.g., phenylpyruvate, branched-chain α-keto acids) are prevented or minimized at the expense of the readily renewable amino group of glutamine, with the concomitant anaplerotic production of α-ketoglutarate, an energetically useful intermediate of the tricarboxylic acid (TCA) cycle.

Closure of the Methionine Salvage Pathway

Glutamine transaminases act as salvage enzymes in yet another context. During polyamine biosynthesis, the carboxyl moiety of methionine is lost as CO_2, the C2-C4 skeleton and the amino group are incorporated into polyamines, and the methyl and sulfur are incorporated into 5′-methylthioadenosine (MTA). If there were no way to salvage MTA, loss of MTA would result in an excessive drain of methyl groups (for 1-carbon and folate metabolism) and reduced sulfur, and a markedly increased requirement for methionine. In the 1990s Abeles and colleagues showed that MTA is converted to α-keto-γ-methiolbutyrate (KMB) by a remarkable series of reactions termed the methionine salvage pathway [15]. The last step in the pathway (i.e., conversion of KMB to methionine) is catalyzed by a transamination reaction. In mammals, and many plants and bacteria, glutamine is the preferred aminotransferase substrate. Thus, the glutaminase II pathway closes the methionine salvage pathway, thereby linking the metabolism of nitrogen from glutamine to that of sulfur from methionine and 1-carbon compounds from folate. Since these reactions are integrated and play a crucial role in providing anaplerotic metabolites, we have aptly entitled these interconnecting pathways as the glutamine-methionine bi-cycle (Fig. 3.2) [10].

Metabolism of Circulating α-Keto Acids: Presence of ω-Amidase and GTK in Epithelial Tissue

Immunohistochemical studies by Stevens and colleagues showed that GTK in rat kidney is markedly enriched in proximal tubules [16], a finding that we later verified [17]. In addition, our immunohistochemical studies showed that in the rat brain, GTK is especially prominent in the choroid plexus [17]. In that same study, we showed that the specific activity of both GTK and ω-amidase in the rat is much higher in the isolated choroid plexus than in a homogenate of the whole brain [17]. As noted above, previous work showed that both GTK and ω-amidase are widely distributed in rat tissues, with liver and kidney exhibiting the highest specific activity for both enzymes [3]. In a separate study, Lin et al. showed by Northern blot analysis that Nit2 mRNA (Nit2 is identical to ω-amidase; see below) is widely distributed in human tissues with highest levels in liver and kidney [18]. Thus, it is likely that the two enzymes of the glutaminase II pathway [i.e., GTK (and possibly GTL) and ω-amidase] are

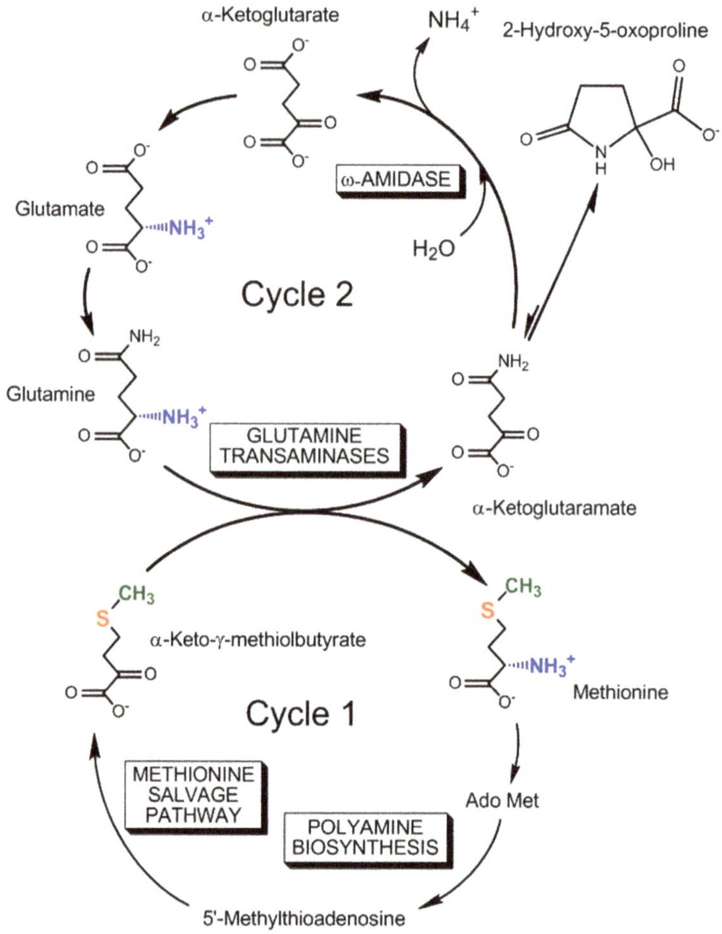

Fig. 3.2 The glutamine-methionine bi-cycle. *Cycle 1*: During polyamine biosynthesis the C1 carbon of L-methionine is lost as CO_2, the amino group is incorporated into polyamines and C2–C4 carbons are incorporated into polyamines. During this process the original methyl group (*green*) and sulfur (*orange*) of L-methionine are incorporated into 5′-methylthioadenosine (MTA). The methyl and sulfur moieties are conserved by a remarkable series of reactions termed the methionine salvage pathway that converts MTA to α-keto-γ-methiolbutyrate (KMB) [15]. This salvage pathway is of ancient lineage and has been conserved, with minor variations, in archaea, bacteria, fungi, plants, and vertebrates. The salvage pathway is closed by transamination of KMB to methionine. In mammals and many other organisms the preferred amino donor is glutamine. In the salvaged methionine the original methyl group (*green*) and the sulfur (*orange*) are retained, the amino group (*blue*) is obtained from the nonessential amino acid glutamine and carbons 1–4 are formed anew from the ribose moiety of MTA. *Cycle 2*: The α-ketoglutarate generated from glutamine by the glutaminase II pathway (KMB as α-keto acid acceptor) is converted to glutamate by the action of glutamate dehydrogenase/α-ketoglutarate-utilizing aminotransferases and thence to glutamine by glutamine synthetase. Modified from ref. [10]

metabolically linked in most (if not all) tissues. As we discuss below, this may be important in the transport of α-keto acids in epithelial tissues.

Much work has been carried out on interorgan trafficking and uptake of amino acids [19], but relatively few studies have focused on the interorgan trafficking of the corresponding α-keto acids. In fact, a recent PubMed search for α-keto acids/transporters brought up only three relevant references, all published more than 25 years ago. The monocarboxylate transporter was shown to be responsible for the uptake of branched-chain α-keto acids into rat liver cells [20], and for the uptake of pyruvate, α-ketoisocaproate, α-ketobutyrate, and KMB across the blood–brain barrier [21]. A mitochondrial transporter for the branched-chain α-keto acids in rat brain has also been described [22]. This paucity of information on α-keto acid transporters is surprising given that (a) excessive accumulation of certain α-keto acids (e.g., phenylpyruvate, branched-chain α-keto acids) is deleterious to brain development, and (b) the concentrations of α-keto acids in blood/plasma are often >10 μM. For example, the concentrations of the keto acid analogues of the branched-chain amino acids in human plasma are in the range of 12–22 μM [23].

The above discussion has prompted us to posit the following hypothesis: Glutaminase II enzymes (i.e., GTK and ω-amidase) are enriched and centrally located in epithelial cells from a wide variety of tissues and are thus poised to transaminate a variety of α-keto acids transported from body fluids using glutamine as the amine donor. Our preliminary evidence has provided support for this hypothesis. Specifically, we have used immunohistochemistry (hNit2/ω-amidase; OriGene; mouse monoclonal) and human hKAT I/GTK (Santa Cruz, goat polyclonal) on sections of human tissues using the Vector ABC immunoperoxidase kit [with 3,3′-diaminobenzidine (DAB) staining] (Fig. 3.3). [All human specimens were from archived tissues. No direct or indirect identifiers were provided.] Immunohistochemical staining indicates that ω-amidase is present in the epithelial cells of normal human prostate (Fig. 3.3a), bladder (Fig. 3.3e), and pancreas (not shown). The staining is much less intense in other areas. Immunohistochemical staining with peroxidase/DAB also illustrates intense localization of GTK in normal human prostate epithelium (Fig. 3.3b), bladder (not shown), and pancreas (not shown). In normal bladder there is intense staining for ω-amidase in the cytoplasm of the urothelial cells (Fig. 3.3e). Interestingly, intense staining for ω-amidase can also be observed in epithelial cells within specimens of human prostate cancer (Fig. 3.3c) and human bladder cancer (Fig. 3.3f). Immunohistochemical staining reveals a similar pattern of epithelial cell staining for GTK in prostate cancer (Fig. 3.3d), bladder cancer (Fig. 3.3g), and pancreatic cancer (Fig. 3.3h).

Taken together these findings strongly suggest that the glutaminase II pathway is poised to metabolize or salvage incoming α-keto acids to the corresponding amino acid with the concomitant conversion of glutamine to anaplerotically useful α-ketoglutarate in epithelial cells in several tissues, including the brain (choroid plexus), prostate, bladder, and pancreas. Moreover, the glutaminase II pathway is well represented in those human cancer tissues that we have investigated thus far. This preliminary work is ongoing to determine whether ω-amidase and GTK are present in epithelial tissues of other normal and cancerous human tissues. As discussed in the next section, the presence of the glutaminase II pathway may be of fundamental importance in cancer biology and progression.

Role of the Glutaminase II Pathway in Tumor Metabolism: Identification of ω-Amidase as a Putative Tumor Suppressor

Two genes in the human genome have been designated *Nit1* (*nit*rilase-like 1) and *Nit2* (*nit*rilase-like 2). In mammals, the gene products are members of branch 10 of the nitrilase superfamily [24]. Nit1 is a tumor suppressor, promoting apoptosis in cancer cells [25]. Nit2 has similarly been identified as a putative tumor suppressor, but in this case the tumor suppressor property appears to be due to interference with the cell cycle [18]. Initially, the substrate specificity of Nit2 was unknown. However, in 2009 our group [10] and Van Schaftingen's group [9] simultaneously reported that Nit2 is identical to ω-amidase. The finding that ω-amidase has tumor suppressor function emphasizes the strong link between glutamine metabolism and cancer progression.

Glutamine is an important energy and nitrogen source for rapidly dividing cells such as fibroblasts [26], colonocytes [27], and jejunal epithelial cells [28]. Metabolism of glutamine yields two

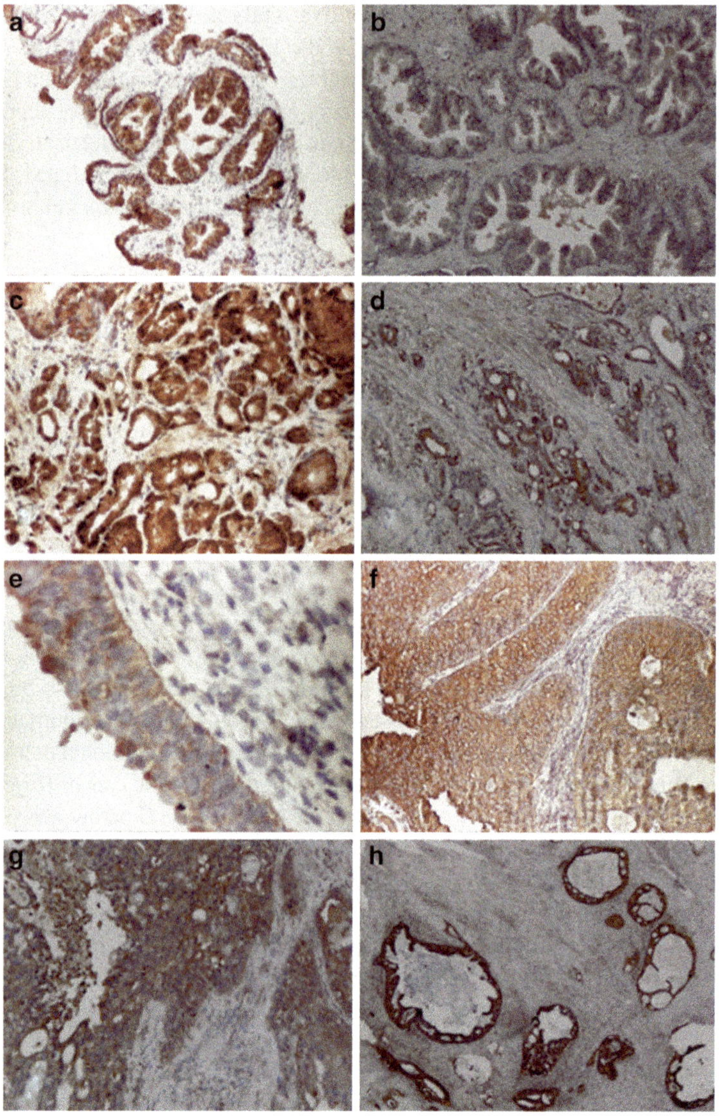

Fig. 3.3 Immunohistochemical localization (peroxidase—DAB staining) of ω-amidase and GTK in human prostate, bladder and pancreatic tissues. (**a**) Normal prostate stained with ω-amidase monoclonal antibody. (**b**) Normal prostate stained with GTK polyclonal antibody. In a and b intense, but diffuse, granular cytoplasmic staining for both ω-amidase and GTK is observed in the luminal epithelial cells. By contrast, no staining is visible for either enzyme in the stromal cells. (**c**) Prostatic carcinoma stained with ω-amidase antibody. (**d**) Prostatic carcinoma stained with GTK antibody. As with normal tissues, the staining within the malignant tissue is limited mostly to luminal epithelial cells. (**e**) Normal bladder stained with ω-amidase antibody. Staining is intense within the cytoplasm of the urothelial cells, whereas some smooth muscle cells exhibit faint staining. (**f**) Bladder carcinoma stained with hNit2/ω-amidase antibody. A complete loss of organized urothelial layer is observed, with invasion of urothelial cells into the stromal cell layer. Invading malignant cells demonstrate intense staining. (**g**) Bladder carcinoma stained with GTK antibody. The staining pattern is remarkably similar to that of ω-amidase in panel f. (**h**) Pancreatic carcinoma stained with GTK antibody. Ducts of different sizes can be seen, with the enlarged duct exhibiting a cribriform (or perforated) pattern, with fusing micropapillaries. The glands are heterogeneous in size and the luminal epithelial cells show very intense staining for GTK. Data are unpublished findings of Dorai and Dorai. [Note that the antibodies sold by the manufacturers for ω-amidase and GTK are designated hNit2 and hKAT I, respectively; GTK is also referred to as CCBL 1. All magnifications are 20×]

equivalents of nitrogen that can be used in DNA and polyamine synthesis, and at the same time the carbon skeleton is easily converted to anaplerotic α-ketoglutarate, an important component of the TCA cycle. Although many rapidly dividing cancer cells have been known for decades to have a high requirement for glutamine [29] it is only recently that this "glutamine addiction" has attracted considerable attention [30–32]. Many cancer cells are also well known to take up considerably more glucose and produce much more lactate than comparable non-cancerous cells, even in the presence of adequate oxygen and well functioning mitochondria (the Warburg Effect) [31, 32]. Thus, much of the energy requirement in cancer cells is derived from anaerobic glycolysis—an important pathway in cancer cells burdened with a limited oxygen supply. In cancer cells the TCA cycle is an important anaplerotic machine for the supply of essential carbon compounds necessary for the replication pathways in rapidly dividing cells [32]. But, how does glutamine carbon enter the TCA cycle? The most thoroughly studied pathway is the glutaminase pathway (Eq. 3.1) that generates glutamate. This glutamate is then converted to the TCA cycle intermediate α-ketoglutarate via the glutamate dehydrogenase reaction (Eq. 3.5) or an aminotransferase reaction (Eq. 3.6):

$$\text{L-Glutamate} + \text{NAD(P)}^{+} \rightleftarrows \alpha\text{-ketoglutarate} + \text{NH}_4^{+} + \text{NAD(P)H} \tag{3.5}$$

$$\text{L-Glutamate} + \alpha\text{-keto acid} \rightleftarrows \alpha\text{-ketoglutarate} + \text{L-amino acid} \tag{3.6}$$

It should be noted that if an α-keto acid is taken up by cancer cells, glutamine can be converted to α-ketoglutarate anaerobically by either (1) coupling the glutaminase reaction (Eq. 3.1) to a glutamate-linked aminotransferase reaction (Eq. 3.6), or (2) the glutaminase II pathway Eqs. (3.2)–(3.4). Utilization of α-keto acids as key partners in aminotransferase reactions, especially if they accumulate in the tumor from elsewhere in the body, would be a distinct advantage to cancer cells under hypoxic conditions. We have detected glutamine transaminase and ω-amidase enzyme activities in a variety of human cancers including breast and prostate cancers (unpublished data), and as noted above, GTK and ω-amidase have been detected immunohistochemically in epithelia of cancerous human prostate, bladder and pancreatic tissues. The following question then arises—Is the glutaminase II pathway a "double-edged sword" for cancer cells? From one perspective, the glutaminase II pathway may serve an anaplerotic function (i.e., provision of α-ketoglutarate) and provide useful nitrogen (for the synthesis of DNA and polyamines), but from another perspective, the pathway may conceal a tumor suppressor function (through the action of Nit2/ω-amidase). Work in our laboratory is ongoing to address the relative importance of these seemingly dichotomous functions.

GTK is a Cysteine *S*-Conjugate β-Lyase: Possible Role in Bioactivation of Halogenated Alkenes

Several pyridoxal 5′-phosphate (PLP)-containing enzymes naturally catalyze β-elimination reactions with amino acids containing a nucleofuge (i.e., a leaving group with electron-withdrawing properties) in the β-position [33]. The product of the enzyme reaction is highly reactive aminoacrylate [$CH_2{=}C(NH_3^+)CO_2^-$], which spontaneously (nonenzymatically) tautomerizes to an imino acid [$CH_3C({=}NH_2^+)CO_2^-$], which in turn nonenzymatically hydrolyzes to pyruvate and ammonia. The net reaction is shown in (Eq. 3.7), where X is the nucleofuge.

$$\text{XCH}_2\text{CH}(\text{NH}_3^{+})\text{CO}_2^{-} + \text{H}_2\text{O} \rightarrow \text{CH}_3\text{C(O)CO}_2^{-} + \text{NH}_4^{+} + \text{XH} \tag{3.7}$$

If an amino acid containing an exceptionally strong nucleofuge (X) binds at the active site, many PLP-containing enzymes (e.g., aminotransferases) that do not normally catalyze a β-elimination

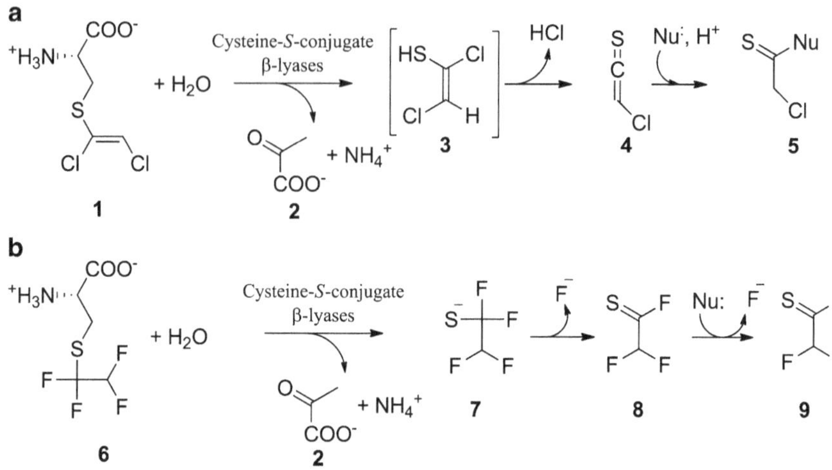

Fig. 3.4 Bioactivation of cysteine *S*-conjugates of halogenated alkenes. (**a**) Bioactivation of *S*-(1,2-dichlorovinyl)-L-cysteine (DCVC) by cysteine *S*-conjugate β-lyases. DCVC (*1*) is converted to pyruvate (*2*), ammonium and a sulfur-containing fragment that has the theoretical structure 1,2-dichloroethylenethiol (*3*). 1,2-Dichloroethylenethiol is unstable and in part loses HCl to form the highly reactive chlorothioketene (*4*). The thioketene reacts with tissue nucleophiles (Nu:) to generate thioacylated products (*5*). (**b**) Bioactivation of *S*-(1,1,2,2-tetrafluoroethyl)-L-cysteine (TFEC) (*6*) by cysteine *S*-conjugate β-lyases. TFEC is converted to pyruvate (*2*), ammonium and a sulfur-containing fragment that has the structure 1,1,2,2-tetrafluoroethanethiolate (*7*). 1,1,2,2-Tetrafluoroethanethiolate is unstable and loses F^- to form difluorothioacetyl fluoride (*8*). Difluorothioacetyl fluoride reacts with tissue nucleophiles (Nu:) to generate thioacylated products (*9*). Based on Dekant et al. [36] and modified from refs. [37–39]

reaction are "coerced" into catalyzing such a reaction. For example, cytosolic aspartate aminotransferase can catalyze β-elimination reactions with β-chloro-L-alanine (X=–Cl) and L-serine *O*-sulfate (X=$-OSO_3H$)) [34]. Owing to the reactivity of aminoacrylate (or aminoacrylate bound to PLP in the active site) the aspartate aminotransferase is eventually syncatalytically inactivated. However, the enzyme may be protected from inactivation if a suitable small-molecular-weight Michael nucleophile, such as thiosulfate or 2-mercaptoethanol is included in the reaction mixture. These reagents add to the double bond of free aminoacrylate (or aminoacrylate in covalent linkage to PLP), preventing a) covalent Michael addition of free aminoacrylate (or aminoacrylate-PLP) to a susceptible group in the vicinity of the active site, or b) reaction between free aminoacrylate and PLP [35].

Cysteine *S*-conjugates possess the structure $XCH_2CH(NH_3^+)CO_2^-$ where X=RS. These conjugates can bind to a number of PLP-containing enzymes. When R is a simple aliphatic group, β elimination is not favorable and transamination is the "preferred" reaction catalyzed by aminotransferases. However, if R is strongly electron withdrawing, the ready polarizability of sulfur makes the RS moiety a good nucleofuge. This phenomenon is observed with toxic cysteine *S*-conjugates derived from many halogenated alkenes. Examples include the cysteine *S*-conjugates derived from trichloroethylene and tetrafluoroethylene, namely *S*-(1,2-dichlorovinyl)-L-cysteine (DCVC) and *S*-(1,1,2,2-tetrafluoroethyl)-L-cysteine (TFEC), respectively. Enzymes that catalyze β-elimination reactions with cysteine *S*-conjugates have been named cysteine *S*-conjugate β-lyases. These enzymes convert DCVC and TFEC to pyruvate, ammonia and a sulfur-containing fragment (RS^-). In both cases, RS^- is unstable and decomposes to products that are potent nucleophiles, subsequently covalently adding to macromolecules (Fig. 3.4) [36]. For reviews see refs. [36–39].

The first cysteine *S*-conjugate β-lyase to be identified in mammalian tissues was GTK [40]. Consequently, the gene for GTK is named *CCBL1* (*c*ysteine *S*-*c*onjugate β-*l*yase isozyme *1*) in human and rodent genomes. In addition, we have recently identified a closely related gene, named *CCBL2*, as coding for KAT III/GTL [5]. In our opinion this is an inappropriate nomenclature as the lyase reaction is not the natural reaction catalyzed by GTK and GTL. Moreover, we and others have identified several other PLP-containing enzymes (mostly aminotransferases, but also cystathionine γ-lyase) that can also catalyze β-lyase reactions with DCVC and/or TFEC (reviewed in ref. [39]). Nevertheless, both GTK and GTL may contribute substantially to the bioactivation (toxification) of halogenated alkenes, some of which are produced on an industrial scale and continue to be environmental contaminants. We shall revisit the ability of GTK and GTL to catalyze β-elimination reactions in a subsequent section that reviews the biochemistry of selenium-containing amino acids.

The Role of Glutamine Transaminases in the Production of Potentially Neuroactive Sulfur-Containing Cyclic Ketimines

As noted above, the glutamine transaminases have broad amino acid specificities. Thus, several sulfur-containing amino acids (e.g., cystathionine, cystine, lanthionine, and thialysine) have been shown to be substrates of glutamine transaminases (reviewed in refs. [12, 41–43]). Figure 3.5 illustrates the metabolic origin of the sulfur-containing amino acids and the importance of the glutamine transaminases in converting these compounds to α-keto acids. These α-keto acids are spontaneously converted to sulfur-containing cyclic ketimines. Naming of these cyclic ketimines is complex and the first authors to describe these compounds assigned these imines trivial names [41], a practice we continue here. Thus, cyclic imines arising via transamination of thialysine (L-aminoethylcysteine), lanthionine, cystathionine, and cystine are named aminoethylcysteine ketimine (AECK), lanthionine ketimine (LK), cystathionine ketimine (CysK), and cystine ketimine (CK), respectively. These compounds exist in equilibrium with their open-chain and enamine forms. The relative concentrations of open-chain-, ketimine- and enamine forms are strongly pH dependent [41–43].

Studies on the functional role of sulfur-containing cyclic ketimines are limited. Nevertheless, some evidence suggests that these compounds may be neuroactive. For example, both the concentration of cystathionine in human brain and glutamine transaminase activity are relatively high in human brain [12]. LK and CysK have been found in human brain and AECK has been found in bovine brain. LK has been shown to increase basal cAMP levels and reversibly bind to brain membranes at concentrations that imply specific neuroreceptor binding. This binding is displaced by other ketimines (AECK and CysK) and also by catecholamines. Several cyclic ketimines have been shown to promote free radical formation by enhancement of NADPH oxidase activity. AECK is a potent inhibitor of D-amino acid oxidase activity and is thus a potential regulator of the concentrations of D-amino acids. In this regard, regulation of D-serine levels is especially important as D-serine is a neurotransmitter and agonist of the NMDA receptor. Finally, a role in neurogenesis is implied by the findings that LK stimulates neurite outgrowth. For original references on the potential neuroactive roles of the cyclic sulfur-containing cyclic ketimines see refs. [42, 43].

The cyclic ketimines formed by glutamine transaminase are subsequently reduced by ketimine reductases, one of which has been identified as the protein μ-crystallin (CRYM) [42, 43]. The activity of this enzyme was shown to be regulated by the thyroid hormone triiodothyronine (T3) and, reciprocally, a role is implied for the enzyme in regulating the bioavailability of intracellular T3 (reviewed in refs. [42, 43]). Mutations in CRYM are associated with non-syndromal deafness. The gene for CRYM is a) upregulated in a murine model of amyotrophic lateral sclerosis, b) downregulated in human glioblastomas, and c) induced by androgens in human prostate cancer. For original references see refs. [42, 43].

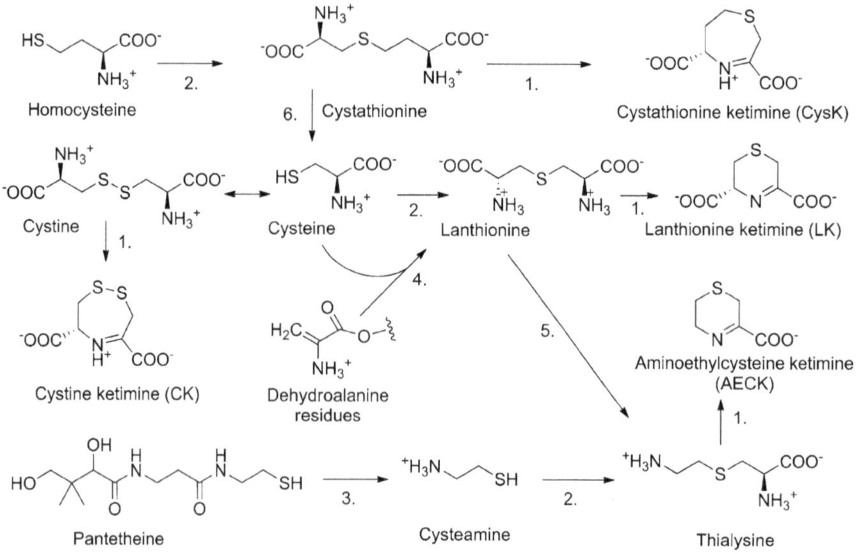

Fig. 3.5 Metabolic pathways leading to the formation of sulfur-containing cyclic ketimines. Enzymes: *1*. Glutamine transaminases; *2*. cystathionine-β-synthase; *3*. pantetheinase; *4*. Michael addition of cysteine/cysteine residues to dehydroalanine residues followed by proteolytic digestion; *5*. uncharacterized decarboxylase; *6*. cystathionine-γ-lyase. For simplicity not all cofactors or reactants are shown. Note the importance of the glutamine transaminases (*1*) in the production of cyclic sulfur-containing imines. Note also that the sulfur-containing imines may be in equilibrium not only with the open-chain form, but in some cases with an enamine (not shown). The ratio of the various forms is strongly dependent on the pH [41–43]. Abbreviations: CysK cystathionine ketimine, LK lanthionine ketimine, CK cystine ketimine, AECK aminoethylcysteine ketimine. From ref. [43] with permission

Possible Role of Glutamine Transaminases in Chemopreventive Action of Selenium-Containing Amino Acids

A large number of cysteine *S*-conjugates [$RSCH_2CH(NH_3^+)CO_2^-$, where R is an aliphatic or aromatic moiety] and selenocysteine *Se*-conjugates [[$RSeCH_2CH(NH_3^+)CO_2^-$, where R is also an aliphatic or aromatic moiety] have been shown to be aminotransferase substrates of highly purified rat kidney GTK [44]. Curiously, the selenocysteine *Se*-conjugates are generally an order of magnitude more effective aminotransferase substrates than are the cysteine *S*-conjugates, possibly as a result of a weaker α C-H bond in the selenocysteine *Se*-conjugates compared to that in the cysteine *S*-conjugates [44]. In the same study, the authors also showed that GTK catalyzes a β-elimination reaction that competes with the transamination reaction when selenocysteine *Se*-conjugates are employed as substrates [44]. The β-elimination reaction is much more favorable with the selenocysteine *Se*-conjugates than with the corresponding cysteine *S*-conjugates. For example, the specific activities of *Se*-methyl-L-selenocysteine (MSC) as an aminotransferase substrate and as a β-lyase substrate of rat kidney GTK were reported to be 7.40 ± 1.55 and 1.61 ± 0.41 μmol/min/mg, respectively. The corresponding values for *S*-methyl-L-cysteine were 1.37 ± 0.25 μmol/min/mg, and below the limit of detection, respectively. The much greater ability of rat kidney GTK to catalyze β-elimination reactions with selenocysteine *Se*-conjugates compared to cysteine *S*-conjugates is presumably due, at least in part, to the weaker strength of the C-Se bond compared to that of the C-S bond [44].

Considerable evidence suggests that seleniferous vegetables, such as members of the allium family, are chemoprotective. These vegetables contain varying levels of organified selenium, mostly in

Table 3.1 Rates of transamination (nmol/min/mg) exhibited by various kynurenine aminotransferases (KAT I, II, III) toward L-selenomethionine (SM) and Se-methyl-L-selenocysteine (MSC)

Amino acid substrate	Recombinant human KAT I/GTK	Recombinant human KAT II/α--aminoadipate aminotransferase	Recombinant mouse KAT III/GTL
SM[a]	162±46	160±59	2000±303
MSC[a]	253±35	172±55	607±44

[a]The rates of transamination were determined at 37 °C in a reaction mixture containing 100 mM potassium phosphate buffer pH 7.4, 1 mM amino acid substrate (SM or MSC) and 0.1 mM KMB as α-keto acid acceptor. At intervals the amount of L-methionine formed from KMB in the reaction mixture was determined by HPLC with coulometric detection as described in ref. [51]. Data are expressed as mean±S.D. of 3 separate determinations

the form of MSC and L-selenomethionine (SM). Numerous studies have reported on the anticancer properties of MSC and SM in breast, prostate and colon (reviewed in refs. [45, 46]). As noted above, rat kidney GTK has been reported to catalyze competing transamination and β-elimination reactions with MSC [44]. We have verified this finding [47]. [Due to the extreme hydrophobicity of the fragment eliminated from MSC (i.e., methylselenol, CH_3SeH) and resulting difficulty in detection, the β-elimination reaction could only be followed by measuring pyruvate formation.] Curiously, MSC is a relatively good aminotransferase substrate of rat kidney GTK, but SM is a relatively poor substrate [47]. We have obtained similar findings with recombinant human KAT I/GTK (Table 3.1). On the other hand, SM is a relatively good aminotransferase substrate of recombinant mouse KAT III/GTL, but MSC is not as effective (Table 3.1; [5]).

The data in Table 3.1 show that both SM and MSC are effective substrates of hGTK and mGTL in the presence of KMB as amine acceptor. In addition, the data show that hKAT II/α-aminoadipate aminotransferase can also catalyze transamination of SM and MSC with KMB. The following question may then be asked: "How relevant are the data in Table 3.1 to the possible in vivo concentrations of SM or MSC (and their α-keto acid metabolites) after ingestion of seleniferous vegetables"? Because aminotransferases catalyze a ping-pong reaction the K_m value for an amino acid will depend on the concentration of the α-keto acid co-substrate. Nevertheless, apparent K_m values for all three enzymes listed in Table 3.1 for glutamine and some of the other most effective amino acid substrates are generally in the range of ~1 to several mM [3, 4, 6]. Thus, it is likely that the apparent K_m for MSC and KMB exhibited by the three aminotransferases evaluated in Table 3.1 will also be in this range (see also ref. [44]). Thus, the concentration of SM and MSC used in the experiments shown in Table 3.1 is probably not saturating. Nevertheless, each of the three aminotransferases exhibits substantial activity with SM and MSC, especially mKAT III/GTL.

Another question may be asked: "Because of the wide amino acid substrate specificity of the aminotransferases listed in Table 3.1 and the relatively high concentration of several of the amino acid substrates in tissues is it possible that the activity exhibited by each of the three aminotransferases toward the seleno amino acids will be severely inhibited in vivo?" In an attempt to answer this question, we conducted similar experiments to those noted in Table 3.1 for MSC except that the reaction mixtures contained from 1 to 100 mM glutamine. Most tissues contain mM amounts of glutamine, but somewhat lower concentrations of methionine, aromatic amino acids and branched-chain amino acids. No significant inhibition of MSC transamination was noted in the presence of 1 mM glutamine. Even in the presence of 100 mM glutamine the rate of transamination of MSC was ~20 % that observed for the control that lacked added glutamine [5]. This finding is significant because it is unlikely that all potential amino acid competitive inhibitors of GTK in the cell added together can reach a combined concentration of 100 mM. In summary, our data suggest that dietary SM and MSC can be converted to the corresponding α-keto acids in vivo despite the presence of a variety of intracellular amino acids that can theoretically compete in aminotransferase reactions involving these seleno amino acids. The importance of the α-keto acids of SM and MSC in chemoprevention is discussed below.

Some evidence suggests that the chemopreventive action of SM and MSC is at least in part due to elimination of methylselenol from these seleno amino acids, which in turn is converted in vivo to a number of metabolites including dimethyldiselenide [$CH_3SeSeCH_3$], methylseleninic acid [$CH_3Se(O)OH$], H_2Se, selenosugars, and trimethylselenonium [$(CH_3)_3Se^+$], some of which may also exhibit intrinsic anticancer properties [48]. The question arises as to how methylselenol is generated from MSC and SM. An enzyme isolated from mouse liver and identified as cystathionine γ-lyase has been shown to catalyze the γ-elimination of methylselenol from SM [49]. The net products are α-ketobutyrate, ammonia, and methylselenol (Eq. 3.8). However, the specific activity with L-selenomethionine as substrate is <1 % that observed with the natural substrate cystathionine [49]:

$$\underset{\text{L-Selenomethionine}}{CH_3SeCH_2CH_2CH\left(NH_3^+\right)CO_2^-} + H_2O \rightarrow \underset{\alpha\text{-ketobutyrate}}{CH_3CH_2C(O)CO_2^-} + NH_4^+ + \underset{\text{methylselenol}}{CH_3SeH} \tag{3.8}$$

In addition, to catalyzing γ-elimination reactions, cystathionine γ-lyase can also catalyze β-elimination reactions [50]. In fact, we have found that highly purified rat liver cystathionine γ-lyase catalyzes the β-elimination of pyruvate from 10 mM MSC at about the same rate as it catalyzes γ-elimination of α-ketobutyrate from cystathionine [5]. Although methylselenol was not measured directly in these experiments, the production of pyruvate must have been accompanied by equimolar production of methylselenol. Moreover, as noted above, MSC is both an aminotransferase and a β-lyase substrate of rat kidney GTK [44, 47]. The formation of methylselenol from MSC is shown in (Eq. 3.9):

$$\underset{Se\text{-Methyl-L-selenocysteine}}{CH_3SeCH_2CH\left(NH_3^+\right)CO_2^-} + H_2O \rightarrow \underset{\text{pyruvate}}{CH_3C(O)CO_2^-} + NH_4^+ + \underset{\text{methylselenol}}{CH_3SeH} \tag{3.9}$$

Inasmuch as many PLP-containing enzymes catalyze β-elimination reactions with amino acids containing a good nucleofuge in the β-position it is highly likely that, in addition to cystathionine γ-lyase and GTK, additional PLP-containing enzymes will catalyze a β-elimination reaction with MSC. In this context it is interesting to note that Suzuki et al. concluded that of the selenium-containing compounds investigated (including SM), MSC is the likely source of methylselenol [48].

In addition to the production of methylselenol, another mechanism by which SM and MSC may be chemoprotective has been identified (Fig. 3.6). We found that both SM and MSC are excellent substrates of snake venom L-amino acid oxidase, quantitatively generating the corresponding α-keto acids, α-keto-γ-methylselenobutyrate (KMSB) and β-methylselenopyruvate (MSP), respectively [45, 46]. Thus, the L-amino acid oxidase reaction afforded us a relatively simple mechanism for generating both KMSB and MSP from their corresponding seleno amino acids, thereby allowing us to study directly their biological properties. We have obtained evidence that both KMSB and MSP are potent inhibitors of histone deacetylases (HDACs), properties that the seleno amino acids do not exhibit [45, 46]. It is interesting to note that both KMSB and MSP are similar in structure to butyrate, a well characterized HDAC inhibitor (Fig. 3.7). The finding that KMSB and MSP are HDAC inhibitors is of considerable interest, particularly in the aftermath of the Selenium and Vitamin E Cancer Prevention Trial (SELECT), the largest prostate cancer prevention study to date (http://www.cancer.gov/clinicaltrials/noteworthy-trials/select/Page1). This Trial was aborted early because it was found that SM supplements alone or in combination with vitamin E did not reduce prostate cancer risk. Understanding the extent of in situ conversion of seleno amino acid to KMSB or MSP by tissue specific glutamine transaminases (GTL or GTK) may reconcile the positive epidemiological data that were obtained using different dietary organoselenium compounds with the disappointing results of the SELECT

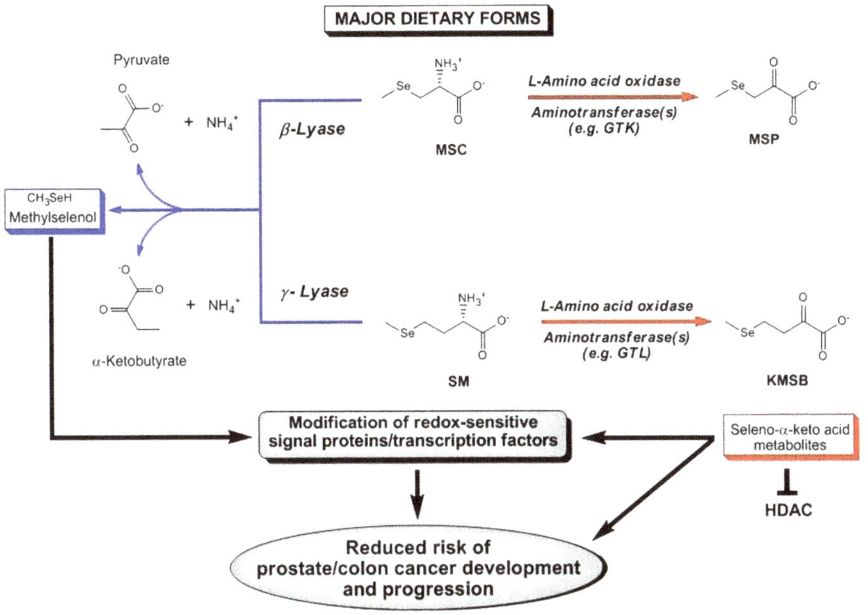

Fig. 3.6 Proposed metabolic pathway for the dietary seleno amino acids *Se*-methyl-L-selenocysteine (MSC) and L-selenomethionine (SM). MSC can undergo enzyme-catalyzed β-elimination, yielding methylselenol, ammonia and pyruvate. SM can undergo enzyme-catalyzed γ-elimination, yielding methylselenol, ammonia and α-ketobutyrate. Both MSC and SM can also undergo transamination (GTK, GTL, KAT II) and L-amino acid oxidase reactions yielding the corresponding seleno α-keto acids. For emphasis pathways to methylselenol and seleno α-keto acids are shown in *blue* and *red*, respectively. Methylselenol is a putative anticancer compound that can react with redox-sensitive signal proteins. The seleno α-keto acids have been shown to inhibit HDACs in human prostate and colon cancer cells. Modified from refs. [46, 51]

Fig. 3.7 Structural similarities of β-methylselenopyruvate (MSP) and α-keto- γ-methylselenobutyrate (KMSB) to the well-documented HDAC inhibitor butyrate

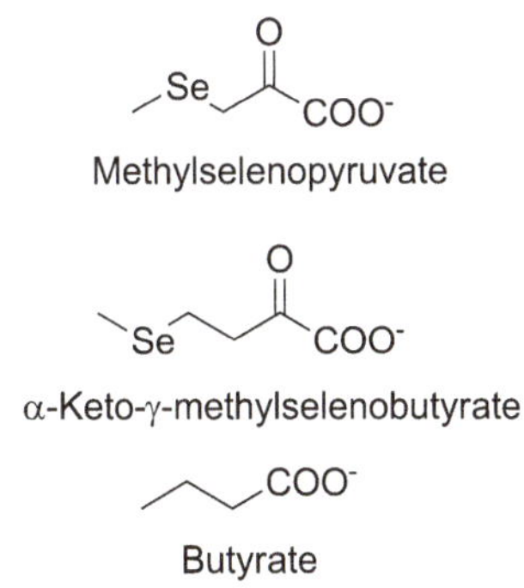

study. For example, our studies [51] show that MSC, *but not SM*, in prostate cancer cells is converted to the corresponding seleno α-keto acid. The α-keto acid generated from MSC (i.e., MSP) exhibits HDAC inhibitory properties and may act to modify DNA and alter pathways controlling cell replication. Future studies need to identify metabolic pathways influenced by intracellular formation of MSP and KMSB by glutamine transaminases (GTK and GTL, respectively) and possibly other aminotransferases. In particular, α-seleno keto acids and their parent seleno amino acids may exhibit differential effects on the glutamine-methionine bi-cycle and glutaminase II. These pathways function at the metabolic "crossroads" that link sulfur, nitrogen, 1-carbon compounds, and selenium for the purpose of maintaining homeostasis and anaplerotic flux of nutrients in normal and cancerous cells.

Conclusions

Unlike glutamate/α-ketoglutarate-linked aminotransferases, whose metabolic importance has been well documented and intensively studied for over 60 years, only a limited number of investigations have focused on glutamine-utilizing transaminases (aminotransferases) and their importance in homeostasis and the control of anaplerotic pathways. Yet, as this chapter attests, the glutamine transaminases are of fundamental importance (1) as repair enzymes (salvage of α-keto acids), (2) in nitrogen and sulfur homeostasis, (3) in 1-carbon metabolism, and (4) in the formation of chemopreventive metabolites of seleno-amino acids. Of relevance to human health and disease, the glutamine transaminases may contribute to the bioactivation (toxification) of halogenated alkenes (and possibly other xenobiotic electrophiles), many of which are environmental contaminants. Finally, the role of the glutaminase II pathway (i.e. glutamine transaminases and ω-amidase) in cancer biology has been little studied. However, the "glutamine addiction" of many tumors suggests that the glutamine transaminases may have a fundamental and influential role in regulating cancer progression.

Acknowledgements Part of the work from our laboratories cited in this chapter was supported by NIH grants CA111842 (to JTP) and ES008421 (to AJLC).

References

1. Meister A, Sober HA, Tice SV, Fraser PE. Transamination and associated deamidation of asparagine and glutamine. J Biol Chem. 1952;197:319–30.
2. Cooper AJL, Meister A. Isolation and properties of a new glutamine transaminase from rat kidney. J Biol Chem. 1974;249:2554–61.
3. Han Q, Li J, Li J. pH dependence, substrate specificity and inhibition of human kynurenine aminotransferase I. Eur J Biochem. 2004;71:4804–14.
4. Han Q, Robinson H, Cai T, Tagle DA, Li J. Biochemical and structural properties of mouse kynurenine aminotransferase III. Mol Cell Biol. 2009;29:784–93.
5. Pinto JT, Krasnikov BF, Alcutt S, Jones ME, Dorai T, Villar MT, Artigues A, Li J, Cooper AJL. Kynurenine aminotransferase III and glutamine transaminase L are identical Enzymes that have cysteine Sconjugate β-lyase activity and can transaminate L-selenomethionine. J Biol Chem. 2014;289:30950–61.
6. Han Q, Cai T, Tagle DA, Robinson H, Li J. Substrate specificity and structure of human aminoadipate aminotransferase/kynurenine aminotransferase II. Biosci Rep. 2008;28:205–15.
7. Cooper AJL, Meister A. Comparative studies of glutamine transaminases from rat tissues. Comp Biochem Physiol. 1981;69B:137–45.
8. Hersh LB. Rat liver ω-amidase: purification and properties. Biochemistry. 1971;10:2884–91.
9. Jaisson S, Veiga-da-Cunha M, Van Schaftingen E. Molecular identification of ω-amidase, the enzyme that is functionally coupled with glutamine transaminases, as the putative tumor suppressor Nit2. Biochimie. 2009;91:1066–71.
10. Krasnikov BF, Chien C-H, Nostramo R, Pinto JT, Nieves E, Callaway M, Sun J, Huebner K, Cooper AJL. Identification of the putative tumor suppressor Nit2 as ω-amidase, an enzyme metabolically linked to glutamine and asparagine transamination. Biochimie. 2009;91:1072–80.
11. Chien CH, Gao QZ, Cooper AJL, Lyu JH, Sheu SY. Structural insights into the catalytic active site and activity of human Nit2/ω-amidase: kinetic assay and molecular dynamics simulation. J Biol Chem. 2012;287:25715–26.
12. Cooper AJL. The role of glutamine transaminase K (GTK) in sulfur and α-keto acid metabolism in the brain, and possible bioactivation of neurotoxicants. Neurochem Int. 2004;44:557–77.

13. Darmaun D, Matthews DE, Bier DM. Glutamine and glutamate kinetics in humans. Am J Physiol. 1986;251:E117–26.
14. Miller JE, Litwack G. Purification, properties, and identity of liver mitochondrial tyrosine aminotransferase. J Biol Chem. 1971;246:3234–40.
15. Wray JW, Abeles RH. The methionine salvage pathway in *Klebsiella pneumoniae* and rat liver. Identification and characterization of two novel dioxygenases. J Biol Chem. 1995;270:3147–53.
16. Jones TW, Qin C, Schaeffer VH, Stevens JL. Immunohistochemical localization of glutamine transaminase K, a rat kidney cysteine conjugate β-lyase, and the relationship to the segment specificity of cysteine conjugate nephrotoxicity. Mol Pharmacol. 1988;34:621–7.
17. Cooper AJL, Abraham DG, Gelbard AS, Lai JC, Petito CK. High activities of glutamine transaminase K (dichlorovinylcysteine β-lyase) and ω-amidase in the choroid plexus of rat brain. J Neurochem. 1993;61:1731–41.
18. Lin CH, Chung MY, Chen WB, Chien CH. Growth inhibitory effect of the human NIT2 gene and its allelic imbalance in cancers. FEBS J. 2007;274:2946–56.
19. Wipf D, Ludewig U, Tegeder M, Rentsch D, Koch W, Frommer WB. Conservation of amino acid transporters in fungi, plants and animals. Trends Biochem Sci. 2002;27:139–47.
20. Patel TB, Waymack PP, Olson MS. The effect of the monocarboxylate translocator inhibitor, α-cyanocinnamate, on the oxidation of branched chain α-keto acids in rat liver. Arch Biochem Biophys. 1980;201:629–35.
21. Steele RD. Blood-brain barrier transport of the α-keto acid analogs of amino acids. Fed Proc. 1986;45:2060–4.
22. Hutson SM, Rannels SL. Characterization of a mitochondrial transport system for branched chain α-keto acids. J Biol Chem. 1985;260:14189–93.
23. Hoffer LJ, Taveroff A, Robitaille L, Mamer OA, Reimer ML. α-Keto and α-hydroxy branched-chain acid interrelationships in normal humans. J Nutr. 1993;123:1513–21.
24. Pace HC, Brenner C. The nitrilase superfamily: classification, structure and function. Genome Biol. 2001;2(1):REVIEWS0001.
25. Huebner K, Saldivar JC, Sun J, Shibata H, Druck T. Hits, fhits and nits: beyond enzymatic function. Adv Enzyme Regul. 2011;51:208–17.
26. Zielke HR, Ozand PT, Tildon JT, Sevdalian DA, Cornblath M. Reciprocal regulation of glucose and glutamine utilization by cultured human diploid fibroblasts. J Cell Physiol. 1978;95:41–8.
27. Roediger WE. Utilization of nutrients by isolated epithelial cells of the rat colon. Gastroenterology. 1982;83:424–9.
28. Mallet RT, Kelleher JK, Jackson MJ. Substrate metabolism of isolated jejunal epithelium: conservation of three-carbon units. Am J Physiol. 1986;250:C191–8.
29. Abou-Khalil WH, Yunis AA, Abou-Khalil S. Prominent glutamine oxidation activity in mitochondria of hematopoietic tumors. Cancer Res. 1983;43:1990–3.
30. Erickson JW, Cerione RA. Glutaminase: a hot spot for regulation of cancer cell metabolism? Oncotarget. 2010;1:734–40.
31. Koppenol WH, Bounds PL, Dang CV. Otto Warburg's contributions to current concepts of cancer metabolism. Nat Rev Cancer. 2011;11:325–37.
32. Ward PS, Thompson CB. Metabolic reprogramming: a cancer hallmark even Warburg did not anticipate. Cancer Cell. 2012;21:297–308.
33. Miles EW. Pyridoxal phosphate enzymes catalyzing β-elimination and β-replacement reactions. In: Dolphin D, Poulson R, Avramović O, editors. Vitamin B_6 pyridoxal phosphate part B. New York, NY: John Wiley and Sons; 1986. p. 253–310.
34. Ueno H, Likos JJ, Metzler DE. Chemistry of the inactivation of cytosolic aspartate aminotransferase by serine O-sulfate. Biochemistry. 1982;21:4387–93.
35. Adams B, Lowpetch K, Thorndycroft F, Whyte SM, Young DW. Stereochemistry of reactions of the inhibitor/substrates L- and D-β-chloroalanine with β-mercaptoethanol catalysed by L-aspartate aminotransferase and D-amino acid aminotransferase respectively. Org Biomol Chem. 2005;3:3357–64.
36. Dekant W, Vamvakas S, Anders MW. Formation and fate of nephrotoxic and cytotoxic glutathione *S*-conjugates: cysteine conjugate β-lyase pathway. Adv Pharmacol. 1994;27:115–62.
37. Anders MW. Chemical toxicology of reactive intermediates formed by the glutathione-dependent bioactivation of halogen-containing compounds. Chem Res Toxicol. 2008;21:145–59.
38. Cooper AJL, Pinto JT. Role of cysteine *S*-conjugate β-lyases in the bioactivation of renal toxicants. In: Elfarra AA, editor. Biotechnology: pharmaceutical aspects. Advances in bioactivation research. New York, NY: Springer; 2008. p. 323–46.
39. Cooper AJL, Krasnikov BF, Niatsetskaya ZV, Pinto JT, Callery PS, Villar MT, Artigues A, Bruschi SA. Cysteine *S*-conjugate β-lyases: Important roles in the metabolism of naturally occurring sulfur and selenium-containing compounds, xenobiotics and anticancer agents. Amino Acids. 2011;7:7–27.

40. Stevens JL, Robbins JD, Byrd RA. A purified cysteine conjugate β-lyase from rat kidney cytosol. Requirement for an α-keto acid or an amino acid oxidase for activity and identity with soluble glutamine transaminase K. J Biol Chem. 1986;261:15529–37.
41. Cavallini D, Ricci G, Duprè S, Pecci L, Costa M, Matarese RM, Pensa B, Antonucci A, Solinas SP, Fontana M. Sulfur-containing cyclic ketimines and imino acids. A novel family of endogenous products in the search for a role. Eur J Biochem. 1991;202:217–23.
42. Hallen A, Cooper AJL, Jamie JF, Haynes PA, Willows RD. Mammalian forebrain ketimine reductase identified as μ-crystallin; potential regulation by thyroid hormones. J Neurochem. 2011;118:379–87.
43. Hallen A, Jamie JF, Cooper AJL. Imine reductases: a comparison of glutamate dehydrogenase to ketimine reductases in the brain. Neurochem Res. 2013;39(3):527–41.
44. Commandeur JNM, Andreadou I, Rooseboom M, Out M, de Leur LJ, Groot E, Vermeulen NPE. Bioactivation of selenocysteine *Se*-conjugates by a highly purified rat renal cysteine conjugate β-lyase/glutamine transaminase K. J Pharmacol Exp Ther. 2000;294:753–61.
45. Nian H, Bisson WH, Dashwood WM, Pinto JT, Dashwood RH. α-Keto acid metabolites of organoselenium compounds inhibit histone deacetylase activity in human colon cancer cells. Carcinogenesis. 2009;30:1416–23.
46. Pinto JT, Lee JI, Sinha R, MacEwan ME, Cooper AJL. Chemopreventive mechanisms of α-keto acid metabolites of naturally occurring organoselenium compounds. Amino Acids. 2011;41:29–41.
47. Cooper AJL, Pinto JT, Krasnikov BF, Niatsetskaya ZV, Han Q, Li J, Vauzour D, Spencer JPE. Substrate specificity of human glutamine transaminase K as an aminotransferase and as a cysteine *S*-conjugate β-lyase. Arch Biochem Biophys. 2008;474:72–81.
48. Suzuki KT, Tsuji Y, Ohta Y, Suzuki N. Preferential organ distribution of methylselenol source *Se*-methylselenocysteine relative to methylseleninic acid. Toxicol Appl Pharmacol. 2008;227:76–83.
49. Okuno T, Motobayashi S, Ueno H, Nakamuro K. Identification of mouse selenomethionine α, γ-elimination enzyme: cystathionine γ-lyase catalyzes its reaction to generate methylselenol. Biol Trace Elem Res. 2005;108:245–57.
50. Cooper AJL, Pinto JT. Aminotransferase, L-amino acid oxidase and β-lyase reactions involving L-cysteine *S*-conjugates found in allium extracts. Relevance to biological activity? Biochem Pharmacol. 2005;69:209–20.
51. Lee JI, Nian H, Cooper AJ, Sinha R, Dai J, Bisson WH, Dashwood RH, Pinto JT. α-Keto acid metabolites of naturally occurring organoselenium compounds as inhibitors of histone deacetylase in human prostate cancer cells. Cancer Prev Res. 2009;2:683–93.

Chapter 4
Glutamine Uptake and Immunomodulation: An Overview

Kenneth Frauwirth

Key Points

- Immune cells require high levels of extracellular glutamine for proper activation.
- The rate of glutamine uptake into leukocytes is likely to be limiting, and is increased by activation.
- Leukocytes can use glutamine as a primary energy source via glutaminolysis.
- Lymphocytes, macrophages, and neutrophils depend on glutamine to maintain specific effector functions.
- Intracellular glutamine levels may regulate uptake of other amino acids and activity of the mTOR signaling pathway.
- Glutamine is a potential precursor for synthesis of antimicrobial ROS and RNS.
- Glutamine metabolism is an important generator of reducing agents, which can protect leukocytes from toxic ROS/RNS products.
- Understanding the regulation of glutamine transport may allow development of novel therapeutic interventions for defective or pathogenic immune responses.

Keywords Glutamine • Lymphocytes • Macrophages • Neutrophils • Transporters • Metabolism • Signaling • Redox

Abbreviations

BCR	B cell antigen receptor
GSH	Reduced glutathione
GSSG	Oxidized glutathione
iNOS	Inducible nitric oxide synthase
MAPK	Mitogen-activated protein kinase
mTOR	Mammalian target of rapamycin
RNS	Reactive nitrogen species
ROS	Reactive oxygen species

K. Frauwirth, Ph.D. (✉)
Department of Cell Biology and Molecular Genetics, University of Maryland, College Park, MD, USA
e-mail: kfrauwir@umd.edu; swingdanceken@yahoo.com

R. Rajendram et al. (eds.), *Glutamine in Clinical Nutrition*, Nutrition and Health,
DOI 10.1007/978-1-4939-1932-1_4, © Springer Science+Business Media New York 2015

SLC	Solute carrier
TCR	T cell antigen receptor
TORC1	mTOR complex 1

Introduction

The vertebrate immune system has evolved to defend against a wide variety of potential pathogens, using multiple complementary mechanisms. Although there are some components that are constitutively present and active, much of the immune response depends on the rapid activation of several different types of immune cells. Activation can involve cellular growth, proliferation, and de novo production of effector molecules. These processes place substantial energetic and biosynthetic demands on the immune system, and the inability to meet these demands may result in immune dysfunction and disease. In order to support the energetic and synthetic needs resulting from activation, immune cells must make large changes in the uptake and metabolism of nutrients, including amino acids. The utilization of glutamine in the immune system has long been an area of particular interest, dating back to early studies of immune cells in tissue culture. More recent studies of both immune cells and cancer cells have also sparked renewed interest in understanding the functions of glutamine in immune cells. This chapter highlights the changes in glutamine uptake and metabolism in cells of the immune system, and discusses potential roles for glutamine in modulating immune responses.

Cells of the Immune System

The cellular portion of the vertebrate immune system is composed of white blood cells, or leukocytes. Leukocytes come in a variety of different cell types with specialized functions for combatting infectious agents. A proper immune response requires the activation and coordination of multiple cell types. Most leukocytes circulate in a relatively quiescent state, and the initiation of an immune response leads to dramatic increases in cellular activity. Cells may grow in size, proliferate, differentiate into effector forms, produce and secrete high levels of effector molecule, and/or generate toxic reactive oxygen and nitrogen species (ROS and RNS, respectively). This chapter focuses on glutamine utilization by three major classes of leukocyte: lymphocytes, macrophages, and neutrophils.

Lymphocytes make up the "adaptive" arm of the immune system, and are responsible for maintaining immune memory. They circulate as small resting cells in the blood and lymphatic system until activated. B lymphocytes (also called B cells) produce antibodies, and are defined by the presence of the B cell antigen receptor (BCR) on their surface. T lymphocytes (also called T cells) are defined by the presence of the T cell antigen receptor (TCR) on their surface, and come in two types, based on the presence of accessory receptors. CD4+ T cells secrete an array of cytokines, which regulate and coordinate the responses of other immune cells, and are thus known as "helper" T cells. CD8+ T cells differentiate into cytotoxic cells that are able to kill virally infected and cancerous body cells. Through the use of somatic DNA recombination, each B or T cell expresses a unique antigen receptor, allowing the immune system to recognize a tremendous diversity of antigens. However, this also means that a given antigen will likely only be recognized by only a few lymphocytes. A strong immune response thus requires the clonal expansion of very small numbers of cells in response to an infectious agent, and so B and T cells must go through many rounds of proliferation in order to mount an effective defense.

Macrophages are phagocytic tissue-resident cells derived from circulating blood monocytes. Upon activation by inflammatory stimuli, macrophages can differentiate further into microbicidal and secretory cells. It is becoming increasingly understood that activated macrophages represent a highly heterogeneous, and possibly plastic, population of cells, with quite different functional properties. Overall, activated macrophages are highly motile and highly phagocytic. Different subpopulations may secrete enzymes, inflammatory lipid mediators, reactive oxygen and nitrogen species, and/or cytokines. The secretory "repertoire" can be modulated by the nature of the stimulus as well as other signals from the environment [1]. After an inflammatory stimulus, large numbers of macrophages can accumulate in the tissue. However, because mature macrophages lose the ability to proliferate, this accumulation is largely due to recruitment of new macrophages from the blood monocyte population.

Neutrophils are the most abundant white blood cells, making up 60–70 % of blood leukocytes in normal individuals. They are characterized by a multi-lobed nucleus (earning them the name "polymorphonuclear leukocytes") and the presence of neutral-staining secretory granules. These are generally the first cells to arrive at the site of an infection, and are highly phagocytic. They also produce toxic ROS and RNS, as well as other antimicrobial substances. Neutrophils are critical for antibacterial defense, and conditions that result in severe neutropenia (low neutrophil counts) lead to recurrent bacterial infections, which can become life threatening. Neutrophils are nondividing cells and are generally short lived, with a circulatory half-life of at most a few days [2]. They must therefore be able to respond very rapidly to initiate inflammatory responses.

Glutamine and the Immune System

The activation of immune cells places significant energetic and biosynthetic demands on these cells. Cellular growth and effector molecule secretion depends on increased protein synthesis, and so increases in amino acid uptake and/or synthesis will also be required. Cells must also increase the generation of ATP and reducing equivalents to power biosynthesis and other energy-consuming processes (signal transduction, phagocytosis, ROS production, cellular migration, etc.). Thus, the nutrient acquisition and metabolism of activated leukocytes must accommodate these new demands.

As with most cells, leukocytes use glucose as a primary energy source, and activation of leukocytes leads to increased glucose consumption [3]. However, studies over the past 20 years have indicated that leukocytes metabolize glutamine at rates that are comparable to, and in some instances higher than, the rates of glucose utilization [4–8]. Thus, it is important to consider glutamine metabolism alongside glucose metabolism in supporting leukocyte activation. In most cases, actual glutamine consumption rates are substantially lower than the capacity of glutamine metabolic enzymes [5, 7, 8], and this suggests that uptake rates may be limiting for glutamine utilization. Depletion of glutamine or inhibition of glutamine metabolism impairs multiple cellular functions in lymphocytes [4, 9, 10], macrophages [11–13], and neutrophils [14–16] (Fig. 4.1), and so glutamine uptake may represent an important point of control for modulating immune responses.

As described earlier in this book, glutamine can be utilized in many metabolic pathways. Although this is likely to be true for leukocytes as well, a dominant metabolic pathway appears to be partial oxidation via the citric acid cycle. This pathway, termed glutaminolysis, results in production of glutamate, aspartate, and lactate. Glutaminolysis can account for greater than 80 % of glutamine consumption by cultured lymphocytes, macrophages, and neutrophils [17]. Cellular activation and differentiation, as well as changes in availability of other nutrients, can influence the relative proportions of the metabolic products [4–6], and can also direct glutamine metabolism toward other pathways, such as arginine synthesis [12]. Thus, the versatility of glutamine as an energy source and biosynthetic precursor is very much on display in the immune system.

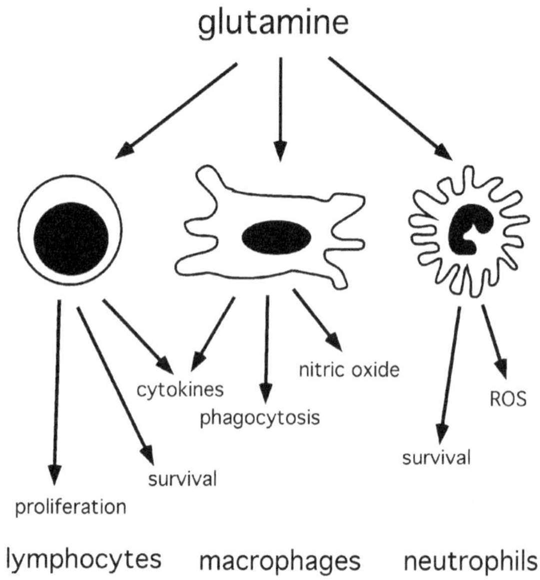

Fig. 4.1 Immune cells depend on glutamine for a wide variety of functions. Lymphocytes require high glutamine levels for proliferation, cytokine secretion, and survival in culture. Macrophages require glutamine for opsonin-dependent phagocytosis and secretion of cytokines and nitric oxide. Neutrophils require glutamine for survival and for production of antimicrobial ROS

Table 4.1 Glutamine transporters: The major glutamine transporters fall into the SLC1 and SLC38 transporter families. Compiled from Kanai et al. (2004) [18] and Mackenzie et al. (2004) [19]

Transport system	Transporter protein	SLC gene name
ASC	ASCT2	SLC1A5
A	SNAT1	SLC38A1
A	SNAT2	SLC38A2
N	SNAT3	SLC38A3
N	SNAT5	SLC38A5

Glutamine Transport

As with all amino acids, glutamine uptake into cells involves a series of transporter proteins from the SoLute Carrier (SLC) superfamily. These transporters are grouped into systems based on their functional properties. Glutamine is a substrate for multiple different systems, with the major importers falling into systems ASC, A, and N [18, 19] (Table 4.1). All of these transporters are sodium-dependent co-transporters, and use the sodium ion electrochemical gradient to drive glutamine uptake. As a result, glutamine can accumulate within cells beyond even the relatively high concentration found in serum, providing a large pool of glutamine for cellular utilization.

The ability of cells to use multiple transport systems (and potentially several different transporters within each system) for glutamine uptake complicates the picture. Different cell types may use distinct subsets of transporters, allowing for cell type-specific regulation. It is also possible that different transporter proteins establish separate intracellular pools of glutamine, as has been suggested for arginine [20]. There has been little characterization of the glutamine transport system(s) used by leukocytes, but we have found that T lymphocytes express members of the SLC38 family (systems A/N transporters) at both the RNA and protein levels [10] (see Fig. 4.2). Transporter mRNA levels and surface protein levels increase with activation, indicating that these transporters may be important for T cell glutamine utilization, but this does not exclude the use of other transporters. A systematic analysis of glutamine transporters in the immune system is needed to determine if there are cell-type differences in uptake mechanisms, and to understand the regulation of glutamine import in activated versus resting leukocytes.

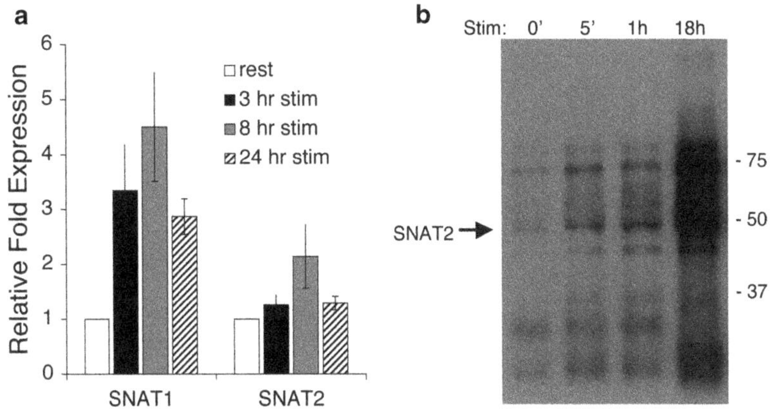

Fig. 4.2 Lymphocytes express SLC38A family members at the RNA and protein levels. (**a**) Purified murine T lymphocytes were stimulated for the indicated times, and SNAT1 and SNAT2 RNA levels were determined by quantitative real-time PCR. (**b**) Purified murine T lymphocytes were stimulated for the indicated times and surface biotinylated. SNAT2 protein was immunoprecipitated and visualized by blot with HRP-linked avidin. Reprinted from Carr et al. [10] with permission. Copyright 2010 The American Association of Immunologists, Inc

Glutamine and Leukocyte Function

High levels of extracellular glutamine are required for proper functioning of lymphocytes, macrophages, and neutrophils. However, the mechanisms by which glutamine modulates the activities of these cells are still not well understood. Notably, it is unknown whether glutamine regulates the various leukocytes via cell type-specific functions, or whether leukocytes possess common glutamine-dependent control points. Because glutamine plays many roles within cells, and because glutamine metabolism interacts and overlaps with the metabolism of other nutrients, it remains difficult to identify the particular points of dependency within the immune system. However, recent work has provided some new insights into both the metabolic and other fates of glutamine in mammalian cells, and these will be discussed in the context of their potential immunological significance.

Glutamine Modulation of Lymphocyte Function

Upon activation, lymphocytes transition from small quiescent cells into rapidly dividing "blasts," and eventually into highly secretory effector cells. Coincident with these functional changes, lymphocytes significantly increase glutamine uptake after antigenic stimulation [4–6, 10]. This is not simply the result of a general increase in amino acid import, but instead represents a selective increase in glutamine import [10] (see Fig. 4.3). This in turn implies that lymphocytes use glutamine for roles beyond protein synthesis. Glutamine serves as a nitrogen donor for the synthesis of nucleotides and NAD, which are important for rapidly growing and dividing cells such as activated lymphocytes. Further, glutamine can easily serve as a precursor for other amino acids and as an energy source. Activated lymphocytes increase expression of key glutamine metabolism enzymes, including glutaminase, glutamate dehydrogenase, and several aminotransferases [10, 21]. This allows glutamine to enter the citric acid cycle and produce other metabolic intermediates, such as lactate and aspartate, and supports a model of glutamine as an important contributor to cellular energetic and biosynthetic processes. However, as noted above, the maximal activities of the metabolic enzymes in lymphocytes are well above glutamine utilization rates [5]. This suggests that lymphocyte metabolism is limited by the rate

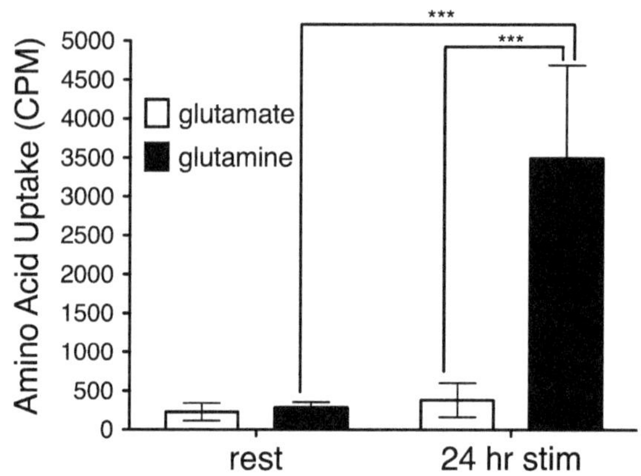

Fig. 4.3 Lymphocytes selectively upregulate glutamine uptake upon activation. Glutamate (*open bars*) and glutamine (*filled bars*) uptake were measured in resting and 24-h-stimulated purified murine T lymphocytes. $^{***}p<0.001$. Reprinted from Carr et al. [10] with permission. Copyright 2010 The American Association of Immunologists, Inc

of glutamine import, and provides a global mechanism for regulation of lymphocyte function, by controlling the expression and/or activity of glutamine transporters.

Metabolism via the citric acid cycle (glutaminolysis) accounts for a substantial fraction of lymphocyte glutamine utilization [17], but it is likely that imported glutamine has additional roles. One key function in the regulation of lymphocytes may be tied to the use of glutamine as an exchange substrate for other amino acid transporters, such as heterodimeric amino acid transporters of the SLC7 family [22]. These transporters are obligate exchangers, and the concentration of the intracellular amino acid appears to be the rate-limiting factor. Glutamine can serve as the exchange partner for uptake of a wide range of neutral amino acids. Thus, the ability to generate a high intracellular glutamine concentration allows the efficient import of other amino acids needed for cell growth, proliferation, and effector molecule synthesis.

The use of glutamine as an exchange substrate to allow import of other amino acids has several important implications. Most obviously, glutamine import contributes to the global control of amino acid levels, with the attendant metabolic consequences. As lymphocyte function is dependent on rapid proliferation and the synthesis of effector molecules (immunoglobulins for B cells, cytokines for CD4+ T cells, and lytic granule components for CD8+ T cells), access to sufficient amino acid supplies is a potential point of regulation. It is also unknown whether the pool of glutamine used for amino acid exchange overlaps with, or is distinct from, the glutamine that is metabolized intracellularly. If there is a common glutamine pool, then interfering with glutamine uptake would impair both metabolism and amino acid import. However, if glutamine is partitioned into separate pools, it may be possible to regulate its functions differentially and selectively by targeting the specific glutamine transporter(s) associated with the function of interest.

How do amino acid levels regulate cellular function? It has become clear that cells express several amino acid sensor systems, with distinct (although possibly overlapping) specificities. The best characterized of these is the mammalian target of rapamycin (mTOR) nutrient sensor system [23]. The nutrient- and rapamycin-sensitive mTOR complex 1 (TORC1) is generally thought to sense essential amino acids, especially leucine and arginine [24–27]. However, there has also been evidence that glutamine may play a role in this pathway [28]. More recent work by Nicklin et al. has been able to connect these observations via the glutamine exchange function [29]. They found that glutamine alone was insufficient to allow activation of mTOR signaling. Instead, import of glutamine via the ASCT2 transporter was required for the subsequent uptake of essential amino acids through the system L transporter LAT1, and activation of mTOR resulted from this exchange. The LAT1 transporter is a heterodimer of the LAT1 protein with the common heavy chain 4F2hc (also known as CD98) [22]. The 4F2hc/CD98 protein is a well-known T cell activation marker [30], and the LAT1 transporter is upregulated during lymphocyte activation [31]. It is therefore likely that increased glutamine import

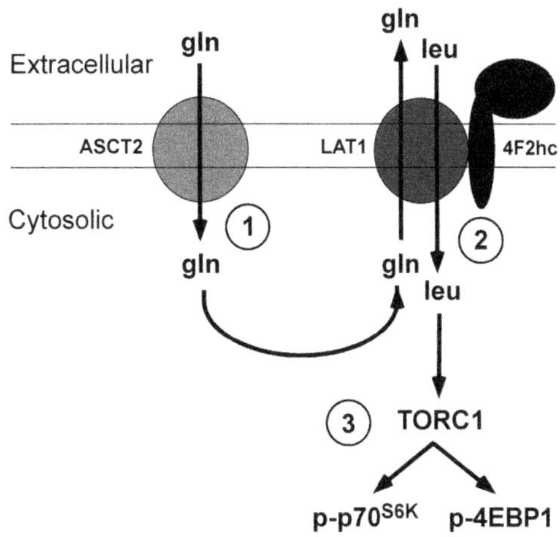

Fig. 4.4 Glutamine uptake regulates mTOR activity. Activation of mTOR signaling depends on uptake of essential amino acids, such as leucine. Extracellular glutamine is imported via the ASCT2 transporter, or possibly via other glutamine transporters (1). Cytoplasmic glutamine is used as an exchange substrate to allow import of leucine (and other essential amino acids) via the LAT1/4F2hc transporter complex (2), allowing for TORC1 signaling (3)

during lymphocyte activation is important for mTOR signaling, via the regulation of essential amino acid uptake (Fig. 4.4).

The regulation of mTOR activity by glutamine uptake is likely to be important for lymphocyte function beyond the role of mTOR in controlling cell growth. It is becoming clear that mTOR is also a central player in directing T cell differentiation into specific cell fates. As an immune response develops, lymphocytes must differentiate into the appropriate effector subtypes in order to best combat the infectious agent. In addition, some cells must differentiate into memory cells in order to be able to respond more rapidly upon a repeat encounter. Recent work has shown that the activity of TORC1 (the amino acid-responsive mTOR complex) is specifically required for differentiation of $CD4^+$ "helper" T cells into the T_H1 and T_H17, subsets [32]. In CD8+ T cells, mTOR signaling is involved in the decision between the effector and memory cell fates [33–35]. The ability of glutamine to facilitate import of mTOR-sensed amino acids therefore ties glutamine uptake to lymphocyte cell fate decisions, and may have an important impact on shaping immune responses.

Glutamine Modulation of Macrophage Function

Macrophages represent a very heterogeneous population and play multiple roles in immune responses, from phagocytosis and killing of microbes to wound healing. These distinct roles involve differentiation of activated macrophages along a continuum of cell fates [1]. External stimuli help to direct this differentiation, and recent work has begun to resolve the signaling pathways involved. Although there has been little analysis of glutamine in macrophage differentiation, it is reasonable to predict that glutamine may play one or more important roles. As with lymphocytes, mTOR signaling appears to be a player, although its exact role is still not fully understood [36]. As described above, glutamine import is closely tied to mTOR activation, and regulation of glutamine uptake may contribute to macrophage differentiation via this mechanism. Signaling through the mitogen-activated protein kinase (MAPK) family members also controls macrophage effector cell fate determination [37]. In T lymphocytes, glutamine uptake is regulated through MAPK signaling [10], suggesting a way that glutamine may serve as a link between the MAPK and mTOR pathways in macrophages. We have also found that glutamine depletion inhibits MAPK signaling in T cells (E. Carr and K. Frauwirth, unpublished results). If a similar relationship exists in macrophages, glutamine may independently regulate MAPK and mTOR signaling.

Once activated, macrophages are dependent on glutamine uptake for a number of specific effector functions. Glutamine metabolism contributes substantially to macrophage ATP production [17], and so glutamine depletion is likely to inhibit processes with high energetic demands. A key role for macrophages is the phagocytosis and killing of invading microbes. Although this would seem to be a highly ATP-consuming process, involving substantial rearrangements of cytoskeletal and plasma membrane components, general phagocytosis by macrophages does not appear to be very sensitive to glutamine levels. However, phagocytosis of opsinized particles is inhibited by low glutamine levels, and this reflects reduced expression of opsonin receptors, such as $F_c\gamma RI$, CR3, and CR4 [38]. Thus, glutamine uptake can control the efficiency of phagocytosis via regulating key cell-surface receptors, but may not be as important in directly supporting the energetics of phagocytosis.

Macrophages also produce numerous toxic substances to allow killing of phagocytosed microbes, including nitric oxide. Upon activation, macrophages can increase expression of inducible nitric oxide synthase (iNOS), which uses arginine as a substrate to generate nitric oxide. Although arginine is abundant in tissue culture medium (>1 mM), it is found at much lower levels in serum. As a result, arginine may become limiting under a range of pathological conditions, including sepsis, trauma, malnutrition, and cancer [39]. Macrophages express the metabolic enzymes required to use glutamine as a precursor for endogenous arginine synthesis (as described in the chapter, "Glutamine and Immunosuppression"), and glutamine is required for nitric oxide secretion under arginine-limited conditions [12]. Given that arginine levels are depleted under the very conditions requiring increased nitric oxide secretion, the high rate of glutamine utilization by activated macrophages may support this critical antimicrobial function.

Glutamine Modulation of Neutrophil Function

Neutrophils are the most numerous blood leukocytes and represent the front line of defense among immune cells. Thus, glutamine may have a sizable impact on immune responses via modulation of neutrophil activity. Neutrophils are terminally differentiated, nondividing, short-lived cells. This means that, unlike with lymphocytes and macrophages, glutamine uptake cannot regulate neutrophil function via long-term processes, such as major changes in gene expression or cell fate. Thus, in contrast to macrophages, glutamine depletion does not reduce expression of cell-surface complement receptors, and does not inhibit phagocytosis [14]. Instead, glutamine's impact is restricted to processes that can respond immediately to the presence of a pathogen.

A key feature of neutrophil antimicrobial activity is the oxidative burst, in which high levels of ROS are produced to kill phagocytosed microbes. Notably, neutrophil production of superoxide depends on glutamine availability [15]. Neutrophils generate the superoxide radical through the non-mitochondrial NADPH oxidase complex, and so depend on high levels of NADPH for superoxide production. Although glucose oxidation via the pentose phosphate shunt is an important pathway for the reduction of NADP+ to NADPH, glutamine is also a potentially significant source for NADPH generation, via the action of NADP-dependent malate dehydrogenase [40, 41] (Fig. 4.5). NADPH is also required for nitric oxide production by iNOS, and so this may represent a second (and parallel) role for glutamine in nitric oxide secretion, in addition to serving as an arginine precursor. Thus, glutamine metabolism may provide not only ATP and biosynthetic substrates for leukocytes, but also NADPH critical for ROS and RNS generation.

The toxic nature of ROS presents a significant problem for neutrophils and macrophages. In order to protect themselves from oxidative damage from their own antimicrobial products, these cells must maintain high levels of antioxidants. Glutamine plays several roles in maintaining cellular redox homeostasis. High intracellular levels of glutamine provide a ready source of glutamate, which in turn is a component of the important antioxidant glutathione. RNAi knockdown of the enzyme

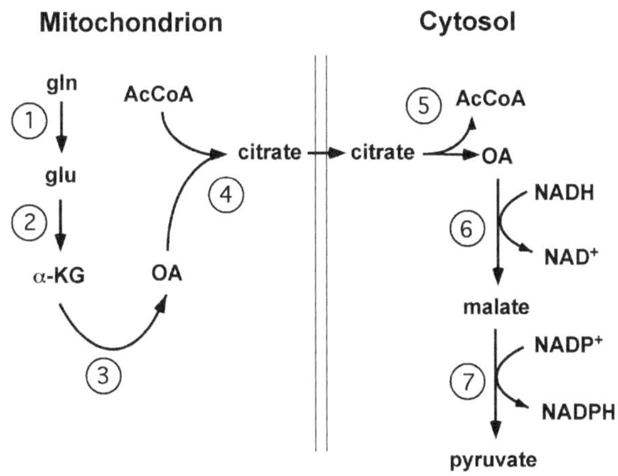

Fig. 4.5 Glutamine metabolism can generate cytoplasmic NADPH. Glutamine is hydrolyzed to glutamate by glutaminase (1), and deaminated to α-ketoglutarate by glutamate dehydrogenase or a transaminase (2). α-ketoglutarate can enter the Krebs cycle to generate oxaloacetate (3). Addition of acetyl-CoA produces citrate, which is transported to the cytosol (4). Citrate lyase cleaves citrate to produce oxaloacetate (5), which is reduced by malate dehydrogenase produces malate (6). Oxidative decarboxylation of malate by malic acid produces pyruvate and generates NADPH (7)

Fig. 4.6 Glutamine can contribute to both sides of redox balance in immune cells. (**a**) NADPH generated from glutamine metabolism (see Fig. 4.5) is required for production of nitric oxide and superoxide. (**b**) Glutaminase hydrolyzes glutamine to glutamate, a precursor for the antioxidant glutathione (1). NADPH generated from glutamine metabolism (see Fig. 4.5) can be used to reduce oxidized glutathione (GSSG), regenerating the antioxidant form (GSH) (2)

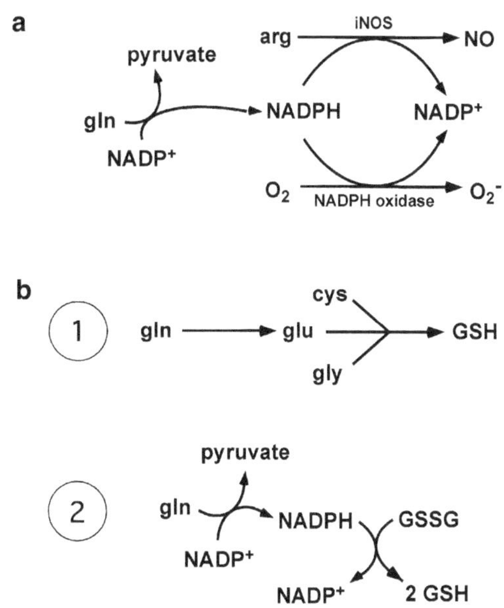

glutaminase, which hydrolyzes glutamine to glutamate, decreases cellular glutathione levels and increases oxidative stress [42–44]. Consistent with its function in glutathione synthesis, glutamine inhibits apoptosis in neutrophils [16].

Beyond the absolute levels of glutathione, redox state is controlled by the ratio of reduced glutathione (GSH) to oxidized glutathione (GSSG). Reduction of GSSG to GSH is catalyzed by glutathione reductase, which requires NADPH as a cofactor. As described above, glutamine metabolism can be used to generate NADPH via NADP-dependent malate dehydrogenase. Thus, glutamine may help provide the reducing power to generate both ROS/RNS to kill microbes and the key antioxidants to protect leukocytes from those same antimicrobial radicals (Fig. 4.6).

Conclusions

Glutamine is a "nonessential" amino acid that is readily synthesized by mammalian cells, and it is the most abundant amino acid in serum. Cells of the immune system appear to be adapted to take advantage of this resource, and they require high levels of extracellular glutamine during activation. Glutamine has the useful property of feeding into a large number of metabolic pathways, serving as a kind of bioenergetic and synthetic hub. Thus, the transport of glutamine into immune cells has the potential to regulate many different functions.

Lymphocytes, macrophages, and neutrophils play distinct roles in immune responses, and have very different functional capabilities. It is therefore intriguing that these cell types have in common the specific dependence on glutamine. One potentially critical use of glutamine in all three cell types is the regulation of redox state. The generation of ROS is a common feature during the activation of lymphocytes, macrophages, and neutrophils, and so limiting the toxic effects of ROS is essential. Glutamine is a precursor for glutathione synthesis, and can also be used for production of the reducing agent NADPH. Given the need to maintain antioxidant levels, leukocytes are dependent on high rates of glutamine uptake. The regulation of glutamine transporter function is therefore likely to play an important common role in controlling oxidative stress in leukocytes during immune responses.

Glutamine transport systems move glutamine into cells against a concentration gradient, allowing cells to accumulate glutamine to high levels intracellularly. A significant consequence of this is the ability to use glutamine as an exchange substrate for other amino acid transporters. The transporters responsible for uptake of a wide range of amino acids, including leucine and other "essential" amino acids, are obligate exchangers, and require export of one amino acid in order to import another. Leukocytes may therefore be importing glutamine through one set of transporters, in part simply to export it again through a different set. While this may seem to be a rather convoluted approach to amino acid uptake, it allows cells to use extracellular glutamine levels as a sensor for general nutrient status. Circulating glutamine is largely synthesized by skeletal muscle and adipose tissue, rather than being derived from dietary protein [45]. Glutamine may therefore act as an integrator for a range of amino acids (and other nutrients), allowing glutamine uptake to serve as a common point of regulation for amino acid import. As long as extracellular glutamine levels remain high, immune cells "know" that conditions are favorable to support an inflammatory response. Conversely, if a pathological condition reduces either local or global glutamine levels, this may be interpreted by the immune system as a more general nutrient-depleted state. As a result, immune responses could be suppressed to maintain nutrient resources for more critical biological functions.

Glutamine has many metabolic fates in cells, and it is likely that no single role is responsible for the glutamine dependence of leukocytes. However, its importance in redox control and regulation of broader amino acid uptake may allow it to act as a critical gatekeeper of immune cell activation. As such, it will be important to gain a more complete understanding of the glutamine transporters used by immune cells, and the regulatory mechanisms that control transporter expression and function. Because of the wide variety of potential cellular fates for glutamine, it will also be necessary to determine how cellular glutamine pools are partitioned. Can all processes access all of the glutamine, or are there separate pools that feed only into specific pathways? If the latter is true, then it is also possible, even likely, that different transporters supply these separate pools. Characterizing the precise roles of individual transporter types will be critical for deciphering how glutamine uptake controls specific immune cell functions. This in turn may allow glutamine transport to become a useful therapeutic target, both to improve suboptimal responses against infectious agents and to reduce harmful immune responses, as in cases of allergy, graft rejection, and autoimmunity.

References

1. Mosser DM, Edwards JP. Exploring the full spectrum of macrophage activation. Nat Rev Immunol. 2008;8(12):958–69.
2. Pillay J, den Braber I, Vrisekoop N, et al. In vivo labeling with 2H2O reveals a human neutrophil lifespan of 5.4 days. Blood. 2010;116(4):625–7.
3. Frauwirth KA, Thompson CB. Regulation of T lymphocyte metabolism. J Immunol. 2004;172(8):4661–5.
4. Ardawi MS, Newsholme EA. Glutamine metabolism in lymphocytes of the rat. Biochem J. 1983;212(3):835–42.
5. Ardawi MS. Glutamine and glucose metabolism in human peripheral lymphocytes. Metabolism. 1988;37(1):99–103.
6. Brand K, Williams JF, Weidemann MJ. Glucose and glutamine metabolism in rat thymocytes. Biochem J. 1984;221(2):471–5.
7. Curi TC, De Melo MP, De Azevedo RB, Zorn TM, Curi R. Glutamine utilization by rat neutrophils: presence of phosphate-dependent glutaminase. Am J Physiol. 1997;273(4 Pt 1):C1124–1129.
8. Newsholme P, Curi R, Gordon S, Newsholme EA. Metabolism of glucose, glutamine, long-chain fatty acids and ketone bodies by murine macrophages. Biochem J. 1986;239(1):121–5.
9. Horig H, Spagnoli GC, Filgueira L, et al. Exogenous glutamine requirement is confined to late events of T cell activation. J Cell Biochem. 1993;53(4):343–51.
10. Carr EL, Kelman A, Wu GS, et al. Glutamine uptake and metabolism Are coordinately regulated by ERK/MAPK during T lymphocyte activation. J Immunol. 2010;185:1037–44.
11. Wallace C, Keast D. Glutamine and macrophage function. Metabolism. 1992;41(9):1016–20.
12. Murphy C, Newsholme P. Importance of glutamine metabolism in murine macrophages and human monocytes to L-arginine biosynthesis and rates of nitrite or urea production. Clin Sci. 1998;95(4):397–407.
13. Murphy C, Newsholme P. Macrophage-mediated lysis of a beta-cell line, tumour necrosis factor-alpha release from bacillus Calmette-Guerin (BCG)-activated murine macrophages and interleukin-8 release from human monocytes are dependent on extracellular glutamine concentration and glutamine metabolism. Clin Sci. 1999;96(1):89–97.
14. Ogle CK, Ogle JD, Mao JX, et al. Effect of glutamine on phagocytosis and bacterial killing by normal and pediatric burn patient neutrophils. JPEN J Parenter Eneral Nutr. 1994;18(2):128–33.
15. Pithon-Curi TC, Levada AC, Lopes LR, Doi SQ, Curi R. Glutamine plays a role in superoxide production and the expression of p47phox, p22phox and gp91phox in rat neutrophils. Clin Sci. 2002;103(4):403. -408.
16. Pithon-Curi TC, Schumacher RI, Freitas JJ, et al. Glutamine delays spontaneous apoptosis in neutrophils. Am J Physiol Cell Physiol. 2003;284(6):C1355–1361.
17. Newsholme P, Curi R, Pithon Curi TC, Murphy CJ, Garcia C, Pires de Melo M. Glutamine metabolism by lymphocytes, macrophages, and neutrophils: its importance in health and disease. J Nutr Biochem. 1999;10(6):316–24.
18. Kanai Y, Hediger MA. The glutamate/neutral amino acid transporter family SLC1: molecular, physiological and pharmacological aspects. Pflugers Arch. 2004;447(5):469–79.
19. Mackenzie B, Erickson JD. Sodium-coupled neutral amino acid (System N/A) transporters of the SLC38 gene family. Pflugers Arch. 2004;447(5):784–95.
20. Morris Jr SM. Arginine: beyond protein. Am J Clin Nutr. 2006;83(2):508S–12S.
21. Ardawi MS, Newsholme EA. Maximum activities of some enzymes of glycolysis, the tricarboxylic acid cycle and ketone-body and glutamine utilization pathways in lymphocytes of the rat. Biochem J. 1982;208(3):743–8.
22. Verrey F, Closs EI, Wagner CA, Palacin M, Endou H, Kanai Y. CATs and HATs: the SLC7 family of amino acid transporters. Pflugers Arch. 2004;447:532–42.
23. Yang X, Yang C, Farberman A, et al. The mammalian target of rapamycin-signaling pathway in regulating metabolism and growth. J Anim Sci. 2008;86(14 Suppl):E36–50.
24. Fox HL, Pham PT, Kimball SR, Jefferson LS, Lynch CJ. Amino acid effects on translational repressor 4E-BP1 are mediated primarily by L-leucine in isolated adipocytes. Am J Physiol. 1998;275(5 Pt 1):C1232–1238.
25. Hara K, Yonezawa K, Weng QP, Kozlowski MT, Belham C, Avruch J. Amino acid sufficiency and mTOR regulate p70 S6 kinase and eIF-4E BP1 through a common effector mechanism. J Biol Chem. 1998;273(23):14484–94.
26. Wang X, Campbell LE, Miller CM, Proud CG. Amino acid availability regulates p70 S6 kinase and multiple translation factors. Biochem J. 1998;334(Pt 1):261–7.
27. Ban H, Shigemitsu K, Yamatsuji T, et al. Arginine and Leucine regulate p70 S6 kinase and 4E-BP1 in intestinal epithelial cells. Int J Mol Med. 2004;13(4):537–43.
28. Iiboshi Y, Papst PJ, Hunger SP, Terada N. L-Asparaginase inhibits the rapamycin-targeted signaling pathway. Biochem Biophys Res Commun. 1999;260(2):534–9.
29. Nicklin P, Bergman P, Zhang B, et al. Bidirectional transport of amino acids regulates mTOR and autophagy. Cell. 2009;136(3):521–34.
30. Gottesdiener KM, Karpinski BA, Lindsten T, et al. Isolation and structural characterization of the human 4 F2 heavy-chain gene, an inducible gene involved in T-lymphocyte activation. Mol Cell Biol. 1988;8(9):3809–19.

31. Nii T, Segawa H, Taketani Y, et al. Molecular events involved in up-regulating human Na+-independent neutral amino acid transporter LAT1 during T-cell activation. Biochem J. 2001;358(Pt 3):693–704.
32. Delgoffe GM, Pollizzi KN, Waickman AT, et al. The kinase mTOR regulates the differentiation of helper T cells through the selective activation of signaling by mTORC1 and mTORC2. Nat Immunol. 2011;12(4):295–303. doi:10.1038/ni.2005.
33. Araki K, Turner AP, Shaffer VO, et al. mTOR regulates memory CD8 T-cell differentiation. Nature. 2009; 460(7251):108–12.
34. Rao RR, Li Q, Odunsi K, Shrikant PA. The mTOR kinase determines effector versus memory CD8+ T cell fate by regulating the expression of transcription factors T-bet and Eomesodermin. Immunity. 2010;32(1):67–78.
35. Li X, Garcia K, Sun Z, Xiao Z. Temporal regulation of rapamycin on memory CTL programming by IL-12. PLoS One. 2011;6(9):e25177.
36. Weichhart T, Costantino G, Poglitsch M, et al. The TSC-mTOR signaling pathway regulates the innate inflammatory response. Immunity. 2008;29(4):565–77.
37. Lucas M, Zhang X, Prasanna V, Mosser DM. ERK activation following macrophage FcgammaR ligation leads to chromatin modifications at the IL-10 locus. J Immunol. 2005;175(1):469–77.
38. Spittler A, Winkler S, Gotzinger P, et al. Influence of glutamine on the phenotype and function of human monocytes. Blood. 1995;86(4):1564–9.
39. Kirk SJ, Barbul A. Role of arginine in trauma, sepsis, and immunity. JPEN J Parenter Eneral Nutr. 1990;14(5 Suppl):226S–9S.
40. Newsholme P, Costa Rosa LF, Newsholme EA, Curi R. The importance of fuel metabolism to macrophage function. Cell Biochem Funct. 1996;14(1):1–10.
41. DeBerardinis RJ, Mancuso A, Daikhin E, et al. Beyond aerobic glycolysis: transformed cells can engage in glutamine metabolism that exceeds the requirement for protein and nucleotide synthesis. Proc Natl Acad Sci U S A. 2007;104(49):19345–50.
42. Lora J, Alonso FJ, Segura JA, Lobo C, Marquez J, Mates JM. Antisense glutaminase inhibition decreases glutathione antioxidant capacity and increases apoptosis in Ehrlich ascitic tumour cells. Eur J Biochem. 2004;271(21):4298–306.
43. Hu W, Zhang C, Wu R, Sun Y, Levine A, Feng Z. Glutaminase 2, a novel p53 target gene regulating energy metabolism and antioxidant function. Proc Natl Acad Sci U S A. 2010;107(16):7455–60.
44. Suzuki S, Tanaka T, Poyurovsky MV, et al. Phosphate-activated glutaminase (GLS2), a p53-inducible regulator of glutamine metabolism and reactive oxygen species. Proc Natl Acad Sci U S A. 2010;107(16):7461–6.
45. Curthoys NP, Watford M. Regulation of glutaminase activity and glutamine metabolism. Annu Rev Nutr. 1995; 15:133–59.

Chapter 5
The Role of Glutamine and Glutamic Acid in the Pituitary Gland Involvement in Thyroid-Stimulating Hormone Release

Sayaka Aizawa, Takafumi Sakai, and Ichiro Sakata

Key Points

- In the central nervous system, glutamate is locally converted in the glutamine/glutamate signaling system and acts as an excitatory neurotransmitter, exerting an important role in the brain functions involved in cognition, memory, and learning functions.
- The high levels of glutamate-binding sites are localized in the peripheral tissues, such as adrenal gland and pituitary glands, and the mRNA expression of many subtypes of glutamate receptors was found in those tissues.
- The administration of excitatory glutamate at very high stimulates the secretion of pituitary hormones, such as prolactin, growth hormone, and cortisol.
- Glutamine/glutamate signaling system including the amino acid transporter A2 known as the glutamine transporter and glutaminase were highly expressed in the pars tuberalis.
- In the pars tuberalis cells, glutamate locally converted from glutamine and induces TSH expression via an ionotropic glutamate receptor KA2 in an autocrine and/or paracrine manner.

Keywords Glutamine • Glutamate • Anterior pituitary • Pars tuberalis • Thyroid-stimulating hormone • Glutamate receptor

Abbreviations

GluR	Glutamate receptor
iGluR	Ionotropic glutamate receptor
mGluR	Metabotropic glutamate receptor
NMDA	*N*-methyl-D-aspartate
AMPA	L-a-Amino-3-hydroxy-5-methylisoxazole-4-propionate
KA	Kainite
KA2 receptor	Ionotropic glutamate receptor KA2

S. Aizawa, Ph.D. • T. Sakai, Ph.D. • I. Sakata, Ph.D. (✉)
Area of Regulatory Biology, Division of Life Science, Graduate School of Science and Engineering, Saitama University, Saitama, Japan
e-mail: saizawa@mail.saitama-u.ac.jp; aizawasayaka@gmail.coms; isakata@mail.saitama-u.ac.jp

R. Rajendram et al. (eds.), *Glutamine in Clinical Nutrition*, Nutrition and Health,
DOI 10.1007/978-1-4939-1932-1_5,

ATA2	Amino acid transporter A2
Gls	Glutaminase
Gls2	Glutaminase 2
ACTH	Adrenocorticotropic hormone
GH	Growth hormone
PRL	Prolactin
FSH	Follicle-stimulating hormone
LH	Luteinizing hormone
TSH	Thyroid-stimulating hormone
MT1	Melatonin receptor type 1

Introduction

Glutamine and glutamate are metabolic intermediates and key links between mammalian carbon and nitrogen metabolism, and in particular between the carbon metabolism of carbohydrates and protein. In general, it is thought that most of the glutamate obtained from food is absorbed and consumed in the intestinal tract as metabolic fuel, while little glutamate enters the bloodstream [1]. A study had shown that 95 % of the dietary glutamate is presented in the gut mucosa layer and is metabolized in a number of mammalian species [2]. Glutamate is the single and most important oxidative substrate for the intestinal mucosa [1, 2]. On the other hand, glutamine is also the most abundant free amino acid found in the body, especially in the muscles and blood [3]. It is also known that glutamine works as brain fuel because it is able to cross the blood–brain barrier [3]. In the central nervous system, glutamate is locally converted from glutamine, which is absorbed into the neurons [4], and acts as a neurotransmitter [5]. The functional molecule that is required for glutamine/glutamate signaling has been identified in neuronal tissues. Therefore, the hypothesis that glutamate is an excitatory amino acid neurotransmitter is now gaining more support because the genes involved in the conversion of glutamine into/from glutamate have been successfully identified in the mammalian central nervous system [5].

Relatively little attention has been paid to the function of glutamine and glutamate as extracellular signal mediators in the autocrine and/or paracrine system of the endocrine tissues. Recently, many studies have suggested that glutamine and glutamate could play a dual role as excitatory neurotransmitters in the central nervous system and as extracellular signaling molecules in endocrine tissues, such as the adrenal gland, pancreas, and testis. In this review, we describe the possible roles of glutamine and glutamate in the pituitary gland.

Glutamine/Glutamate Signaling Molecules and Glutamate Receptor

Glutamine/glutamate signaling as excitatory neurotransmitter is well established and it is involved in higher nervous activities such as cognitive, memory, and learning functions [6, 7].

Figure 5.1 shows the neurochemical mechanisms of glutamatergic signaling and glutamate-glutamine recycling. In the synaptic cleft, presynaptic cells intake extracellular glutamine and convert it into glutamate through glutaminase (glutamine + $H_2O \rightarrow$ glutamate + NH_3). The sources of glutamine are (1) extracellular circulating glutamine and (2) conversion from α-ketoglutarate in the tricarboxylic acid (TCA) cycle into glutamine. Then, glutamate is released from the presynaptic terminal via a small clear vesicle into the synaptic gap, and the released glutamate binds to the glutamate receptor located in the postsynaptic cell and acts as an excitatory neurotransmitter [5]. On the other hand, high concentrations of extracellular glutamate induce neuronal death caused by the

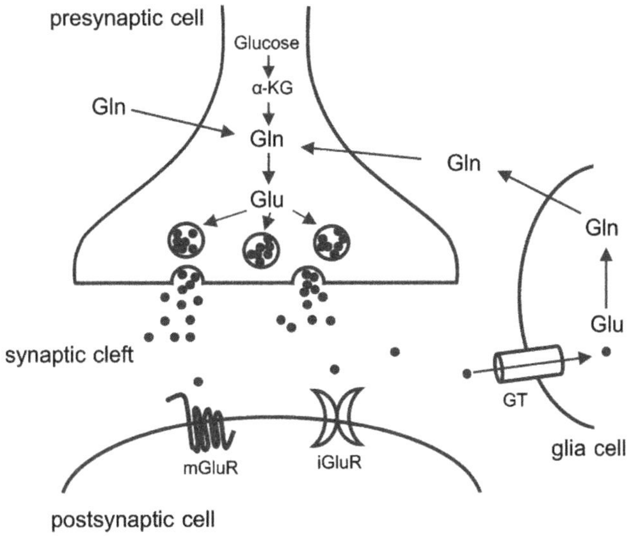

Fig. 5.1 Glutamine/glutamate signaling molecules as excitatory neurotransmitters. In the synaptic cleft, presynaptic cells intake extracellular glutamine (Gln) and convert it into glutamate (Glu) through glutaminase, or conversion from α-ketoglutarate (KG) in the TCA cycle into Gln. Then, Glu is released via a small clear vesicle into the synaptic gap, and it binds to the glutamate receptor mGluR (metabotropic glutamate receptor) and/or iGluR (ionotropic glutamate receptor) located in the postsynaptic cell, where it acts as an excitatory neurotransmitter. Glu is also transferred into glial cells through the glutamate transporter (GT), and converted into Gln by the action of glutamine synthetase

overstimulation of the excitatory amino acid receptors [8, 9]. Therefore, extracellular glutamate is transferred into glial cells through the excitatory amino acid transporter and glutamate transporter, which are present on the cell membrane of the glial cells. In the glial cells, glutamate is converted into glutamine by the action of glutamine synthetase (glutamate + $NH_3 \rightarrow$ glutamine). Finally, glutamine converted from glutamate in the glial cells is released extracellularly, and converted again into glutamate in the presynaptic cell (Fig. 5.1).

The receptors for glutamate (GluRs) are categorized into two classes, ionotropic receptor (iGluR) and G protein-coupled receptor (GPCR; also called metabotropic receptor, mGluR), according to their molecular structure and the different intracellular signal transduction mechanisms [10–12]. To date, 14 types of iGluR and 8 types of mGluR have been identified in the mammalian central nervous system [13]. On the basis of agonist studies, iGluR is further classified into *N*-methyl-D-aspartate (NMDA) receptors, L-a-amino-3-hydroxy-5-methylisoxazole-4-propionate (AMPA) receptors [14], and kainate (KA) receptors [13]. iGluRs are ligand-gated cation channels that allow the flow of K^+, Na^+, and Ca^{2+} in response to glutamate binding. NMDA receptors are permeable to Ca^{2+}, while AMPA receptors and KA receptors are permeable to Na^+. mGluRs are GPCRs containing seven transmembrane domains and are further subdivided into three distinct subtypes: group I (mGluR1 and mGluR5), group II (mGluR2 and mGluR3), and group III (mGluR4, mGluR6, mGluR7, and mGluR8), in line with each receptor's exogenous agonists and intracellular second messengers [15, 16]. The mGluR group I subtype induces the formation of inositol-1,4,5-triphosphate and increases the intracellular Ca^{2+} concentrations [15, 16]. Both group II and III subtypes induce the inhibition of adenylate cyclase and reduction of intracellular cyclic adenosine monophosphate (cAMP) [15, 16]. In the central nervous system, glutamate is locally converted in the glutamine/glutamate signaling system, as described above, and acts as an excitatory neurotransmitter, exerting an important role in the brain functions involved in cognition, memory, and learning.

Effect of Glutamine and Glutamate on Endocrine Organs

Relatively little attention has been paid to the glutamine/glutamate signaling and the functions of glutamine and glutamate in peripheral tissues. It has been reported that high levels of glutamate binding sites are localized in the rat adrenal gland [17] and pituitary glands [18], and that the mRNA expression of many subtypes of iGluRs and mGluRs was found in those tissues. For example, high-affinity [3H] glutamate-binding sites were found in rat adrenal medulla, and it was shown that AMPA and NMDA receptors are expressed in the adrenal cortex and adrenal medulla, respectively [17]. The role of glutamate in adrenal glands has been investigated not only using glutamate but also iGluR (NMDA, AMPA, and KA) agonists and an mGluR agonist, and it was found that all stimulate catecholamine release from the adrenal gland [19]. On the other hand, the membrane-binding assay revealed that [3H] glutamate-binding sites are widely spread in the rat brain, not only in the nervous system but also in the pituitary gland and pineal glands [20, 21]. In the pineal gland, 1 mM exogenous glutamate leads to the inhibition of the activation of norepinephrine-induced *N*-acetyltransferase and hydroxyindole-*O*-methyltransferase activation, which are enzymes involved in the day/night rhythmic production of melatonin by the modification of serotonin, in a dose-dependent manner in cultured rat pineal glands, consequently suppressing both the synthesis and secretion of melatonin [22]. Interestingly, there are many reports showing the effects of glutamate and glutamine on the pituitary gland. In this chapter, we focus on the effect of glutamine and glutamate on the pituitary gland.

The Pituitary Gland

The pituitary gland is the endocrine gland that is located at the base of the brain and is composed of three lobes: anterior lobe, intermediate lobe, and posterior lobe. The posterior pituitary is composed of neurons and it collects the nerve terminals from the hypothalamus. The hypothalamic neurosecretory cells produce the hormone oxytocin, which targets the mammary glands causing milk release and causes the contractions of the smooth uterine muscles. The hypothalamic neurosecretory cells also produce vasopressin, which targets the kidney tubules and increases water retention; these cells transmit these hormones through the axons to the posterior pituitary [23], where secretory vesicles containing the hormone are stored and released through the hypophyseal vein in response to the nerve impulses from the hypothalamus [24].

The anterior pituitary has been known as the major organ of the endocrine system, producing six different anterior pituitary hormones: adrenocorticotropic hormone (ACTH), growth hormone (GH), prolactin (PRL), follicle-stimulating hormone (FSH), luteinizing hormone (LH), and thyroid-stimulating hormone (TSH). The regulatory mechanisms for these anterior pituitary hormones have been well studied, and they were found to be mainly regulated by the molecules produced in the hypothalamus and by the negative feedback from the organs targeted by these hormones. The anterior pituitary receives the releasing and/or inhibiting hormones from the hypothalamic neurosecretory cells through a hypothalamic-hypophyseal portal system, and these hypothalamic hormones regulate the cells of the anterior pituitary gland responsible for hormone production and secretion.

The anterior pituitary gland is divided into two parts: pars distalis and pars tuberalis. The pars distalis comprises the majority of the anterior pituitary and is the bulk of the pituitary hormone production. The pars tuberalis exists as a thin cell layer extending from the pars distalis and covering around the pituitary stalk and median eminence. In general, the mammalian pars tuberalis consists of two cell types, folliculo-stellate cells and glycoprotein hormone-producing cells, such as thyrotropes (TSH-producing cells) and gonadotropes (FSH/LH-producing cells) [25]. Notably, a high density of melatonin-binding sites has been observed in the pars tuberalis of many species [26], and melatonin receptor type 1 (MT1) is expressed in the mammalian pars tuberalis [27]. Melatonin is exclusively secreted from the pineal gland during the dark period, and its signal corresponds to the duration of the dark period, thereby providing photoperiodic information to the melatonin receptor-producing target sites. Although the function of the pars tuberalis is poorly understood, it might play an important role in the mediation of seasonal and/or circadian signals.

On the other hand, attention has been paid to the function of glutamine and/or glutamate in the anterior pituitary gland, both pars distalis and pars tuberalis. Interestingly, the circadian changes of the concentration of glutamine and glutamate in the rat anterior pituitary were reported [28]. Both glutamine and glutamate have a peak at the Zeitgeber time 15 (3 h later than light off; lights-on time defined as ZT0 (08:00) and lights-off time defined as ZT12 (20:00)) in the anterior pituitary, and the concentration is much higher than that in the posterior pituitary (neurohypophysis) [28].

Glutamine and Glutamate in the Pars Distalis

Many subtypes of glutamine and glutamate receptors are expressed in the pars distalis. Earlier, it has been shown using binding assays that glutamate strongly binds to the pituitary gland homogenate in addition to the brain homogenate [18]. Molecular biological and immunohistochemical analyses have demonstrated the presence of glutamate receptors such as non-NMDA [29, 30] and NMDA iGluRs in the pituitary gland [31]. In addition, Hinoi et al. demonstrated that [^{3}H] kinate binds to the rat pituitary gland and showed that an intraperitoneal injection of KA increased the DNA-binding activity of the nuclear transcription factor activator protein-1 (AP1) in the hippocampus and the pituitary gland of the rat, suggesting that glutamate may regulate the pituitary hormone production at the transcriptional level [21]. In isolated rat pituitary melanotropes, glutamate induced a marked increase in the cytosolic free Ca^{2+} concentration [32]. Collectively, these findings indicate that particular subtypes of glutamate receptors are functionally expressed and glutamate might induce several physiological effects on the pars distalis.

It has been reported that glutamate plays an important role in the regulation of pituitary hormone secretion in the pars distalis. Several studies have demonstrated the direct regulation of hormone secretion by glutamate in primary pars distalis cell cultures. In the agonist study, it was reported that NMDA and KA induced the secretion of GH in several mammalian species in vitro and in vivo [33]. In rat somatotropes, glutamate increased the cytosolic Ca^{2+} concentration and increased GH release [34]. It has been well known that the growth hormone-releasing hormone (GHRH) and growth hormone-inhibiting hormone (GHIH or somatostatin) from the hypothalamus mainly control GH secretion. Therefore, the stimulatory effect of glutamate on GH secretion seems to be additive to the regulation of hypothalamic hormones, suggesting that glutamate might play a role in basal GH secretion [33]. In addition, the effect of glutamate on prolactin release has been reported. An in vitro study showed that high concentrations of glutamate (1 mM) increased the calcium concentration in the prolactin-producing cells, stimulating prolactin secretion [35], while its effect was blocked by MK-801, an antagonist of NMDA iGluRs [36]. Furthermore, KA, the agonist of glutamate receptor KA, stimulated LH and FSH release at low concentrations (1 μM) in the rat anterior pituitary gland in vitro, and this effect disappeared with progression of age; this effect might be exerted both through NMDA and non-NMDA receptor subtypes [37]. According to a study conducted on monkeys, the administration of excitatory glutamate at very high doses or active agonist for glutamate receptors has been reported to stimulate the secretion of pituitary hormones, such as prolactin, GH, ACTH (cortisol), and LH and/or FSH [38–40, 42].

The Effect of Glutamine and Glutamate on the Pars Tuberalis

The relationship between glutamine and/or glutamate and hormone production in the pars tuberalis has been recently studied. The mammalian pars tuberalis consists of folliculo-stellate cells and glycoprotein hormone-producing cells (i.e., thyrotropes and gonadotropes) [25]. In rats, the majority of the hormone-producing cells in the pars tuberalis are small and oval-shaped TSH-producing cells that are characterized by spot-like TSH immunoreactivity in the Golgi apparatus [41]. The regulatory mechanisms of the TSHβ subunit and α-glycoprotein subunit (αGSU) mRNA expression and TSH release in the pars tuberalis are believed to be different from those in the pars distalis cells because the TSH-producing cells in the pars tuberalis do not express the receptor for the thyrotropin-releasing hormone (TRH) and thyroid hormone receptor beta 2 (TR-β2) that are needed for the negative feedback regulation from the target organ, the thyroid gland [42]. As the notable characteristics of the pars tuberalis, it is known that MT1 is highly expressed in the pars tuberalis [27]. Melatonin, known as the "hormone of darkness," is secreted from the pineal gland, and its signal corresponds to the duration of the dark period, thereby providing photoperiodic information to the melatonin receptor-producing target sites and mediating the circadial and/or seasonal physiological functions, such as seasonal reproduction. Therefore, the pars tuberalis is thought to play an important role in the mediation of the seasonal and/or circadian signals. In fact, the mRNA expression and protein secretion of the TSH in the pars tuberalis are inhibited by melatonin, and the TSH expression and production have a circadian rhythm [43].

Recently, another regulatory mechanism of TSH in the pars tuberalis has been elucidated and it has been shown that glutamine and glutamate stimulate the TSH mRNA expression and secretion [44]. In the rat pars tuberalis, the KA2 receptor, which is one of the iGluR subtype, is highly expressed and its expression level is higher than that of MT1 (Fig. 5.2a, b). Furthermore, amino acid transporter A2 (ATA2) (Fig. 5.2c), which is also known as glutamine transporter [45], glutaminase (Gls), and glutaminase 2 (Gls2) [4] are highly expressed in the pars tuberalis (Fig. 5.2d, e). Moreover, slice culture experiments using rat brain showed that 1 mM L-glutamic acid significantly enhanced the TSHβ subunit mRNA expression within 2 h. Furthermore, 1 mM glutamine also increased the TSHβ mRNA expression in 4 and 8 h in a time-dependent manner after stimulation. Since the ATA2, which acts as glutamine transporter, and glutaminase and glutaminase 2, which convert glutamine to glutamate, were also highly expressed in the pars tuberalis, it was suggested that the converted glutamate in the pars tuberalis increased the TSHβ subunit mRNA expression and secretion [44] in an autocrine and/or paracrine manner and that it might be necessary for the maintenance of TSHβ expression and secretion in the pars tuberalis [44] (Figs. 5.3 and 5.4).

The Effect of Glutamine and Glutamate on the Human Pituitary Gland

In humans, the studies of the effect of glutamine and glutamate on the pituitary hormones are limited, but the significant effect of oral glutamate intake on prolactin and cortisol secretion has been reported. Oral administration of 10 g of glutamate (high dose) stimulated the secretion of prolactin and cortisol to approximately twice the baseline values [46]. However, this result is thought to be unwarranted, and another study on healthy men who received oral glutamate in the morning after overnight fasting reported no significant effect of the oral intake of glutamate on the pituitary hormone. In particular, although the plasma concentration of the glutamate immediately increased from 50 nmol/mL (fasting plasma glutamate concentration) to 11-fold within 60 min after high-dose oral glutamate intake (12.7 g), the plasma prolactin concentration was so very little stimulated that it failed to reach

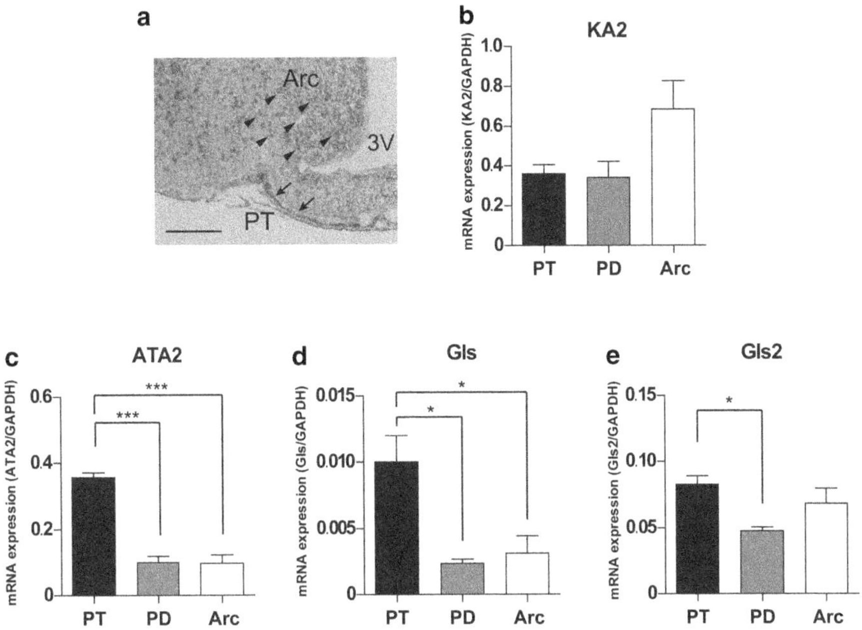

Fig. 5.2 Glutamate signaling components in the pars tuberalis, pars distalis, and arcuate nucleus. (**a**) Microphotograph of iGluR kinate receptor cells expressing KA2 mRNA, detected by in situ hybridization. KA2 (kinate receptor 2) mRNA-expressing cells were observed not only in the rat PT (*arrows*) but also in the hypothalamus, including the Arc (*arrowheads*). Scale bar: 200 μm. (**b**) qPCR analysis of KA2 mRNA expression in the PT, PD, and Arc. The KA2 mRNA level in the PT was similar to that in the PD. Although there was no statistically significant difference in the mRNA levels between the PT and Arc, the KA2 mRNA level tended to be lower in the PT. (**c**) Glutamine transporter ATA2 mRNA expression in the PT, PD, and Arc. The ATA2 mRNA level was significantly higher in the PT than in the PD and Arc. (**d**) Glutaminase (Gls) and (**e**) Glutaminase2 (Gls2) mRNA expression in the PT, PD, and Arc. Gls mRNA expression was higher in the PT than in the PD and Arc. Gls2 mRNA expression in the PT was significantly higher than that in the PD but comparable to that in the Arc. PT, pars tuberalis; Arc, arcuate nucleus; and 3 V, third ventricle. Values are the means ± S.E.M. ($n=3$). $^*P<0.05$ and $^{***}P<0.001$

significance [47]. To clarify the effects of glutamate on prolactin secretion, further human studies are needed in the future, as well as the description of the mechanisms of the influence of glutamate on hormone secretion in the pituitary gland.

On the other hand, it has been shown that oral administration of glutamine influences the physiological functions controlled by the pituitary gland hormones. For example, orally administrated glutamine acts on the anterior pituitary gland and increases the production of GH at the pituitary level, resulting in an increase in the plasma GH levels in humans [48, 49]. Although there is no direct evidence, the glutamine/glutamate signaling might be active in the human pituitary and through the stimulation of the pituitary hormone secretion by glutamate in an autocrine and/or paracrine manner, similar to the TSH secretion from the pars tuberalis in animals.

The number of studies concerning the effects of glutamine and glutamate on human pituitary gland is small. Recently, using animal models, researches have been gradually proceeding in elucidating the functions of glutamate and glutamine. By conducting the same experiments on humans, it might be possible to discover novel functions of glutamate and glutamine in some physiological and pathological conditions.

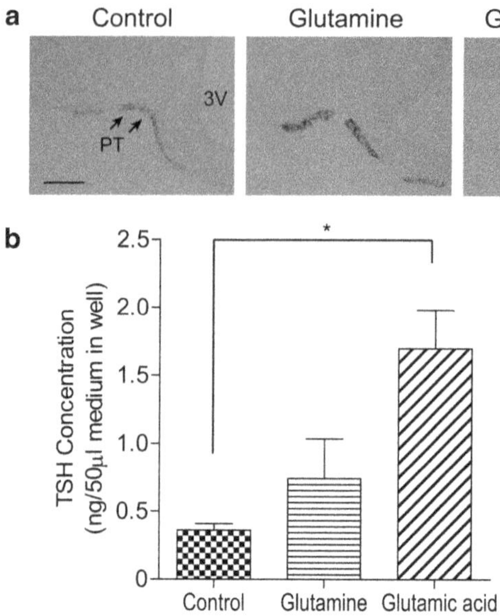

Fig. 5.3 Effects of glutamine and L-glutamic acid on TSHβ subunit mRNA expression and secretion in the rat pars tuberalis. (**a**) Microphotographs of in situ hybridization for TSHβ subunit mRNA. The staining densities of TSHβ subunit mRNA were altered by treatment with glutamine (*middle column*) or L-glutamic acid (*right column*) compared to the control (*left column*). Scale bar = 200 µm. PT, pars tuberalis; 3 V, third ventricle. (**b**) Concentration of TSH secreted into the medium from brain slices that included the pars tuberalis, measured by ELISA. Treatment with 1 mM L-GLUTAMIC acid for 4 h significantly increased the TSH secretion compared to the control. $*P<0.05$. Values are the means ± S.E.M. ($n=3$)

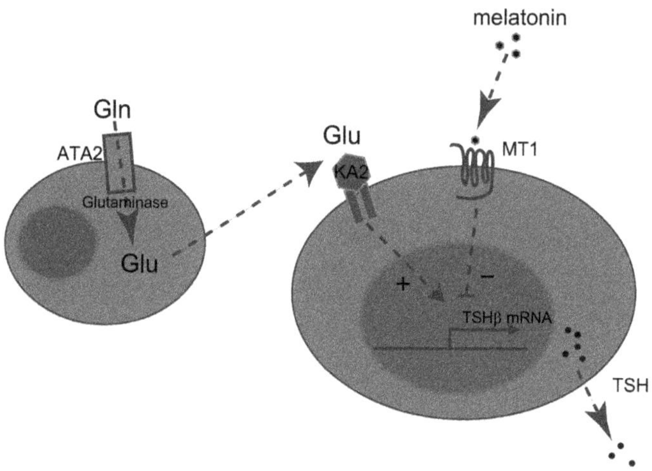

Fig. 5.4 Model of the glutamine/glutamate signaling in the pars tuberalis. PT cells intake extracellular glutamine (Gln) through glutamine transporter ATA2. Glutaminase and glutaminase 2 convert Gln to glutamate (Glu). The converted Glu acts on iGluR kinate receptor KA2 in an autocrine and/or paracrine manner and induces TSHβ subunit mRNA expression and TSH secretion, while melatonin inhibits the TSHβ subunit mRNA expression via melatonin receptor MT1

Conclusions

The hypothesis of glutamine and glutamate as extracellular signaling molecules in peripheral tissues is gaining more support after the successful cloning of a number of genes coding for the machinery required for this glutamine/glutamate signaling, including glutamine transporter, glutaminase, glutamate transporter, glutamine synthetase, and glutamate receptor. Many reports have shown that glutamate plays the role of excitatory neurotransmitter in the central neuroendocrine system and as an extracellular signal in the peripheral endocrine organs, including the pituitary gland. In general, glutamate obtained from food is absorbed and consumed in the intestinal tract as metabolic fuel, while little glutamate enters the blood stream. The concentration of serum glutamate seems to be low, impeding the access to the glutamate receptor. On the other hand, glutamine is the most abundant free amino acid in the blood stream and it could pass the blood–brain barrier, where the neuronal system can interact with the glutamate converted from glutamine through the glutamine/glutamate signaling. In the peripheral endocrine tissues as well as the neuronal system, the source of glutamate might be the circulating glutamine. Based on these observations, although inconclusive, it has been proposed that glutamate is locally converted from glutamine and then acts as extracellular signal in an autocrine and/or paracrine manner in the pituitary gland.

References

1. Reeds PJ et al. Enteral glutamate is almost completely metabolized in first pass by the gastrointestinal tract of infant pigs. Am J Physiol. 1996;270(3 Pt 1):E413–8.
2. Reeds PJ et al. Intestinal glutamate metabolism. J Nutr. 2000;130(4S Suppl):978S–82.
3. Lee WJ et al. Glutamine transport by the blood-brain barrier: a possible mechanism for nitrogen removal. Am J Physiol. 1998;274(4 Pt 1):C1101–7.
4. de la Rosa V et al. A novel glutaminase isoform in mammalian tissues. Neurochem Int. 2009;55(1–3):76–84.
5. Fonnum F. Glutamate: a neurotransmitter in mammalian brain. J Neurochem. 1984;42(1):1–11.
6. Schwartz TL, Sachdeva S, Stahl SM. Glutamate neurocircuitry: theoretical underpinnings in schizophrenia. Front Pharmacol. 2012;3:195.
7. Pittenger C, Bloch MH, Williams K. Glutamate abnormalities in obsessive compulsive disorder: neurobiology, pathophysiology, and treatment. Pharmacol Ther. 2011;132(3):314–32.
8. Albin RL, Greenamyre JT. Alternative excitotoxic hypotheses. Neurology. 1992;42(4):733–8.
9. Sattler R, Tymianski M. Molecular mechanisms of glutamate receptor-mediated excitotoxic neuronal cell death. Mol Neurobiol. 2001;24(1–3):107–29.
10. Dingledine R et al. The glutamate receptor ion channels. Pharmacol Rev. 1999;51(1):7–61.
11. De Blasi A et al. Molecular determinants of metabotropic glutamate receptor signaling. Trends Pharmacol Sci. 2001;22(3):114–20.
12. Hinoi E et al. Glutamate signaling in peripheral tissues. Eur J Biochem. 2004;271(1):1–13.
13. Hollmann M et al. Cloning by functional expression of a member of the glutamate receptor family. Nature. 1989;342(6250):643–8.
14. Nakanishi N, Shneider NA, Axel R. A family of glutamate receptor genes: evidence for the formation of heteromultimeric receptors with distinct channel properties. Neuron. 1990;5(5):569–81.
15. Masu M et al. Sequence and expression of a metabotropic glutamate receptor. Nature. 1991;349(6312):760–5.
16. Tanabe Y et al. A family of metabotropic glutamate receptors. Neuron. 1992;8(1):169–79.
17. Yoneda Y, Ogita K. Localization of [3H]glutamate binding sites in rat adrenal medulla. Brain Res. 1986;383(1–2):387–91.
18. Yoneda Y, Ogita K. [3H]glutamate binding sites in the rat pituitary. Neurosci Res. 1986;3(5):430–5.
19. Gonzalez MP et al. Effect of glutamate receptor agonists on catecholamine secretion in bovine chromaffin cells. Neuroendocrinology. 1998;67(3):181–9.
20. Meeker RB, Greenwood RS, Hayward JN. Glutamate receptors in the rat hypothalamus and pituitary. Endocrinology. 1994;134(2):621–9.
21. Hinoi E, Yoneda Y. Expression of GluR6/7 subunits of kainate receptors in rat adenohypophysis. Neurochem Int. 2001;38(6):539–47.

22. Govitrapong P, Ebadi M. The inhibition of pineal arylalkylamine n-acetyltransferase by glutamic acid and its analogues. Neurochem Int. 1988;13(2):223–30.
23. Acher R. Molecular evolution of fish neurohypophysial hormones: neutral and selective evolutionary mechanisms. Gen Comp Endocrinol. 1996;102(2):157–72.
24. Hatton GI. Pituicytes, glia and control of terminal secretion. J Exp Biol. 1988;139:67–79.
25. Gross DS. The mammalian hypophysial pars tuberalis: a comparative immunocytochemical study. Gen Comp Endocrinol. 1984;56(2):283–98.
26. Williams LM, Morgan PJ. Demonstration of melatonin-binding sites on the pars tuberalis of the rat. J Endocrinol. 1988;119(1):R1–3.
27. Klosen P et al. The mt1 melatonin receptor and RORbeta receptor are co-localized in specific TSH-immunoreactive cells in the pars tuberalis of the rat pituitary. J Histochem Cytochem. 2002;50(12):1647–57.
28. Caride A et al. Daily pattern of pituitary glutamine, glutamate, and aspartate content disrupted by cadmium exposure. Amino Acids. 2010;38(4):1165–72.
29. Kiyama H, Sato K, Tohyama M. Characteristic localization of non-NMDA type glutamate receptor subunits in the rat pituitary gland. Brain Res Mol Brain Res. 1993;19(3):262–8.
30. Mahesh VB et al. Characterization of ionotropic glutamate receptors in rat hypothalamus, pituitary and immortalized gonadotropin-releasing hormone (GnRH) neurons (GT1-7 cells). Neuroendocrinology. 1999;69(6):397–407.
31. Bhat GK et al. Localization of the N-methyl-D-aspartate R1 receptor subunit in specific anterior pituitary hormone cell types of the female rat. Neuroendocrinology. 1995;62(2):178–86.
32. Giovannucci DR, Stuenkel EL. Glutamate receptor agonists modulate [Ca2+]i in isolated rat melanotropes. Neuroendocrinology. 1995;62(2):111–22.
33. Niimi M et al. Effect of excitatory amino acid receptor agonists on secretion of growth hormone as assessed by the reverse hemolytic plaque assay. Neuroendocrinology. 1994;60(2):173–8.
34. Lindstrom P, Ohlsson L. Effect of N-methyl-D, L-aspartate on isolated rat somatotrophs. Endocrinology. 1992;131(4):1903–7.
35. Pampillo M et al. Effect of ionotropic and metabotropic glutamate agonists and D-aspartate on prolactin release from anterior pituitary cells. Exp Clin Endocrinol Diabetes. 2002;110(3):138–44.
36. Login IS. Direct stimulation of pituitary prolactin release by glutamate. Life Sci. 1990;47(24):2269–75.
37. Zanisi M et al. The anterior pituitary gland as a possible site of action of kainic acid. Proc Soc Exp Biol Med. 1994;206(4):431–7.
38. Arslan M et al. Possible modulation of N-methyl-D, L-aspartic acid induced prolactin release by testicular steroids in the adult male rhesus monkey. Life Sci. 1991;49(15):1073–7.
39. Medhamurthy R, Gay VL, Plant TM. Repetitive injections of L-glutamic acid, in contrast to those of N-methyl-D, L-aspartic acid, fail to elicit sustained hypothalamic GnRH release in the prepubertal male rhesus monkey (Macaca mulatta). Neuroendocrinology. 1992;55(6):660–6.
40. Urbanski HF et al. Alpha-adrenergic receptor antagonism and N-methyl-D-aspartate (NMDA) induced luteinizing hormone release in female rhesus macaques. Brain Res. 1997;744(1):96–104.
41. Sakai T, Inoue K, Kurosumi K. Light and electron microscopic immunocytochemistry of TSH-like cells occurring in the pars tuberalis of the adult male rat pituitary. Arch Histol Cytol. 1992;55(2):151–7.
42. Bockmann J et al. Thyrotropin expression in hypophyseal pars tuberalis-specific cells is 3,5,3′-triiodothyronine, thyrotropin-releasing hormone, and pit-1 independent. Endocrinology. 1997;138(3):1019–28.
43. Aizawa S et al. Diurnal change of thyroid-stimulating hormone mRNA expression in the rat pars tuberalis. J Neuroendocrinol. 2007;19(11):839–46.
44. Aizawa S, Sakai T, Sakata I. Glutamine and glutamic acid enhance thyroid-stimulating hormone beta subunit mRNA expression in the rat pars tuberalis. J Endocrinol. 2012;212(3):383–94.
45. Sugawara M et al. Cloning of an amino acid transporter with functional characteristics and tissue expression pattern identical to that of system A. J Biol Chem. 2000;275(22):16473–7.
46. Carlson HE et al. Stimulation of pituitary hormone secretion by neurotransmitter amino acids in humans. Metabolism. 1989;38(12):1179–82.
47. Fernstrom JD. Pituitary hormone secretion in normal male humans: acute responses to a large, oral dose of monosodium glutamate. J Nutr. 2000;130(4S Suppl):1053S–7.
48. Wales PW et al. Human growth hormone and glutamine for patients with short bowel syndrome. Cochrane Database Syst Rev. 2010;6, CD006321.
49. Buchardt J et al. Transglutaminase-mediated methods for site-selective modification of human growth hormone. Biopolymers. 2010;94(2):229–35.

Chapter 6
Glucose-Independent Glutamine-Driven TCA Cycle in Cancer Cells

Brad Poore, Nicholas Siegel, Joshua K. Park, Benjamin Jung Hwang, Iman Afif, and Anne Le

Key Points

- Human lymphoma B cells display a glucose-independent glutamine-driven TCA cycle.
- Persistence of glutamine oxidation via the TCA cycle under hypoxia.
- Glutamine metabolism contributes to bioenergetics and redox homeostasis.
- Glutaminase inhibition diminishes in vitro and in vivo tumor cell growth.

Keywords TCA cycle • Glutaminolysis • Glucose-independent glutamine-driven TCA cycle • Targeting glutamine metabolism • Glucose-deficient microenvironment

Abbreviations

TCA	Tricarboxylic acid cycle
PDC	Pyruvate dehydrogenase complex
GLS	Glutaminase
GLDH	Glutamate dehydrogenase
OAA	Oxaloacetate
ME	Malic enzyme
BPTES	Bis-2-(5 phenylacetamido-1 2, 4-thiadiazol-2-yl) ethyl sulfide
GLS1	Kidney-type glutaminase isoform
SDH	Succinate dehydrogenase
TTFA	2-Thenoyltrifluoroacetone
AOA	Aminooxyacetate
TRAIL	Tumor necrosis factor-related apoptosis-inducing ligand

B. Poore, B.S. • N. Siegel, B.S. • J.K. Park, B.S. • B.J. Hwang, B.A. • I. Afif, B.A. • A. Le, M.D. (✉)
Department of Pathology, Division of Gastrointestinal and Liver Pathology, Johns Hopkins University School of Medicine, Baltimore, MD, USA
e-mail: annele@jhmi.edu

R. Rajendram et al. (eds.), *Glutamine in Clinical Nutrition*, Nutrition and Health,
DOI 10.1007/978-1-4939-1932-1_6, © Springer Science+Business Media New York 2015

Introduction

Since the discovery of the Warburg effect, it has been known that cancer can meet its metabolic needs in a different manner from that of normal cells. In order to grow and survive in the harsh hypoxic, and nutrient-deprived, conditions of the tumor microenvironment, cancer cells must generate additional metabolic energy and be able to synthesize the necessary biosynthetic precursors of proteins, nucleic acids and membrane lipids in order to make new cells. Studies in recent years have documented differences in the metabolism of cellular nutrients, such as glucose and glutamine, between cancer cells and normal cells [1]. Under aerobic conditions, normal cells will convert glucose to pyruvate and then use pyruvate to run the tricarboxylic acid cycle (TCA). In the absence of oxygen, glucose is instead converted to lactate to regenerate NAD+as a means of producing ATP from glycolysis [2] (Fig. 6.1). However, in cancer cells, the conversion of pyruvate to lactate occurs even in the presence of oxygen. This aberrant process is called aerobic glycolysis or the "Warburg effect" [3, 4]. The altered nature of the Warburg effect suggests that the sources of the carbon for the TCA cycle may differ between normal and cancerous cells. Recently, research by Le et al. demonstrated that human lymphoma B cells maintain the TCA cycle by exclusively relying on glutamine in the absence of glucose. When subjecting cancer cells to hypoxic conditions, glutamine metabolism also contributes to bioenergetics. The TCA cycle provides cellular energy and metabolites through a series of chemical reactions, is a key part of aerobic respiration, and is classically regarded as the dominant pathway for glucose oxidation. However, the study by Le et al. found that glutamine plays a prominent role in cancer cells, as it can provide the TCA cycle intermediates, thereby promoting cell growth and survival in the absence of glucose [5] (Fig. 6.2).

Cancer defines a broad category of diseases involving genetic alterations, which result in direct alterations to the regulation of cellular metabolism. This reprogramming of cellular metabolic

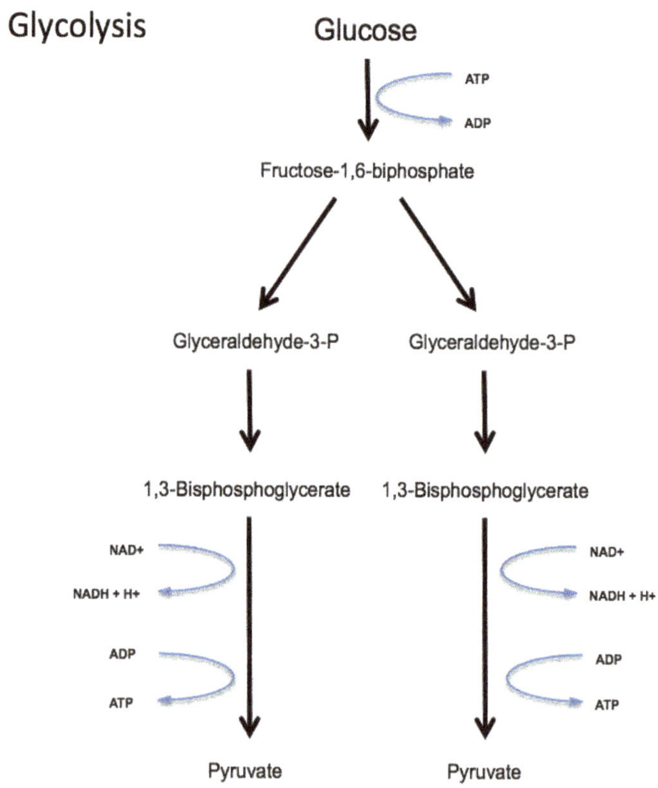

Fig. 6.1 Glycolysis. Diagram of glycolysis depicting the conversion of glucose into pyruvate. For every molecule of glucose, 2 molecules of pyruvate are produced through a series of reactions, producing a number of intermediates. Glycolysis occurs in both aerobic and anaerobic conditions and produces a net of 2 ATP and 2 NADH. In the presence of oxygen, pyruvate is decarboxylated into acetyl-CoA and enters tri-carboxylic acid cycle

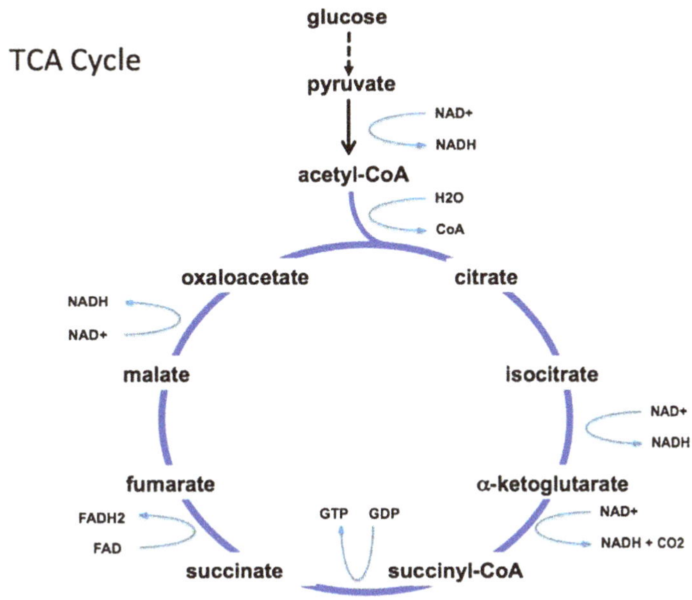

Fig. 6.2 The tricarboxylic acid (TCA) cycle

processes ensures adequate nourishment for the unusually resilient and proliferative cancer cells despite their hypoxic and nutrient-deprived microenvironments.

The Tricarboxylic Acid (TCA) Cycle

The tricarboxylic acid (TCA) cycle—also known as the Krebs cycle, or the citric acid cycle—is a series of enzyme-catalyzed reactions that play a key role in aerobic respiration and cellular metabolism in order to generate energy through the oxidization of acetate. Acetate can be derived from a wide variety of sources including carbohydrates, fats, and proteins. Taking place in the mitochondrial matrix, the cycle produces precursors needed to synthesize a range of biological molecules. The TCA cycle is a component of cellular respiration and acts as the link between the decarboxylation of pyruvate and oxidative phosphorylation [2]. Cellular respiration begins when glucose, a carbohydrate, is reduced into pyruvate through glycolysis. Pyruvate is then transported into the mitochondria and is decarboxylated into acetyl CoA, the starting product of the TCA cycle. The conversion of pyruvate into acetyl-CoA, referred to as pyruvate decarboxylation, is catalyzed by the pyruvate dehydrogenase complex (PDC). Acetyl CoA consists of an acetyl group attached to a coenzyme A molecule. Acetyl CoA then undergoes a condensation reaction with oxaloacetate (OAA), a TCA cycle intermediate, to form citric acid. The addition of water releases coenzyme A from the PDC and forms citrate. Citrate is subsequently transformed into several TCA intermediates that include isocitrate, α-ketoglutarate, succinyl-CoA, succinate, fumarate, and malate through oxidative and decarboxylative reactions, which concomitantly generate NADH. Acetyl-CoA and OAA each loses carbons in the reaction, and therefore generates CO_2 as a by-product. The conversion of succinyl-CoA to succinate by succinyl-CoA synthetase generates GTP, which is used by diphospho kinase in a trans-phosphorylation reaction to produce ATP from ADP. The GDP regenerated from GTP allows for the continued operation of succinyl-CoA synthetase. The 3 moles of NADH and 1 mole of FADH2 generated during each round of the cycle feed into the oxidative phosphorylation pathway. Each mole of NADH generates 3 moles of ATP and each mole of FADH2 leads to 2 moles of ATP via oxidative phosphorylation.

Therefore, for each mole of pyruvate which enters the TCA cycle, 12 moles of ATP can be generated. Between 30 and 38 molecules of ATP are obtained after the complete oxidation of one molecule of glucose in glycolysis, the citric acid cycle, and oxidative phosphorylation [6].

The TCA cycle plays an essential role in the metabolism of normal cells, providing energy and molecules necessary for cell survival. However, could the TCA cycle be driven in the absence of glucose?

Glucose-Independent Glutamine-Driven TCA for Human Lymphoma B Cell Survival and Proliferation

Using isotopically labeled carbon and nitrogen to trace glutamine in human lymphoma B cells grown in the absence of glucose, the study by Le et al. documented that TCA cycle intermediates can be derived solely from glutamine in the lymphoma B cells. They observed a range of citrate isotopologues produced: ^{13}C3- ($m+3$), ^{13}C4- ($m+4$), ^{13}C5- ($m+5$), and ^{13}C6-citrate ($m+6$) (Figs. 6.3, 6.4, and 6.5).

First, ^{13}C6,^{15}N2-labeled glutamine is converted into ^{13}C5,^{15}N1-labeled glutamate via the enzyme glutaminase (GLS) and then into ^{13}C5-labeled α-ketoglutarate via glutamate dehydrogenase (GLDH). The ^{13}C5-citrate can be directly derived from ^{13}C5- α- ketoglutarate (which is from ^{13}C6-glutamine) via reductive carboxylation [7] (purple circles, Fig. 6.3).

Another possibility for the ^{13}C5-citrate (orange circles, Fig. 6.4) is that ^{13}C5-citrate is produced from ($m+2$) acetyl-CoA and ($m+3$) OAA. First, ^{13}C5-labeled α-ketoglutarate goes to the forward reactions of the cycle to make ($m+4$) malate, which then converts into ($m+3$) pyruvate via the oxidative decarboxylation by the malic enzyme (ME, blue). This $m+3$ pyruvate pool ($m+3$) can serve as a precursor for both ($m+2$) acetyl-CoA, by the pyruvate dehydrogenase complex (PDC, light blue), and ($m+3$) OAA, by pyruvate carboxylase (PC, green) (Fig. 6.4).

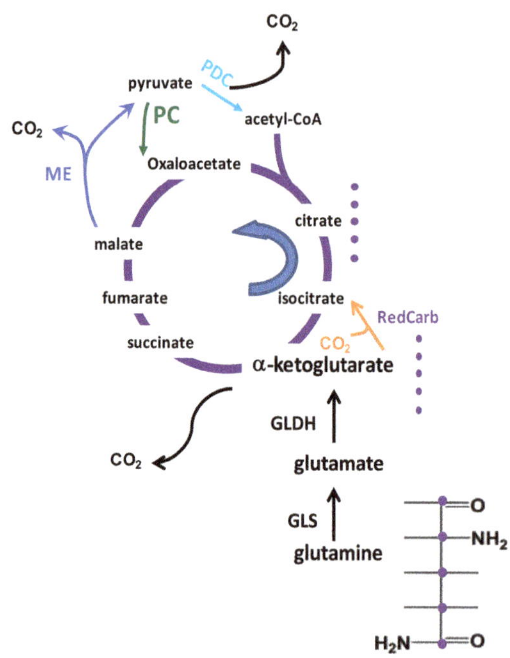

Fig. 6.3 ^{13}C5-citrate can be directly derived from ^{13}C5- α-ketoglutarate (which is from ^{13}C5-glutamine) via reductive carboxylation. ME: malic enzyme; PC: pyruvate carboxylase; PDC: pyruvate dehydrogenase complex; GLS: glutaminase; GLDH: glutamate dehydrogenase (GLDH). CO_2 indicates where carbon dioxide is released

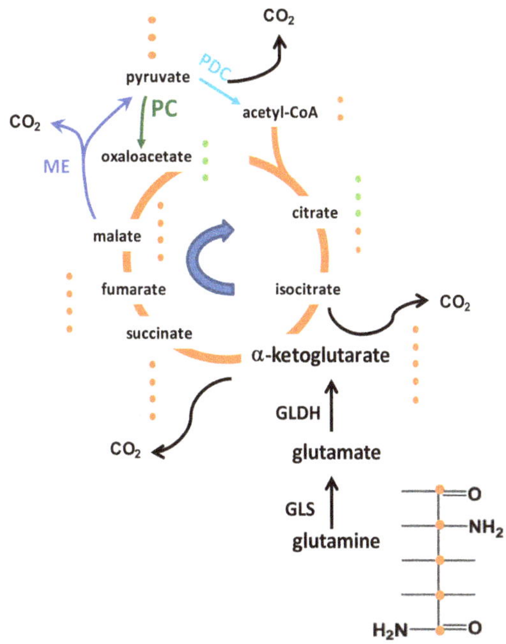

Fig. 6.4 ^{13}C5-citrate from $(m+2)$ acetyl-CoA and $(m+3)$ OAA via GLS-GLDH-ME-PC- PDC pathway. ME: malic enzyme; PC: pyruvate carboxylase; PDC: pyruvate dehydrogenase complex; GLS: glutaminase; GLDH: glutamate dehydrogenase (GLDH). CO_2 indicates where carbon dioxide is released

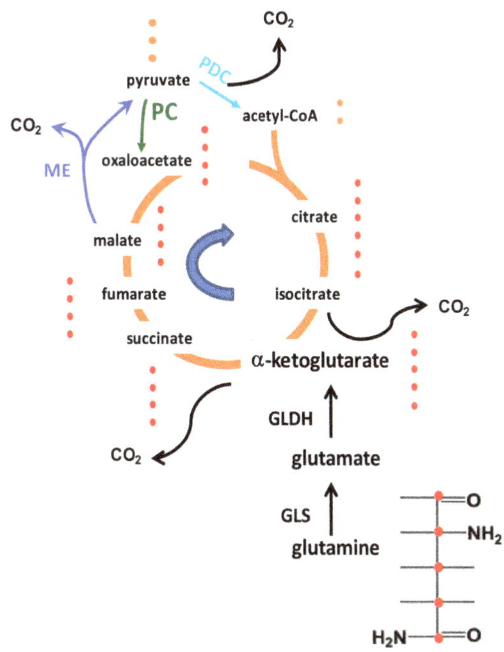

Fig. 6.5 ^{13}C6-citrate from $(m+2)$ acetyl-CoA and $(m+4)$ OAA via GLS-GLDH-ME-PC- PDC pathway. ME: malic enzyme; PC: pyruvate carboxylase; PDC: pyruvate dehydrogenase complex; GLS: glutaminase; GLDH: glutamate dehydrogenase (GLDH). CO_2 indicates where carbon dioxide is released

The $(m+4)$ malate pool can also continue the forward reactions of the cycle to produce $(m+4)$-OAA, which then combines with $(m+2)$ acetyl-CoA to yield ^{13}C6-citrate $(m+6)$ (red, Fig. 6.5). This ^{13}C6-citrate (m+6) can proceed via backward reactions to produce acetyl CoA and OAA via the cytoplasmic ATP-citrate lyase (ACL, red), concomitantly generates ADP (Fig. 6.6).

The presence of the ^{13}C6-citrate isotopologue is the result of fully labeled acetyl CoA produced from the glutamine tracer via the ACL-ME-PDH pathway.

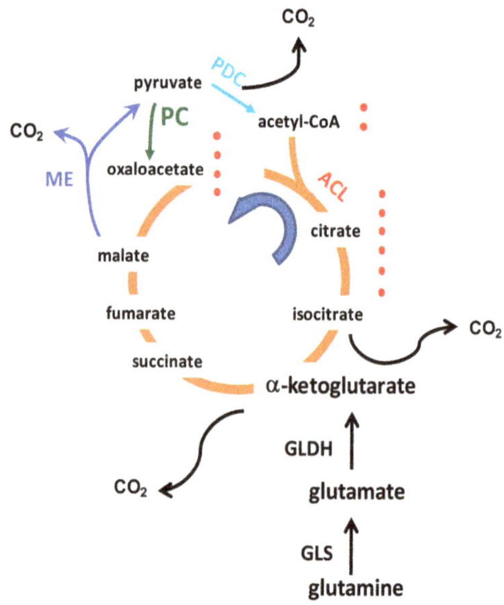

Fig. 6.6 The cytoplasmic ATP-citrate lyase (ACL) pathway

These citrate isotopologues will continue the forward reactions of the TCA cycle to make ^{13}C3-succinate, -fumarate, and -malate, which cannot be formed from labeled glutamine via the TCA cycle activity alone. Notably, ^{13}C,^{15}N-labeled glutamine only forms ^{13}C4-succinate, -fumarate, and -malate via TCA cycle activity. The ^{13}C4-citrate ($m+4$) can come from the combination of ^{13}C3-OAA and^{13}C1-acetyl CoA. The ^{13}C3-citrate ($m+3$) can come from ^{13}C2-OAA and^{13}C1-acetyl CoA or from ^{13}C3- OAA and non-labeled acetyl. The unlabeled acetyl-CoA is potentially the product of either fatty acid oxidation or the oxidation of amino acids.

Overall, the relative abundance of the $m+5$ is less than $m+3$, $m+4$, and $m+6$ citrate isotopologues, which are characteristic of the forward reactions in the Krebs cycle plus pyruvate carboxylation.

The malic enzyme (ME) is a key component in running the TCA cycle when it is dependent upon glutamine. ME converts malate to pyruvate, which is then converted to OAA via pyruvate carboxylation. These processes subsidize the TCA cycle with OAA and acetyl-CoA, making the cycle independent from glucose-derived metabolites, which would be advantageous for cancer cells subjected to glucose deficiency in the tumor microenvironment. In the absence of glucose, P493 cells remained viable, and still able to maintain cell populations, as compared to cells under glucose-replete conditions. This can be explained by the ability of glutamine metabolism to meet the energy demands of the cells and to maintain redox homeostasis. Specifically, the citrate produced through pathways of glutaminolysis also serves as a precursor for glutathione synthesis, which is critical in alleviating oxidative stress.

Using this glutamine dependent TCA cycle, cancer cells can produce 17.5 moles of ATP for every mole of glutamine. This process is much more efficient than the canonical glutaminolysis pathways, which convert glutamine to lactate, CO_2, and 5 moles of ATP, and completely bypass the TCA cycle [8–10]. These processes are critical for the survival and proliferation of cancer cells and are consistent with the fact that interruption of glutamine conversion by the means of a drug-tool glutaminase inhibitor, BPTES, increased ROS production and slowed cell growth. Genetic alterations, in addition to being the fundamental drivers of tumorigenesis, give rise to a variety of adaptive metabolic changes that further the extraordinary and characteristic capacity of cancer cells to reprogram the TCA cycle by depending on glutamine. This metabolic change demonstrates the flexibility of cancer cells' ability to utilize alternative fuel sources in order to generate energy, an important factor for tumor adaptation. More practically, therapeutic approaches that target metabolism must consider these adaptive strategies.

Glutamine Metabolism as a Target for Cancer Therapy

The recent elucidation of glutamine's more consequential involvement in cancer metabolism provides an attractive array of potential targets for therapeutic intervention. Given the evidence suggesting glutamine's novel role in a glucose-independent and glutamine-driven TCA cycle, a scheme to inhibit this alternative pathway of energy production so as to disrupt cancer progression is not only realistic and appealing, but is, in fact, already contributing promising results. The activation of the oncogene MYC facilitates glutamine uptake and an increase in glutaminolysis through a coordinated transcriptional program. The excessive intake of glutamine in cancer cells, along with its necessary role in glucose-independent glutamine metabolism via TCA cycling, demonstrates that increased aerobic glycolysis is not sufficient to drive the bioenergetics requirements that rapidly proliferating cancer cells demand [11]. Therefore, this specific, alternative energy-generating glutaminolysis pathway via TCA cycling is an attractive target of focus for therapy. Methods to regulate the level of glutamine and its metabolism can offer great promise in the prevention and treatment of cancer.

As shown in Fig. 6.7, one primitive test of this concept involves BPTES [bis-2-(5 phenylacetamido-1, 2, 4-thiadiazol-2-yl) ethyl sulfide]. This uncompetitive inhibitor has been elucidated to inhibit human glutaminase [12]. Studies have revealed that BPTES, a small molecule, binds to an allosteric site at the dimer interface of KGA—a kidney-type glutaminase isoform (GLS1)—and leads to a conformational change near the catalytic site, which inactivates the enzyme [13]. Thus, the interruption of glutamine metabolism by this inhibitor has shown to be a promising area of focus. In fact, the inhibition of glutaminase by BPTES activity in hypoxic conditions has shown to result in a killing effect on pancreatic cancer cells [5].

A member of the benzo[a]phenanthridinone family, compound 968 is a small molecule inhibitor that exploits a regulatory connection between NF-kB phosphorylating GAC, the slicing isoform of GLS1, and NF-kB, the latter of which is activated by Rho GTPases. Rho GTPases have previously been observed to be overexpressed and/or hyperactivated in a variety of cancers [14–16]. The treatment of human breast cancer cells with the small molecule 968 has been shown to reduce growth, density, and invasiveness of malignant cells [17]. Moreover, an additional effect was observed when cancer cells were dosed with 968 and BPTES simultaneously, suggesting that these inhibitors act via different mechanisms. This information could provide a realistic avenue for therapeutic intervention [18].

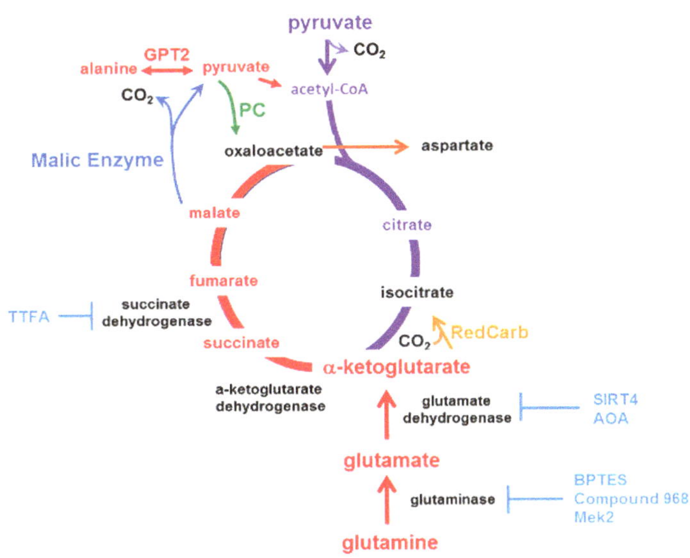

Fig. 6.7 The glucose-independent and glutamine-driven TCA Cycle relies on key enzymes to catalyze the production of ATP, nucleotides, lipids, and glutathione from glutamine. Efforts to inhibit glutaminase (GLS), which prepares glutamate and α-ketoglutarate for the TCA cycle, has led to the development and investigation of BPTES, compound 968, and Mek2-K101A. Similarly, SIRT4 has been studied for its inhibitory effect on glutamine dehydrogenase

Similar multidrug approaches toward the inhibition of target enzymes involved in glutamine metabolism have been explored. The combined inhibitory effect of Mek2 and BPTES on KGA and cell proliferation has been reported, and has introduced the potential for more effective designs and strategies to inhibit KGA- and Mek2-linked pathways to target glutamine metabolism [13]. Glutamate dehydrogenase has also been targeted as a means to indirectly inhibit glutamine metabolism. The inhibition of GLDH by SIRT4, a mitochondrial NAD-dependent ADP-ribosyltransferase encoded by the SIRT4 gene, has been shown to reduce the production of α-ketoglutarate, which in turn reduces the level of ATP production from the TCA cycle [19].

Key enzymes of the TCA cycle are also viable targets for the inhibition of glutamine metabolism. One such enzyme is succinate dehydrogenase (SDH), a critical component of the TCA cycle that catalyzes the conversion of succinate to fumarate. The inhibition of SDH by 2-thenoyltrifluoroacetone (TTFA) as a possible pathway for the disruption of glutamine metabolism has yet to be confirmed [20]. Aminooxyacetate (AOA), an inhibitor of glutamate-dependent transaminase, has also been shown to target glutamine metabolism, as well as to sensitize melanoma cells to tumor necrosis factor-related apoptosis inducing-ligand (TRAIL), while sparing normal cells [21].

Depending on their genetic makeup, cancer cells can become dependent on either glucose or glutamine to such an extent that they cannot survive without it. Exploitation of this dependence via inhibition of these pathways in some cancer cells provides therapeutic potential. However, this approach introduces great complexities, as cancer cells can exhibit unique metabolic pathways in addition to the classic metabolic pathways of normal cells. This plasticity makes it difficult to specifically target the metabolic enzymes in cancer cells while sparing those in normal cells.

Conclusion

A convergence of studies identify glutamine metabolism as a crucial component in the reprogramming of cancer cell metabolism. In this chapter, a glucose-independent, glutamine-driven TCA cycle is highlighted as an alternative energy-generating pathway for the survival and growth of tumor cells despite hypoxic and nutrient-deprived microenvironments. Through analysis of various labeled isotopologues of TCA cycle intermediates, the continued function of the TCA cycle in the absence of glucose, and sole presence of glutamine, provides substantial evidence that glutamine is a viable alternative source of energy for glucose-deprived cancer cells.

This alteration of cellular metabolism in cancer cells is linked with the oncogene MYC, which is involved in regulating glutamine metabolism. When this oncogene is induced, the enzyme glutaminase is expressed, and thus stimulates glutamine metabolism via the TCA cycle.

Given the importance of the glucose-independent and glutamine-driven TCA cycle in proliferating tumor cells, inhibitors like BPTES and 968 are being investigated to effectively exploit cancer's reliance on glutamine catabolism to meet its demanding bioenergetics needs. The coupled application of some of these inhibitors has already shown promise in vitro; therefore, future investigation to better design and develop drugs in order to disrupt the glucose-independent and glutamine-driven TCA cycle holds tremendous value for the advancement of preventing and treating cancer.

Acknowledgments The Sol Goldman Pancreatic Cancer Research Fund 80028595, Lustgarten Fund 90049125, and R21CA169757 (to A. Le). Special thanks to Michel Soudée and Laura Shingleton for their helpful comments.

Conflict of Interest The authors disclose no financial conflict of interest.

References

1. Dang CV. Links between metabolism and cancer. Genes Dev. 2012;26:877–90.
2. Sadava DE, Louis A. Duhring Fund. Life: the science of biology. 10th edition. 2012 Sunderland, MA: Sinauer Associates.
3. Vander Heiden MG, Cantley LC, Thompson CB. Understanding the Warburg effect: the metabolic requirements of cell proliferation. Science. 2009;324:1029–33.
4. Warburg O. On the origin of cancer cells. Science. 1956;123:309–14.
5. Le A, Lane AN, Hamaker M, et al. Glucose-independent glutamine metabolism via TCA cycling for proliferation and survival in B cells. Cell Metab. 2012;15:110–21.
6. Berg JM, Tymoczko JL, Stryer L, Clarence J. Marshall memorial library fund. Biochemistry. 5th ed. New York: W.H. Freeman; 2002.
7. Mullen AR, Wheaton WW, Jin ES, et al. Reductive carboxylation supports growth in tumour cells with defective mitochondria. Nature. 2011;481:385–8.
8. Helmlinger G, Schell A, Dellian M, Forbes NS, Jain RK. Acid production in glycolysis- impaired tumors provides new insights into tumor metabolism. Clin Cancer Res. 2002;8:1284–91.
9. Newsholme EA, Crabtree B, Ardawi MSM. Glutamine-Metabolism in Lymphocytes—Its Biochemical, Physiological and Clinical Importance. Q J Exp Physiol. 1985;70:473–89.
10. Newsholme EA, Crabtree B, Ardawi MSM. The role of high-rates of glycolysis and glutamine utilization in rapidly dividing cells. Biosci Rep. 1985;5:393–400.
11. Appleyard MV, O'Neill MA, Murray KE, et al. Seliciclib (CYC202, R-roscovitine) enhances the antitumor effect of doxorubicin in vivo in a breast cancer xenograft model. Int J Cancer. 2009;124:465–72.
12. Hartwick EW, Curthoys NP. BPTES inhibition of hGA(124-551), a truncated form of human kidney-type glutaminase. J Enzyme Inhib Med Chem. 2011;27:861–7.
13. Thangavelu K, Pan CQ, Karlberg T, et al. Structural basis for the allosteric inhibitory mechanism of human kidney-type glutaminase (KGA) and its regulation by Raf-Mek-Erk signaling in cancer cell metabolism. Proc Natl Acad Sci U S A. 2012;109:7705–10.
14. Suwa H, Ohshio G, Imamura T, et al. Overexpression of the rhoC gene correlates with progression of ductal adenocarcinoma of the pancreas. Br J Cancer. 1998;77:147–52.
15. Mira JP, Benard V, Groffen J, Sanders LC, Knaus UG. Endogenous, hyperactive Rac3 controls proliferation of breast cancer cells by a p21-activated kinase-dependent pathway. Proc Natl Acad Sci U S A. 2000;97:185–9.
16. Fritz G, Brachetti C, Bahlmann F, Schmidt M, Kaina B. Rho GTPases in human breast tumours: expression and mutation analyses and correlation with clinical parameters. Br J Cancer. 2002;87:635–44.
17. Wang JB, Erickson JW, Fuji R, et al. Targeting mitochondrial glutaminase activity inhibits oncogenic transformation. Cancer Cell. 2010;18:207–19.
18. Katt WP, Ramachandran S, Erickson JW, Cerione RA. Dibenzophenanthridines as inhibitors of glutaminase C and cancer cell proliferation. Mol Cancer Ther. 2012;11:1269–78.
19. Haigis MC, Mostoslavsky R, Haigis KM, et al. SIRT4 inhibits glutamate dehydrogenase and opposes the effects of calorie restriction in pancreatic beta cells. Cell. 2006;126:941–54.
20. Cervera AM, Bayley JP, Devilee P, McCreath KJ. Inhibition of succinate dehydrogenase dysregulates histone modification in mammalian cells. Mol Cancer. 2009;8:89.
21. Qin JZ, Xin H, Nickoloff BJ. Targeting glutamine metabolism sensitizes melanoma cells to TRAIL-induced death. Biochem Biophys Res Commun. 2010;398:146–52.

Chapter 7
The Role of Glutamine Synthetase in the Glutamine Independence in Mammary Tissue

Hsiu-Ni Kung and Jen-Tsan Chi

Key Points

- Glutamine is an essential nutrient that feeds into multiple metabolic pathways of tumor cells.
- There are significant heterogeneity of glutamine metabolisms between the basal vs. luminal breast cancer cells.
- Basal breast cancer cells are addicted to exogenous glutamine while luminal breast cancer cells are independent of exogenous glutamine.
- The distinct glutamine metabolism and dependence are mediated by their distinct expression patterns of genes and enzymes that involved in glutamine metabolisms.
- The glutamine addiction of basal-type breast cancer cells is triggered by c-myc and presents therapeutic opportunities.
- The glutamine independence of luminal-type breast cancer cells is mediated by the cell-type-specific expression of glutamine synthetase triggered by GATA3.
- Significant metabolic interaction and symbiosis between the adjacent luminal and basal breast cancers.
- Control of glutamine availability and metabolism represents a promising therapeutic strategy.

Keywords Glutamine • Glutamate • Breast cancer • Luminal • Basal • Glutaminase • Glutamine synthetase • GATA3

Abbreviations

ALL	Acute lymphoblastic leukemia
ALT	Alanine transaminase
ASCT2	Neutral amino acid transporter

H.-N. Kung, Ph.D. (✉)
Department of Anatomy and Cell Biology, School of Medicine, National Taiwan University, 1-1 Jen-Ai Road, Taipei 10051, Taiwan
e-mail: kunghsiuni@gmail.com

J.-T. Chi, M.D., Ph.D. (✉)
Department of Molecular Genetics & Microbiology, Center for Genomics and Computational Biology, Duke Medical Center, 101 Science Drive, DUMC 3382, CIEMAS 2177A, Durham, NC, USA
e-mail: jentsan.chi@duke.edu

R. Rajendram et al. (eds.), *Glutamine in Clinical Nutrition*, Nutrition and Health, DOI 10.1007/978-1-4939-1932-1_7,

AST	Aspartate transaminase
DNA	Deoxyribonucleic acid
FAS	Fatty acid synthase
GCL	Glutamate cysteine ligase
Gln (Q)	Glutamine
GLS	Glutaminase
Glu (E)	Glutamate
GLUL	Glutamate-ammonia ligase
GS	Glutamine synthetase
mRNA	Messenger ribonucleic acid
mTOR	Mammalian target of rapamycin complex 1
NADPH	Nicotinamide adenine dinucleotide phosphate
NF-κB	Nuclear factor κ light-chain enhancer of activated B cells
TCA	Tricarboxylic acid
TNBC	Triple-negative breast cancer

Introduction

Treatment for breast cancer has advanced significantly in recent years and is at least partly responsible for the recent improvement in disease outcome. Even with these advances, the American Cancer Society estimated that 39,620 US women will die of the disease in 2013. Continual improvements in chemo, hormonal, and molecular targeted therapies will continue to chip away at these numbers, although likely only with incremental benefit. Triple negative breast cancer (TNBC) is the subset of breast tumors that are negative for ER, PR and HER2 amplification [1]. The treatment for TNBC has been challenging due to the lack of well-defined molecular targets and heterogeneity of the disease. TNBC tumors tend to be larger, respond less well to chemotherapeutics and exhibit higher propensity for metastasis. Detailed characterizations of cancer genomes have revealed how genetic dysregulation contributes to tumor heterogeneity [2]. However, few effective therapeutic targets have emerged, especially for TNBC. For example, recent analysis of the gene expression of a large number of TNBC tumors have identified at least six different subtypes of TNBC that show significant differences in the biological behaviors and response to various therapeutic agents [3].

One possible ways to treat TNBC is to exploit the distinct metabolic requirements between normal and cancerous cells. Different types of cells have distinct ways of utilizing nutrients and generating energy, thus resulting in diverse nutrient needs or addictions. Among different differentiated cells, such cell-type-specific metabolic differences may preserve during the oncogenic transformations to exhibit similar differences in the corresponding transformed cells. For example, glutamine is recognized as an important and essential nutrient that contributes to various metabolic processes and signaling events of oncogenesis in human cancers. Therefore, the therapeutic targeting of glutamine metabolism has been proposed to have significant potential. However, the mechanisms of glutamine dependence and likely response and resistance of such glutamine-targeting strategies among cancers are largely unknown. Recently, we have found a systematic variation in the glutamine dependence among breast tumor subtypes associated with mammary differentiation: basal- but not luminal-type breast cells are more glutamine-dependent and may be susceptible to glutamine-targeting therapeutics [4]. Glutamine independence of luminal-type cells is associated mechanistically with lineage-specific expression of glutamine synthetase (GS). Luminal cells can also rescue basal cells in co-culture without glutamine, indicating a potential for glutamine symbiosis within breast ducts. The luminal-specific expression of GS is directly induced by GATA3 and represses glutaminase expression. Such distinct glutamine dependency and metabolic symbiosis is coupled with the acquisition of the GS and glutamine independence during the mammary differentiation program. Understanding the genetic circuitry governing distinct metabolic patterns is relevant to many symbiotic relationships among different cells and organisms. In addition, the ability of GS to predict patterns of glutamine metabolism and dependency among tumors is also crucial in the rational design and application of glutamine and other metabolic pathway targeted therapies.

Dysregulated Metabolism as Potential Therapeutic Targets in Cancers

Dysregulation of basic metabolic processes is often associated with oncogenic progression. Therefore a detailed knowledge of cancer biochemistry may be of critical importance to understand the disease [5, 6]. The metabolic changes of cancer cells create specific therapeutic windows, or "metabolic Achilles' heels," some of which have already provided treatment opportunities for certain types of cancer, such as the use of asparaginase to treat acute lymphoblastic leukemia (ALL). However, very few ongoing efforts focus on realizing the "metabolic Achilles' heel" potential in breast cancer. While metabolic pathways of most untransformed cells usually exhibit great flexibility, which can become significantly limited during oncogenic transformation. The Warburg effect remains a central concept of tumor physiology: the use of glycolysis for energy renders cancer cells addicted to glucose and therefore sensitive to inhibition by glucose analogues. Similarly, different oncogenic mutations limit cellular metabolic flexibility by altering requirements for certain amino acids. Glutamine is reported to be essential for cancer cells harboring oncogenic events including c-myc activation [7–9]. Recently, we found that inflexible tumor metabolic dysregulation is manifest in basal-type breast cancer cells which both exhibit a robust hypoxia program [10] and require exogenous glutamine for survival [4]. Several recent reports have also revealed that exogenous glutamine is essential under hypoxia or lactic acidosis in the presence of an IDH1 mutation for lipid biogenesis [11–13]. Therefore, glutamine metabolism has been considered an attractive target for the significant number of tumors that appear to be addicted to this nutrient [14, 15]. In addition, other amino acids can also be essential for tumor cells. Asparagine is required to maintain the viability of acute lymphoblastic leukemia (ALL), providing a rational basis for asparaginase treatment [16]. Also, leucine deprivation causes the apoptotic death of melanoma cells [17]. Other studies have highlighted the essentiality of arginine, [18] methionine, [19] and valine [20] in various biological contexts. These data indicate that amino acid addiction is a common cancer phenomenon. While systematic information that links amino acid addictions and cancer genetics remains largely absent, understanding this connection is now feasible with current biochemical and genetic methods.

The Role of Glutamine in the Metabolisms and Signaling of Cancer Cells

Glutamine is the most abundant amino acid in plasma and has long been recognized to play a unique role in the metabolism of proliferating cells. While first reported in 1970s, the essential role of glutamine in cancer metabolisms is not well understood until recent studies using the modern biochemical and genetic tools. Glutamine plays several important metabolic roles, including as carbon source for energy production, contributes carbon and nitrogen to biosynthetic reactions, regulates lipid generation, and adjusts redox homeostasis (Fig. 7.1). Glutamine availability and metabolism also tightly intersected with signal transduction pathways involved in oncogenesis. Each of these following functions of glutamine supports different aspects of the metabolic requirement of cell growth and proliferation.

Glutamine as carbon sources: While non-proliferating cells can completely oxidize glucose-derived carbon in the TCA cycle to support their energy needs, proliferating cells use nutrients to support

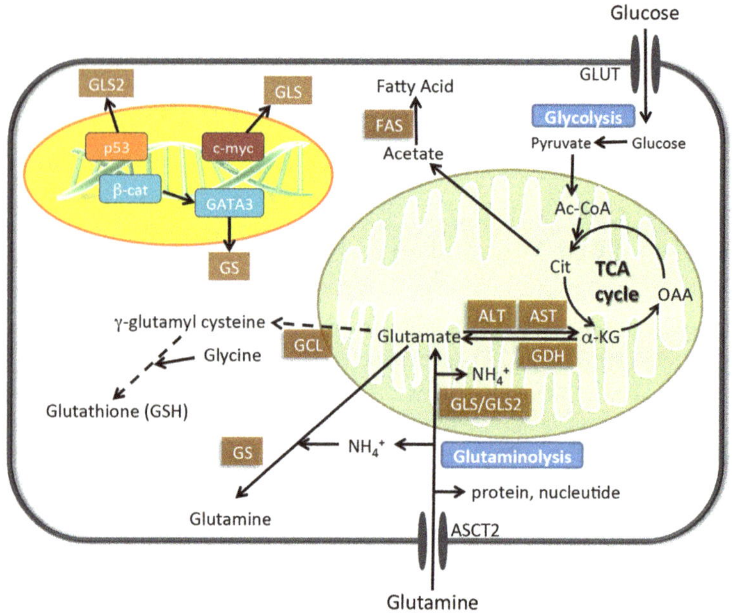

Fig. 7.1 Glutamine and glucose metabolism. The import and metabolisms of glucose and glutamine metabolisms in the cytosol, mitochondria, TCA cycle, GSH synthesis, and fatty acid synthesis. The transcriptional regulation of several genes involved in glutamine metabolism, including glutaminase (GLS1 and GLS2) and glutamine synthetase (GS) in the nuclei

biosynthesis of macromolecules for proliferation. To support lipid biosynthesis from acetyl-CoA in the cytoplasm, citrate is exported out of the mitochondria to generate acetyl-CoA (Fig. 7.1). This will deplete the metabolic metabolites in TCA and require additional source to replenish the TCA cycle in processes called anapleurosis. Glutamine serves as an important anaplerotic substrate in most proliferating cells to generate oxaloacetate that will combine with acetyl-CoA to replenish citrate. Glutamine's role as a carbon source is critical for many cancer cells which are glutamine addicted. The cellular viability can be restored by supplementing cells with TCA cycle intermediates, such as pyruvate, oxaloacetate, or α-ketoglutarate. Under hypoxia or mitochondria dysfunction, glutamine can also directly supply acetyl-CoA for lipogenesis by converting malate into pyruvate, by malic enzyme, which re-enters the TCA cycle as acetyl-CoA. The α-ketoglutarate can undergo reductive carboxylation to generate isocitrate, which is then converted into citrate by a process termed "reductive carboxylation." [11, 12]

Glutamine as nitrogen sources: The amido and amino groups of glutamine contribute to multiple biosynthetic pathways, including synthesis of nonessential amino acids, nucleotides, and hexosamines, especially during proliferation. K-ras-transformed fibroblasts cultured in glutamine-depleted media exhibit decreased cellular proliferation and abortive S phase entrance, which could be restored by addition of the four deoxyribonucleotides. Interestingly, the expression of glutaminase 1 (GLS1) and the glutamine consumption is tightly regulated within the process of cell cycle—highly expressed during S phase and decreases as cells progress into G2/M. This cell-cycle regulation is due to its targeted by APC/C (anaphase-promoting complex/cyclosome)-Cdh1, the ubiquitin ligase that controls G1- to S-phase transition. A decrease in the activity of APC/C-Cdh1 in mid-to-late G1 releases GLS1 and simultaneously increases glutamine utilization during cell proliferation. Thus, the function of glutamine during DNA synthesis contributes to its role in supporting cell proliferation.

Glutamine as signaling molecules and redox homeostasis: In addition to serving metabolic needs, glutamine has also been implicated in modulating cell-signaling pathways to promote growth. These signaling events include mammalian target of rapamycin complex 1 (mTORC1) [21], mitochondrial ROS production [22] and ERK signaling [23]. Glutamine metabolism also plays a key role in the cellular redox homeostasis by its role in synthesis of glutathione, an endogenous antioxidant comprised of glutamate, cysteine, and glycine. The high level of glutathione (GSH) makes it the predominant cellular anti-oxidants that neutralize the ROS by donating electrons and becoming oxidized (GSSG). The regeneration of GSH from GSSG requires NADPH, which can be produced by glutamine metabolism through malic enzyme [24, 25].

The Heterogeneity of Tumor Metabolisms in Breast Cancers

It is now well established that significant heterogeneity of metabolism exists among human breast cancers. This heterogeneity is observable at every level of examination from the macroscopic to the molecular. Recent large-scale efforts to measure and describe human breast tumor heterogeneity include the Cancer Genome Atlas (TCGA) where a number of high-throughput "omic" technologies were systemically applied to hundreds of primary cancer specimens [26]. Mutations, germ line polymorphisms, DNA copy number, RNA expression, DNA methylation, and protein expression analyses were performed in parallel on a large and carefully curated set of breast cancer specimens to produce the most comprehensive molecular portrait of the disease to date.

One significant metric that was not included in TGCA was an unbiased analysis of tumor metabolism. While metabolic flux cannot be measured in fixed or frozen specimens, steady-state levels of numerous key metabolites may provide insight into these fundamental phenotypic traits. A number of studies in cancer have uncovered relationships between genetic abnormalities and various metabolic reprogramming suggesting that key metabolic process can be altered as a result of specific transformation events [27–29]. Relatively nonspecific cancer related events such as increased proliferation may also underlie some of the inferred/observed metabolic remodeling. Glucose uptake, serine and glutamine auxotrophy, and mitochondrial oxidative phosphorylation all appear to have roles in defining breast cancer metabolism [10]. However, it is not clear whether these regulatory relationships can be observed in all or subsets of human tumors.

Breast cancers are broadly categorized as luminal versus basal types possibly derived from different precursor cells or at least different committed parental lineages [30, 31]. Within these broad categories, alterations in specific driver genes are believed to produce the heterogeneity observed amongst and within breast tumor subtypes. While the identity and frequency of driver alterations are generally different in basal and luminal cancers, there is still considerable overlap. For example, TP53 mutations are very common in basal tumors and so as PI3KCA mutations in luminal cancer, but neither is subtype exclusive. In contrast, MYC (8q24) amplification can be seen in both types. Each of these genetic drivers has been associated with specific changes in cellular metabolism and therefore may have dominant effects that can be observed across tumor types. Metabolomic profiling via mass spectrometry or NMR is now an established approach that has been employed in several studies to analyze primary human breast tissues (normal and cancer) [32–34]. Building upon transcriptional profiling of breast cancer, there have also been several efforts to integrate steady-state metabolite levels with specific breast cancer subtypes defined by mRNA expression. Expression subtypes are dominated by estrogen receptor and ERBB2 status and thus, metabolic profiling was performed to seek an additional level of information to refine these existing classifications. These analyses identified a subclassification of luminal A type cancers based on metabolite levels and found higher levels of Warburg-associated metabolites in more aggressive cancer types [35, 36].

Glutamine Addiction vs. Independence in Breast Cancers

The metabolism in cancer cells is different from normal cells, and they uptake more nutrients from the environment to survive and even spread. Two nutrients, glucose and glutamine, are main sources of energy production for tumor cells. Although high glucose consumption (Warburg effect) is recognized

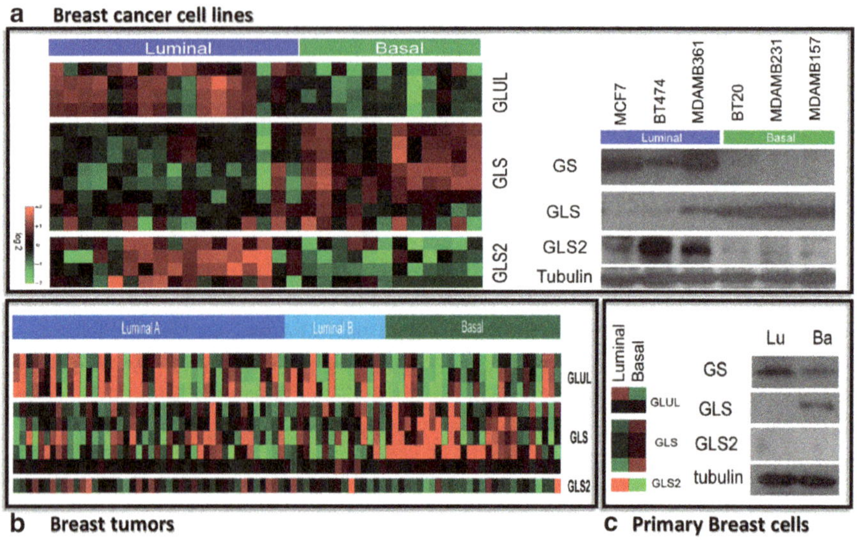

Fig. 7.2 The differential expression of GLS1, GLS2 and GS (GLUL) in the luminal vs. basal cancer cell lines (**a**), primary breast tumor (**b**) and isolated primary breast cells (**c**)

as a selective marker for tumor cells, the glutamine need in tumor cells is getting noticed and under huge amount of investigations by scientists. Glutamine for tumors not only serves as a nitrogen donor, in nucleotide and amino acid biosynthesis, but also a primary mitochondrial substrate, for maintenance of mitochondrial membrane potential and integrity, NADPH production, and glutathione production (Fig. 7.1). Researchers revealed that different breast cancer cells have various glutamine dependencies. The glutamine-dependent cells cannot survive or grow in glutamine-free condition, such as MDAMB231 and SUM149, and the growth of glutamine-independent cells is not limited in glutamine free environment, such as MCF10A and MCF7 [37].

There are two key enzymes directly involve in the metabolism of glutamine, glutaminase (GLS/GLS2) and glutamine synthetase (GS). These two enzymes help controlling the intracellular glutamine homeostasis. GLS is the first enzyme in the glutamine utilizing pathway that transfers glutamine into glutamate and amine group. Glutamate can be used as the blocks of DNA, RNA, or protein synthesis or further metabolized into α-ketoglutarate and thus included into the TCA cycle for ATP production. In order to avoid the toxicity of glutamate and amine group inside cells, these two components can be joined by GS to form glutamine again.

The expression pattern of glutamine-related enzymes, including GS, GLS, and GLS2, is conspicuously different between luminal and basal breast cancer cells (Fig. 7.2a), as well in breast tumor samples (Fig. 7.2b) and normal breast cells (Fig. 7.2c), and this distinguishing expression pattern may be related to the glutamine preference in breast cancer cells.

Glutamine Addiction of the "Basal"-Type Breast Cancer Tumors

The high rate of glutamine uptake and glutamine utilization exhibited by glutamine-dependent cells is called "glutamine addiction." [15] Since this type of cells uses and uptakes more glutamine as the main energy resource, they should have higher GLS to get more glutamate for TCA cycle. The expression of GLS is controlled by Myc protein, which suppresses the GLS inhibitor, miR-23a/b [9, 38]. Myc is frequently overexpressed in aggressive breast cancers, drive poor prognosis gene expression signature, and a marker for tumor malignancy [39–42]. Myc is also found to distinguish basal-type

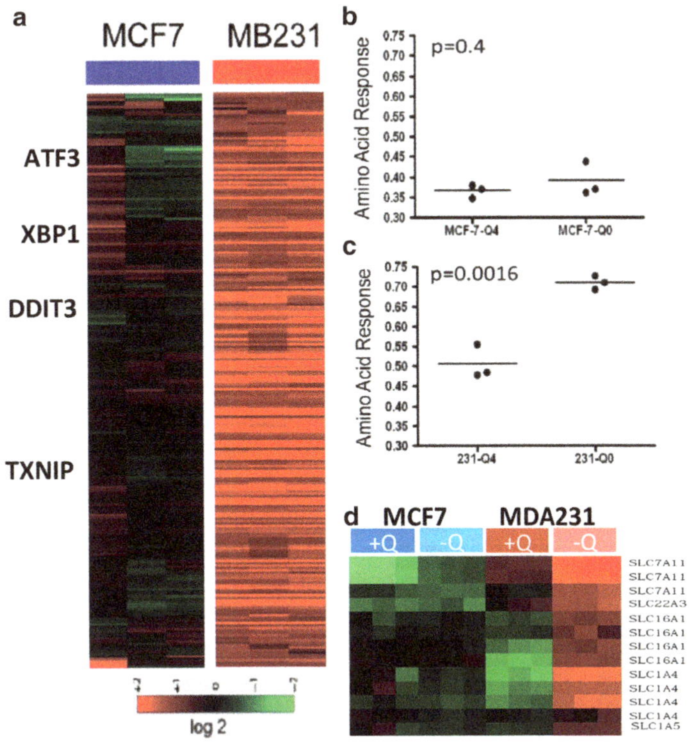

Fig. 7.3 The differential transcriptional response of MCF-7 and MDA-MB231 to glutamine deprivation (**a**) and the amino acid response in the MCF-7 (**b**) and MDA-MB231 (**c**). Induction of several glutamine transporters by glutamine deprivation in MDA-MB231 but not MCF-7. The relative expressions of various glutamine transporters in both MCF7 and MDAMB231 cells with or without glutamine (**d**)

breast cancer from luminal-type breast cancer [41, 43, 44]. It is also obvious that GLS level is significantly higher in basal type of cells [4]. From all the researches mentioned above, glutamine addiction can be positively linked to basal-type breast tumor, with higher myc and glutaminase levels (Fig. 7.2). Furthermore, this phenomenon can be observed in breast tumors and primary breast cells (Fig. 7.2). Under glutamine deprivation environment, the DNA synthesis is stopped [45] and the amino acid response (AAR) genes are activated [4, 46], including TXNIP, XBP1, and ATF3, in glutamine-addicted tumor cells (Fig. 7.3a–c). The expression levels of various glutamine transporters were also dramatically induced by glutamine deprivation in basal breast cancer cells, but not in luminal-type breast cancer cells (Fig. 7.3d, unpublished data).

Unlike the expression position of kidney type of glutaminase (GLS), there is another subtype of glutaminase, the liver-type glutaminase (GLS2), which expressed in different organs. GLS2 expression is induced in response to DNA damage or oxidative stress in a p53-dependent manner, and overexpression of GLS2 reduces the growth of tumor cells and colony formation. GLS2 level is lower in basal-type breast tumors [4] (Fig. 7.2), showing that basal breast tumors use GLS as the key enzyme transferring glutamine to glutamate for energy production and other functions. Among these two enzymes, GLS has been demonstrated to be correlated to tumor cell growth and be regulated by oncogenes, while GLS2 behaves more like a tumor suppressor by glutathione-dependent antioxidant defense. Thus, modulation of glutaminase function may be a new therapeutic target for cancer treatment [47].

Glutamine Independence of the "Luminal"-Type Breast Tumors

Except glutamine-addicted basal-type breast cancer cells, luminal-type breast cancer cells are more glutamine independent [4, 45]. Luminal cells have higher glutamine synthetase (GS) and lower GLS in cells [4] (Fig. 7.2). The higher GS level is regulated by GATA3 [4] (Fig. 7.1), which promotes luminal cell differentiation in luminal breast cancers [48]. GATA3 is also a downstream signaling element in β-catenin pathway [49]; thus the GS expression level could also be controlled by β-catenin. In addition, GATA3 causes the downregulation of GLS, which the mechanism is still unclear [4] and need further investigations. GS can generate glutamine from glutamate and amine group, while the usage of glutamine is reduced by the downregulation of GLS, thus indicating that luminal breast cancer cells can resist extracellular glutamine deprivation [4].

Glutamine Synthetase and Glutaminase as Determinants of Glutamine Dependence Phenotypes

The differential expression of glutamine-metabolizing enzymes among luminal and basal breast cancers correlate to the distinct glutamine requirement, and are consistent with the genetic circuitry governing breast cancer subtypes [4, 45]. Basal-type breast tumor usually exhibit a more malignant phenotype with few current therapeutic options, they may benefit from glutamine-targeting therapies with the feature of glutamine addiction [14, 15]. Although GS and GLS cannot perfectly distinguish the subtypes within basal-type breast tumors [45], such as claudin-low, their expression still can be determinants of glutamine dependence phenotypes in the breast tumor analysis. Since glutamine metabolism could be a potential therapeutic target, researchers now focus on searching more promising targets in the glutamine metabolism. A potential target, xCT antiporter, is recently found to be a therapeutic target in triple-negative breast tumors [45].

Metabolic Symbiosis Between Different Breast Cancer Cells

When facing glutamine deprivation condition, intracellular GS level increased to produce more glutamine supporting the cell survival and regular functions in luminal cells (Figs. 7.4a and 7.5a). They even can export the excess glutamine to the environment to sustain the survival of adjacent cells, including basal-type breast cells [4]. With transwell co-culture technique, we observe that the survival of basal-type breast cancer cell, MDAMB231, is increased by the co-culture of MCF7 under glutamine deprivation (Fig. 7.4b). Since higher GS leads cells become more glutamine independent, and GS is regulated by GATA3, MDAMB231 cells can produce more glutamine with GS or GATA3 overexpression (Fig. 7.4c-right panel). The survival of MDAMB231 cell is upregulated by co-culturing with GS or GATA3 overexpression MDAMB231 (Fig. 7.4c-lower panel), which means the increase of GS in cells helps MDAMB231 cells to generate glutamine and export to the environment and the glutamine can support the critical survival of glutamine addicted basal-type breast cancer cells under glutamine deprivation situation (Fig. 7.5a). This nutritional and metabolic symbiosis can be seen in many organisms and cell types, for example the symbiotic nitrogen fixation in the root nodules on legumes of plants, the mutualistic symbiosis between bacteria and insects, and the shuttle glutamine-glutamate transport between neuron cell and glial cells (Fig. 7.5b).

Since basal-type breast tumor is more sensitive to glutamine withdrawal, targeting glutamine metabolisms may present potential target therapy for TNBC with few therapeutic choices. In the process of glutamine denudation, luminal-type breast cells or other non-tumor cells, such as fibroblast and macrophages, might synthesize glutamine and export glutamine to extracellular environment or into the blood circulation to provide the survival of basal-type breast and to reduce the effect of glutamine targeting therapy. Therefore, GS inhibition should be combined into the glutamine targeting therapy to improve the efficiency and reduce the resistance in treating basal-type breast tumors with glutamine-targeting therapies.

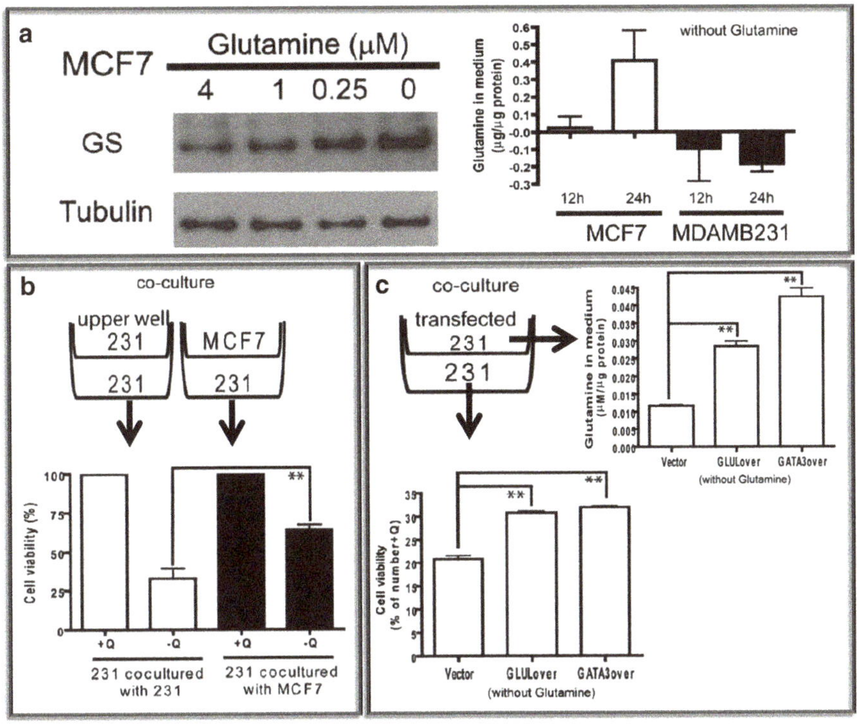

Fig. 7.4 Co-culture of basal and luminal breast cells in glutamine symbiosis. (**a**) The induction of GS protein and medium glutamine levels in MCF7 (**b**) A diagram illustrating the co-culture systems and increased viability of 231 cells when co-cultured with MCF7. (**c**) The co-culture system of MDAMB231 cells (base) with GLUL- or GATA3-overexpression MDAMB231 cells (transwell membrane). The glutamine concentration in the medium and the survival of MDAMB231 cells (base) were both increased significantly

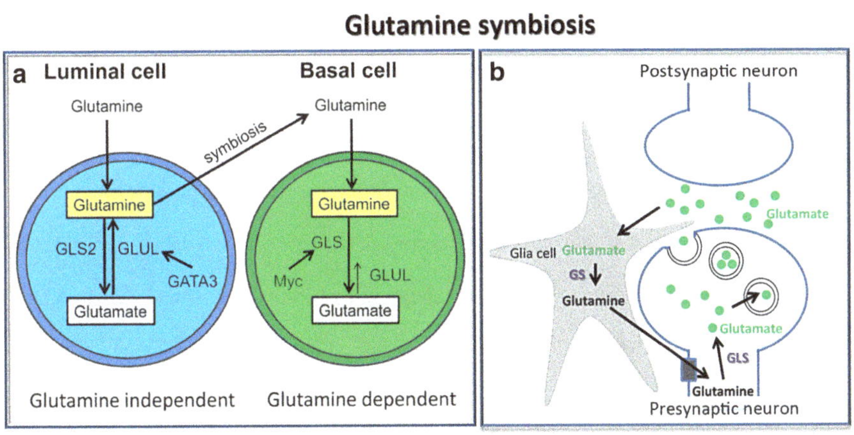

Fig. 7.5 (**a**) Model of distinct glutamine metabolism and symbiosis between luminal and basal breast cancer cells. (**b**) Similar glutamine symbiosis between glial and neuron cells by GS

Conclusion

With all the therapies in the clinic for now, breast tumor, especially the TNBC or basal-type breast cancers, is still a great threaten among various tumors. Finding a new and promising therapeutic strategy is urgent and demands immediate attention. The glutamine dependency can be a potential target for treating breast cancers. Although not in a perfect correlation, the glutamine metabolic enzymes, GS and GLS, controlled the glutamine dependency. With the glutamine addiction phenotype, drugs targeting glutaminase is thought to be a good way to inhibit the growth of basal-type breast tumors with few therapeutic options. But with higher GS levels, luminal breast cancer cells are more glutamine independent. They even can export excess glutamine to support the cells in the neighborhood, which could lower the efficiency of glutamine targeting therapy on basal-type breast cancer cells. Combine with the glutamine symbiosis between luminal and basal-type breast cancer cells, GS inhibition should be combined with glutamine-targeting therapy to increase the effect and decrease the resistance of therapy.

References

1. Foulkes WD, Smith IE, Reis-Filho JS. Triple-negative breast cancer. N Engl J Med. 2010;363(20):1938–48.
2. The Cancer Genome Atlas Network. Comprehensive molecular portraits of human breast tumours. Nature. 2012;490(7418):61–70.
3. Lehmann BD, Bauer JA, Chen X, et al. Identification of human triple-negative breast cancer subtypes and preclinical models for selection of targeted therapies. J Clin Invest. 2011;121(7):2750–67.
4. Kung HN, Marks JR, Chi JT. Glutamine synthetase is a genetic determinant of cell type-specific glutamine independence in breast epithelia. PLoS Genet. 2011;7(8):e1002229.
5. Sreekumar A, Poisson LM, Rajendiran TM, et al. Metabolomic profiles delineate potential role for sarcosine in prostate cancer progression. Nature. 2009;457(7231):910–4.
6. Dang L, White DW, Gross S, et al. Cancer-associated IDH1 mutations produce 2-hydroxyglutarate. Nature. 2010;465(7300):966.
7. Yuneva M, Zamboni N, Oefner P, Sachidanandam R, Lazebnik Y. Deficiency in glutamine but not glucose induces MYC-dependent apoptosis in human cells. J Cell Biol. 2007;178(1):93–105.
8. Wise DR, DeBerardinis RJ, Mancuso A, et al. Myc regulates a transcriptional program that stimulates mitochondrial glutaminolysis and leads to glutamine addiction. Proc Natl Acad Sci U S A. 2008;105(48):18782–7.
9. Gao P, Tchernyshyov I, Chang TC, et al. c-Myc suppression of miR-23a/b enhances mitochondrial glutaminase expression and glutamine metabolism. Nature. 2009;458(7239):762–5.
10. Gatza ML, Kung HN, Blackwell KL, Dewhirst MW, Marks JR, Chi JT. Analysis of tumor environmental response and oncogenic pathway activation identifies distinct basal and luminal features in HER2-related breast tumor subtypes. Breast Cancer Res. 2011;13(3):R62.
11. Metallo CM, Gameiro PA, Bell EL, et al. Reductive glutamine metabolism by IDH1 mediates lipogenesis under hypoxia. Nature. 2012;481(7381):380–4.
12. Mullen AR, Wheaton WW, Jin ES, et al. Reductive carboxylation supports growth in tumour cells with defective mitochondria. Nature. 2012;481(7381):385–8.
13. Lamonte G, Tang X, Chen JL, et al. Acidosis induces reprogramming of cellular metabolism to mitigate oxidative stress. Cancer Metab. 2014;1:23.
14. Wang JB, Erickson JW, Fuji R, et al. Targeting mitochondrial glutaminase activity inhibits oncogenic transformation. Cancer Cell. 2010;18(3):207–19.
15. Wise DR, Thompson CB. Glutamine addiction: a new therapeutic target in cancer. Trends Biochem Sci. 2010;35(8):427–33.
16. Clavell LA, Gelber RD, Cohen HJ, et al. Four-agent induction and intensive asparaginase therapy for treatment of childhood acute lymphoblastic leukemia. N Engl J Med. 1986;315(11):657–63.
17. Sheen JH, Zoncu R, Kim D, Sabatini DM. Defective regulation of autophagy upon leucine deprivation reveals a targetable liability of human melanoma cells in vitro and in vivo. Cancer Cell. 2011;19(5):613–28.
18. Scott L, Lamb J, Smith S, Wheatley DN. Single amino acid (arginine) deprivation: rapid and selective death of cultured transformed and malignant cells. Br J Cancer. 2000;83(6):800–10.
19. Kreis W, Baker A, Ryan V, Bertasso A. Effect of nutritional and enzymatic methionine deprivation upon human normal and malignant cells in tissue culture. Cancer Res. 1980;40(3):634–41.
20. Ohtawa K, Ueno T, Mitsui K, et al. Apoptosis of leukemia cells induced by valine-deficient medium. Leukemia. 1998;12(10):1651–2.
21. Marc Rhoads J, Wu G. Glutamine, arginine, and leucine signaling in the intestine. Amino Acids. 2009;37(1):111–22.
22. Reid MA, Wang WI, Rosales KR, Welliver MX, Pan M, Kong M. The B55alpha subunit of PP2A drives a p53-dependent metabolic adaptation to glutamine deprivation. Mol Cell. 2013;50(2):200–11.

23. Thangavelu K, Pan CQ, Karlberg T, et al. Structural basis for the allosteric inhibitory mechanism of human kidney-type glutaminase (KGA) and its regulation by Raf-Mek-Erk signaling in cancer cell metabolism. Proc Natl Acad Sci U S A. 2012;109(20):7705–10.
24. Moreadith RW, Lehninger AL. The pathways of glutamate and glutamine oxidation by tumor cell mitochondria. Role of mitochondrial NAD(P)+-dependent malic enzyme. J Biol Chem. 1984;259(10):6215–21.
25. Sauer LA, Dauchy RT, Nagel WO. Identification of an NAD(P)+-dependent 'malic' enzyme in small-intestinal-mucosal mitochondria. Biochem J. 1979;184(1):185–8.
26. Cancer Genome Atlas Network. Comprehensive molecular portraits of human breast tumours. Nature. 2012; 490(7418):61–70.
27. Levine AJ, Puzio-Kuter AM. The control of the metabolic switch in cancers by oncogenes and tumor suppressor genes. Science. 2010;330(6009):1340–4.
28. Reitman ZJ, Jin G, Karoly ED, et al. Profiling the effects of isocitrate dehydrogenase 1 and 2 mutations on the cellular metabolome. Proc Natl Acad Sci U S A. 2011;108(8):3270–5.
29. Yuneva MO, Fan TW, Allen TD, et al. The metabolic profile of tumors depends on both the responsible genetic lesion and tissue type. Cell Metab. 2012;15(2):157–70.
30. Perou CM, Sorlie T, Eisen MB, et al. Molecular portraits of human breast tumours. Nature. 2000;406(6797):747–52.
31. Lim E, Vaillant F, Wu D, et al. Aberrant luminal progenitors as the candidate target population for basal tumor development in BRCA1 mutation carriers. Nat Med. 2009;15(8):907–13.
32. Tang X, Lin CC, Spasojevic I, Iversen ES, Chi JT, Marks JR. A joint analysis of metabolomics and genetics of breast cancer. Breast Cancer Res. 2014 Aug 5;16(4):415.
33. Sitter B, Lundgren S, Bathen TF, Halgunset J, Fjosne HE, Gribbestad IS. Comparison of HR MAS MR spectroscopic profiles of breast cancer tissue with clinical parameters. NMR Biomed. 2006;19(1):30–40.
34. Budczies J, Denkert C, Muller BM, et al. Remodeling of central metabolism in invasive breast cancer compared to normal breast tissue - a GC-TOFMS based metabolomics study. BMC Genomics. 2012;13:334.
35. Borgan E, Sitter B, Lingjaerde OC, et al. Merging transcriptomics and metabolomics–advances in breast cancer profiling. BMC Cancer. 2010;10:628.
36. Brauer HA, Makowski L, Hoadley KA, et al. Impact of tumor microenvironment and epithelial phenotypes on metabolism in breast cancer. Clin Cancer Res. 2013;19(3):571–85.
37. Singh B, Tai K, Madan S, et al. Selection of metastatic breast cancer cells based on adaptability of their metabolic state. PLoS One. 2012;7(5):e36510.
38. Dang CV. MYC, microRNAs and glutamine addiction in cancers. Cell Cycle. 2009;8(20):3243–5.
39. Nair R, Roden DL, Teo WS, et al. c-Myc and Her2 cooperate to drive a stem-like phenotype with poor prognosis in breast cancer. Oncogene. 2014;33(30):3992–4002.
40. Horiuchi D, Kusdra L, Huskey NE, et al. MYC pathway activation in triple-negative breast cancer is synthetic lethal with CDK inhibition. J Exp Med. 2012;209(4):679–96.
41. Xu J, Chen Y, Olopade OI. MYC and breast cancer. Genes Cancer. 2010;1(6):629–40.
42. Ben-Porath I, Thomson MW, Carey VJ, et al. An embryonic stem cell-like gene expression signature in poorly differentiated aggressive human tumors. Nat Genet. 2008;40(5):499–507.
43. Chandriani S, Frengen E, Cowling VH, et al. A core MYC gene expression signature is prominent in basal-like breast cancer but only partially overlaps the core serum response. PLoS One. 2009;4(8):e6693.
44. Chen Y, Olopade OI. MYC in breast tumor progression. Expert Rev Anticancer Ther. 2008;8(10):1689–98.
45. Timmerman LA, Holton T, Yuneva M, et al. Glutamine sensitivity analysis identifies the xCT antiporter as a common triple-negative breast tumor therapeutic target. Cancer Cell. 2013;24(4):450–65.
46. Kilberg MS, Shan J, Su N. ATF4-dependent transcription mediates signaling of amino acid limitation. Trends Endocrinol Metab. 2009;20(9):436–43.
47. Mates JM, Segura JA, Martin-Rufian M, Campos-Sandoval JA, Alonso FJ, Marquez J. Glutaminase isoenzymes as key regulators in metabolic and oxidative stress against cancer. Curr Mol Med. 2013;13(4):514–34.
48. Kouros-Mehr H, Bechis SK, Slorach EM, et al. GATA-3 links tumor differentiation and dissemination in a luminal breast cancer model. Cancer Cell. 2008;13(2):141–52.
49. Grote D, Boualia SK, Souabni A, et al. Gata3 acts downstream of beta-catenin signaling to prevent ectopic metanephric kidney induction. PLoS Genet. 2008;4(12):e1000316.

Chapter 8
Glutamine Addiction of Cancer Cells

Enrico Desideri and Maria Rosa Ciriolo

Key Points

- Cancer cells show alterations in metabolic pathways to fulfill their energetic and biosynthetic requirements.
- Glutamine is the most abundant amino acid in plasma and it is taken up by cancer cells at higher rates that all other amino acids.
- As with glucose, glutamine can provide both ATP and precursors for biosynthetic pathways.
- Alterations of glutamine metabolism favor glutamine uptake and catabolism.
- Most of the alterations of glutamine metabolism are driven by oncogenes.
- Exploit glutamine addiction is a feasible strategy for therapeutic purposes.
- Glutamine deprivation chemopotentiates the efficacy of monocarboxylated anticancer drugs like 3-bromopyruvic acid and dichloroacetate.

Keywords Cancer • Glutamine • Metabolism • Glutaminase • Chemotherapy • Oncogene • Chemopotentiation • 3-Bromopyruvic acid

Abbreviation

αKG	α-Ketoglutarate
3-BrPA	3-Bromopyruvic acid
ALL	Acute lymphoblastic leukemia
BECN1	Beclin 1 autophagy related
BPTES	Bis-2-(5-phenylacetamido-1,2,4-thiadiazol-2-yl)ethyl sulfide
CRC	Colorectal adenocarcinoma
DCA	Dichloroacetate
DON	6-Diazo-5-oxo-L-norleucine
EEAs	Essential amino acids
ErbB2	v-erb-b2 erythroblastic leukemia viral oncogene homolog 2 neuro/glioblastoma-derived oncogene homolog (avian)

E. Desideri, Ph.D. • M.R. Ciriolo, Ph.D. (✉)
Department of Biology, University of Rome "Tor Vergata", Rome, Italy
e-mail: Desideri.enrico@fastwebnet.it; ciriolo@bio.uniroma2.it

R. Rajendram et al. (eds.), *Glutamine in Clinical Nutrition*, Nutrition and Health,
DOI 10.1007/978-1-4939-1932-1_8, © Springer Science+Business Media New York 2015

ETC	Electron transport chain
FDG-PET	[^{18}F]-fluorodeoxyglucose positron emission tomography
G6PD	Glucose-6-phosphate dehydrogenase
GAPDH	Glyceraldehyde-3-phosphate dehydrogenase
GDH	Glutamate dehydrogenase
GLS	Glutaminase
GLUL	Glutamate-ammonia ligase
GLUT	Glucose transporter
GPNA	Gamma-L-glutamyl-*p*-nitroanilide
GS	Glutamine synthetase
GSH	Glutathione reduced
GSSS	Glutathione oxidized
HCC	Hepatocellular carcinoma
HK2	Hexokinase 2
IDH1	Isocitrate dehydrogenase 1
LDH	Lactate dehydrogenase
MCT-1	Monocarboxylate transporter 1
ME1	Malic enzyme 1
mTORC1	Mammalian target of rapamycin complex 1
NADPH	Nicotinamide adenine dinucleotide phosphate reduced
OXPHOS	Oxidative phosphorylation
PA	Phenylacetate
PB	Phenylbutyrate
RFTA	Radiofrequency thermal ablation
ROS	Reactive oxygen species
SDH	Succinate dehydrogenase
SLC1A5	Solute carrier family 1 (neutral amino acid transporter) member 5
SLC7A5	Solute carrier family 7 (amino acid transporter light chain L system), member 5
TCA	Tricarboxylic acid

Introduction

Most cancer cells show a higher rate of glucose uptake and consumption and lactate production than their normal counterparts. In 1920s, Otto Warburg observed that cancer cells preferentially utilize glycolysis with respect to oxidative phosphorylation (OXPHOS) to produce ATP, even in the presence of normal oxygen tension, the so-called "Warburg effect" or "aerobic glycolysis" [1] (Fig. 8.1). The increased glucose uptake of cancer cells has been successfully exploited for diagnostic purposes through [^{18}F]-fluorodeoxyglucose (FDG) positron emission tomography (FDG-PET). Indeed, FDG is taken-up mainly by tumor cells, resulting in a "hot" spot on PET imaging and providing a powerful tool for the diagnosis of solid tumors [2]. Although Warburg effect was initially thought to be due to defects in the mitochondrial electron transport chain (ETC), later studies showed that many cancer cells do not present defects in oxidative metabolism and the tricarboxylic acid (TCA) cycle is completely functional. However, if we consider that glycolysis is far less efficient than OXPHOS in terms of ATP production (36 versus 2 mol ATP/mol glucose), the advantage conferred by such metabolic switch must be searched beyond the need of ATP. This apparent paradox can be explained taking into consideration that cancer cells, in addition to ATP, require a continuous supply of biosynthetic precursors and reducing equivalents for the synthesis of nucleotides, proteins, and lipids, necessary for sustaining their fast proliferation rate. Intermediates of glucose degradation can, indeed, be used for the synthesis of ribose, glycerol, and NADPH [3]. Moreover, an extensive lactate production and extrusion towards

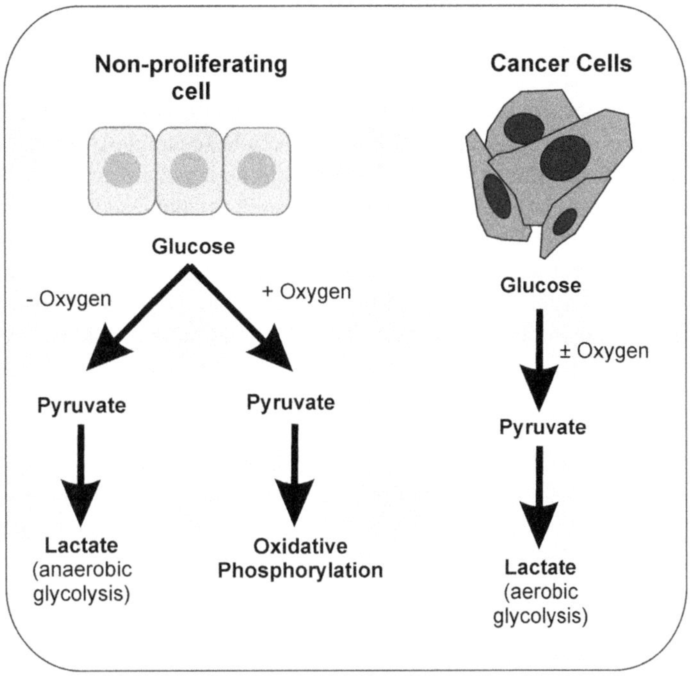

Fig. 8.1 Cancer cells exhibit Warburg Effect. In presence of normal oxygen tension, non-proliferating cells (*left panel*) preferentially utilize oxidative metabolism, a far more efficient mechanism than glycolysis (up to 36 mol ATP/mol glucose *vs.* 2 mol ATP/mol glucose), to produce ATP. When oxygen tension is low, pyruvate produced from glycolysis is converted to lactate (anaerobic glycolysis) to regenerate NAD^+ required for glycolysis. Lactate is extruded towards the extracellular environment. Many cancer cells (*right panel*) preferentially utilize glycolysis regardless of oxygen tension (Warburg Effect), even in the presence of a fully functional TCA cycle

the extracellular environment lowers the pH of the extracellular space and allows cancer cells survival by favoring blood vessel invasion in response to angiogenic stimuli [4]. Although glucose is a crucial nutrient for the growth of cancer cells, it is not the sole nutrient that cells can consume. The bloodstream, indeed, supplies cells with a broad range of compounds that can be used to satisfy both the energetic and biosynthetic requirements. This is the case of glutamine, the most abundant amino acid in plasma, whose consumption is much greater (up to tenfold) than that of all other amino acids [5]. Although glutamine is a nonessential amino acid that can be synthesized from glutamate by glutamate-ammonia ligase (GLUL), also known as glutamine synthetase (GS), the extreme sensitivity of many cancer cells to fluctuations of glutamine availability highlights the importance of this amino acid in tumor metabolism. In fact, similarly to glucose, glutamine can serve as a substrate for both bioenergetics and anabolic pathways. The discovery that proteins responsible for oncogenic transformation, such as Myc, akt, and ras [6], can drive tumor metabolic reprogramming has boosted both the interest in this research area and the attempts to exploit tumor-specific metabolic features for the development of novel anticancer therapies.

Glutamine Fuels Cancer Cell Growth

As with glucose, glutamine can satisfy the need of both energy (ATP) and intermediates for the synthesis of macromolecules. Glutamine is taken up and consumed at higher rates with respect to all other amino acids. Within the cell, glutamine plays a broad range of metabolic and non-metabolic roles [7]. As soon as it enters the cell, it can be promptly extruded through the antiporter solute carrier family 7 (amino acid transporter light chain, L system), member 5 (SLC7A5), to allow the uptake of essential amino acids (EAAs), including leucine, which has been recently characterized as an activator of the mammalian target of rapamycin (mTOR) complex 1 (mTORC1), a potent positive regulator of protein translation and cell growth [8]. Glutamine also provides both nitrogen, derived from both its amido and amino groups, and carbon from its carbon skeleton for anabolic processes. Indeed, nitrogen derived from glutamine amido group is required for the de novo synthesis of both purines and pyrimidines. This function of glutamine may be at the basis of the reduced proliferation and the abortive S-phase entry observed in K-Ras-transformed fibroblasts deprived of glutamine [9]. Glutamine amido group is also important for the synthesis of hexosamines, which are involved in cellular signaling and can influence tumor growth. Other biosynthetic reactions use the amino group of glutamate produced from glutamine through a deamination process catalyzed into the mitochondria by glutaminase (GLS), which has been reported to be upregulated in some tumor types [10]. In this process ammonia (NH_4^+) is also produced. Ammonia is an extremely toxic compound, which is massively released by cancer cells toward the extracellular environment. Although ammonia can diffuse through the plasma membrane, many lines of evidence reported that ammonia could be extruded via some transporters, which have not yet been completely characterized. These putative transporters could be attractive targets to trap ammonia inside the cells and exploit its high toxicity to induce cancer cells death. Although it is extremely toxic, recent findings demonstrated that ammonia derived from glutamine is also able to stimulate basal autophagy, which may confer cancer cells resistance to nutrient shortage or chemotherapeutics [11]. Glutamine-derived glutamate can be further metabolized by glutamate dehydrogenase (GDH) to α-ketoglutarate (αKG), a metabolic intermediate of the TCA cycle. TCA cycle is critical for fast proliferating cancer cells. Actually, in these cells, TCA cycle intermediates are continuously drained to sustain biosynthetic pathways, in particular lipid synthesis. Glutamine-derived αKG refuels TCA cycle (anaplerosis) and maintains constant levels of biosynthetic precursors. GDH activity is positively regulated by the direct binding of leucine, which leads to an increased production of αKG [12]. Leucine uptake is directly regulated by glutamine availability through the glutamine/leucine antiport SLC7A5, thus providing a finely regulated mechanism to increase or decrease glutaminolysis in response to glutamine concentration. The rate of αKG production in cancer cells may exceed the need of metabolic intermediates [13]; thus αKG could be involved in other cellular processes. In a recent paper by Duran et al. a role for αKG in the regulation of autophagy has emerged. In fact, αKG activates mTORC1-mediated pathways by favoring Rag GTPase-dependent mTORC1 sequestration to lysosomes [14]. As indicated before, mTORC1 stimulates cell growth. Moreover, mTORC1 has been known for long time to be also a negative regulator of autophagy. Autophagy is an evolutionarily conserved mechanism that is crucial for the maintenance of cellular homeostasis, and alteration of autophagy regulation contributes to a great number of pathological conditions, including cancer [15]. The role of autophagy in cancer is dual: on the one hand, autophagy can preserve cancer cell viability in condition of nutrient deprivation, hypoxia or in presence of chemotherapeutics; on the other hand, it strongly interferes with tumorigenesis in several ways (see Box 8.1); thus it can be considered a tumor suppressor mechanism.

Box 8.1 Autophagy Counteracts Tumorigenesis by Multiple Mechanisms

Macroautophagy, commonly known as autophagy, is a catabolic mechanism consisting in the degradation of cellular components through the lysosomal pathway. Initially known for its role in providing ATP when nutrients are limited, it is now considered pivotal for the maintenance of cellular homeostasis. Autophagy is a finely regulated mechanism whose alteration contributes to the onset of many diseases, including cancer. The evidence that a high percentage of human cancers harbors a Beclin-1 monoallelical deletion [16] contributed to the current thought of autophagy as a tumor suppressor mechanism. The role of autophagy as a tumor suppressor is carried out through multiple mechanisms. The most relevant of these are (I) the preservation of DNA integrity through the selective digestion of damaged proteins and organelles, which could

(continued)

Box 8.1 (continued)

otherwise give rise to an increase in detrimental oxidative stress; (II) in apoptosis-deficient cells, autophagy can prevent necrotic cell death, which is known to trigger an inflammatory response, a condition that favors tumorigenesis [17]. Moreover, an excessive autophagic rate can give rise to autophagic cell death, or type II cell death, which, unlike necrosis, does not trigger an inflammatory response.

A fast proliferation rate is often associated with an increased production of reactive oxygen species (ROS), which can be detrimental for cell, being able to damage all cellular structures (e.g., membranes, proteins, nucleic acids). To cope with the deleterious effects of ROS, cancer cells must be equipped with an antioxidant defense. In this context, glutathione (GSH), a tripeptide-like molecule consisting of glutamate, cysteine, and glycine, with its intracellular concentration in the millimolar range, is considered pivotal to maintain the intracellular redox homeostasis and to counteract ROS-induced oxidative damages [18]. Recently, we have demonstrated that GSH participates in the modulation of autophagy induced by nutrient deprivation. Under this experimental conditions, ROS are produced, likely by mitochondria, and are indispensable for the activation of autophagy [19]. In this context, GSH modulates the autophagic response, preventing an excessive activation of this process, which may result to be detrimental and lead to cell death [20]. Deprivation of glutamine affects intracellular GSH concentration in two different ways, (I) by reducing the availability of glutamate and (II) by limiting the uptake of cysteine that is mediated by the glutamate/cystine antiporter system X_c^-, which transports cystine (the dimer of cysteine) with the concomitant extrusion of glutamate [21]. The maintenance of the proper redox environment also relies on the availability of reducing equivalents, supplied by reduced nicotinamide adenine dinucleotide phosphate (NADPH). NADPH is, indeed, the cofactor required for reductions, such as the reduction of oxidized glutathione (GSSG) by glutathione reductase (GR). NADPH is also required for biosynthetic reactions, in particular for the synthesis of lipids. A robust source of NADPH derives from the activity of glucose-6-phosphate dehydrogenase. However, glutamine contributes to maintain NADPH pool through the activity of $NADP^+$-dependent cytosolic malic enzyme 1 (ME1), which is under the control of the tumor suppressor p53 [22]. ME1 converts the TCA cycle intermediate malate to pyruvate, with the concomitant production of NADPH. Pyruvate produced by ME1 is converted to lactate by lactate dehydrogenase (LDH) and it is finally extruded toward the extracellular milieu through monocarboxylate transporters (MCTs) [23].

Alterations of Glutamine-Related Enzymes in Cancer Cells

To adapt glutamine metabolism to their needs, cancer cells display several alterations that favor glutamine uptake and catabolism (glutaminolysis) (Table 8.1). Many alterations of glutamine metabolism have been found to be driven by oncogenes responsible for oncogenic transformation, highlighting the

Table 8.1 Oncogenes-driven alterations of glutamine metabolism in cancer cells

Oncogene	Target	Tumor type
Myc	Glutaminase 1 (GLS1)	Breast Cancer
	SLC1A5 (glutamine transport)	Hepatocellular Carcinoma
	SLC38A5 (glutamine transport)	Colon Cancer
β-catenin	Glutamine synthetase (GS)	Hepatocellular Carcinoma
Rho-GTPase	Glutaminase 1 (GLS1)	Breast Cancer
Erbb2	Glutaminase 1 (GLS1)	Breast Cancer

importance of metabolic reprogramming in tumorigenesis. A key player in the alteration of glutamine metabolism is the oncogene Myc, which is overexpressed in a plethora of human cancers. Myc has been known for long time as one of the responsible for the Warburg effect. In fact, Myc stimulates the expression of several enzymes that favors glucose uptake and glycolysis, including glucose transporters (GLUTs), hexokinase 2 (HK2) and lactate dehydrogenase (LDH) [24]. More recently, Myc has been found to be profoundly involved also in the modulation of glutamine metabolism. Myc, indeed, favors glutamine uptake and glutaminolysis [25]. One of the direct target genes of Myc is the solute carrier family 1 (neutral amino acid transporter), member 5 (SLC1A5), also known as ASCT2. This plasma membrane-localized protein is responsible for glutamine incorporation inside the cell. SLC1A5/ASCT2 has been found to be overexpressed in a great number of cancerous tissues, as well as in several cancer cell lines, like colorectal adenocarcinomas (CRC) and human hepatocellular carcinomas (HCCs) [26], and its expression levels are often associated with an aggressive biological behavior [27]. Glutaminase (GLS) catalyzes the first step of glutamine degradation within the cell. The evidence that GLS is upregulated in some tumor types raised the interest in this protein as a possible therapeutic target for the treatment of cancer. As with SLC1A5/ASCT2, Myc positively regulates GLS expression. Indeed, although GLS is not a direct target of Myc, its expression levels are modulated by two microRNA, miR-23a and miR-23b, which reduce GLS expression. It has been recently demonstrated by Gao et al. that Myc is able to repress the transcription of these two microRNAs, thus leading to the upregulation of GLS [28]. The influence of Myc on cancer cell metabolism is reflected by the extreme dependence of cell overexpressing Myc on glutamine [29]. In fact, many lines of evidence showed that glutamine removal preferentially induces cell death in this type of cells. Beyond Myc, other oncogenes can modulate the expression of GLS. Worthwhile citing is the reported involvement of the oncogene ErbB2 in the regulation of GLS. The oncogene ErbB2 is overexpressed in almost 30 % of human breast cancers, as well as in other tumor types, including ovarian and lung carcinomas [30], and it is associated with a more aggressive tumor behavior and with a poor prognosis. ErbB2 regulates GLS through the activation of NF-κB signaling pathway [30]. The NF-κB signaling pathway is also involved in the modulation of GLS activity induced by Rho-GTPases, which influence a wide range of cellular processes and are involved in malignant transformation [31]. Although many cancer cells depends on exogenous glutamine, they can synthesize glutamine from glutamate and ammonia through the activity of glutamine synthetase (GS), whose expression levels are regulated by the Wnt/β-catenin signaling pathway. GS is increased in some cancer types like HCCs, where it has been found to be abnormally expressed in the majority of the cases. The high frequency of GS overexpression in HCCs could make this protein a potential biomarker for early diagnosis of HCCs, as already speculated [32]. Cells expressing high levels of GS should possess a metabolic advantage with respect to cell expressing low levels of GS, since they are less dependent on exogenous glutamine. This may be crucial for HCCs survival, since glutamine concentration is generally low in the parenchyma of cirrhotic liver in which HCC occurs [33]. A study published in 2000s shows that GS expression could be associated with a higher metastatic potential of HCCs and an high risk of recurrence [34]. On the contrary, a more recent paper shows that patients with HCCs showing GS-positive immunostaining have a better survival rate after radiofrequency thermal ablation (RFTA) [35]. Overall, the limited availability of experimental data caused by the reduced interest received by GS with respect to other enzymes involved in glutamine metabolism, such as GLS, leaves the question about GS role in tumor formation and progression still open and cloudy.

Targeting Glutamine Metabolism for Anticancer Therapy

The higher dependence of many tumors on glutamine supply than normal cells makes glutamine metabolism a potentially ideal target for the development of anticancer strategies. The attempts to exploit glutamine addiction for therapeutic purposes can be dated back of several decades, when glutamine analogs, such as 6-diazo-5-oxo-L-norleucine (DON) and acivicin showed a promising antitumor activity, both in preclinical and in clinical studies [36]. However, the use of these compounds has been progressively suspended due to their severe side effects and toxicity. A high selectivity for a compound that targets glutamine metabolism is critical to avoid the severe side effect a plasma reduction of glutamine could cause. In fact, as the main storage of glutamine is the skeletal muscle, cancer patients often (up to 50 % of the cases) suffer cachexia, i.e., a loss of skeletal muscle mass, caused by the avid consumption of glutamine by tumor cells [37]. Thus, a systemic glutamine deprivation could worsen this condition, which is already known to be responsible for a high percentage of deaths of cancer patients. Moreover, several pieces of evidence showed that glutamine supplementation has beneficial effect in cancer patients, including a reduced risk of chemo- and radiotherapy, as well as protection against radiotherapy-induced oxidative stress [38]. Nowadays, a deeper comprehension of signaling pathways involved in cellular functions and the discovery of the importance of metabolic pathways for cancer cell proliferation led to a renewed interest in cancer cell metabolism and provided the possibility to develop more selective strategies aimed at selectively killing cancer cells, with no or reduced effects for non-transformed cells. A great number of compounds targeting enzymes involved in glutamine metabolism have been developed and tested in both preclinical and clinical studies, Fig. 8.2 and Table 8.2, some of them showing promising effects.

L-Asparaginase

Asparaginase is an anticancer agent successfully used in chemotherapy protocols for the treatment of pediatric acute lymphoblastic leukemia (ALL) [44]. Asparaginase catalyzes the conversion of asparagine to aspartate, thus limiting asparagine plasma concentration. Moreover, asparaginase also possesses glutaminase activity, catalyzing the conversion of glutamine to glutamate and ammonia, leading to reduced level of glutamine in the plasma. Some of the effects of asparaginase could be attributed to its glutaminase activity. Although asparaginase showed a great efficacy towards ALL, it resulted in some degree of toxicity and little efficacy against other types of tumor, in particular solid ones [45].

Phenylbutyrate/Phenylacetate

Phenylbutyrate (PB) is a modified fatty acid that is rapidly oxidized to its active metabolite phenylacetate (PA). PA conjugates with plasma glutamine to form phenylacetylglutamine, which is excreted in the urine, resulting in a net decrease of glutamine plasma levels [46]. PA has been tested for its anticancer activity in a great number of cancer cell lines, showing efficacy in reducing cancer cell growth [47]. PA underwent some Phase I studies in patients with advanced solid tumors showing no toxicity and some anticancer effects. Unfortunately, a Phase II study in patients with recurrent malignant glioma showed that PA had very little efficacy [41].

Gamma-L-Glutamyl-p-Nitroanilide

Gamma-L-Glutamyl-*p*-Nitroanilide (GPNA) is a pharmacological inhibitor of the glutamine transporter SLC1A5, which is a direct target of the oncogene Myc and it is upregulated in some cancer types. Preclinical studies showed that inhibition of SLC1A5 by GPNA resulted in a reduced growth and viability of lung cancer cell lines, at least in part dependent on the inactivation of mTORC1-mediated pathways [39]. At the moment, neither in vivo nor clinical studies are available about the efficacy of GPNA in cancer treatment as single agent.

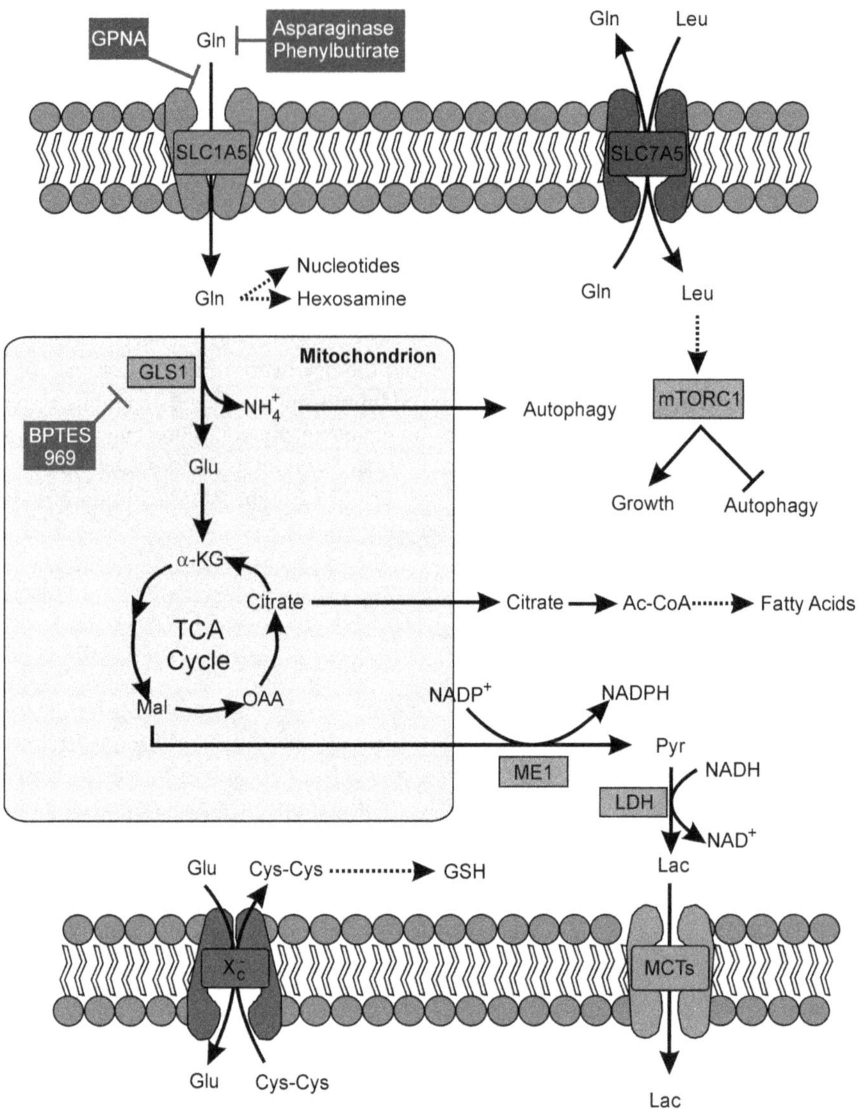

Fig. 8.2 Glutamine metabolism fuels cancer cell proliferation and offers potential therapeutic targets. Cancer cells avidly consume glutamine. Administration of asparaginase and phenylbutyrate lowers plasma level of glutamine, triggering anti-tumor effects. Glutamine is taken up by the solute carrier family 1 (neutral amino acid transporter), member 5 (SLC1A5) and can be extruded by solute carrier family 7 (amino acid transporter light chain, L system), member 5 (SLC7A5) to favor the uptake of leucin, an essential amino acid and an activator of the mammalian target of rapamycin (mTOR) complex 1 (mTORC1), a positive regulator of cell growth and an inhibitor of autophagy. SLC1A5 is inhibited by Gamma-l-Glutamyl-p-Nitroanilide (GPNA). Glutamine deamination by mitochondrial glutaminase (GLS) converts glutamine to glutamate and ammonia (NH_4^+), which triggers basal autophagy. Mitochondrial GLS is a target of many novel anticancer drugs, such as the small molecules 968 and BPTES. Glutamate derived from glutamine can supply TCA cycle after conversion to α-ketoglutarate (α-KG). Citrate is continuously drained from TCA cycle for fatty acid synthesis. Malate is converted to pyruvate by cytosolic malic enzyme 1 (ME1) to produce nicotinamide adenine dinucleotide phosphate reduced (NADPH). Pyruvate is converted to lactate by lactate dehydrogenase (LDH) and then extruded through monocarboxylate transporters (MCTs) towards the extracellular environment. Glutamine contributes to glutathione (GSH) synthesis by mediating the uptake of cystine through the X_c^- cystine/glutamate antiporter system

Table 8.2 Compounds targeting glutamine metabolism in preclinical/clinical studies

Compound	Target	Stage	References
GPNA	SLC1A5 (glutamine transport)	Pre-clinical	Hassanein M et al. [39]
Asparaginase	Plasma Asparagine/glutamine	Approved agent for ALL	Cory and Cory [40]
Phenylacetate	Plasma glutamine	Phase II	Chang SM et al. [41]
968	Glutaminase 1 (GLS1)	Pre-clinical	Wang et al. [42]
BPTES	Glutaminase 1 (GLS1)	Pre-clinical	Seltzer et al. [43]

Glutaminase Inhibitors

Most glutamine roles in cell metabolism requires its deamination by glutaminase (GLS). It is then obvious that GLS has been identified as a good potential therapeutic target. In the last few years, a lot of compounds targeting this enzyme have been developed and tested. However, although inhibition of GLS showed promising anticancer effects, not one result derives from clinical studies. In fact, all the available information comes from cell or mouse models, such as in the case of the small molecule 968, a dibenzophenanthridine, which inhibits Rho-GTPase. The small molecule 968 has been showed to blocks Rho GTPase-dependent transformation, as well as the growth of human cancer cells, both in vitro and mouse xenograft models [42]. Another piece of paper showed the efficacy of an additional small-molecule inhibitor of glutaminase, bis-2-(5-phenylacetamido-1,2,4-thiadiazol-2-yl)ethyl sulfide (BPTES), which showed efficacy in reducing growth of glioma cells harboring mutant isocitrate dehydrogenase 1 (IDH1) [43]. Both these papers, although of reduced clinical value, support the idea that glutaminase could be a good target for cancer treatments and show the potentiality of the use of small-molecule inhibitors to selectively target a protein.

Glutamine Deprivation Opens the Door to Monocarboxylic Drugs: The Case of 3-Bromopyruvate

Another intriguing possibility to exploit glutamine addiction of cancer cells derives from the evidence that glutamine deprivation enhances the efficacy of anticancer agents. Our group has recently demonstrated that glutamine deprivation chemopotentiates the efficacy of 3-bromopyruvate (3-BrPA) [48, 49], a halogenated analog of pyruvic acid (Fig. 8.3). 3-BrPA possesses alkylating properties and exhibits a great anticancer effect, as demonstrated by a great number of in vitro and in vivo studies [50] and it is currently under clinical investigation [51]. 3-BrPA has been shown to possess multiple targets within the cell, including many enzymes involved in cell metabolism, such as hexokinase-II (HKII), succinate dehydrogenase (SDH), and glyceraldehyde-3-phosphate dehydrogenase (GAPDH) [50]. The inhibitory effect of 3-BrPA triggers a metabolic stress with a reduction of anabolic precursors and ATP, which finally results in the induction of cell death. 3-BrPA is incorporated in the cell through the monocarboxylate transporter-1 (MCT-1). MCT-1 stability is directly influenced by glutamine availability. In fact, in the presence of normal glutamine concentrations, MCT-1 levels are maintained low by a high protein turnover through proteasome-dependent degradation. When glutamine is lacking, or when its uptake is inhibited by GPNA, the turnover rate of MCT-1 is reduced, resulting in higher protein levels and localization at the plasma membrane. The increased levels of MCT-1 allow the entry of greater concentrations of monocarboxylate drugs, such 3-BrPA, potentiating their anticancer effect (Fig. 8.4). Although still in preclinical stages, the combined use of glutamine deprivation, or the inhibition of glutamine uptake, and monocarboxylated drugs showed promising results in in vitro, as well as in mouse xenograft studies, without showing any apparent toxicity or side-effect. In fact, an evident

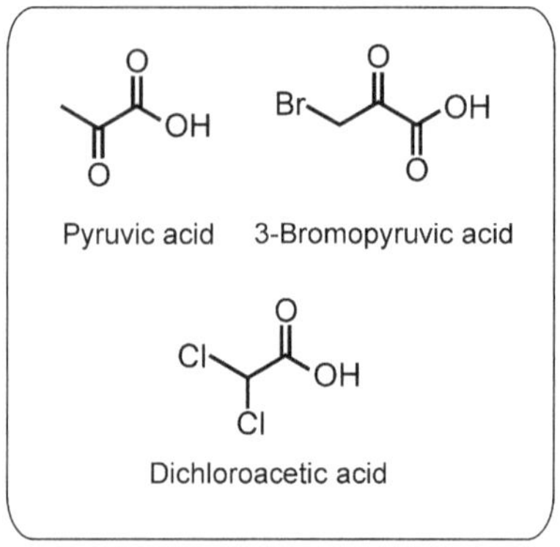

Fig. 8.3 The pyruvic acid analog 3-bromopyruvic acid and dichloroacetate, two monocarboxylic drugs with anticancer properties. Structure of pyruvic acid (*left*). Structure of 3-bromopyruvic acid (3-BrPA) (*middle*), a halogenated derivative of pyruvic acid with alkylating properties. Dichloroacetate (DCA), an analogue of acetic acid. 3-BrPA and DCA showed both in vitro and in vivo anticancer properties

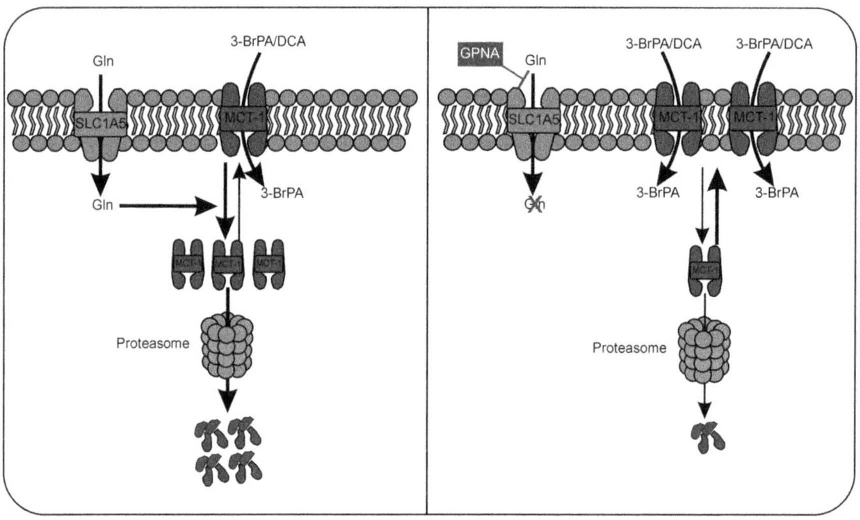

Fig. 8.4 Glutamine deprivation opens the door to monocarboxylate drugs. (*left panel*) Under normal glutamine concentration, the monocarboxylate transporter 1 (MCT-1) is degraded in a proteasome-dependent mechanism, resulting in a reduced amount of protein localized at the plasma membrane and limiting the uptake of monocarboxylate drugs 3-bromopyruvic acid (3-BrPA) and dichloroacetate (DCA). (*right panel*) When glutamine concentration is low or glutamine transporter solute carrier family 1 (neutral amino acid transporter), member 5 (SLC1A5) is inhibited by gamma-l-glutamyl-p-nitroanilide (GPNA), the turnover of the MCT-1 transporter is reduced, resulting in an increased localization of MCT-1 at the plasma membrane. Increased expression of MCT-1 favors the delivery of 3-BrPA and DCA inside the cells, thus increasing their anticancer properties

advantage of the chemopotentiating effect of glutamine deprivation is to maintain the efficacy of the drugs at lower concentrations, thus limiting its toxic effect towards non-transformed cells. The results obtained can be extended to other available monocarboxylated drugs, like dichloroacetate (DCA), whose effects are also potentiated by a reduced glutamine availability and opens the door to a potentially winning strategy through the development of other monocarboxylated drugs, which may benefit of glutamine deprivation to enhance their delivery inside the cell.

Conclusions

Cancer cells have been known for long time to possess peculiar metabolic requirements to sustain their fast proliferation rate. As with glucose, glutamine can play a plethora of functions within the cells and satisfy all cancer cells needs, being able to provide both ATP and intermediates for anabolic reactions. Many cancer cells have adapted their metabolism to enhance glutamine uptake and catabolism. In this way, cancer cells can sustain an extremely high proliferation rate. On the other hand, this glutamine addiction renders these cells extremely more sensitive to fluctuation in glutamine availability with respect to non-transformed cells. This metabolic feature can be exploited to selectively kill cancer cells, without detrimental effects to normal cells. During the past 50 years, a great number of compounds have been developed and tested as anticancer agents. Unfortunately, only few of them underwent clinical studies, not always with positive results. In fact, it must be taken into big consideration that glutamine is involved in many cellular functions also in normal cells and that depriving organism of glutamine could have severe deleterious effects. This is particularly true for cancer patients, which often suffer a depletion of glutamine caused by its avid usage by cancer cells, resulting in a loss of skeletal muscle mass, where the majority of glutamine is localized. A further reduction of glutamine levels could be detrimental rather than beneficial for this type of patients. Thus, a deep comprehension of the pathways in which glutamine is involved and the alterations that favor these pathways is mandatory for the development of chemotherapeutics with a high degree of specificity and low degree of toxicity. In this chapter, we reported several proteins abnormally expressed in cancer cells (most of which are under the control of oncogenes) that may represent good therapeutics targets (e.g., GLS and SLC1A5) and that are subject of intensive studies from several research groups. Finally, the chemopotentiation of monocarboxylic drugs by glutamine deprivation offers an intriguing strategy aimed at increasing the delivery of anticancer compounds, enhancing their efficacy and offering the possibility to reduce their concentrations, with enormous beneficial effects for the entire organism. So far, MCT-1 is the sole transporter identified to be upregulated by glutamine shortage, thus limiting the possibility to develop new compounds to monocarboxylic derivatives. However, the possible discovery of other transporters like MCT-1 but with other substrate specificities would open the door to the development of a great variety of anticancer drugs with different chemical and biological properties, and with an increased specificity.

Acknowledgements This work was partially funded by grants from AIRC (# IG 10636) and from Ministero dell'Università e della Ricerca (MIUR).

References

1. Warburg O. On respiratory impairment in cancer cells. Science. 1956;124(3215):269–70.
2. Kelloff GJ, Hoffman JM, Johnson B, et al. Progress and promise of FDG-PET imaging for cancer patient management and oncologic drug development. Clin Cancer Res. 2005;11(8):2785–808.
3. Tennant DA, Duran RV, Gottlieb E. Targeting metabolic transformation for cancer therapy. Nat Rev. 2010; 10(4):267–77.
4. Jensen JA, Hunt TK, Scheuenstuhl H, Banda MJ. Effect of lactate, pyruvate, and pH on secretion of angiogenesis and mitogenesis factors by macrophages. Lab Investig. 1986;54(5):574–8.
5. Eagle H. Nutrition needs of mammalian cells in tissue culture. Science. 1955;122(3168):501–14.
6. Levine AJ, Puzio-Kuter AM. The control of the metabolic switch in cancers by oncogenes and tumor suppressor genes. Science. 2010;330(6009):1340–4.
7. DeBerardinis RJ, Cheng T. Q's next: the diverse functions of glutamine in metabolism, cell biology and cancer. Oncogene. 2010;29(3):313–24.
8. Nicklin P, Bergman P, Zhang B, et al. Bidirectional transport of amino acids regulates mTOR and autophagy. Cell. 2009;136(3):521–34.

9. Gaglio D, Soldati C, Vanoni M, Alberghina L, Chiaradonna F. Glutamine deprivation induces abortive s-phase rescued by deoxyribonucleotides in k-ras transformed fibroblasts. PLoS One. 2009;4(3):e4715.
10. Yuneva MO, Fan TW, Allen TD, et al. The metabolic profile of tumors depends on both the responsible genetic lesion and tissue type. Cell Metab. 2012;15(2):157–70.
11. Eng CH, Yu K, Lucas J, White E, Abraham RT. Ammonia derived from glutaminolysis is a diffusible regulator of autophagy. Sci Signal. 2010;3(119):ra31.
12. Erecinska M, Nelson D. Activation of glutamate dehydrogenase by leucine and its nonmetabolizable analogue in rat brain synaptosomes. J Neurochem. 1990;54(4):1335–43.
13. DeBerardinis RJ, Mancuso A, Daikhin E, et al. Beyond aerobic glycolysis: transformed cells can engage in glutamine metabolism that exceeds the requirement for protein and nucleotide synthesis. Proc Natl Acad Sci U S A. 2007;104(49):19345–50.
14. Duran RV, Oppliger W, Robitaille AM, et al. Glutaminolysis activates Rag-mTORC1 signaling. Mol Cell. 2012; 47(3):349–58.
15. Choi AM, Ryter SW, Levine B. Autophagy in human health and disease. N Engl J Med. 2013;368(7):651–62.
16. Yue Z, Jin S, Yang C, Levine AJ, Heintz N. Beclin 1, an autophagy gene essential for early embryonic development, is a haploinsufficient tumor suppressor. Proc Natl Acad Sci U S A. 2003;100(25):15077–82.
17. Mathew R, Karantza-Wadsworth V, White E. Role of autophagy in cancer. Nat Rev. 2007;7(12):961–7.
18. Meister A. Metabolism and function of glutathione: an overview. Biochem Soc Trans. 1982;10(2):78–9.
19. Filomeni G, Desideri E, Cardaci S, Rotilio G, Ciriolo MR. Under the ROS…thiol network is the principal suspect for autophagy commitment. Autophagy. 2010;6(7):999–1005.
20. Desideri E, Filomeni G, Ciriolo MR. Glutathione participates in the modulation of starvation-induced autophagy in carcinoma cells. Autophagy. 2012;8(12):1769–81.
21. Lo M, Wang YZ, Gout PW. The x(c)- cystine/glutamate antiporter: a potential target for therapy of cancer and other diseases. J Cell Physiol. 2008;215(3):593–602.
22. Jiang P, Du W, Mancuso A, Wellen KE, Yang X. Reciprocal regulation of p53 and malic enzymes modulates metabolism and senescence. Nature. 2013;493(7434):689–93.
23. Hertz L, Dienel GA. Lactate transport and transporters: general principles and functional roles in brain cells. J Neurosci Res. 2005;79(1–2):11–8.
24. Yeung SJ, Pan J, Lee MH. Roles of p53, MYC and HIF-1 in regulating glycolysis - the seventh hallmark of cancer. Cell Mol Life Sci. 2008;65(24):3981–99.
25. Wise DR, DeBerardinis RJ, Mancuso A, et al. Myc regulates a transcriptional program that stimulates mitochondrial glutaminolysis and leads to glutamine addiction. Proc Natl Acad Sci U S A. 2008;105(48):18782–7.
26. Fuchs BC, Bode BP. Amino acid transporters ASCT2 and LAT1 in cancer: partners in crime? Semin Cancer Biol. 2005;15(4):254–66.
27. Witte D, Ali N, Carlson N, Younes M. Overexpression of the neutral amino acid transporter ASCT2 in human colorectal adenocarcinoma. Anticancer Res. 2002;22(5):2555–7.
28. Gao P, Tchernyshyov I, Chang TC, et al. c-Myc suppression of miR-23a/b enhances mitochondrial glutaminase expression and glutamine metabolism. Nature. 2009;458(7239):762–5.
29. Yuneva M, Zamboni N, Oefner P, Sachidanandam R, Lazebnik Y. Deficiency in glutamine but not glucose induces MYC-dependent apoptosis in human cells. J Cell Biol. 2007;178(1):93–105.
30. Yu D, Hung MC. Overexpression of ErbB2 in cancer and ErbB2-targeting strategies. Oncogene. 2000;19(53): 6115–21.
31. Vega FM, Ridley AJ. Rho GTPases in cancer cell biology. FEBS Lett. 2008;582(14):2093–101.
32. Long J, Wang H, Lang Z, Wang T, Long M, Wang B. Expression level of glutamine synthetase is increased in hepatocellular carcinoma and liver tissue with cirrhosis and chronic hepatitis B. Hepatol Int. 2011;5(2):698–706.
33. Medina MA. Glutamine and cancer. J Nutrit. 2001;131(9 (suppl)):2539S–42. discussion 2550S-2531S.
34. Osada T, Nagashima I, Tsuno NH, Kitayama J, Nagawa H. Prognostic significance of glutamine synthetase expression in unifocal advanced hepatocellular carcinoma. J Hepatol. 2000;33(2):247–53.
35. Dal Bello B, Rosa L, Campanini N, et al. Glutamine synthetase immunostaining correlates with pathologic features of hepatocellular carcinoma and better survival after radiofrequency thermal ablation. Clin Cancer Res. 2010; 16(7):2157–66.
36. Ahluwalia GS, Grem JL, Hao Z, Cooney DA. Metabolism and action of amino acid analog anti-cancer agents. Pharmacol Ther. 1990;46(2):243–71.
37. Tisdale MJ. Pathogenesis of cancer cachexia. J Supportive Oncol. 2003;1(3):159–68.
38. Savarese DM, Savy G, Vahdat L, Wischmeyer PE, Corey B. Prevention of chemotherapy and radiation toxicity with glutamine. Cancer Treat Rev. 2003;29(6):501–13.
39. Hassanein M, Hoeksema MD, Shiota M, et al. SLC1A5 mediates glutamine transport required for lung cancer cell growth and survival. Clin Cancer Res. 2013;19(3):560–70.
40. Cory JG, Cory AH. Critical roles of glutamine as nitrogen donors in purine and pyrimidine nucleotide synthesis: asparaginase treatment in childhood acute lymphoblastic leukemia. In Vivo. 2006;20(5):587–9.

41. Chang SM, Kuhn JG, Robins HI, et al. Phase II study of phenylacetate in patients with recurrent malignant glioma: a North American Brain Tumor Consortium report. J Clin Oncol. 1999;17(3):984–90.
42. Wang JB, Erickson JW, Fuji R, et al. Targeting mitochondrial glutaminase activity inhibits oncogenic transformation. Cancer Cell. 2010;18(3):207–19.
43. Seltzer MJ, Bennett BD, Joshi AD, et al. Inhibition of glutaminase preferentially slows growth of glioma cells with mutant IDH1. Cancer Res. 2010;70(22):8981–7.
44. Narta UK, Kanwar SS, Azmi W. Pharmacological and clinical evaluation of L-asparaginase in the treatment of leukemia. Crit Rev Oncol. 2007;61(3):208–21.
45. Lessner HE, Valenstein S, Kaplan R, DeSimone P, Yunis A. Phase II study of L-asparaginase in the treatment of pancreatic carcinoma. Cancer Treat Rep. 1980;64(12):1359–61.
46. Darmaun D, Welch S, Rini A, Sager BK, Altomare A, Haymond MW. Phenylbutyrate-induced glutamine depletion in humans: effect on leucine metabolism. Am J Physiol. 1998;274(5 Pt 1):E801–7.
47. Franco OE, Onishi T, Umeda Y, et al. Phenylacetate inhibits growth and modulates cell cycle gene expression in renal cancer cell lines. Anticancer Res. 2003;23(2B):1637–42.
48. Cardaci S, Rizza S, Filomeni G, et al. Glutamine deprivation enhances antitumor activity of 3-bromopyruvate through the stabilization of monocarboxylate transporter-1. Cancer Res. 2012;72(17):4526–36.
49. Cardaci S, Ciriolo MR. Deprive to kill: glutamine closes the gate to anticancer monocarboxylic drugs. Autophagy. 2012;8(12):1830–2.
50. Cardaci S, Desideri E, Ciriolo MR. Targeting aerobic glycolysis: 3-bromopyruvate as a promising anticancer drug. J Bioenerg Biomembr. 2012;44(1):17–29.
51. Ko YH, Verhoeven HA, Lee MJ, Corbin DJ, Vogl TJ, Pedersen PL. A translational study "case report" on the small molecule "energy blocker" 3-bromopyruvate (3BP) as a potent anticancer agent: from bench side to bedside. J Bioenerg Biomembr. 2012;44(1):163–70.

Chapter 9
L-[5-^{11}C]-Glutamine and Metabolic Imaging in Cancer Cells

Karl Ploessl, Brian P. Lieberman, Seok Rye Choi, Lin Zhu, and Hank F. Kung

Key Points

- By modifying different genes required for changing cellular energy production, tumor metabolism is significantly different from the normal cells.
- Changes in cellular metabolism, "aerobic glycolysis" plays an essential role in maintaining tumor growth and proliferation.
- Glutamine, which is the most abundant nonessential amino acid in the human body, is an alternative nutrient for tumor growth.
- In vivo imaging of metabolism with L-[5-^{11}C]-glutamine and [^{18}F]-(2S,4R)4-fluoro-L-glutamine will provide a tool for mapping the location and proliferation status of tumors, which may be "addicted" to use glutamine for survival.
- Imaging of glutamine, as an essential nutrient for metabolism, may be useful for diagnosis and treatment of tumor cells, which may be re-programmed and adapted for various tumor microenvironments.
- Recent advances in developing anti-cancer treatment, based on modulating tumor metabolism, may also be benefited by mapping tumor metabolism prior to or during the anti-metabolism drug treatment.

Keywords Tumor • Proliferation • Positron Emission Tomography • In vivo Imaging • Glutaminolysis

Abbreviations

PET Positron emission tomography

K. Ploessl, Ph.D. (✉) • B.P. Lieberman • S.R. Choi, Ph.D. • H.F. Kung, Ph.D.
Department of Radiology, University of Pennsylvania School of Medicine, Philadelphia, PA, USA
e-mail: ploessl@sunmac.spect.upenn.edu

L. Zhu, Ph.D.
Department of Radiology, University of Pennsylvania School of Medicine, Philadelphia, PA, USA

College of Chemistry, Beijing Normal University, Beijing, China

R. Rajendram et al. (eds.), *Glutamine in Clinical Nutrition*, Nutrition and Health,
DOI 10.1007/978-1-4939-1932-1_9, © Springer Science+Business Media New York 2015

Introduction

Recently, strong emerging evidence suggests that glutamine, which is the most abundant nonessential amino acid in the human body, may be an alternative nutrient for tumor growth [1, 2]. Glutamine transporters play an important role in mammalian cell biology, and these include SNAT1, SNAT3, SNAT5, SLC6A19, and ASCT2 [3, 4]. Among these, ASCT2 appears to be the glutamine transporter most commonly utilized in actively growing tumors. ASCT2 is up-regulated in tumor cells in a manner analogous to the up-regulation of the glucose transporter, GLUT1, in tumors utilizing aerobic glycolysis. Increased uptake of glutamine may result in enhanced accumulation of labeled glutamine tracers in tumors, thereby enabling their imaging. Adaption to tumor microenvironment plays an essential role in maintaining tumor growth and proliferation. Exploring the changes occurred in tumor metabolism under a changing microenvironment was first reported by Warburg [5]. Cancer cells preferentially use glucose without active participation of the glycolytic Krebs cycle. This leads to an overproduction of lactate, even when oxygen supply is plentiful. This increased glycolysis is commonly called the "Warburg effect" [6–9]. Boosted by genetic alterations, cancer cells often display up-regulations of the PI3K/Akt/mTor and related pathways. The up-regulation leads to an increase in glucose transporters and hexokinase 2. Both enhance the uptake and phosphorylation of glucose and its close analog 2-fluoro-2-deoxy-glucose (FDG) inside the cell. They serve as the biochemical basis of using [^{18}F]FDG-PET as a diagnostic tool for the detection of human cancers [10–12]. Beyond detecting tumor location, FDG-PET is also useful for: staging and assessing the extent of the disease, targeting and delineating radiation therapy treatment, and predicting and evaluating response to therapy [4, 13–15].

Glutamine, which is the most abundantly available nonessential amino acid in the human body, is an alternative nutrient for tumor growth. In cancer patients it becomes a conditioned essential amino acid for tumor growth. It enters the mitochondria via α-ketoglutarate and can be used to replenish Krebs cycle intermediates [16, 17]. Glutamine also serves as a precursor to produce more pyruvate through the action of malic enzymes. As part of the process, the c-Myc gene induces cancer cell metabolic changes in favor of using glutamine as the energy source [7, 8, 18–20]. In contrast to FDG-PET studies of glycolysis, the association between different oncogenic pathways and glutamine metabolism is less well known. Since the 1950s, glutamine has been recognized as an important tumor nutrient that contributes to key metabolic processes in proliferating cancer cells [21, 22]. Glutamine participates in bioenergetics, supports cell defenses against oxidative stress, complements glucose metabolism, and is an obligate nitrogen donor for nucleotide and amino acid synthesis [23–28]. Glutamine also influences a number of signaling pathways that contribute to tumor growth, in part through maintaining the activation of mTOR [29]. Although the myc gene appears to play a key role in promoting glutaminolysis in cancer cell lines, its role in tumor metabolism in vivo is less clearly defined. In addition, the relationship between glutamine uptake, metabolism, and other oncogenic pathways remains unexplored.

Figure 9.1 A simplified schematic drawing of intracellular metabolism of glucose and glutamine is presented to show the possible metabolic changes in tumor cells using "glycolysis" or "glutaminolysis." The tumor cells may utilize both pathways to generate energy and intermediate metabolites for survival and growth. However, tumor cells may switch the energy source to glutamine and thus, enhance their survival and proliferation.

Positron emission tomography (PET) imaging is an important tool, which could facilitate the diagnosis and treatment planning of glioblastoma and other tumors. Currently, [^{18}F]FDG/PET has been approved for the diagnosis of cancer. There is a growing infrastructure of local radiopharmacies supplying [^{18}F]FDG, thus circumventing the need for an on-site cyclotron in nuclear medicine clinics. [^{18}F]FDG is currently the most widely available PET imaging agent. Most of the FDG/PET studies are designed for the detection of tumors, based on the fact that tumor tissues often exhibit a higher glucose metabolism. A normal brain is one of the organs in the body that actively metabolizes glucose.

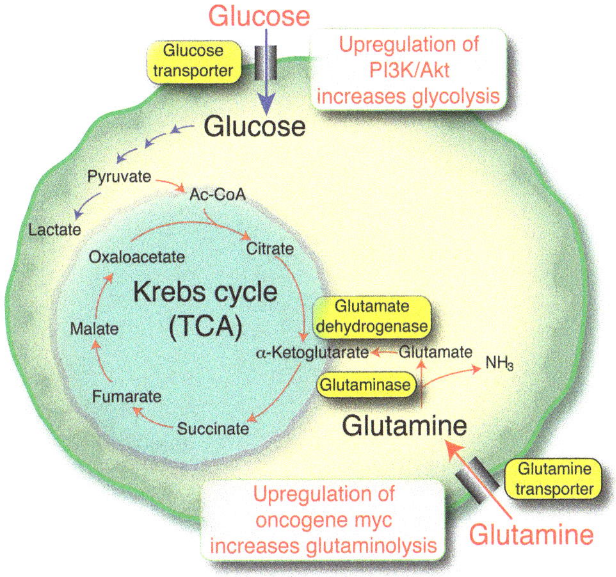

Fig. 9.1 Intracellular metabolism of glucose and glutamine (reprinted with permission from *J Nucl Med.* Jan 2012; 53(1):98–105)

Due to high background activity in a normal brain, FDG/PET is not useful for glioblastoma imaging. As such, alternative tracers, which show higher tumor uptakes and can distinguish between glioma and normal brain tissue, are needed [30]. The rationale for using labeled glutamine and its related derivatives is evident. However, it is likely that using [^{11}C]L-glutamine in PET imaging to study the glutaminolysis may measure the additive effects of up-regulation of glutamine transport and glutamine utilization. Similar to the mechanisms of tumor cell trapping of FDG, based on up-regulations of membrane-bound glucose transporter 1 and cytosol hexokinase, glutamine may be utilized via glutamine transporter (ASCT2) and glutaminases located in the cytosol [2, 11, 31]. Previously, [^{13}N] glutamine imaging of various spontaneous canine tumors showed that the imaging agent displayed positive correlation with postmortem findings [32, 33].

L-[5-^{11}C]-Glutamine for Pet Imaging

Recently, a convenient procedure to prepare L-[5-^{11}C]-glutamine, **5**, was reported [34]. The synthesis of ^{11}C-labeled L-glutamine was performed as described in Scheme 1. The radiolabeling process started from converting [^{11}C]CO_2 to a [^{11}C]cyanide ion according to a previously reported method [35]. This method for preparation of L-[5-^{11}C]-glutamine, **5**, is more efficient than the previously reported enzymatic preparation [36].

Figure 9.2 Scheme for synthesis of precursor and radiolabeling of [^{11}C]L-glutamine, **5**. Reagents and conditions: (a) p-Toluenesulfonyl chloride, triethylamine, dimethylaminopyridine, DCM, r.t.; (b) KI, acetone, reflux; (c) K^{11}CN, DMF, KOH, 5 min, 120 °C; (d) TFA/H_2SO_4, 10 min, 120 °C.

Time-dependent uptake of L-[5-^{11}C]-glutamine, **5**, in PBS was determined in rat glioma 9 L and human glioblastoma SF188 (Fig. 9.3). L-[5-^{11}C]-glutamine, **5**, demonstrated high uptake and linear incremental uptake within 60 min in both cell lines. Uptake in the SF188 cell line, which has shown a 25-fold amplification of the oncogene, myc, was higher than in 9 L cells. The maximum uptake of L-[5-^{11}C]-glutamine, **5**, reached 17.9 and 22.5 % uptake/100 μg protein at 60 min in 9 L and SF188 cells, respectively. In the dual isotope studies, uptake of [^{3}H]L-glutamine was similar to that of

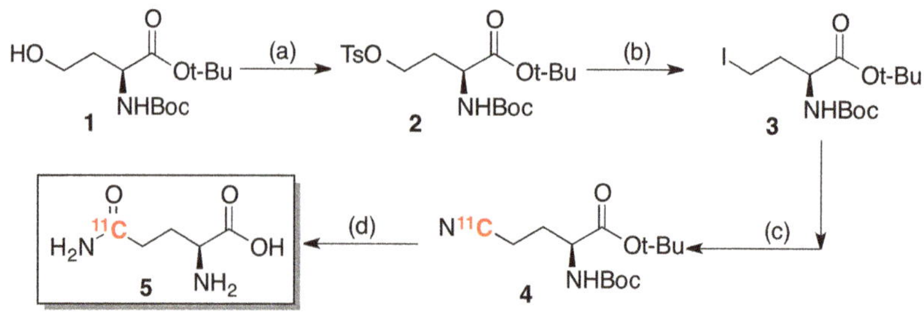

Fig. 9.2 Synthesis of L-[5-^{11}C]-glutamine

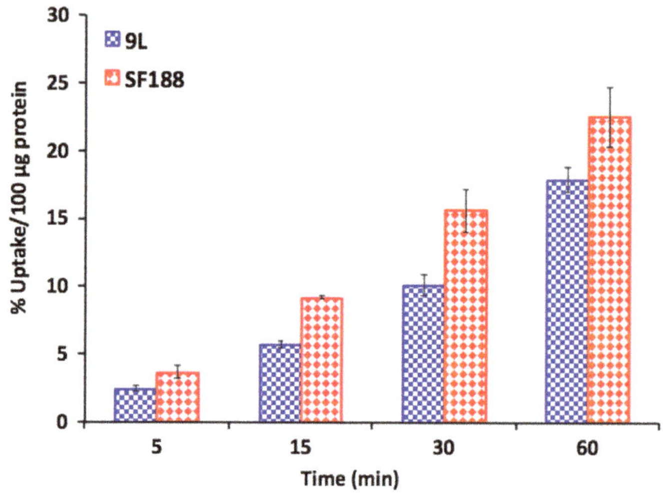

Fig. 9.3 Uptake of [^{11}C] L-glutamine in 9 L and SF188 glioma cell lines (reprinted with permission from *J Nucl Med*. Jan 2012; 53(1):98–105)

Table 9.1 Protein incorporation of L-glutamine

Cells	Protein incorporation (%) of L-[5-^{11}C]-glutamine, 5	Protein incorporation (%) of [^{3}H]L-glutamine
9L	44.1 ± 2.28	53.7 ± 3.18
SF188	26.7 ± 0.48	35.5 ± 2.77

L-[5-^{11}C]-glutamine, **5**, under the same condition (e.g., [^{3}H]L-glutamine had 13.5 % uptake/100 µg protein at 30 min in SF188 cells, which was comparable to 15.6 % uptake/100 µg protein for L-[5-^{11}C]-glutamine). A comparable experiment using [^{3}H]L-glutamic acid showed one-tenth of the cell uptake (1–2 % uptake/100 µg protein, data not shown).

Figure 9.3 Uptake of [^{11}C]L-glutamine, **5**, in 9 L and SF188 glioma cell lines. The uptake value is represented as % uptake/100 µg protein, mean ± standard deviation (SD), $n=3$.

To study the metabolism of this tracer in tumor cells, incorporation of L-[5-^{11}C]-glutamine, **5**, into protein in 9 L and SF188 cell lines was measured at 30 min after incubation (Table 9.1). In this dual-isotope experiment L-[5-^{11}C]-glutamine, **5**, and [^{3}H]L-glutamine, were incorporated with comparable values into protein as measured by the trichloroacetic acid precipitation method. The percent incorporation in the 9 L cells was 44.1 ± 2.28 % and 53.7 ± 3.18 %, respectively, while the protein incorporation in the SF188 tumor cells was 26.7 ± 0.48 % and 35.5 ± 2.77 %, respectively. The results further suggest that the tumor cells promptly used L-glutamine as the source of energy. It is likely that the L-glutamine was rapidly introduced inside the cytosol and incorporated into protein and other macromolecules.

Table 9.1 Protein incorporation of [^{11}C]L-glutamine, **5**, and [^{3}H]L-glutamine in glioma cells after 30-min incubation period (% incorporation TCA precipitated fraction, mean ± SD, $n=3$).

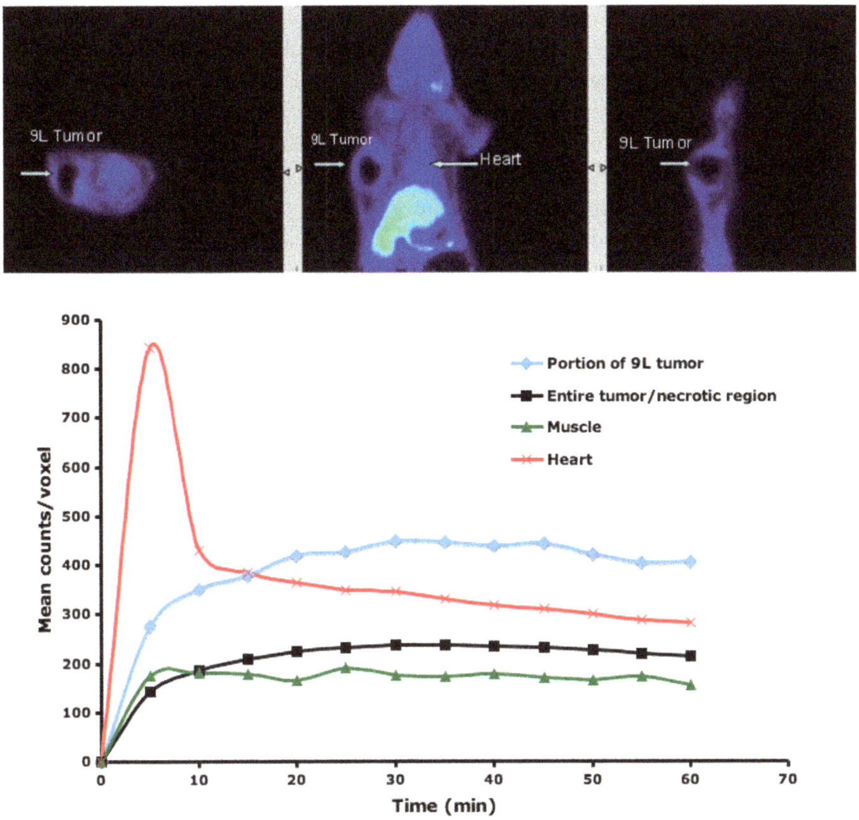

Fig. 9.4 Small animal APET images of [^{11}C]L-glutamine (reprinted with permission from *J Nucl Med* Jan 2012; 53(1):98–105)

The in vivo biodistribution of L-[5-^{11}C]-glutamine, **5**, showed the expected behavior of a radiolabeled amino acid with significant pancreas uptake (7.37 % dose/g at 15 min) in male ICR mice (20–25 g), most likely due to the exocrine function and high protein turnover within the pancreas. Pancreatic function requires the use of various amino acids as precursors for protein and peptide synthesis. Heart uptake and retention drops rapidly after 15 min post-injection, showing lower activity at 60 min postinjection (3.34 % dose/g). Initial lung and kidney uptake was prominent, although quickly washing out at 60 min post-injection. Rapid uptake of the tracer is observed within the kidneys but is quickly excreted through the urinary bladder. L-[5-^{11}C]-glutamine, **5**, showed moderate liver uptake with a relatively slow washout rate. The brain exhibited moderate uptake of 1.49 % dose/g at 15 min post-injection and rapidly washed out to 0.89 % dose/g at 60 min [34].

Small animal PET studies on rats bearing 9 L tumor xenograft tumors were carried out with L-[5-^{11}C]-glutamine, **5** (Fig. 9.4). Animal PET images of summed 60-min coronal, transverse and sagittal sections were selected for visualization. As the images demonstrate, clear tumor uptake is visualized, despite the necrotic tissue observed within the F344 rat tumor (Fig. 9.4). Region-of-interest analysis was performed on the reconstructed images in order to generate the time activity curves for L-[5-^{11}C]-glutamine, **5**. The kinetics indeed confirmed that the tracer exhibited higher tumor uptake compared to the background (muscle) regions. After 15 min post-injection, tumor washout is rapid through the 60-min scan time. Within the F344 animal model, maximum tumor uptake was reached within the first 20 min after injection. Tumor uptake then remains consistent throughout the 60-min scan time, with little to no washout observed, suggesting that the radioactivity was taken up and trapped in the tumor tissue (Fig. 9.4).

Figure 9.4 (Upper) Small animal APET images of [^{11}C]L-glutamine, **5**, in xenografted 9 L tumor of a F344 rat after an intravenous injection. Data represent images from a summed 60-min scan. The images are shown in transverse, coronal, and sagittal views. Note areas of necrosis within the 9 L tumor (donut shape). Arrows correspond to organs and tissues of interest.

(Lower) Small animal PET time activity curve for [^{11}C]L-glutamine, **5**, after iv injection into a F344 rat. The xenografted 9 L tumor was clearly visualized; however, there was necrotic tissue located in the middle region of the tumor, which does not show glutamine uptake (donut shape). The heart, liver, and pancreas uptake was also prominent, which is consistent with the biodistribution data.

This new tracer, L-[5-^{11}C]-glutamine, **5**, may serve as a metabolic imaging agent for probing glutamine-addicted tumors not detected by FDG-PET. The development of a convenient synthesis of L-[5-^{11}C]-glutamine, **5**, may provide an exciting opportunity for advancing diagnosis and treatment of tumor. This novel tumor metabolic imaging agent may lead to new methods to appraise the metabolic status of tumor growth in human cancer by PET imaging. In the future, this agent may be a useful tool for monitoring the efficacy of chemotherapeutics, which alter the metabolism of cancer cells.

[^{18}F](*2S,4R*)4-Fluoro-Glutamine for Pet Imaging

Recently, ^{11}C- and ^{18}F-labeled amino acids have been used as PET tumor imaging agents [34, 37]. Logistically, ^{18}F tracers are more suitable to be prepared from an off-site cyclotron (half-life of ^{18}F is 110 min). The manufacturing and distribution of ^{18}F tracers can be centralized, which will significantly simplify the manufacturing, distribution and clinical application. A novel chemical synthesis and characterization of four isomers of 4-fluoroglutamine have been reported [38]. One of the isomers, [^{18}F](*2S,4R*)4-fluoro-glutamine, was fully identified and a detailed radiochemistry preparation was successfully implemented. This tracer appeared to be a suitable candidate showing high tumor cell uptake and retention [38].

Figure 9.5 Representative radiolabeling reaction and an HPLC profile (Chirex 3126 (d)-penicillamine, 1 mM $CuSO_4$ solution, 1 mL/min) for [^{18}F](*2S,4R*)4-fluoro-glutamine.

The radiosynthesis for [^{18}F](*2S,4R*)4-fluoroglutamine was accomplished by a method as described before (Fig. 9.5) [38]. The radiochemical and stereochemical purity of the final product was determined by chiral HPLC (Chirex 3126 (d)-penicillamine, 1 mM $CuSO_4$ solution, 1 mL/min). The radiochemical yield was 8.4 ± 3.4 % (non-decay corrected). The radiochemical purity was 98 ± 1 %; optical purity$>91 \pm 8$ %; $n = 10$).

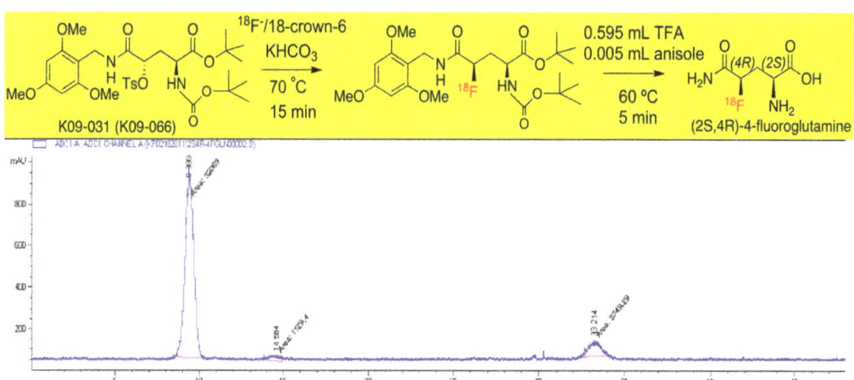

Fig. 9.5 HPLC profile of [^{18}F](*2S,4R*)4-fluoroglutamine

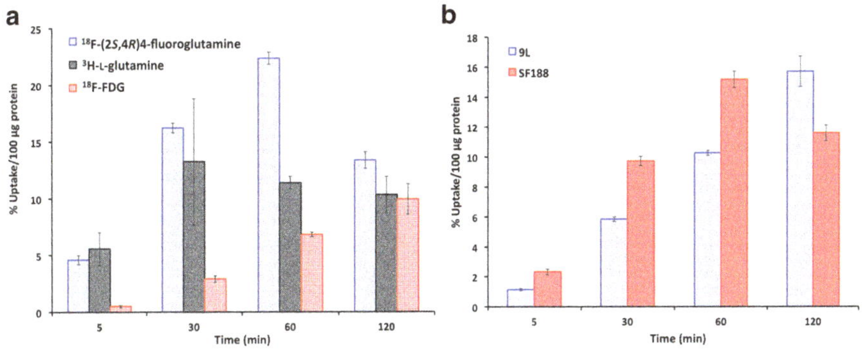

Fig. 9.6 (**a**) In vitro uptake of [^{18}F](*2S,4R*)4-fluoroglutamine (*blue*), [^{3}H]L-glutamine (*black*) and [^{18}F]FDG (*red*); (**b**) [^{18}F](*2S,4R*)4-fluoroglutamine in 9 L and SF188 cells (reprinted with permission from *J Nucl Med.* Dec 2011; 52(12):1947–1955)

Results of in vitro and in vivo evaluations of this novel metabolic tracer, an optically pure [^{18}F](*2S,4R*)4-fluoroglutamine, for positron emission tomography (PET) imaging of glutamine-addicted tumors: time-dependent uptake of [^{18}F](*2S, 4R*)4-fluoroglutamine in PBS was determined in rat glioma 9 L, a commonly used proliferative cell line for the evaluation of tumor imaging agents [39, 40]. A second type of tumor cell line SF188, derived from human glioblastoma, displays a 25-fold amplification of oncogene c-Myc [24]. It has been demonstrated that elevated levels of c-Myc lead to glutamine addiction and increased uptake of glutamine. Results demonstrated high cell uptakes of [^{18}F](*2S,4R*)4-fluoroglutamine in both tumor cell lines. In 9 L cells, this new tracer showed a linear increasing uptake and reached a maximum of 15.7 ± 1.0 % ID/100 µg protein at 120 min. This value is comparable or little higher than that reported for [^{18}F]FACBC (1-amino-3-^{18}F-fluorocyclobutane-carboxylic acid), another ^{18}F labeled amino acid for tumor imaging developed under a totally different uptake mechanism [39, 41, 42]. In SF188 cells, uptake of [^{18}F](*2S,4R*)4-fluoroglutamine exhibited different kinetics from that in 9 L cells and reached maximum around 60 min, and then decreased. Within the first 60 min, rate of the uptake was higher in SF188 cells and the uptake value in SF188 at 60 min was 1.5 fold higher than the corresponding uptake in 9 L cells.

Figure 9.6a In vitro uptake studies of [^{18}F](*2S,4R*)4-fluoroglutamine (blue) in SF188$_{bcl\text{-}xL}$cell line. [^{3}H]L-glutamine (black) and [^{18}F]FDG (red) were used as reference ligands. (Adopted from [38]). (b) Uptake of [^{18}F](*2S,4R*)4-fluoroglutamine in 9 L and SF188 cells. Values are represented as mean ± SD, $n = 3$.

We have compared the cell uptake of [^{18}F](*2S,4R*)4-fluoroglutamine to [^{18}F]FDG in SF188 using [^{3}H]L-glutamine (GLN) as the internal reference (Fig. 9.5). Results indicate that the uptake of [^{18}F](*2S,4R*)4-fluoroglutamine was significantly higher than that of [^{18}F]FDG. The maximum uptake of [^{18}F](*2S, 4R*)4-fluoroglutamine was more than twofold higher than that of [^{18}F]FDG. Since the experiments were performed under the same condition using two tracers at the same time, the results of these dual-isotope experiments strongly suggest that the cell uptake of this new tracer, [^{18}F](*2S,4R*)4-fluoroglutamine, is likely associated with the up-regulation of c-myc in SF188 cells.

To investigate the transport mechanisms involved in the uptake of [^{18}F](*2S,4R*)4-fluoroglutamine, we have conducted a series of competitive inhibition studies in 9 L cells using specific inhibitors for system A, ASC, L, and N. These are major amino acid transport systems in mammalian cells and are potentially responsible for the uptake of glutamine and its analogs [3, 43]. The result showed that system A inhibitor MeAIB (methylaminoisobutyric acid) had no inhibitory effect on the uptake of [^{18}F](*2S,4R*)4-fluoroglutamine, which suggests that system A amino acid transport was not involved in the uptake of this new tracer. System L inhibitor BCH, System ASC inhibitor L-serine (L-Ser) and System ASC, N inhibitor L-glutamine (L-Gln) exhibited similar concentration-dependent reduction of cell uptake, thus indicating potential involvement of system L, ASC, and N in the uptake of [^{18}F](*2S,4R*)4-fluoroglutamine. Further examination of transport mechanism by Na^+ and pH dependence studies showed that the uptake of [^{18}F](*2S,4R*)4-fluoroglutamine was reduced by 78 % in Na^+ free medium and was insensitive to pH change from 6 to 8. Since activity of system N is highly pH sensitive and is almost inactive in pH 6 [44], this might suggest that system N did not play an important role in the transport. Moreover, system ASC is sodium dependent, while system L is sodium independent [45]. These results indicate that system L might be responsible for sodium-independent uptake of [^{18}F](*2S,4R*)4-fluoroglutamine, while sodium-dependent uptake of the tracer was predominately through system ASC. We also differentiated the roles of two subtypes of amino acid transport systems (ASCT1 and ASCT2) [46], in the uptake of [^{18}F](*2S,4R*)4-fluoroglutamine. ASCT2 is over-expressed in a variety of cancer cells and is important for tumor growth and survival [47, 48]. To examine the selectivity of [^{18}F](*2S,4R*)4-fluoroglutamine towards ASCT2, we compared the inhibitory effect of L-γ-glutamyl-p-nitroanilide (GPNA), a potent ASCT2 inhibitor [49], to its close analog L-γ-glutamyl-anilide (GA) that is inactive towards ASCT2. It was found that GPNA had more impact on the uptake: 1 mM GPNA could reduce the uptake by 77 % compared to 44 % when 1 mM GA was present. The result suggests that the transport of [^{18}F](*2S,4R*)4-fluoroglutamine might prefer ASCT2 to ASCT1. Results of the transport studies suggest that the transport of [^{18}F](*2S,4R*)4-fluoroglutamine may be predominantly through system ASC and may prefer its subtype ASCT2.

Incorporation of [^{18}F](*2S,4R*)4-fluoroglutamine into protein at 30 and 120 min in 9 L and SF188 cells was measured (Fig. 9.7). [^{3}H]L-glutamine, the native glutamine, was used as the reference ligand in this experiment. [^{18}F](*2S,4R*)4-fluoroglutamine demonstrated a similar incorporation profile as observed for [^{3}H]L-glutamine. A significant percentage of [^{18}F](*2S,4R*)4-fluoroglutamine was incorporated into protein after 2 h. At 30 and 120 min, the protein incorporation of [^{18}F](*2S,4R*)4-fluoroglutamine in 9 L cells was 29 % and 72 % and 12 % and 62 % in SF188 cells, respectively (Fig. 9.6).

Figure 9.7 Incorporation of [^{18}F](*2S,4R*)4-fluoroglutamine and [^{3}H]L-glutamine into protein in 9 L and SF-188 tumor cells. The comparison of cellular uptake of [^{18}F](*2S,4R*)4-fluoroglutamine and [^{3}H]L-glutamine was performed using dual-isotope experiments at 30 and 120 min incubation time periods.

In vivo biodistribution of [^{18}F](*2S,4R*)4-fluoroglutamine in mice showed the expected behavior of a radiolabeled amino acid with significant pancreas uptake (19.7 % dose/g at 30 min), most likely due to the exocrine function and high protein turnover within the pancreas. Pancreatic function requires the use of various amino acids as precursors for protein and peptide synthesis. Blood levels drop fairly quickly with time, showing low blood activity at 240 min post injection (0.48 % dose/g). There was no significant uptake within the lung, along with no significant retention within the first

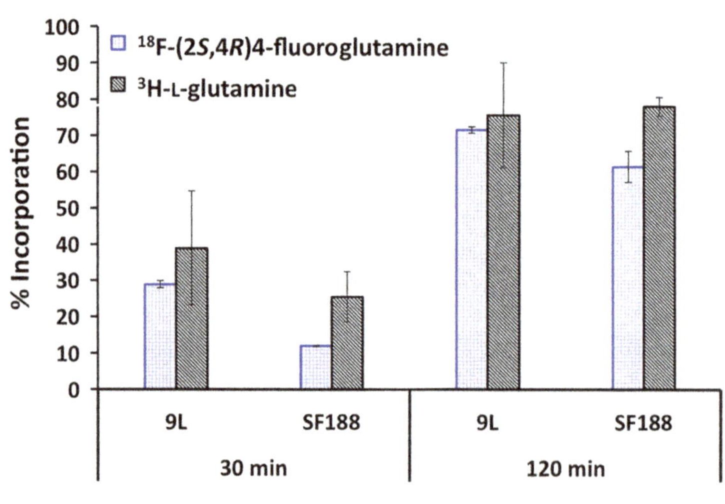

Fig. 9.7 Incorporation of [^{18}F](*2S,4R*)4-fluoroglutamine and [^{3}H] L-glutamine into protein in 9 L and SF-188 tumor cells (reprinted with permission from *J Nucl Med.* Dec 2011; 52(12):1947–1955)

arteriovenous capillary bed. This suggests that [^{18}F](*2S,4R*)4-fluoroglutamine is fairly hydrophilic and water-soluble. Rapid uptake is observed within the kidneys but is quickly excreted through the urinary bladder. [^{18}F](*2S,4R*)4-fluoroglutamine showed a moderate liver uptake with a relatively slow wash-out rate. Brain uptake exhibited a relatively low, but consistent, uptake of 0.54 % dose/g at 2 min post-injection and remained consistent with little to no washout throughout the 240 min experiment. Lastly, bone (femur) showed rapid uptake and increased with time implying that in vivo de-fluorination may be occurring after injection.

Use and production of 9 L xenografts in F344 rats is a well-known and established animal model that represents typical glioblastomas that would be found within a clinical setting [39, 50]. Uptake of [^{18}F](*2S,4R*)4-fluoroglutamine showed respectable 9 L tumor uptake values (1.03 % dose/g uptake at 30 min post injection). 9 L tumor/muscle ratio (target/background) decreased slightly from 2.78 at 30 min to a ratio of 2.00 at 60 min post-injection. Results of biodistribution studies also showed a high pancreas uptake, again due to the various amino acid precursors used for protein and peptide synthesis. Bone uptake (femur) slightly rose from 0.78 % dose/g at 30 min to 1.03 % dose/g at 60 min post-injection, suggesting in vivo de-fluorination of the compound may be occurring.

Dynamic small animal PET studies on rats bearing 9 L tumor xenograft tumors were carried out with [^{18}F](*2S,4R*)4-fluoroglutamine. A-PET images of summed 2-h coronal sections were selected for visualization. As the images demonstrate, clear tumor uptake is visualized within each animal model. Reconstructed images were used to generate time activity curves for [^{18}F](*2S,4R*)4-fluoroglutamine. The kinetics indeed confirmed that the tracer exhibited higher tumor uptake compared to the muscle (background) regions. Rapid tumor uptake is visualized in each animal model within the first 20 min. Tumor uptake remains rather constant throughout the 2-h scan time, with a slow washout rate observed. High kidney and bladder uptake was observed (see Fig. 9.8).

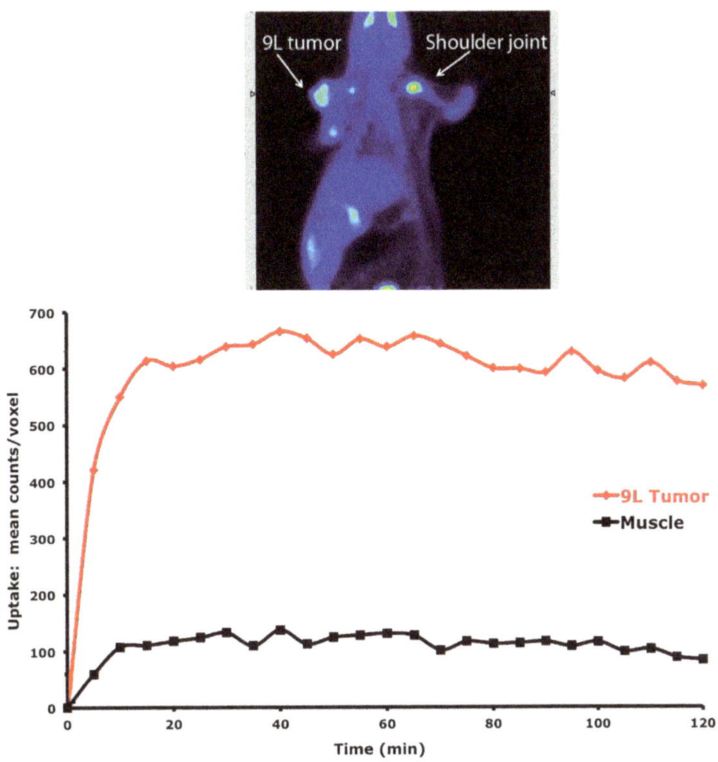

Fig. 9.8 Small animal APET images of [^{18}F](*2S,4R*)4-fluoroglutamine in F344 9 L rat (reprinted with permission from *J Nucl Med.* Dec 2011; 52(12):1947–1955)

Figure 9.8 (Upper) Small animal APET images of [^{18}F]*(2S,4R)*4-fluoroglutamine in F344 9 L rat after an iv injection. Data represent images from a summed 2-h scan. Images are shown in transverse, coronal, and sagittal views. Arrows represent the location of tumors. (Lower) Small animal APET time activity curve for [^{18}F](2*S*,4*R*)4-fluoroglutamine after iv injection into F344 rat bearing a xenografted 9 L tumor on the left shoulder.

It has been demonstrated that animal PET imaging studies using [^{18}F]*(2S,4R)*4-fluoroglutamine exhibited the expected high uptake and retention in the tumor models in rats (9 L xenografted tumor). The 9 L xenografted tumor model is well known in the literature for studying novel tumor imaging agents [39, 50, 51]. The imaging studies in this rat tumor model clearly confirmed that the agent is highly sequestered in tumor tissue and the trapping was highly persistent—suggesting that the tracer was taken up and incorporated into protein, other cytosol macromolecules, and the large intracellular glutamic acid pool. However, the linkage between c-myc and quantitative PET imaging of glutaminolysis is not yet fully established. One obstacle not easy to overcome is that the size of the tumor varies under different c-myc gene expression levels; thus obtaining quantitative data of tumor uptake by animal PET imaging studies is difficult to accomplish. Correction for tumor size might alleviate some of the variations, but the quantitative correlation of c-myc gene expression and glutamine uptake may be a challenge not yet easily resolved.

Conclusions

In summary, it was demonstrated that in vitro tumor cell uptake of [^{18}F](2*S*,4*R*)4-fluoroglutamine is higher than those of [^{3}H]L-glutamine and [^{18}F]FDG. In vivo PET imaging studies showed significant tumor uptake and trapping inside tumor tissue in two different tumor models. The results support the feasibility of PET imaging for the study of a fundamental change in tumor metabolism—high-rate glutaminolysis.

Previously published works on [^{18}F]*(2S,4R)*4-fluoroglutamine [37] and L-[5-^{11}C]-glutamine [34] have contributed to the completion of this chapter. Human studies of [^{18}F](2*S*,4*R*)4-fluoroglutamine are ongoing at Memorial Sloan Kettering Cancer Center and the clinical trial of L-[5-^{11}C]-glutamine has been planned for the near future.

Acknowledgments This work was supported in part by grants from Stand-Up 2 Cancer (SU2C), PA Health, and NIH CA-0164490.

References

1. Rajagopalan KN, Deberardinis RJ. Role of glutamine in cancer: therapeutic and imaging implications. J Nucl Med. 2011;52(7):1005–8.
2. Erickson J, Cerione R. Glutaminase: A hot spot for regulation of cancer cell metabolism? Oncotarget. 2010;1(8):734–40.
3. McGivan JD, Bungard CI. The transport of glutamine into mammalian cells. Front Biosci. 2007;12:874–82.
4. Plathow C, Weber WA. Tumor cell metabolism imaging. J Nucl Med. 2008;49 Suppl 2:43S–63.
5. Warburg O. On the origin of cancer cells. Science. 1956;123(3191):309–14.
6. Koppenol WH, Bounds PL, Dang CV. Otto Warburg's contributions to current concepts of cancer metabolism. Nat Rev Cancer. 2011;11(5):325–37.
7. Mattaini KR, Vander Heiden MG. Cancer. Glycosylation to adapt to stress. Science. 2012;337(6097):925–6.
8. Metallo CM, Vander Heiden MG. Understanding metabolic regulation and its influence on cell physiology. Mol Cell. 2013;49(3):388–98.
9. Vander Heiden M, Cantley L, Thompson C. Understanding the Warburg effect: The metabolic requirements of cell proliferation. Science. 2009;324(5930):1029–33.

10. Ong LC, Jin Y, Song IC, Yu S, Zhang K, Chow PK. 2-[^{18}F]-2-Deoxy-D-Glucose (FDG) Uptake in Human Tumor Cells Is Related to the Expression of GLUT-1 and Hexokinase II. Acta Radiologica. 2008;31:1–10.
11. Gillies RJ, Robey I, Gatenby RA. Causes and consequences of increased glucose metabolism of cancers. J Nucl Med. 2008;49 Suppl 2:24S–42.
12. Gambhir SS. Molecular imaging of cancer: from molecules to humans. Introduction. J Nucl Med. 2008;49 Suppl 2:S1–4.
13. Buerkle A, Weber WA. Imaging of tumor glucose utilization with positron emission tomography. Cancer Metastasis Rev. 2008;27(4):545–54.
14. van Baardwijk A, Dooms C, van Suylen RJ, et al. The maximum uptake of (18)F-deoxyglucose on positron emission tomography scan correlates with survival, hypoxia inducible factor-1alpha and GLUT-1 in non-small cell lung cancer. Eur J Cancer. 2007;43(9):1392–8.
15. Busk M, Horsman MR, Kristjansen PE, van der Kogel AJ, Bussink J, Overgaard J. Aerobic glycolysis in cancers: implications for the usability of oxygen-responsive genes and fluorodeoxyglucose-PET as markers of tissue hypoxia. Int J Cancer. 2008;122(12):2726–34.
16. Kaelin Jr WG, Thompson CB. Q&A: Cancer: clues from cell metabolism. Nature. 2010;465(7298):562–4.
17. Wise DR, Ward PS, Shay JE, et al. Hypoxia promotes isocitrate dehydrogenase-dependent carboxylation of alpha-ketoglutarate to citrate to support cell growth and viability. Proc Natl Acad Sci U S A. 2011;108(49):19611–6.
18. Daye D, Wellen KE. Metabolic reprogramming in cancer: Unraveling the role of glutamine in tumorigenesis. Semin Cell Dev Biol. 2012;23(4):362–9.
19. Dang CV, Hamaker M, Sun P, Le A, Gao P. Therapeutic targeting of cancer cell metabolism. J Mol Med. 2011;89(3):205–12.
20. Dang CV. Glutaminolysis: supplying carbon or nitrogen or both for cancer cells? Cell Cycle. 2010;9(19):3884–6.
21. Kvamme E, Svenneby G. Effect of anaerobiosis and addition of keto acids on glutamine utilization by Ehrlich ascites-tumor cells. Biochim Biophys Acta. 1960;42:187–8.
22. Eagle H. The specific amino acid requirements of a human carcinoma cell (Stain HeLa) in tissue culture. J Exp Med. 1955;102(1):37–48.
23. Yang C, Sudderth J, Dang T, Bachoo RM, McDonald JG, DeBerardinis RJ. Glioblastoma cells require glutamate dehydrogenase to survive impairments of glucose metabolism or Akt signaling. Cancer Res. 2009;69(20): 7986–93.
24. Wise D, DeBerardinis R, Mancuso A, et al. Myc regulates a transcriptional program that stimulates mitochondrial glutaminolysis and leads to glutamine addiction. Proc Natl Acad Sci U S A. 2008;105(48):18782–7.
25. DeBerardinis RJ, Mancuso A, Daikhin E, et al. Beyond aerobic glycolysis: transformed cells can engage in glutamine metabolism that exceeds the requirement for protein and nucleotide synthesis. Proc Natl Acad Sci U S A. 2007;104(49):19345–50.
26. DeBerardinis RJ, Lum JJ, Hatzivassiliou G, Thompson CB. The biology of cancer: metabolic reprogramming fuels cell growth and proliferation. Cell Metab. 2008;7(1):11–20.
27. Deberardinis RJ, Sayed N, Ditsworth D, Thompson CB. Brick by brick: metabolism and tumor cell growth. Curr Opin Genet Dev. 2008;18(1):54–61.
28. DeBerardinis R, Cheng T. Q's next: the diverse functions of glutamine in metabolism, cell biology and cancer. Oncogene. 2010;29(3):313–24.
29. Nicklin P, Bergman P, Zhang B, et al. Bidirectional transport of amino acids regulates mTOR and autophagy. Cell. 2009;136(3):521–34.
30. Klasner BD, Krause BJ, Beer AJ, Drzezga A. PET imaging of gliomas using novel tracers: a sleeping beauty waiting to be kissed. Expert Rev Anticancer Ther. 2010;10(5):609–13.
31. Robey IF, Stephen RM, Brown KS, Baggett BK, Gatenby RA, Gillies RJ. Regulation of the Warburg effect in early-passage breast cancer cells. Neoplasia. 2008;10(8):745–56.
32. Conlon KC, Bading JR, DiResta GR, Corbally MT, Gelbard AS, Brennan MF. Validation of transport measurements in skeletal muscle with N-13 amino acids using a rabbit isolated hindlimb model. Life Sci. 1989;44(13):847–59.
33. Gelbard AS, Christie TR, Clarke LP, Laughlin JS. Imaging of spontaneous canine tumours with ammonia and L-glutamine labeled with N-13. J Nucl Med. 1977;18(7):718–23.
34. Qu W, Oya S, Lieberman BP, et al. Preparation and Characterization of L-[5-11C]-Glutamine for Metabolic Imaging of Tumors. J Nucl Med. 2012;53:98–105.
35. Iwata R, Ido T, Takahashi T, Nakanishi H, Iida S. Optimization of [11C]HCN production and no-carrier-added [1-11C]amino acid synthesis. Int J Rad Appl Instrum A. 1987;38(2):97–102.
36. Antoni G, Omura H, Ikemoto M, Moulder R, Watanabe Y, Langstrom B. Enzyme catalyzed synthesis of L-[4-11C] aspartate and L-[5-11C]glutamate. J Labelled Compd Rad. 2001;44(4):287–94.
37. Lieberman BP, Ploessl K, Wang L, et al. PET imaging of glutaminolysis in tumors by [18]F-(2S,4R)4-fluoroglutamine. J Nucl Med. 2011;52:1947–55.
38. Qu W, Zha Z, Ploessl K, et al. Synthesis of optically pure 4-fluoro-glutamines as potential metabolic imaging agents for tumors. J Am Chem Soc. 2011;133(4):1122–33.

39. Yu W, Williams L, Camp V, Olson J, Goodman M. Synthesis and biological evaluation of anti-1-amino-2-[^{18}F]fluoro-cyclobutyl-1-carboxylic acid (anti-2-[^{18}F]FACBC) in rat 9 L gliosarcoma. Bioorg Med Chem Lett. 2010;20(7):2140–3.
40. Martarello L, McConathy J, Camp VM, et al. Synthesis of syn- and anti-1-amino-3-[^{18}F]fluoromethyl-cyclobutane-1-carboxylic acid (FMACBC), potential PET ligands for tumor detection. J Med Chem. 2002;45(11):2250–9.
41. Schuster DM, Savir-Baruch B, Nieh PT, et al. Detection of recurrent prostate carcinoma with anti-1-amino-3-^{18}F-fluorocyclobutane-1-carboxylic acid PET/CT and 111In-capromab pendetide SPECT/CT. Radiology. 2011; 259(3):852–61.
42. McConathy J, Goodman MM. Non-natural amino acids for tumor imaging using positron emission tomography and single photon emission computed tomography. Cancer Metastasis Rev. 2008;27(4):555–73.
43. Wasa M, Wang HS, Okada A. Characterization of L-glutamine transport by a human neuroblastoma cell line. Am J Physiol Cell Physiol. 2002;282(6):C1246–53.
44. Hatanaka T, Nakanishi T, Huang W, et al. Na+- and Cl– -coupled active transport of nitric oxide synthase inhibitors via amino acid transport system B(0,+). J Clin Invest. 2001;107(8):1035–43.
45. Bodoy S, Martin L, Zorzano A, Palacin M, Estevez R, Bertran J. Identification of LAT4, a novel amino acid transporter with system L activity. J Biol Chem. 2005;280(12):12002–11.
46. Kekuda R, Prasad PD, Fei YJ, et al. Cloning of the sodium-dependent, broad-scope, neutral amino acid transporter Bo from a human placental choriocarcinoma cell line. J Biol Chem. 1996;271(31):18657–61.
47. Fuchs BC, Bode BP. Amino acid transporters ASCT2 and LAT1 in cancer: partners in crime? Semin Cancer Biol. 2005;15(4):254–66.
48. Okudaira H, Shikano N, Nishii R, et al. Putative Transport Mechanism and Intracellular Fate of Trans-1-Amino-3-^{18}F-Fluorocyclobutanecarboxylic Acid in Human Prostate Cancer. J Nucl Med. 2011;52(5):822–9.
49. Esslinger CS, Cybulski KA, Rhoderick JF. N-gamma-aryl glutamine analogues as probes of the ASCT2 neutral amino acid transporter binding site. Bioorg Med Chem. 2005;13(4):1111–8.
50. Lee TS, Ahn SH, Moon BS, et al. Comparison of ^{18}F-FDG, ^{18}F-FET and ^{18}F-FLT for differentiation between tumor and inflammation in rats. Nucl Med Biol. 2009;36(6):681–6.
51. Yu W, Williams L, Camp V, Malveaux E, Olson J, Goodman M. Stereoselective synthesis and biological evaluation of syn-1-amino-3-[^{18}F]fluorocyclobutyl-1-carboxylic acid as a potential positron emission tomography brain tumor imaging agent. Bioorg Med Chem. 2009;17(5):1982–90.

Chapter 10
Endotoxemia and Glutamine

François Blachier, Xiangfeng Kong, Guoyao Wu, Daniel Tomé, Antonio Lancha Jr., Mireille Andriamihaja, and Yulong Yin

Key Points

- Endotoxemia markedly modifies glutamine metabolism in tissues with a decrease of intestinal glutamine uptake and metabolism.
- In liver, endotoxemia increases glutamine uptake and utilization but decrease glutamine endogenous synthesis.
- In skeletal muscles, endotoxemia increases synthesis and release of glutamine for other tissues, resulting in decrease of muscle glutamine content.
- In lungs, endotoxemia results in a decrease of glutamine uptake with increased glutamine endogenous synthesis and release.
- Supplementation with glutamine allows to mitigate in endotoxemic situation the increment of intestinal permeability and bacterial translocation, and, in intestine and lung, to decrease inflammation and injury.

Keywords Endotoxemia • Glutamine • Glutamine metabolism • Glutamine supplementation • Lung • Liver • Intestine

Abbreviations

ALI	Acute lung Injury
ARDS	Adult Respiratory Distress Syndrome
BCAA	Branched-Chain Amino Acid

F. Blachier, Ph.D. (✉) • D. Tomé, Ph.D. • M. Andriamihaja, Ph.D.
INRA/AgroParisTech, UMR 914 Nutrition Physiology and Ingestive Behavior, Paris, France
e-mail: francois.blachier@agroparistech.fr

X. Kong, Ph.D. • Y. Yin, Ph.D.
Key Laboratory of Agro-ecological Processes in Subtropical Region, Institute of Subtropical Agriculture, Chinese Academy of Sciences, Changsha, Hunan, China

G. Wu, Ph.D.
Department of Animal Science, Texas A&M University, College Station, TX, USA

A. Lancha Jr., Ph.D.
Laboratory of Applied Nutrition and Metabolism, School of Physical Education and Sports, University of Sao Paulo, Brazil, Sao Paulo, Brazil

R. Rajendram et al. (eds.), *Glutamine in Clinical Nutrition*, Nutrition and Health,
DOI 10.1007/978-1-4939-1932-1_10,

GS	Glutamine Synthetase
GSH	Glutathione
HSP	Heat Shock Protein
IL	Interleukin LPS: Lipopolysaccharide
MAPK	Mitogen-Activated Protein Kinase
MPEC	Microvascular Pulmonary Endothelial Cells
NO	Nitric Oxide
PAEC	Pulmonary Artery Endothelial Cells
TLR	Toll-Like Receptor
TNF	Tumor Necrosis Factor

Introduction

Endotoxemia is defined as the presence of endotoxin in blood and may result from a transfer of a pathological amount of endotoxin (also currently called bacterial lipopolysaccharide LPS) from the intestinal lumen to the bloodstream due to impaired gut selective barrier function. Major endotoxemia can lead to sepsis defined as a medical condition characterized by a whole-body inflammatory state (also called systemic inflammatory response syndrome or SIRS) [1]. Septic shock is another medical condition which results from severe infection and sepsis. Sepsis may begin with a localized infection which can reach the bloodstream. Septic shock can lead to the multiple organ dysfunction syndrome. Patients suffering from septic shock are taken in charge in intensive care units with a mortality rate being as high as 20–50 % [2, 3]. Although the pathogenesis of septic shock is much complicated and not entirely understood, it involves events including the release of cytokines, the activation of macrophages, neutrophils, and microvascular endothelial cells, as well as coagulation disorders and severe metabolic alterations [1, 4]. In critically ill patients, the gastrointestinal tract is believed to play a central role in the pathogenesis of septic shock [5, 6]. Indeed, increased gut permeability and bacterial translocation play an active role in multiple organ failure by inducing a vicious cycle of increased intestinal permeability, leading to increased transfer of luminal compounds to the bloodstream. In this way, the gut can be seen as both an instigator and a victim of post-injury multiple organ failure [5]. This idea was already present in the pioneering work of Deitch et al. [7] showing that intraperitoneal injection of endotoxin to mice was able to promote the translocation of bacteria from the gut.

In this general context, the aim of this chapter is to present an overview on (1) the effect of endotoxemia and sepsis on glutamine metabolism in tissues and (2) the effects of glutamine supplementation in endotoxemia and sepsis.

Endotoxemia and Glutamine Metabolism in Intestine

It is well known that one of the major roles of the small intestine is to absorb the nutrients (including amino acids) from the intestinal lumen to the bloodstream. However, a significant part of luminal amino acids are metabolized by enterocytes in the process of absorption. This is particularly true for several amino acids including glutamine which are very largely metabolized by the enterocytes during their transcellular journey [8]. Glutamine metabolism corresponds to energy supply in a context of rapid renewal of the epithelium (and thus intense ATP-consuming anabolic metabolism) and to sodium extrusion at the basolateral membrane through the action of the Na/K ATPase. As noted previously, glutamine also provides nitrogen for nucleotide synthesis, and is a precursor for several amino acids produced in enterocytes. Lastly, glutamine has been shown to be able to preserve protein synthesis in Caco-2 cells submitted to "luminal fasting." [9]

Sepsis considerably alters the intestinal barrier functions, which in turn modifies the absorption and bioavailability of nutrients [10]. In septic patients, sodium-dependent glutamine transport is decreased in both jejunum and ileon when compared to control surgical healthy patients [11]. In addition, gut glutamine and oxygen consumption are markedly diminished in these patients [12]. In rats treated by intraperitoneal injection of LPS, transport data indicated decreases in both sodium-dependent jejunal glutamine uptake and glutaminase activity [11–13] suggesting that less glutamine is available for enterocyte metabolism. In the model of sepsis induced by cecal ligation and puncture, the capacity of enterocytes for glutamine oxidation and the intestinal mucosa glutaminase activity are decreased [14, 15] with a concomitant negative nitrogen balance. In contrast, in vivo, LPS treatment increases the activity of small intestine glutamine synthetase (GS) by 250 % [16]. However, experimental works by another group using the cecal ligation and puncture model of sepsis have shown that the effects of sepsis on glutamine transport may be biphasic with an initial increase followed by a decrease [17]. Simultaneously, intestinal extraction of glutamine from the bloodstream fell by 56 %. This latter reduction in the uptake of circulating glutamine cannot be accounted for by a fall in the arterial concentration. Thus, immediately after endotoxemia, brush border glutamine uptake is increased while consumption of glutamine entering across the basolateral membrane is decreased.

Although the mechanisms involved in the decreased glutamine metabolism in enterocytes recovered from septic animals remain unclear, interleukin-1 (IL-1) has been shown to act as a mediator of the alterations in gut glutamine metabolism in endotoxemia and sepsis [18, 19]. Karinch et al. [20] suggested that IGF-1 has a direct effect on the stimulation of the glutamine transport. However, the effect of endotoxemia and sepsis on glutamine metabolism in the intestinal mucosa appears rather unspecific since absorption of several other amino acids (including leucine, proline, glutamate, arginine) are also affected [11, 21–24]. Indeed, following endotoxemia, almost all circulating amino acids (including amino acids like citrulline and ornithine which are not incorporated in alimentary proteins but are derived from amino acid precursors) are markedly decreased suggesting a marked decrease of the intestinal functions [25]. In addition, endotoxemia affects the morphology of the intestinal mucosa [26, 27], and decreases the mucosal oxygen consumption [28, 29], reinforcing the view that endotoxemia affects the intestinal functions. The main alterations of glutamine metabolism in intestine due to endotoxemia are presented in Fig. 10.1.

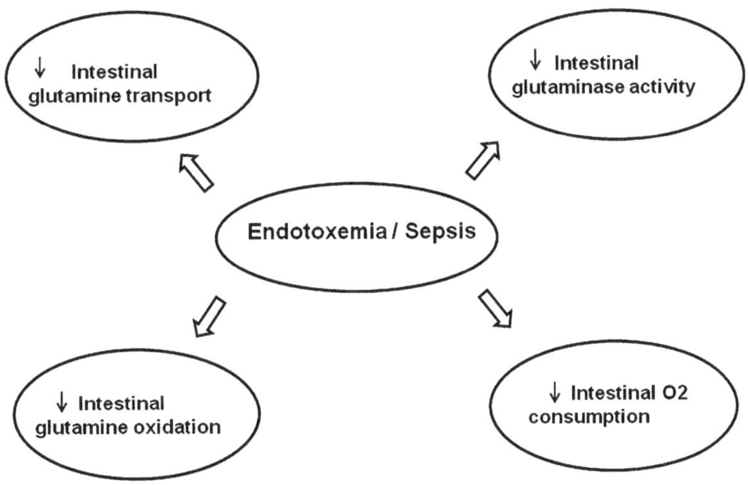

Fig. 10.1 Main alterations of glutamine metabolism in intestine due to endotoxemia

Glutamine Supplementation and Intestinal Functions in Endotoxemia and Sepsis

Clinical and preclinical studies have suggested that glutamine supplementation may be beneficial to humans with altered intestinal functions. Using a gastrostomy-fed rat infant "pup-in-a-cup" model, the effects of glutamine supplementation on the proinflammatory response induced by LPS given before dietary supplementation via the gastrostomy tube were examined [30]. Using a 3.5 g/kg/day dose of glutamine, a decrease of the expression of the intestinal cytokine-induced neutrophil chemoattractant and a decrease of the myeloperoxidase activity (used as a parameter indicating neutrophil accumulation in intestinal mucosa), as well as a decrease of intestinal and plasma TNF-α concentrations occurred in endotoxemic animals when compared with control (untreated) animals. In a model of infant rats treated with intraperitoneal injection of LPS and receiving at the same time a supplementation of glutamine (2 mmol/g) by the same intraperitoneal way, glutamine supplementation was able to counteract the fast decrease of the circulating glutamine concentration and to partly prevent the increase of circulating TNF-α provoked by the LPS treatment. In rats receiving LPS by the subcutaneous way, supplementation with 2 % glutamine given in the drinking water before and following injection of LPS was able to prevent gut mucosal injury and to improve the mucosal recovery in terms of bowel weight and mucosal weight as well as villus height in the jejunum [31]. Ding and Li [32] found that prophylactic treatment with glutamine could minimize the increment of intestinal permeability and bacterial translocation caused by endotoxemia in rats treated with total parenteral nutrition. Uehara et al. [33] reported that glutamine pretreatment significantly ameliorated intestinal tissue injury and the survival of rats following LPS treatment.

When given before LPS administration, glutamine treatment significantly ameliorated LPS-induced mucosal injury, inflammation, and apoptotic cell death in the ileum and the colon, as judged by significant decreases in TNF-α gene expression and ameliorated histologic damage scores. In adult humans, glutamine pretreatment decreases the production of the proinflammatory cytokines IL-6 and IL-8 by the intestinal mucosa [34, 35]. Accordingly, glutamine deprivation enhanced IL-8 production by Caco-2 colonic human adenocarcinoma cells after LPS stimulation [36, 37]. In human fetal and adult intestinal epithelium, it has been shown that glutamine modulates LPS-induced IL-8 production through IκB/NFκB transduction pathways [38]. Zhou et al. [39] revealed that an oral preventive supply of combined glutamine and arginine before endotoxemia induction significantly decreases TNF-α and IL-1β mRNA abundance in both the jejunum and ileum, while they also significantly decrease anti-inflammatory IL-10 in the ileum. In the model of rats treated intravenously with LPS, supplementation with glutamine (0.75 g/kg) and with L-alanyl-L-glutamine dipeptide (same amount of glutamine than glutamine alone) before and after LPS injection prevented the LPS-induced decrease of the functional capillary density of the intestinal muscular and mucosal layers as well as the number of adherent leukocytes in the submucosal venules, indicating that glutamine supplementation is able to improve the intestinal microcirculation [40]. In the rat model injected with LPS via the intraperitoneal way and supplemented with glutamine in drinking water (2 %), it was reported that glutamine supplementation was able to downregulate the Toll-like receptor TLR-4 as well as the myeloid differentiation factor 88; and to ameliorate the intestinal mucosal injury caused by endotoxemia [41]. In the model of rats receiving LPS via intravenous administration and concomitantly glutamine at the dose of 0.75 g/kg by the same way, it was found that glutamine supplementation can efficiently attenuate the increase in circulating proinflammatory cytokines and protect against organ damage as assessed by histological examination, and decrease mortality from endotoxemia [42].

In rats receiving continuous intravenous injection of LPS, glutamine supplementation at a dose of 2 % was able to ameliorate the nitrogen balance and to increase the intestinal mucosal glutaminase activity [43]. In addition, the morphological aspect of the jejunal mucosa was ameliorated in glutamine-supplemented animals as judged from the villus height, crypt depth and wall thickness. Higashiguchi et al. [44] studied the effect of sepsis and the regulation by glutamine of protein synthesis in enterocytes isolated from the small intestine of rats. Sixteen hours after endotoxemia induction, protein synthesis was increased by 65 %, 89 %, and 137 %, respectively, in enterocytes from the tips and mid-portions of the villi and from the crypts. Addition of glutamine to incubated enterocytes stimulates protein synthesis in a dose-dependent manner. In the study by Okuma et al. [45], the authors induced sepsis in rats by continuous intraperitoneal administration of endotoxin, and supplemented the animals with 2 % L-alanyl-L-glutamine by total parenteral nutrition. Under such experimental conditions, they found that the supplementation with the dipeptide did not ameliorate neither the nitrogen balance nor bacterial translocation from the gut to the mesenteric lymph nodes. However, the supplementation with the dipeptide containing glutamine was able to increase the intestinal mucosal weight, and the villus height. In a study aiming at evaluating the effect of a supplementation with glutamine (0.75 g/kg, in its free form or in the form of the dipeptide L-alanyl-L-glutamine) on the microcirculation in the endotoxemic rat model, Sheibe et al. [46] found that glutamine supplementation before LPS challenge was able to reduce leukocyte adherence and mesenteric plasma extravasation, indicating that glutamine diminish the detrimental impact of endotoxemia on the mesenteric microcirculation. In endotoxemic rats treated with intraperitoneal injection of LPS followed by food deprivation for 24 h and then receiving glutamate supplementation (4 g/kg/d), glutamine concentration was increased in the jejunum and the intestinal villus height was higher in the jejunum of supplemented animals when compared to control [26].

In the early weaning piglet model, supplementation with glycyl-glutamine dipeptide (0.15 %) in LPS-treated animals is able to partly alleviate the suppression of growth and immune functions [47]. In the study by Dugan and McBurney [48], a segment of distal ileum was isolated from anesthetized piglets and perfused without or with 2 % glutamine before treatment with endotoxin. By using such an experimental design, the authors found that endotoxin-induced permeability changes (as measured using the plasma-to-lumen clearances of Cr-EDTA) can be partly prevented by supplying luminal glutamine. In the study of Haynes et al. [49], enterocytes from neonatal pigs were cultured in the presence of LPS with or without millimolar concentrations of glutamine in its free form or as the dipeptide L-alanyl-L-glutamine. The results obtained indicate that glutamine is able to reduce the LPS-induced cell death. In the same study, the authors gave an oral supplementation of glutamine or L-alanyl-L-glutamine to 7-day-old piglets before intraperitoneal administration of LPS, and found that the dietary supplementation with glutamine is able to ameliorate the LPS-induced intestinal injury, to enhance growth performance, and to reduce the intestinal expression of the LPS Toll-like receptor-4, of the active caspase 3, and of the transcription factor NF-κB. The main effects of glutamine supplementation on intestinal functions in endotoxemia are presented in Fig. 10.2.

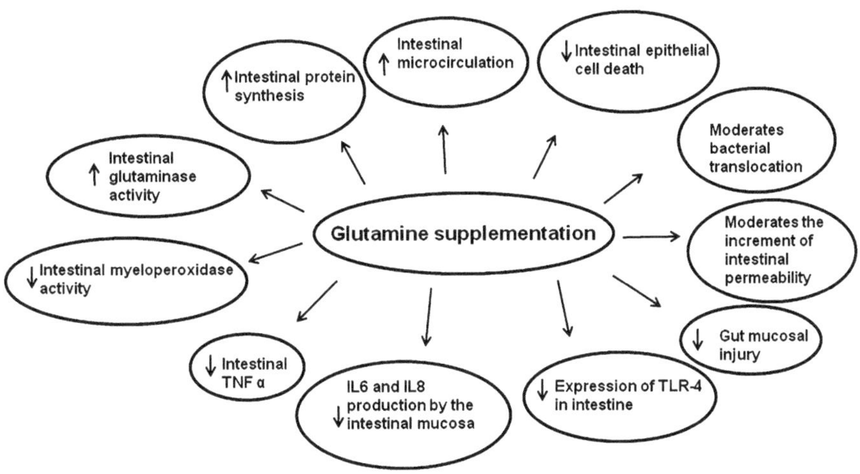

Fig. 10.2 Main effects of glutamine supplementation on intestine in endotoxemia

Endotoxemia and Glutamine Metabolism in Liver

Endotoxin treatment in rats results in a tenfold increase of hepatic glutamine uptake owing to both an increase in hepatic blood flow and in glutamine extraction from the bloodstream [18]. This marked increase in metabolic activity is concomitant with signs of hepatocellular injury. Thus in this experimental model, the liver becomes the major organ for glutamine consumption [18]. In the study by Pacitti et al. [50], hepatic glutamine consumption is accordingly increased 11-fold after LPS-induced endotoxemia in rats. Glutamine uptake by the liver is markedly accelerated during endotoxemia, and this is due to an increase in hepatocyte plasma membrane transport activity. System N transporters in hepatocytes play a major role in hepatic glutamine transport. Studies in endotoxemic rodents have shown net hepatic glutamine uptake to be markedly increased, a result which is due partially to a three- to fourfold increase in hepatocyte transport System N activity [20]. LPS administration resulted in a time- and dose-dependent two- to threefold increase in Na^+-dependent glutamine transport activity [51, 52] secondary to an increase in the transport maximal velocity (V_{max}), consistent with the appearance of an increased numbers of corresponding transporter proteins in the hepatocyte plasma membrane vesicles. Maximal increases in transport was observed 4 h after exposure to endotoxin. This increase in transport activity represents an important mechanism regulating the accelerated hepatic glutamine uptake that occurs during severe infection. Wang et al. [53] investigated the changes of hepatic transporters in early endotoxemic rats provoked by intraperitoneal injection of LPS. They showed that both the mRNA and protein expression of SNAT3 and SNAT5 are enhanced by LPS in a time- and dose-dependent manner. Fischer et al. [54] showed that LPS treatment administered intraperitoneally in fed and fasted (48 h) rats increased transport activity 2.6- and 6-fold, respectively. This effect in endotoxemic starved rats is mediated by both an increase in System N V_{max} and the induction of a high affinity System A amino acid carrier which transports glutamine. In this latter study, starvation and endotoxemia appear to regulate hepatocyte glutamine transport independently and synergistically. The authors propose that the hepatic response allows to provide glutamine to support key metabolic pathways in the liver during critical illness. However, the effect of endotoxemia on glutamine transport is not restricted to glutamine since rats treated with a single injection of endotoxin are characterized by a stimulation of arginine transport [55]. Vejchapipat et al. [56] showed that early stages of endotoxemia induced by LPS injection significantly decrease neonatal hepatic level of glutamine. The increase in liver glutamine utilization is associated with increases in parenchymal DNA and glutathione levels, as well as glutathione and urea release into the systemic circulation. This accelerated utilization provides carbons for energy and gluconeogenesis, and substrate for nucleotide and glutathione biosynthesis in order to support cell repair [18].

Glutamine synthetase (GS) in the liver is restricted to a small perivenous hepatocyte population and plays an important role in the scavenging of ammonia that has escaped the periportal urea-synthesizing compartment. Görg et al. [57] showed that LPS single intraperitoneal injection impairs hepatic ammonia detoxification by both downregulation of GS and its inactivation through tyrosine nitration. GS protein expression 24 h after LPS injection was decreased by approximately 20 %, whereas the corresponding enzymatic activity was lowered by 40–50 %. In line with GS inactivation, glutamine synthesis from ammonia in perfused livers obtained from LPS-treated rats is decreased by approximately 50 %. The resulting defect of the perivenous scavenger cell function with regard to ammonia elimination may partly contribute to sepsis-induced development of hyperammonemia. In rats treated with LPS, glutaminase activity and flux through glutaminase in intact mitochondria are markedly increased by the endotoxin treatment. The effect is associated with an increase in the sensitivity of glutaminase flux to the enzyme activator phosphate [58]. In the liver, glutamine plays an important role in ammonia detoxication and the regulation of pH homeostasis ("intercellular glutamine-glutamate cycle"). In addition, glutamine regulates liver metabolism by mechanisms that cannot be attributed to its metabolism. Examples include the stimulation of protein and glycogen synthesis, bile acid secretion, and inhibition of proteolysis in liver. A major trigger for such effects is an increased hepatocyte hydration due to the cumulative uptake of glutamine into the cells, which activates osmo-signaling pathways involving mitogen-activated protein kinases (MAPK). Glutamine- and hypoosmolarity-induced cell swelling activates extracellular signal-regulated kinases (ERK) and p38 (MAPK). Also, the antiproteolytic effect of glutamine is largely due to glutamine-induced cell swelling, which activates osmosignaling pathways. The glutamine-induced p38 (MAPK) activation mediates the inhibition of autophagic proteolysis at the level of autophagosome formation [59].

Surgical neonates are at risk of sepsis with associated liver dysfunction. Hydrogen peroxide (H_2O_2) and nitric oxide (NO) are important mediators of sepsis, which impair neonatal hepatic metabolism. Glutamine by itself or in the form of dipeptides, have been shown to have beneficial effects on the altered hepatocyte metabolism and liver damage during neonatal sepsis. The study from Babu et al. [60] found that glutamine and its dipeptides are indeed efficient in reversing the effects of septic mediators on hepatic oxidative metabolism in neonatal rats.

Markley et al. [61] determined the effects of glutamine on hepatocyte energy metabolism under conditions of neonatal endotoxemia, and concluded that glutamine reverses the inhibition of mitochondrial metabolism observed in endotoxemia, which is primarily at the level of ATP synthesis. The addition of glutamine to hepatocytes from endotoxemic rats restored intramitochondrial oxygen consumption to control levels. Although glutamine did not reverse the inhibition of the thermogenic proton leak observed in endotoxemia, it significantly increased oxygen consumption due to mitochondrial ATP synthesis. Glutamine significantly increases the hepatocyte ATP/ADP ratio compared with hepatocytes from endotoxemic rats. Electron microscopy reveals morphological damage to the mitochondria of hepatocytes from endotoxemic rats, and evidences a return to a normal appearance with the addition of glutamine. Intramitochondrial O_2 consumption is inhibited in isolated hepatocytes from suckling septic rats and this impairment can be reversed by glutamine. Kim et al. [62] showed that glutamine significantly increased fatty acid oxidation in hepatocytes from control and endotoxemic animals, suggesting that it may promote substrate oxidation during endotoxemia. In the pig model, after endotoxin-induced sepsis, the net protein synthesis is rapidly increased in the liver [63]. In the endotoxemic dog model, the net hepatic glucose output is increased approximately twofold [64], with an increase in the net hepatic glycogenolysis accounting for the majority of the increased hepatic glucose production. The main alterations of glutamine metabolism in liver due to endotoxemia is presented in Fig. 10.3.

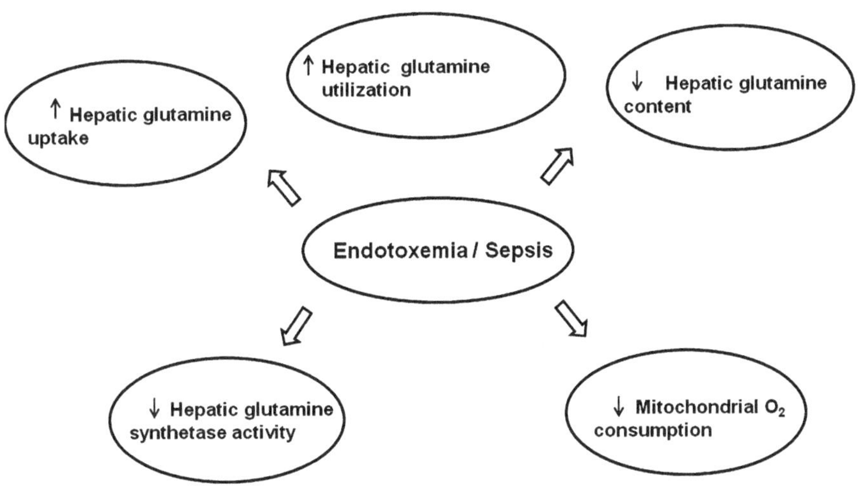

Fig. 10.3 Main alterations of glutamine metabolism in liver due to endotoxemia

Endotoxemia and Glutamine Metabolism in Skeletal Muscle

Skeletal muscle, the major repository of glutamine, plays a crucial role in maintaining nitrogen homeostasis during health and critical illness by synthesizing and exporting glutamine. Glutamine is both synthesized and degraded in skeletal muscle, and the balance of this intracellular cycle determines the net synthesis and release of glutamine from the tissue [65]. Skeletal muscles exhibit a twofold increase in glutamine release during infection, which is associated with a significant increase in endogenous glutamine biosynthesis. Skeletal muscle glutaminase activity is unchanged by endotoxemia, but expression of glutamine synthetase (GS) mRNA and specific activity increase in a time-dependent fashion. Despite an increase in GS activity in skeletal muscle, the intracellular glutamine pool becomes depleted, indicating that release rates likely exceed synthesis rates [20]. As a consequence, the muscle glutamine concentration fell in the endotoxin-treated animals by 25–40 %, an event that is apparent as early as 2 h after endotoxin treatment [66] and remains still visible 2 days after LPS injection [25]. This glutamine depletion is caused by accelerated muscle glutamine release [67] rather than by an increase in intracellular degradation or a fall in intracellular biosynthesis. The adaptive increase in GS expression requires de novo RNA and protein synthesis and may be designed to prevent complete depletion of the intracellular glutamine pool [66]. Simultaneously, the circulating pool of glutamine does not increase, suggesting accelerated uptake by other organs [20].

Ardawi and Majzoub [15] found that there is an enhanced rate of production of glutamine from skeletal muscle of septic rats in the cecal ligation and puncture model, which may be due to changes in efflux and/or increased intracellular formation of glutamine. Sepsis results in decreases of the concentrations of skeletal muscle glutamine, glutamate, 2-oxoglutarate, and adenosine monophosphate. Hindlimb blood flow showed no marked change in response to sepsis, but was accompanied by an enhanced net release of glutamine and alanine. The maximal activity of GS was increased only in quadriceps muscles of septic rats, whereas that of glutaminase was decreased in all muscles studied.

The expression of GS is induced in rat skeletal muscle cells (L-6) in response to treatment with the inflammatory cytokine TNF-α. Chakrabarti [68] demonstrated that the rat GS gene is transcriptionally regulated by TNF-α and identifies a TNF-α-responsive region at the 5′ flanking sequence of the GS gene. Lukaszewicz et al. [69] reported that induction of GS expression in skeletal muscle after endotoxin administration is adrenal gland dependent. Treatment of normal rats with LPS results in a marked increase in GS mRNA that appears dose and time dependent, and precedes the increase in GS protein. The increase in muscle GS mRNA observed in normal rats in response to LPS is abrogated in adrenalectomized rats at 3 h after treatment with a high dose of LPS. These and other studies implicate glucocorticoid hormones as a key, but not exclusive, regulator of GS expression in skeletal muscle after a catabolic insult.

Suojaranta-Ylinen et al. [70] reported that glutamine cannot prevent endotoxemia during or after cardiac surgery. However, Meador and Huey [71] suggested that glutamine supplementation provides an effective, novel, clinically applicable means of preserving muscle force during acute inflammation. LPS treatment is associated with a 33 % reduction in maximal plantarflexor isometric force and elevated serum TNF-α and IL-6. Glutamine completely prevents this LPS-induced force decrement and reduces muscle heat shock protein HSP-70 and IL-6. The main alterations of glutamine metabolism in skeletal muscles in endotoxemia are presented in Fig. 10.4.

Endotoxemia and Glutamine Metabolism in Lung

Severe infection alters lung glutamine metabolism. Insufficient glutamine for the lungs during sepsis may contribute to an impairment of lung function. Lung glutamine metabolism is supported by both blood glutamine uptake and de novo biosynthesis using circulating BCAA and glutamate as precursors.

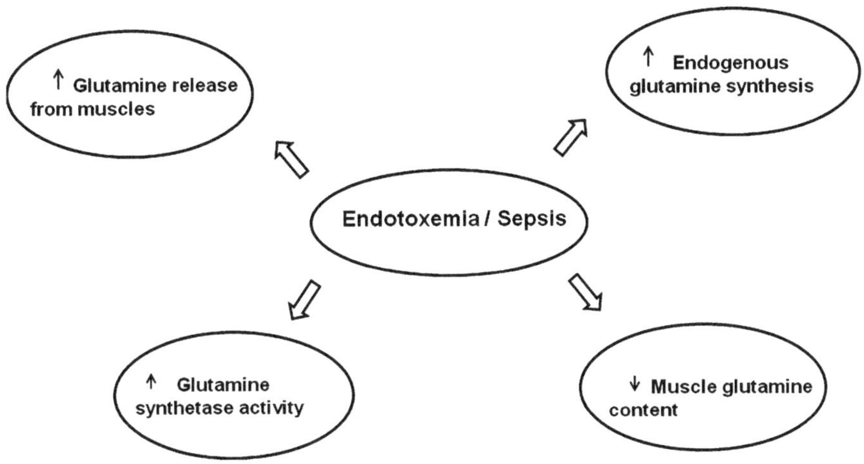

Fig. 10.4 Main alterations of glutamine metabolism in skeletal muscles in endotoxemia

Pan et al. [72] isolated lung plasma membrane vesicles from control and LPS-treated rats and assayed glutamine transport activity in these vesicles. They showed that 80 % of glutamine uptake in lung vesicles is mediated via the high affinity Na^+-dependent carrier system ASC, while 19 % occurred via the Na^+-independent System ASC. Treatment of rats with LPS resulted in a decrease in System ASC and X_{AG-} activity in lung plasma membrane vesicles, which may contribute to reduced glutamate uptake, reduced lung glutamine availability, and impaired cellular metabolism and function during septic states.

During sepsis, the lung responds by exporting increased amounts of glutamine. This response is accompanied by increased enzymatic activity of GS. Austgen et al. [73] studied the alterations in lung glutamine metabolism that occurs in the endotoxin-injured lung in rats and subsequently correlated with flux changes that occur in patients with the adult respiratory distress syndrome (ARDS). In healthy control rats, net amounts of glutamine are released by the lungs into the systemic circulation. The rate of glutamine release from the lung doubled 30 min after intravenous endotoxin. This accelerated fractional release of glutamine by the lungs is no longer detected 2 h after endotoxin treatment. By the 12-h time point, a more than twofold increase in GS activity is recorded. Simultaneously, lung weights are increased by 21 % and histologic examination shows an interstitial infiltrate and pulmonary edema. Similar observations were made in patients with "early" sepsis which exhibited a marked increase in lung glutamine release. During septic states, efflux of glutamine from the lung increases, a response thus sustained by an increase in GS activity. Abcouwer et al. [74] have used rat epithelial cell line of pulmonary origin (L2 cells) to study the effect of several hormones and cytokines (which mediate the septic shock response) on GS expression. They found that GS expression, as determined by measurement of mRNA and protein contents, increases rapidly and severalfold in response to physiologically relevant levels of the synthetic glucocorticoid dexamethasone (Dex). In contrast, GS expression is not markedly induced by LPS, cytokines, activated complement C5a, or prostaglandins. The results of this study are consistent with a regulation of lung GS expression via a direct glucocorticoid receptor-mediated response. In addition, GS mRNA decay in L2 cells seems to be regulated by two independent mechanisms, one being sensitive to the protein synthesis inhibitor cycloheximide, and the other being sensitive to actinomycin D. It is also known that GS expression in the rat lung can be induced by glucocorticoid hormones. Lukaszewicz et al. [75] characterized the induction of GS expression during LPS-induced endotoxemia in normal, neutropenic, and adrenalectomized rats, and showed that GS gene induction during sepsis is only partially mediated by adrenal-derived glucocorticoid hormones. Normal rats exhibited a time- and dose-dependent induction of GS mRNA levels after a single intraperitoneal dose of LPS. In response to endotoxemia, GS mRNA levels in the lung of adrenalectomized rats increased twofold compared with sixfold in sham-operated control rats.

Herskowitz et al. [76] incubated pulmonary artery endothelial cells (PAECs) with endotoxin (1 μg/ml) and showed a significant increase in System ASC-mediated glutamine transport which was maximal after 12 h of exposure. Kinetic studies indicated that the increase in carrier-mediated activity was not due to a change in K_m, but rather to a 73 % increase in V_{max}. The increase in glutamine uptake by PAECs was completely blocked by actinomycin D and cycloheximide, indicating that the accelerated glutamine transport was most probably due to an increase in transporter synthesis. During septic states, the lungs produce increased amounts of glutamine, an event that is likely mediated by both LPS and glucocorticoid hormones and is presumed to be due to accelerated intracellular glutamine biosynthesis. Because enhanced net glutamine release in vivo could also be due to a decrease in cellular uptake, Pan et al. [77] determined glutamine transport in cultured rat microvascular pulmonary endothelial cells (MPECs), and showed that dexamethasone (0.1 μmol/L) and LPS (1 μg/mL) inhibited glutamine uptake by decreasing the V_{max} of system ASC transporter (which mediates more than 90 % of glutamine transport) in a time- and dose-dependent manner. There was no synergistic or additive effect when both compounds were added together.

Acute lung injury (ALI) is a critical syndrome associated with respiratory dysfunction. It has been reported that glutamine can attenuate ALI after sepsis. Nakamura et al. [78] showed that glutamine added to the solution for total parenteral nutrition improved endotoxin-induced acute lung injury in rats. The survival rate and the nitrogen balance were significantly improved at 48 h after endotoxin administration as a result of glutamine treatment; the arterial oxygen partial pressure being significantly increased.

Neutrophils are considered to be central for the pathogenesis of ALI. It is noteworthy that Zhang et al. [79] indicated that glutamine could prevent neutrophil recruitment and infiltration, protect the alveolar barrier, and attenuate inflammatory injury during sepsis. These results may be related to enhanced glutathione (GSH) synthesis. Indeed, glutamine supplementation reduced the total protein concentration and total cell and neutrophil counts in bronchoalveolar lavage fluid after LPS challenge. Glutamine enhanced GSH synthesis and attenuated IL-8 release and myeloperoxidase activity in lung tissues. Glutamine also decreased CD11b expression in blood neutrophils and prevented lung histologic changes. L-buthionine-(S,R)-sulfoximine (BSO, a blocker of GSH synthesis) abolished the effects of glutamine and attenuated its protection on ALI.

Septic shock leads to alterations of cellular metabolism. Glutamine can enhance lung HSP70 expression which can preserve cellular metabolism after lethal endotoxemia and other forms of cellular stress. Singleton et al. [80] reported that a single dose of glutamine can enhance HSP70 in pulmonary epithelial cells and macrophages, and attenuate lung metabolic dysfunction by improving the ratio of adenosine triphosphate to adenosine diphosphate in the lung after sublethal endotoxemia. This beneficial effect on lung tissue may be mediated in part by enhanced expression of HSP70. Furthermore, Zhang et al. [81] investigated the role of GSH synthesis in the regulation on nuclear factor NF-κ activity and TNF-α released by glutamine in LPS-stimulated alveolar type II (AT-II) epithelial cells of rat lungs, and showed that glutamine can prevent the NF-kappaB activation and attenuate the release of TNF-α in LPS-stimulated AT-II cells, an effect that may be mediated via GSH synthesis.

Lung epithelial cells are important barriers in the respiratory system that can prevent pathogens from invading the body after nuclear factor NF-κB activation. LPS is a common pathogen-associated stimulus that activates IκB kinase (IKK) to regulate NF-κB-mediated inflammation through modulating nuclear translocation and phosphorylation of NF-κB. Previously, it has been shown that Akt and mTOR are involved in the phosphorylation of IKK to activate NF-κB. Hou et al. [82] demonstrated that glutamine modulated LPS-induced activation of NF-κB through the Akt/mTOR/IKK pathway in BEAS-2B cells. Glutamine deprivation induces phosphorylation of Akt/mTOR/IKK signaling, increases the level of NF-κB nuclear translocation and phosphorylated NF-κB, and upregulates NF-κB-dependent transcriptional activity, which is suppressed by glutamine administration. These findings provide potential mechanisms for the modulation by glutamine of LPS-induced NF-κB

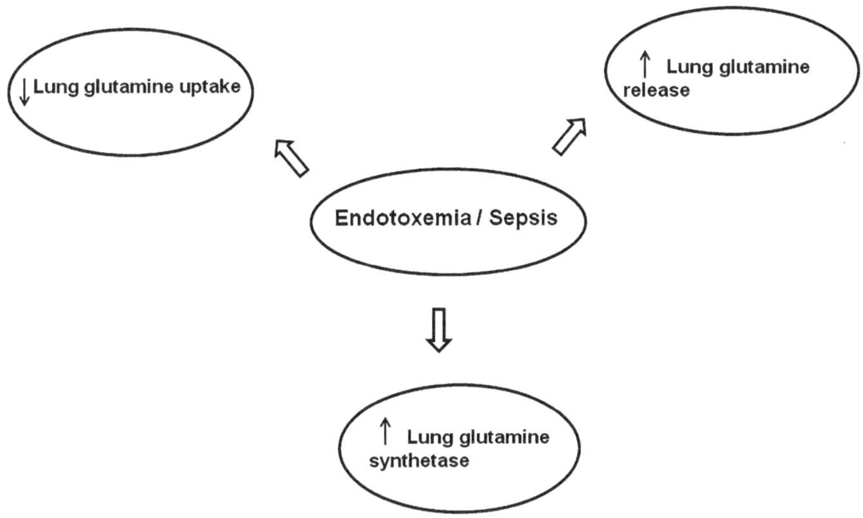

Fig. 10.5 Main alterations of glutamine metabolism in lung due to endotoxemia

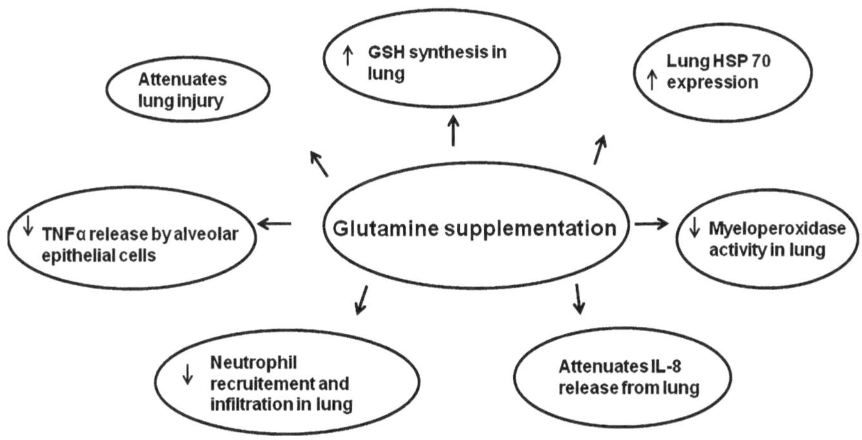

Fig. 10.6 Main effects of glutamine supplementation on lung in endotoxemia

activation in lung epithelial cells and strongly suggest that maintaining a physiological concentration of glutamine is essential in preventing LPS-induced lung inflammation. The main alterations of glutamine metabolism in lung due to endotoxemia is presented in Fig. 10.5; and the main effects of glutamine supplementation on lung functions in endotoxemia are summarized in Fig. 10.6.

Conclusions

Major endotoxemia can lead to sepsis, to septic shock and to multiple organ dysfunction syndrome. From experiments with animal models of endotoxemia, and (much less frequently) from clinical studies, it has been shown that endotoxemia markedly modifies glutamine metabolism in tissues with a decrease of intestinal glutamine uptake and metabolism, and decrease of oxygen consumption. However, this decrease is not specific for glutamine since numerous other amino acids are less absorbed in endotoxemia as a result of decreased intestinal functions. In liver, endotoxemia increases glutamine uptake and utilization while diminishing the glutamine synthetase activity, coinciding with decreased hepatic glutamine content and decreased mitochondrial oxygen consumption. In skeletal muscles, endotoxemia increases endogenous glutamine synthesis and release resulting in a decrease of the muscle glutamine content. In lungs, endotoxemia results in a decrease of glutamine uptake with increased glutamine endogenous synthesis and release. Supplementation with glutamine in its free form or in its dipeptide form allows to moderate in endotoxemic situation the increment of intestinal permeability and bacterial translocation, to decrease intestinal inflammation (and more generally of gut mucosal injury), and to increase the intestinal microcirculation and intestinal protein synthesis. In the lung, glutamine supplementation attenuates pulmonary inflammation and injury.

Mostly from experimental works with animal models, it thus appears that the rationale for glutamine supplementation in endotoxemia by the enteral way appears thus relatively strong, as long as a sufficient intestinal capacity for the absorption of this amino acid is preserved. Future works in experimental and clinical studies should consider, in endotoxemic/septic situation, supplementation with glutamine together with other conditionally essential amino acids to help in the nutritional management of this pathology.

Acknowledgments The authors wish to warmly thank INRA, AgroParisTech and the National Natural Science Foundation of China (#31110103909), the China Basic Research Program (#2013CB127301), the National Science and Technology Support Program Funding (#2012BAD39B03) and the University of Sao Paulo (Brazil, FAPESP grant 2012/07319-0) for their support.

References

1. Tsiotou AG, Sakorafas GH, Anagnostopoulos G, et al. Septic shock: current pathogenetic concepts from a clinical perspective. Med Sci Monit. 2005;11:RA76–85.
2. Nardi O, Polito A, Aboab J, et al. StO(2) guided early resuscitation in subjects with severe sepsis or septic shock: a pilot randomized trial. J Clin Monit Comput. 2013;27(3):215–21.
3. Venkatesh AK, Avula U, Bartimus H, et al. Time to antibiotics for septic shock: evaluating a proposed performance measure. Am J Emerg Med. 2013;31(4):680–3.
4. Pulido D, Nogues MV, Boix E, et al. Lipopolysaccharide neutralization by antimicrobial peptides: a gambit in the innate host defense strategy. J Innate Immun. 2012;4:327–36.
5. Hassoun HT, Kone BC, Mercer DW, et al. Post-injury multiple organ failure: the role of the gut. Shock. 2001;15:1–10.
6. Swank GM, Deitch EA. Role of the gut in multiple organ failure: bacterial translocation and permeability changes. World J Surg. 1996;20:411–7.
7. Deitch EA, Berg R, Specian R. Endotoxin promotes the translocation of bacteria from the gut. Arch Surg. 1987;122:185–90.
8. Blachier F, Boutry C, Bos C, et al. Metabolism and functions of L-glutamate in the epithelial cells of the small and large intestines. Am J Clin Nutr. 2009;90:814S–21.
9. Le Bacquer O, Laboisee C, Darmaun D. Glutamine preserves protein synthesis and paracellular permeability in Caco-2 cells submitted to « luminal fasting ». Am J Physiol. 2003;285:G128–36.
10. Elwafi F, Curis E, Zerrouk N, et al. Endotoxemia affects citrulline, arginine and glutamine bioavailability. Eur J Clin Invest. 2012;42:282–9.
11. Salloum RM, Copeland EM, Souba WW. Brush border transport of glutamine and other substrates during sepsis and endotoxemia. Ann Surg. 1991;213:401–9.
12. Souba WW, Herskowitz K, Klimberg VS. The effects of sepsis and endotoxemia on gut glutamine metabolism. Ann Surg. 1990;211:543–51.
13. Haque SM, Chen K, Usui N, et al. Effects of endotoxin on intestinal hemodynamics, glutamine metabolism, and function. Surg Today. 1997;27:500–5.
14. Ardawi MS, Jamal YS, Ashy AA, et al. Glucose and glutamine metabolism in the small intestine of septic rats. J Lab Clin Med. 1990;115:660–8.
15. Ardawi MS, Majzoub MF. Glutamine metabolism in skeletal muscle of septic rats. Metabolism. 1991;40:155–64.

16. Sarantos P, Abouhamze A, Chakrabarti R, et al. Glucocorticoids regulate intestinal glutamine synthetase gene expression in endotoxemia. Arch Surg. 1994;129:59–65.
17. Niu L, Qiao W, Li G, et al. Different alterations in rat intestinal glutamine transport during the progression of CLP- and LPS-induced sepsis. J Surg Res. 2011;169:284–91.
18. Austgen TR, Chen MK, Flynn TC, et al. The effects of endotoxin on the splanchnic metabolism of glutamine and related substrates. J Trauma. 1991;31:742–51.
19. Mester M, Tompkins RG, Gelfand JA, et al. Intestinal production of interleukin-1 alpha during endotoxemai in the mouse. J Surg Res. 1993;54:584–91.
20. Karinch AM, Pan M, Lin CM. Glutamine metabolism in sepsis and infection. J Nutr. 2001;131:2535S–8.
21. Abad B, Mesonero JE, Salvador MT, et al. Effect of lipopolysaccharide on small intestinal L-leucine transport in rabbit. Dig Dis Sci. 2001;46:1113–9.
22. Gardiner KR, Gardiner RE, Barbul A. Reduced intestinal absorption of arginine during sepsis. Crit Care Med. 1995;23:1227–32.
23. Gardiner KR, Ahrendt GM, Gardiner RE, et al. Failure of intestinal amino acid absorptive mechanisms in sepsis. J Am Coll Surg. 1995;181:431–6.
24. Gardiner K, Barbul A. The role of the imino transporter protein in sepsis-impaired intestinal proline absorption. JPEN J Parenter Enteral Nutr. 1993;17:507–12.
25. Boutry C, Matsumoto H, Bos C, et al. Decreased glutamate, glutamine and citrulline concentrations in plasma and muscle in endotoxemia cannot be reversed by glutamate or glutamine supplementation: a primary intestinal defect? Amino Acids. 2012;43:1485–98.
26. Chambon-Savanovitch C, Farges MC, Raul F, et al. Can a glutamate-enriched diet counteract glutamine depletion in endotoxemic rats? J Nutr Biochem. 1999;10:331–7.
27. Crouser ED, Julian MW, Weinstein DM, et al. Endotoxin-induced ileal mucosal injury and nitric oxide dysregulation are temporally dissociated. Am J Respir Crit Care Med. 2000;161:1705–12.
28. King CJ, Tytgat S, Delude RL, et al. Ileal mucosal oxygen consumption is decreased in endotoxemic rats but is restored toward normal by treatment with aminoguanidine. Crit Care Med. 1999;27:2518–24.
29. Crouser ED, Julian MW, Dorinski PM. Ileal VO(2)-O(2) alterations induced by endotoxin correlate with severity of mitochondrial injury. Am J Respir Crit Care Med. 1999;160:1347–53.
30. Li N, Liboni K, Fang MZ, et al. Glutamine decreases lipopolysaccharide-induced intestinal inflammation in infant rats. Am J Physiol. 2004;286:G914–21.
31. Sukhotnik I, Agam M, Shamir R, et al. Oral glutamine prevents gut mucosal injury and improves mucosal recovery following lipopolysaccharide endotoxemia in a rat. J Surg Res. 2007;143:379–84.
32. Ding LA, Li JS. Effects of glutamine on intestinal permeability and bacterial translocation in TPN-rats with endotoxemia. World J Gastroenterol. 2003;9:1327–32.
33. Uehara K, Takahashi T, Fujii H, et al. The lower intestinal tract-specific induction of heme oxygenase-1 by glutamine protects against endotoxemic intestinal injury. Crit Care Med. 2005;33:381–90.
34. Coeffier M, Miralles-Barrachina O, Le Pessot F, et al. Influence of glutamine on cytokine production by human gut in vitro. Cytokine. 2001;13:148–54.
35. Coeffier M, Marion R, Leplingard A, et al. Glutamine decreased interleukin-8 and interleukin-6 but not nitric oxide and prostaglandins E2 production by human gut in vitro. Cytokine. 2002;18:92–7.
36. Huang Y, Li N, Liboni K, et al. Glutamine decreases lipopolysaccharide-induced IL-8 production in Caco-2 cells through a non-NFκB p50 mechanisms. Cytokine. 2003;22:77–83.
37. Liboni KC, Li N, Neu J. Mechanism of glutamine-mediated amelioration of lipopolysaccharide- induced IL-8 production in Caco-2 cells. Cytokine. 2004;26:57–65.
38. Liboni KC, Li N, Scumpia PO, et al. Glutamine modulates LPS-induced IL-8 production through IκB/NF-κB in human fetal and adult intestinal epithelium. J Nutr. 2005;135:245–51.
39. Zhou X, Wu X, Yin Y, et al. Preventive oral supplementation with glutamine and arginine has beneficial effects on the intestinal mucosa and inflammatory cytokines in endotoxemic rats. Amino Acids. 2012;43:813–21.
40. Lehmann C, Pavlovic D, Zhou J, et al. Intravenous free and dipeptide-bound glutamine maintains intestinal microcirculation in experimental endotoxemia. Nutrition. 2012;28:588–93.
41. Kessel A, Toubi E, Pavlotzky E, et al. Treatment with glutamine is associated with down-regulation of Toll-like receptor-4 and myeloid differentiation factor 88 expression and decrease in intestinal mucosal injury caused by lipopolysaccharide endotoxaemia in a rat. Clin Exp Immunol. 2008;151:341–7.
42. Wischmeyer PE, Kahana M, Wolfson R, et al. Glutamine induces heat shock protein and protects against endotoxin shock in the rat. J Appl Physiol. 2001;90:2403–10.
43. Chen K, Okuma T, Okamura K, et al. Glutamine-supplemented parenteral nutrition improves gut mucosa integrity and function in endotoxemic rats. JPEN J Parenter Enteral Nutr. 1994;18:167–71.
44. Higashiguchi T, Noguchi Y, Meyer T, et al. Protein synthesis in isolated enterocytes from septic or endotoxaemic rats: regulation by glutamine. Clin Sci (Lond). 1995;89:311–9.
45. Okuma T, Kaneko H, Chen K, et al. Total parenteral nutrition supplemented with L-alanyl-L-glutamine and gut structure and protein metabolism in septic rats. Nutrition. 1994;10:241–5.

46. Scheibe R, Schade M, Grundling M. Glutamine and alanyl-glutamine dipeptide reduce mesenteric plasma extravasation, leukocyte adhesion and tumor necrosis factor-α (TNF-α) release during experimental endotoxemia. J Physiol Pharmacol. 2009;60:S19–24.
47. Jiang ZY, Sun LH, Lin YC. Effects of dietary glycyl-glutamine on growth performance, small intestinal integrity, and immune responses of weaning piglets challenged with lipopolysaccharide. J Anim Sci. 2009;87:4050–6.
48. Dugan ME, McBurney MI. Luminal glutamine perfusion alters endotoxin-related changes in ileal permeability of the piglet. JPEN J Parenter Enteral Nutr. 1995;19:83–7.
49. Haynes TE, Li P, Li XL. L-Glutamine or L-alanyl-L-glutamine prevents oxidant- or endotoxin-induced death of neonatal enterocytes. Amino Acids. 2009;37:131–42.
50. Pacitti AJ, Austgen TR, Souba WW. Mechanisms of increased hepatic glutamine uptake in the endotoxin-treated rat. J Surg Res. 1992;53:298–305.
51. Inoue Y, Pacitti AJ, Souba WW. Endotoxin increases hepatic glutamine transport activity. J Surg Res. 1993;54: 393–400.
52. Plumley DA, Watkins K, Bode BP, et al. Cyclo-oxygenase blockade abrogates the endotoxin-induced increase in Na(+)-dependent hepatic amino acid transport. JPEN J Parenter Enteral Nutr. 1995;19:9–14.
53. Wang W, Li Y, Zhang W, et al. Changes of plasma glutamine concentration and hepatocyte membrane system N transporters expression in early endotoxemia. J Surg Res. 2011;166:290–7.
54. Fischer CP, Bode BP, Souba WW. Starvation and endotoxin act independently and synergistically to coordinate hepatic glutamine transport. J Trauma. 1996;40:688–93.
55. Inoue Y, Bode BP, Souba WW. Hepatic Na(+)-independent amino acid transport in endotoxemic rats: evidence for selective stimulation of arginine transport. Shock. 1994;2:164–72.
56. Vejchapipat P, Eaton S, Fukumoto K, et al. Hepatic glutamine metabolism during endotoxemia in neonatal rats. Nutrition. 2002;18:293–7.
57. Görg B, Wettstein M, Metzger S, et al. Lipopolysaccharide-induced tyrosine nitration and inactivation of hepatic glutamine synthetase in the rat. Hepatology. 2005;41:1065–73.
58. Ewart HS, Qian D, Brosnan JT. Activation of hepatic glutaminase in the endotoxin-treated rat. J Surg Res. 1995;59:245–9.
59. Häussinger D, Graf D, Weiergräber OH. Glutamine and cell signaling in liver. J Nutr. 2001;131:S2509–14.
60. Babu R, Eaton S, Drake DP, et al. Glutamine and glutathione counteract the inhibitory effects of mediators of sepsis in neonatal hepatocytes. J Pediatr Surg. 2001;36:282–6.
61. Markley MA, Pierro A, Eaton S. Hepatocyte mitochondrial metabolism is inhibited in neonatal rat endotoxaemia: effects of glutamine. Clin Sci. 2002;102:337–44.
62. Kim SC, Pierro A, Zamparelli M, Spitz L, Eaton S. Fatty acid oxidation in neonatal hepatocytes: effects of sepsis and glutamine. Nutrition. 2002;18:298–300.
63. Bruins MJ, Soeters PB, Deutz NE. Endotoxemia affects organ protein metabolism differently during prolonged feeding in pigs. J Nutr. 2000;130:3003–13.
64. Meinz H, Lacy DB, Ejiofor J, et al. Alterations in hepatic gluconeogenic amino acid uptake and gluconeogenesis in the endotoxin treated conscious dog. Shock. 1998;9:296–303.
65. Wu G, Thompson JR, Baracos VE. Glutamine metabolism in skeletal muscle from the broiler chick (Gallus domesticus) and the laboratory rat (Rattus norvegicus). Biochem J. 1991;274:769–74.
66. Austgen TR, Chakrabarti R, Chen MK, et al. Adaptive regulation in skeletal muscle glutamine metabolism in endotoxin-treated rats. J Trauma. 1992;32:600–6.
67. Vesali RF, Klaude M, Rooyackers O, et al. Amino acid metabolism in led muscle after an endotoxin injection in healthy volunteers. Am J Physiol. 2005;288:360–4.
68. Chakrabarti R. Transcriptional regulation of the rat glutamine synthetase gene by tumor necrosis factor-alpha. Eur J Biochem. 1998;254:70–4.
69. Lukaszewicz GC, Souba WW, Abcouwer SF. Induction of muscle glutamine synthetase gene expression during endotoxemia is adrenal gland dependent. Shock. 1997;332–338.
70. Suojaranta-Ylinen R, Ruokonen E, Pulkki K. Preoperative glutamine loading does not prevent endotoxemia in cardiac surgery. Acta Anaesthesiol Scand. 1997;41:385–91.
71. Meador BM, Huey KA. Glutamine preserves skeletal muscle force during an inflammatory insult. Muscle Nerve. 2009;40:1000–7.
72. Pan M, Fischer CP, Wasa M, et al. Characterization of glutamine and glutamate transport in rat lung plasma membrane vesicles. J Surg Res. 1997;69:418–24.
73. Austgen TR, Chen MK, Salloum RM, et al. Glutamine metabolism by the endotoxin- injured lung. J Trauma. 1991;31:1068–74.
74. Abcouwer SF, Lukaszewicz GC, Souba WW. Glucocorticoids regulate glutamine synthetase expression in lung epithelial cells. Am J Physiol. 1996;270:L141–51.
75. Lukaszewicz GC, Abcouwer SF, Labow BI, et al. Glutamine synthetase gene expression in the lungs of endotoxin-treated and adrenalectomized rats. Am J Physiol. 1997;273:L1182–90.

76. Herskowitz K, Bode BP, Block ER, et al. The effects of endotoxin on glutamine transport by pulmonary artery endothelial cells. J Surg Res. 1991;50:356–61.
77. Pan M, Wasa M, Ryan U, et al. Inhibition of pulmonary microvascular endothelial glutamine transport by glucocorticoids and endotoxin. JPEN J Parenter Enteral Nutr. 1995;19:477–81.
78. Nakamura T, Yamakawa M, Maeda J, et al. Effect of glutamine on acute lung injury in rats with endotoxemia. Clin Nutr. 1997;16:79–83.
79. Zhang F, Wang X, Pan L, et al. Glutamine attenuates lipopolysaccharide-induced acute lung injury. Nutrition. 2009;25:692–8.
80. Singleton KD, Serkova N, Banerjee A, et al. Glutamine attenuates endotoxin-induced lung metabolic dysfunction: potential role of enhanced heat shock protein 70. Nutrition. 2005;21:214–23.
81. Zhang F, Wang X, Wang W, et al. Glutamine reduces TNF-alpha by enhancing glutathione synthesis in lipopolysaccharide-stimulated alveolar epithelial cells of rats. Inflammation. 2008;31:344–50.
82. Hou YC, Chiu WC, Yeh CL, et al. Glutamine modulates lipopolysaccharide-induced activation of NF-κB via the Akt/mTOR pathway in lung epithelial cells. Am J Physiol. 2012;302:L174–83.

Part II
Glutamine Use in Critically Ill Patients and Their Diagnosis

Chapter 11
Plasma Glutamine and Its Levels in Metabolic Stress

Jan Wernerman

Key Points

- Glutamine constitutes 1/3 of the total amino acid concentration in plasma.
- Low plasma glutamine in critical illness is associated with an unfavorable outcome.
- High plasma glutamine in critical illness is probably associated with an unfavorable outcome.
- Plasma glutamine concentration is not related to endogenous de novo glutamine synthesis.
- The entire free glutamine pool is tuned over in 24 h.

Keywords Critical illness • Skeletal muscle • Inter-organ flux • First-pass elimination • Compartmentalization

Introduction

Plasma glutamine concentration is a reflection of a number of processes. In metabolic stress and in particular in critical illness the plasma level may deviate from the normal range, which is associated with an unfavorable outcome. The underlying mechanisms are still obscure. This chapter merely deals with the empirically finding of plasma glutamine concentration in humans in health and disease.

Glutamine and the Plasma Compartment

Free glutamine holds the highest amino acid concentration in plasma in man and is the most abundant free amino acid in man (Fig. 11.1). Normally 0.5–0.8 mmol/L out of a total free amino acid concentration in plasma of around 2.0–2.5 mmol/L. Glutamine is also the most abundant free amino acid over all in man, which to a large extent relates to the very high intracellular concentration in skeletal

J. Wernerman, M.D., Ph.D. (✉)
Karolinska University Hospital Huddinge, Karolinska Institutet, Stockholm, Sweden
e-mail: jan.wernerman@karolinska.se

R. Rajendram et al. (eds.), *Glutamine in Clinical Nutrition*, Nutrition and Health,
DOI 10.1007/978-1-4939-1932-1_11, © Springer Science+Business Media New York 2015

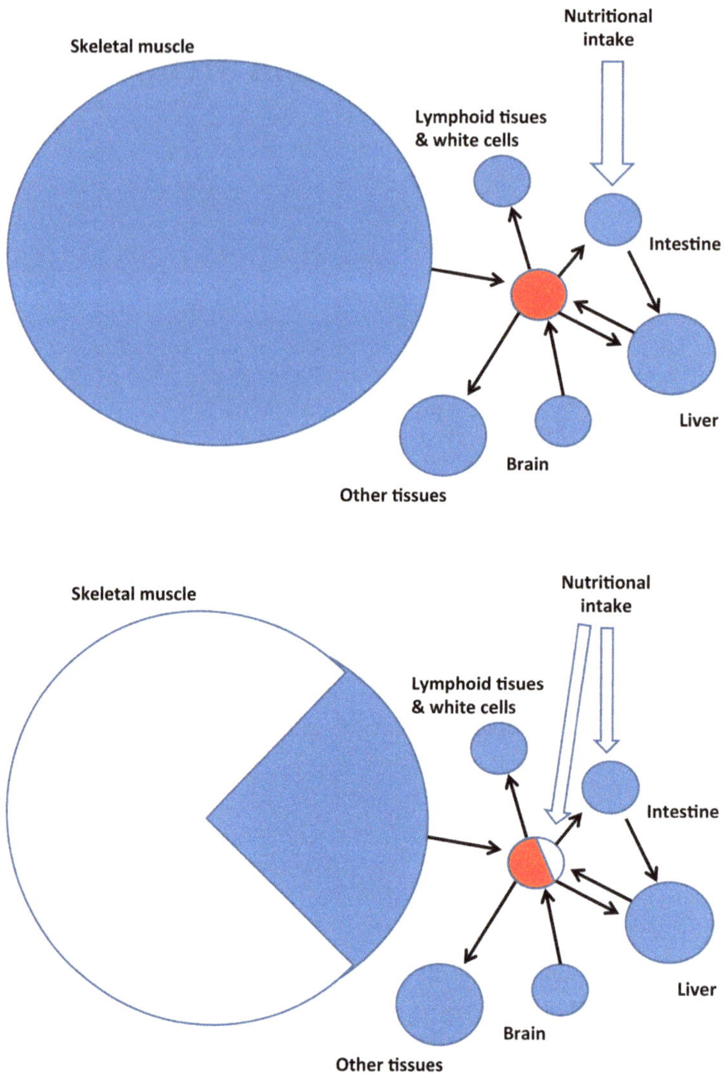

Fig. 11.1 A schematic illustration of the pool sizes of free glutamine in individual tissues. (**a**) The *upper panel* illustrates conditions in healthy adult subjects. The *red pool* is plasma, and the *arrows* indicate the directions of fluxes between the pools. In healthy subjects nutritional intake will come through the intestine as indicated. (**b**) The *lower panel* illustrates typical conditions in critical illness, when muscle pool and plasma pool are diminished, and intake may come through intestine or intravenously

muscle, in healthy man 12–18 mmol/L intracellular water [1]. This corresponds to a gradient between the intracellular and extracellular fluid of around 30. In other tissues the gradient is less pronounced: for liver 4–5 [2], for intestinal mucosa around 2 [3, 4].

Besides the relative high concentration of free glutamine there is also a high turnover of glutamine. Measurements of glutamine rate of appearance employing isotopic labels report values of 50–80 g per 24 h [5–8]. In rough figures this means that the total pool of free glutamine in the human body turns over every 24 h. The extracellular glutamine pool is in total less than 2 g, and it has a rapid turnover, whilst the intracellular glutamine pool of more than 50 g, turns over slower. This is illustrated by the fact that equilibration of an injected tracer takes several days [8].

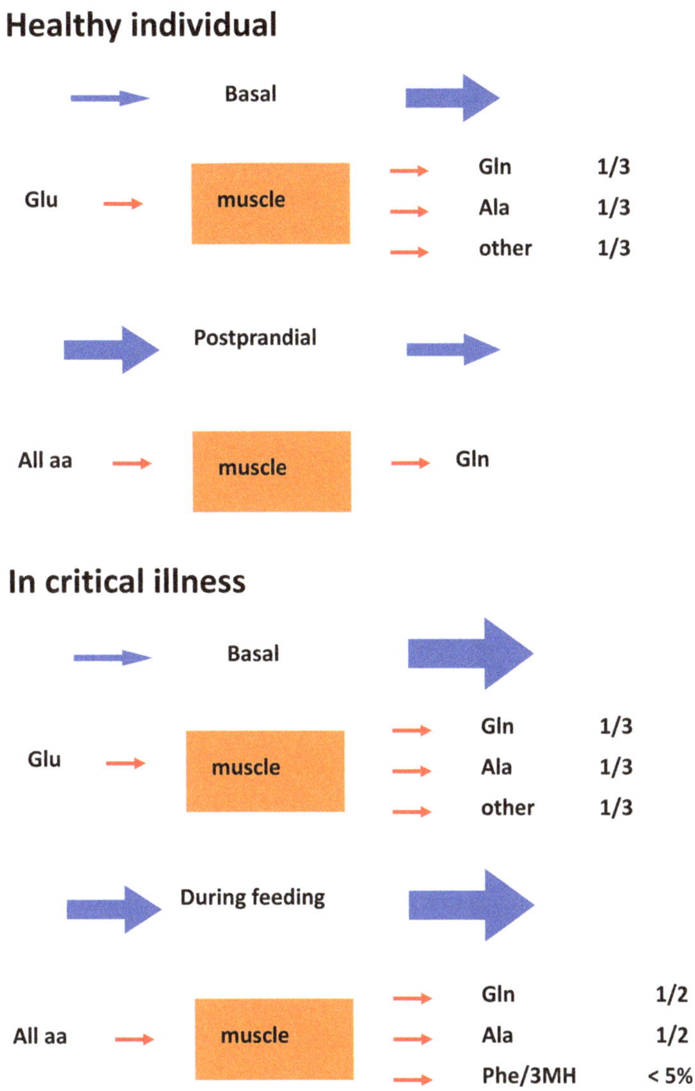

Fig. 11.2 Schematic illustrations of the relative size of amino acid fluxes across skeletal muscle in healthy subjects (*upper panels*) and in critical illness (*lower panels*). The differences in fluxes related to feeding are illustrated. (Gln—glutamine, Ala—alanine, Glu—glutamate, Phe—phenylalanine, 3MH—3-methylhistidine)

Many other chapters of this volume give insight into how the availability and turnover of glutamine relates to functions in cells. Plasma glutamine concentration discussed here is a reflection of all those processes integrated and the transport in between organs (Fig. 11.2). The perspective of this transport function is necessary to discuss why measurement of plasma glutamine may be useful. In particular muscle tissue holds a high free glutamine concentration, and it is the major site of de novo glutamine synthesis in health as well as in critical illness [5, 9, 10]. It is obvious that plasma glutamine is the accessible sampling site, but the interpretation of a singular determination of plasma glutamine may not be obvious.

Plasma concentration of glutamine is related to the multiple functions that glutamine serve, each of which may influence the level. Taken all potential influences into account, the plasma level of glutamine is remarkably constant in a given individual in a given health state.

Glutamine and Feeding

In response to feeding, glutamine levels change only marginally [11–13]. This is particularly true for enteral feeding, also when the enteral food given has a high content of glutamine (Fig. 11.2). There are no reports that this is different in various stressed states. So the first pass elimination through the splanchnic area is high [14]. Commonly a high enteral intake of glutamine results in an increase of plasma glutamate concentration and an elevated flux of glutamate from the splanchnic area to skeletal muscle. Furthermore any high protein intake by the enteral route is associated with an increase of plasma concentrations of a number of amino acids, in particular the branched-chain amino acids, which have a comparatively low first-pass elimination following an enteral protein intake. Consequently the branched-chain amino acids are transported to skeletal muscle. The uptake of glutamate and the branched-chain amino acids in muscle result in oxidation and transamination reactions and an elevated efflux of glutamine from skeletal muscle [15, 16]. This is one example of the function of glutamine as an inter-organ carrier of nitrogen or amino-groups.

Glutamine and Critical Illness

In stressed states, in particular in critical illness, a depletion of glutamine is reported [17–19]. Empirically the plasma glutamine concentration at ICU admission is related to mortality [20, 21]. Primarily low plasma concentrations of glutamine are predictive of an unfavorable outcome. However, there are reports of an U-shaped curve, where also high glutamine levels out of the normal range are associated with an unfavorable outcome in critical illness [21]. Overall, a plasma glutamine concentration out of the normal range at ICU admission is a mortality predictor independent of the standard scoring systems APACHE II and SAPS 2. The plasma level of glutamine is remarkably constant over time in the individual ICU patient [22, 23].

In the Amsterdam study a plasma glutamine concentration <0.42 mmol/L at ICU admission was associated with a higher hospital mortality [20]. The standard mortality ratio for patients with glutamine level <0.42 mmol/L was around 1.00, while the standard mortality ratio for those with a level >0.42 mmol/L was around 0.60. Prediction for a low glutamine level was found for high age and for a high level of creatine phosphokinase in plasma at admission. In the Stockholm study a more or less identical cutoff level for low plasma glutamine concentration as a mortality predictor was found [21]. The elevated mortality was not ICU mortality, but rather post-ICU mortality, a finding probably more reflecting ICU discharge criteria than a difference in epidemiology. In addition the Stockholm material identified the small group with high plasma glutamine levels being at risk. In the Amsterdam study a few individuals had high levels, but the authors did not find reason to comment upon that. Also in the Stockholm study the number of patients with high glutamine admittance level were few, and the interpretation must therefore be done with caution.

Both these studies including consecutive patients identifies approximately 1/3 of patients having low admittance plasma glutamine concentration without any relation to outcome predictors such as APACHE II or organ failure scores such as SOFA. In a recent large multicentre study of selected critically ill patients with ≥2 organ failures a fraction of approximately 1/3 was also reported to have a low plasma glutamine concentration, at least in a subset of the patients studied [24].

Furthermore in the Stockholm study the mortality associated with a low admittance plasma glutamine concentration was most pronounced as post-ICU mortality. This may to some degree be related to hospital organization of critical care; if intermediate care/high dependency is organized as a part of intensive care medicine or if it is organized separately. It may be speculated if the predictive value of low glutamine is a reflection of a risk of limited metabolic or nutritional reserves. Unfortunately the generally applied risk scores for malnutrition and/or metabolic depletion in hospitalized patients are of limited relevance for the critical care population [25].

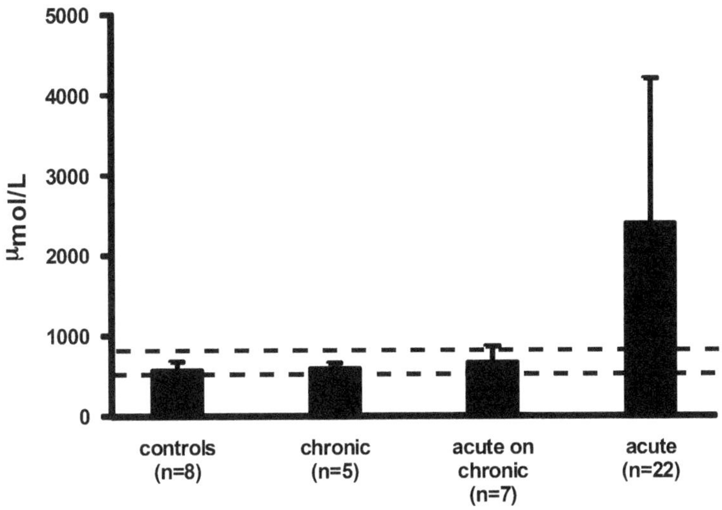

Fig. 11.3 Data from Tjader et al. [22] illustrating that plasma glutamine concentrations may be restored to normal level (500–800 µmol/L) by intravenous glutamine supplementation in all critically ill patients by providing 20 g (–40 g)/24 h as a continuous infusion

Hyperglutaminemia

The only patient group with high plasma glutamine concentrations reported are acute hepatic insufficiency [26]. This only applies for the group of individuals without an underlying chronic liver disease (Fig. 11.3). Patients with acute-on-chronic hepatic insufficiency as well patients with chronic hepatic insufficiency have normal or low plasma glutamine concentrations. There are only few publications in this field, and therefore it is not clear if hyperglutaminemia in acute hepatic failure has a prognostic implication. In chronic liver failure glutamine may be involved in the pathogenesis of hepatic encephalopathy [27]. The rational behind it that glutamate is an excitatory transmitter substance in the central nervous system and that clearance of glutamate is by re-uptake in nerve endings and by uptake into astroglia cells and metabolization to glutamine to be exported out of the central nervous system. Also the capture of ammonia is considered to be an important role of glutamine in hepatic encephalopathy [28]. The oral glutamine challenge is sometimes used to diagnose the susceptibility of an individual with liver cirrhosis to develop encephalopathy [29].

The significance of hyperglutaminemia in other conditions than acute hepatic failure is obscure. There are no systematic reports on this issue. Inborn errors of metabolism such as urea-cycle disorders may present with hyperglutaminemia [30], but there are also cases with very high plasma glutamine concentrations during critical illness without any obvious explication and which return to normal levels as patients recover [31].

Glutamine and Surgical Trauma

Following surgery plasma glutamine is most often unaltered, although the glutamine concentration in skeletal muscle decreases in proportion to the extent of trauma [32, 33]. This is a decrease that evolves slowly over time with a nadir at approximately 72 h, the greater the trauma the later the nadir. After that there is a slow recovery back to normal levels in muscle over a 3–4-week period [34, 35]. A

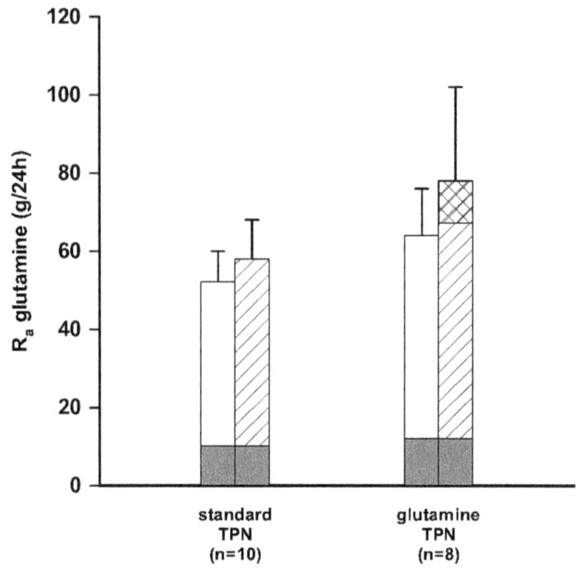

Fig. 11.4 Data from van Acker et al. [10] demonstrating the absence of a feedback mechanism on endogenous glutamine production when exogenous glutamine is provided intravenously. Metabolically healthy patients scheduled for elective surgery were investigated preoperatively before and during provision of TPN with or without glutamine supplementation. Glutamine production was estimated by the rate of glutamine appearance calculated from a constant infusion of ^{13}C-glutamine. *Open bars* depict basal state, hatched bars fed state. The *grey* zones depict contribution from protein degradation and cross-hatched zone the contribution from exogenous supplementation

similar depletion of muscle free glutamine with only a marginal influence on plasma concentrations is seen in healthy volunteers given an infusion of stress hormones [36, 37]. It applies to a triple combination of adrenaline, cortisol and glucagon, but it is also seen after adrenalin alone. Typically the decrease starts after 3–6 h and continues for at least 24 h, and the decline continues also after the stress hormone infusion is stopped [36]. A similar delayed decrease is also reported after an endotoxin challenge to healthy volunteers following the same time pattern [38].

The relation between plasma glutamine concentration and the de novo glutamine synthesis is poorly elucidated. In the limited existing literature no clear relation between plasma glutamine concentration and glutamine Ra is found [9, 10]. Unfortunately, the subjects investigated so far have concentrations mainly within the normal range, and the number of individuals investigated with levels outside the normal range are too few to allow for any conclusions (Fig. 11.4). For critically ill patients the plasma glutamine level is not related to the concentration in muscle and also not the level of efflux out of skeletal muscle [22]. Several authors have speculated over how the de novo synthesis of glutamine and the inter-organ flux of glutamine may be regulated [39]. Secondarily to this come the possible regulators of plasma level and tissue level. A fair summary for today is that this is insufficiently known.

Plasma Glutamine and Exogenous Supply

Now, how do critically ill patients respond to exogenous glutamine supply in terms of plasma concentration (Fig. 11.5)? In cases of intravenous administration of crystalline glutamine or a glutamine-containing dipeptide there is a prompt increase in concentration [31]. With a high infusion rate the time needed to reach a steady state is variable [40]. Likewise the concentration returns back to basal fairly

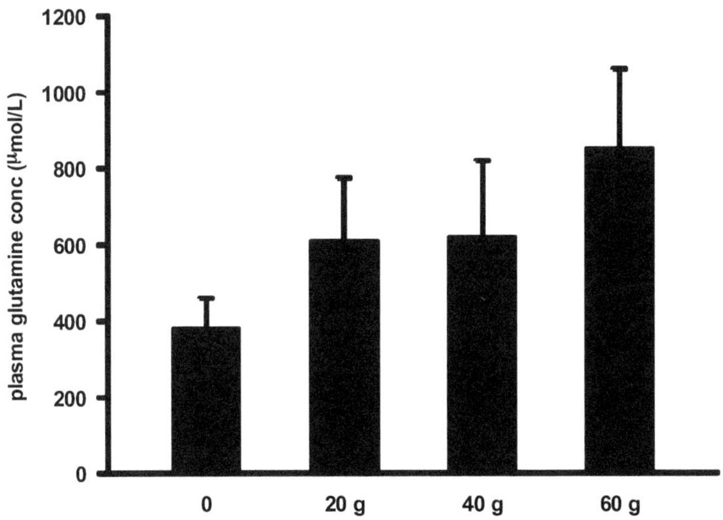

Fig. 11.5 Data from Clemmensen et al. [26], illustrating plasma glutamine concentration in patients with different types of liver insufficiency. Chronic liver insufficiency, whether compensated or not, is accompanied by a normal plasma glutamine concentration, while acute fulminant liver insufficiency may be accompanied by a very high plasma glutamine concentration. The normal interval of glutamine concentration (500–800 μmol/L) is indicated by the hatched lines

quick after stopping the administration, the decay-curve is mostly a reflection of redistribution to tissue compartments. After enteral administration, the situation for critically ill patients is very similar to that of healthy individuals, with a high first-pass elimination [14]. So the effect of enteral glutamine supplementation on plasma glutamine levels is marginal in the critically ill [41]. Still the upper part of the gastrointestinal tract and the liver, where the extraction corresponding to the first-pass elimination takes place, may benefit from glutamine supplementation even if the plasma concentrations is unaltered. There are reports of beneficial effect of enteral glutamine supplementation to clinically ill subjects [42, 43], but in general the results of enteral administration are inconsistent as compared to the results reported when glutamine supplementation is given by the intravenous route [44].

Glutamine supplementation is reported to be beneficial to critically ill patients only by parenteral route and in combination with parenteral nutrition [44, 45]. The beneficial effect of parenteral administration of glutamine may be attributed to the elevation or normalization of plasma glutamine concentration by that route of administration. The beneficial effect being confined only to patients on parenteral nutrition is more difficult to understand mechanistically. Does it correspond to that the intestinal tract is depleted by the absence of enteral glutamine, or does it relate to that patients on parenteral nutrition are in general more sick, or at least more glutamine depleted?

Until now outcome studies of glutamine supplementation in critically ill patients are designed to fit a pharmaco-nutritional perspective than a depletion perspective. Patients are given supplementation as a standard dose [46] or in relation to body size [24, 47, 48], with little concern for the actual plasma concentration. The relation between pretreatment level, the dose given, and the level during treatment have so far not been recorded in any major study. At least with intravenous administration the plasma glutamine concentration is related to the dose given [22, 31]. A dose-response relationship of clinical or outcome parameters related to glutamine depletion is therefore possible. Such a dose-response relationship should also be considered if glutamine overdosing is associated with toxic effects. The association between a high plasma glutamine concentration at ICU admittance and unfavorable outcomes, may not be a direct relation, but rather a signal of an inability to clear glutamine from the plasma compartment is cases of metabolic susceptibility. If so, it is the inability to deal with nitrogen overloading in general, rather than glutamine specifically that is the problem. This is clearly a field where more mechanistic research is desperately needed. This is particularly true as the larger multicenter study over combined enteral and parenteral glutamine supplementation demonstrated a mortality disadvantage when a large dose of glutamine dipeptide was given early in critical illness separated from nutrition [24]. The study result may be most relevant in patients with ≥3 organ failures, as the treatment groups turned out not to be comparable for these high-risk patients. Therefore, if the elevated mortality risk reported is relevant for patients outside this limited patient population is not clear, but the finding is alarming and it motivates mechanistic studies to settle the background to the detrimental effect in that particular study.

In general the major criticism of the available studies of glutamine supplementation in the critically ill, is the absence of characterization of the glutamine status of the individual patients, not even by an admission value of plasma glutamine concentration. Without a characterization of glutamine status, the supplementation with glutamine is totally blind without knowledge of if a possible depletion is at hand or if so, if the dosage given is adequate. The historical pilot studies are excused, but more in recent well-sponsored studies omitting this basic information are more difficult to comprehend. Future studies over exogenous glutamine supplementation should be seriously advised to include characterization of glutamine status as part the protocol.

Plasma Glutamine Concentration and Glutamine Deficiency

Still the question remains if restoration of the glutamine plasma level to normal should be the target of exogenous glutamine supplementation? Or is the association between admission plasma glutamine level and outcomes just an epiphenomenon? To answer these questions a number of studies in critically ill patients are needed. The endogenous production of glutamine should be better characterized, as well as the relation between feeding, plasma glutamine concentration, and glutamine de novo synthesis [49, 50].

Conclusions

Plasma glutamine concentration mirrors a number of metabolic events. Today the glutamine level is usually not available in routine hospital chemistry. With a better understanding of the underlying mechanisms behind the plasma glutamine concentration, this may become a valuable tool to evaluate nutritional status, metabolic status, and the risk for an unfavorable outcome in metabolic stress and in critical illness.

References

1. Bergstrom J, Furst P, Noree LO, Vinnars E. The effect of peritoneal dialysis on intracellular free amino acids in muscle from uraemic patients. Proc Eur Dial Transplant Assoc. 1972;9:393–401. PubMed PMID: 4668917. Epub 1972/01/01. eng.
2. Barle H, Ahlman B, Nyberg B, Andersson K, Essen P, Wernerman J. The concentrations of free amino acids in human liver tissue obtained during laparoscopic surgery. Clin Physiol. 1996;16(3):217–27. PubMed PMID: 8736710. Epub 1996/05/01. eng.
3. Ahlman B, Ljungqvist O, Persson B, Bindslev L, Wernerman J. Intestinal amino acid content in critically ill patients. JPEN J Parenter Enteral Nutr. 1995;19(4):272–8. PubMed PMID: 8523625.

4. Ollenschlager G, Langer K, Steffen HM, Schrappe-Bacher M, Schmitt H, Allolio B, et al. Intracellular free amino acid patterns in duodenal and colonic mucosa. Clin Chem. 1990;36(2):378–81. PubMed PMID: 2302784. Epub 1990/02/01. eng.
5. Mori M, Rooyackers O, Smedberg M, Tjader I, Norberg A, Wernerman J. Endogenous glutamine production in critically ill patients: the effect of exogenous glutamine supplementation. Crit Care. 2014;18(2):R72.
6. Darmaun D, Matthews DE, Bier DM. Glutamine and glutamate kinetics in humans. Am J Physiol. 1986;251(1 Pt 1):E117–26. PubMed PMID: 2873746.
7. Matthews DE, Marano MA, Campbell RG. Splanchnic bed utilization of glutamine and glutamic acid in humans. Am J Physiol. 1993;264(6 Pt 1):E848–54. PubMed PMID: 8101428.
8. van Acker BA, Hulsewe KW, Wagenmakers AJ, Soeters PB, von Meyenfeldt MF. Glutamine appearance rate in plasma is not increased after gastrointestinal surgery in humans. J Nutr. 2000;130(6):1566–71. PubMed PMID: 10827211.
9. Rooyackers O, Prohn M, Van Riel N, Wernerman J. Bolus injection on 13C-glutamine to study glutamine metabolism in humans. Clin Nutr. 2005;24:575–6.
10. van Acker BA, Hulsewe KW, Wagenmakers AJ, von Meyenfeldt MF, Soeters PB. Response of glutamine metabolism to glutamine-supplemented parenteral nutrition. Am J Clin Nutr. 2000;72(3):790–5. PubMed PMID: 10966901.
11. Marliss EB, Aoki TT, Pozefsky T, Most AS, Cahill Jr GF. Muscle and splanchnic glutmine and glutamate metabolism in postabsorptive andstarved man. J Clin Invest. 1971;50(4):814–7. PubMed PMID: 5547277. Pubmed Central PMCID: 291995. Epub 1971/04/01. eng.
12. Abumrad NN, Rabin D, Wise KL, Lacy WW. The disposal of an intravenously administered amino acid load across the human forearm. Metabolism. 1982;31(5):463–70. PubMed PMID: 7043179. Epub 1982/05/01. eng.
13. Aoki TT, Brennan MF, Muller WA, Soeldner JS, Alpert JS, Saltz SB, et al. Amino acid levels across normal forearm muscle and splanchnic bed after a protein meal. Am J Clin Nutr. 1976;29(4):340–50. PubMed PMID: 1266783. Epub 1976/04/01. eng.
14. Dechelotte P, Darmaun D, Rongier M, Hecketsweiler B, Rigal O, Desjeux JF. Absorption and metabolic effects of enterally administered glutamine in humans. Am J Physiol. 1991;260(5 Pt 1):G677–82. PubMed PMID: 1903599. Epub 1991/05/01. eng.
15. Darmaun D, Dechelotte P. Role of leucine as a precursor of glutamine alpha-amino nitrogen in vivo in humans. Am J Physiol. 1991;260(2 Pt 1):E326–9. PubMed PMID: 1996635. Epub 1991/02/01. eng.
16. Eriksson LS, Olsson M, Bjorkman O. Splanchnic metabolism of amino acids in healthy subjects: effect of 60 hours of fasting. Metabolism. 1988;37(12):1159–62. PubMed PMID: 3193901. Epub 1988/12/01. eng.
17. Roth E, Funovics J, Muhlbacher F, Schemper M, Mauritz W, Sporn P, et al. Metabolic disorders in severe abdominal sepsis: Glutamine deficiency in skeletal muscle. Clin Nutr. 1982;1(1):25–41. PubMed PMID: 16829366.
18. Gamrin L, Andersson K, Hultman E, Nilsson E, Essen P, Wernerman J. Longitudinal changes of biochemical parameters in muscle during critical illness. Metabolism. 1997;46(7):756–62. PubMed PMID: 9225828.
19. Gamrin L, Essen P, Forsberg AM, Hultman E, Wernerman J. A descriptive study of skeletal muscle metabolism in critically ill patients: free amino acids, energy-rich phosphates, protein, nucleic acids, fat, water, and electrolytes. Crit Care Med. 1996;24(4):575–83. PubMed PMID: 8612406.
20. Oudemans-van Straaten HM, Bosman RJ, Treskes M, van der Spoel HJ, Zandstra DF. Plasma glutamine depletion and patient outcome in acute ICU admissions. Intensive Care Med. 2001;27(1):84–90. PubMed PMID: 11280678.
21. Rodas PC, Rooyackers O, Hebert C, Norberg A, Wernerman J. Glutamine and glutathione at ICU admission in relation to outcome. Clin Sci (Lond). 2012;122(12):591–7. PubMed PMID: 22248298. Pubmed Central PMCID: 3294430. Epub 2012/01/18. eng.
22. Tjader I, Rooyackers O, Forsberg AM, Vesali RF, Garlick PJ, Wernerman J. Effects on skeletal muscle of intravenous glutamine supplementation to ICU patients. Intensive Care Med. 2004;30(2):266–75. PubMed PMID: 14722645.
23. Vesali RF, Klaude M, Rooyackers OE, TJader I, Barle H, Wernerman J. Longitudinal pattern of glutamine/glutamate balance across the leg in long-stay intensive care unit patients. Clin Nutr. 2002;21(6):505–14. PubMed PMID: 12468371. Epub 2002/12/07. eng.
24. Heyland D, Muscedere J, Wischmeyer PE, Cook D, Jones G, Albert M, et al. A randomized trial of glutamine and antioxidants in critically ill patients. N Engl J Med. 2013;368(16):1489–97. PubMed PMID: 23594003. Epub 2013/04/19. eng.
25. Kondrup J, Allison SP, Elia M, Vellas B, Plauth M. ESPEN guidelines for nutrition screening 2002. Clin Nutr. 2003;22(4):415–21. PubMed PMID: 12880610. Epub 2003/07/26. eng.
26. Clemmesen JO, Kondrup J, Ott P. Splanchnic and leg exchange of amino acids and ammonia in acute liver failure. Gastroenterology. 2000;118(6):1131–9. PubMed PMID: 10833488.
27. Rama Rao KV, Jayakumar AR, Norenberg MD. Glutamine in the pathogenesis of acute hepatic encephalopathy. Neurochem Int. 2012;61(4):575–80. PubMed PMID: 22285152. Epub 2012/01/31. eng.
28. Ytrebo LM, Sen S, Rose C, Ten Have GA, Davies NA, Hodges S, et al. Interorgan ammonia, glutamate, and glutamine trafficking in pigs with acute liver failure. Am J Physiol Gastrointest Liver Physiol. 2006;291(3):G373–81. PubMed PMID: 16782695.

29. Oppong KN, Al-Mardini H, Thick M, Record CO. Oral glutamine challenge in cirrhotics pre- and post-liver transplantation: a psychometric and analyzed EEG study. Hepatology. 1997;26(4):870–6. PubMed PMID: 9328307. Epub 1997/10/27. eng.
30. Lee B, Yu H, Jahoor F, O'Brien W, Beaudet al, Reeds P. In vivo urea cycle flux distinguishes and correlates with phenotypic severity in disorders of the urea cycle. Proc Natl Acad Sci U S A. 2000;97(14):8021–6. PubMed PMID: 10869432. Pubmed Central PMCID: 16663. Epub 2000/06/28. eng.
31. Berg A, Rooyackers O, Norberg A, Wernerman J. Elimination kinetics of L-alanyl-L-glutamine in ICU patients. Amino Acids. 2005;29(3):221–8. PubMed PMID: 16049639.
32. Vinnars E, Bergstom J, Furst P. Influence of the postoperative state on the intracellular free amino acids in human muscle tissue. Ann Surg. 1975;182(6):665–71. PubMed PMID: 1190870.
33. Askanazi J, Carpentier YA, Michelsen CB, Elwyn DH, Furst P, Kantrowitz LR, et al. Muscle and plasma amino acids following injury. Influence of intercurrent infection. Ann Surg. 1980;192(1):78–85. PubMed PMID: 7406567. Pubmed Central PMCID: 1344810. Epub 1980/07/01. eng.
34. Petersson B, Waller SO, Vinnars E, Wernerman J. Long-term effect of glycyl-glutamine after elective surgery on free amino acids in muscle. JPEN J Parenter Enteral Nutr. 1994;18(4):320–5. PubMed PMID: 7933438.
35. Petersson B, Vinnars E, Waller SO, Wernerman J. Long-term changes in muscle free amino acid levels after elective abdominal surgery. Br J Surg. 1992;79(3):212–6. PubMed PMID: 1555085. Epub 1992/03/01. eng.
36. Wernerman J, Hammarqvist F, Botta D, Vinars E. Stress hormones alter the pattern of free amino acids in human skeletal muscle. Clin Physiol. 1993;13(3):309–19. PubMed PMID: 8519166. Epub 1993/05/01. eng.
37. Wernerman J, Brandt R, Strandell T, Allgen LG, Vinnars E. The effect of stress hormones on the interorgan flux of amino acids and on the concentration of free amino acids in skeletal muscle. Clin Nutr. 1985;4(4):207–16. PubMed PMID: 16831734. Epub 1985/11/01. eng.
38. Vesali RF, Klaude M, Rooyackers O, Wernerman J. Amino acid metabolism in leg muscle after an endotoxin injection in healthy volunteers. Am J Physiol Endocrinol Metab. 2005;288(2):E360–4. PubMed PMID: 15367399.
39. Wilmore DW, Schloerb PR, Ziegler TR. Glutamine in the support of patients following bone marrow transplantation. Curr Opin Clin Nutr Metab Care. 1999;2(4):323–7. PubMed PMID: 10453314.
40. Van Acker BA, Hulsewe KW, Wagenmakers AJ, Deutz NE, Van Kreel BK, Halliday D, et al. Absence of glutamine isotopic steady state: implications for the assessment of whole-body glutamine production rate. Clin Sci (Lond). 1998;95(3):339–46. PubMed PMID: 9730854.
41. Melis GC, Boelens PG, van der Sijp JR, Popovici T, De Bandt JP, Cynober L, et al. The feeding route (enteral or parenteral) affects the plasma response of the dipetide Ala-Gln and the amino acids glutamine, citrulline and arginine, with the administration of Ala-Gln in preoperative patients. Br J Nutr. 2005;94(1):19–26. PubMed PMID: 16115328. Epub 2005/08/24. eng.
42. Garrel D, Patenaude J, Nedelec B, Samson L, Dorais J, Champoux J, et al. Decreased mortality and infectious morbidity in adult burn patients given enteral glutamine supplements: a prospective, controlled, randomized clinical trial. Crit Care Med. 2003;31(10):2444–9. PubMed PMID: 14530749.
43. Houdijk AP, Rijnsburger ER, Jansen J, Wesdorp RI, Weiss JK, McCamish MA, et al. Randomised trial of glutamine-enriched enteral nutrition on infectious morbidity in patients with multiple trauma. Lancet. 1998;352(9130):772–6. PubMed PMID: 9737282.
44. Bollhalder L, Pfeil AM, Tomonaga Y, Schwenkglenks M. A systematic literature review and meta-analysis of randomized clinical trials of parenteral glutamine supplementation. Clin Nutr. 2013;32(2):213–23. PubMed PMID: 23196117. Epub 2012/12/01. eng.
45. Novak F, Heyland DK, Avenell A, Drover JW, Su X. Glutamine supplementation in serious illness: a systematic review of the evidence. Crit Care Med. 2002;30(9):2022–9. PubMed PMID: 12352035.
46. Andrews PJ, Avenell A, Noble DW, Campbell MK, Croal BL, Simpson WG, et al. Randomised trial of glutamine, selenium, or both, to supplement parenteral nutrition for critically ill patients. BMJ. 2011;342:d1542. PubMed PMID: 21415104. Epub 2011/03/19. eng.
47. Griffiths RD, Jones C, Palmer TE. Six-month outcome of critically ill patients given glutamine-supplemented parenteral nutrition. Nutrition. 1997;13(4):295–302. PubMed PMID: 9178278.
48. Wernerman J, Kirketeig T, Andersson B, Berthelson H, Ersson A, Friberg H, et al. Scandinavian glutamine trial: a pragmatic multi-centre randomised clinical trial of intensive care unit patients. Acta Anaesthesiol Scand. 2011;55(7):812–8. PubMed PMID: 21658010. Epub 2011/06/11. eng.
49. Wernerman J. Glutamine – from conditionally essential to totally dispensable? Crit Care. 2014;18(4):162.
50. Wernerman J. Glutamine supplementation to critically ill patients? Crit Care. 2014;18(2):214.

Chapter 12
Glutamine Supplementation in Major Surgery and Intensive Care

Luca Gianotti, Massimo Oldani, Sara Coppola, Luca Nespoli, Marco Zanello, and Marco Braga

Key Points

- Glutamine is an essential substrate for several key metabolic pathways.
- Glutamine supplementation is able to modulate the inflammatory and immune response after injury.
- Glutamine effectively protects the gut function during critical illness.
- Glutamine plays a crucial role in attenuating the oxidative stress.
- The effect of glutamine on clinically relevant outcomes in both elective surgical patients and critically ill patients is under intensive investigation.
- The results of recent randomized clinical trials in intensive care patients with shock and multiple organ dysfunction suggest no benefit or even harm of high dose of glutamine supplementation.
- Additional trials are needed to investigate dose-finding and the effect of glutamine in more defined patient populations.

Keywords Glutamine • Surgery • Critical illness • Outcome • Intensive care • Complications • Length of stay • Mortality • Nutritional support • Artificial nutrition

Abbreviations

GLN	Glutamine
ICU	Intensive care unit
MODS	Multiple organ dysfunction syndrome
RCTs	Randomized controlled trials
TPN	Total parenteral nutrition
LOS	Length of stay
HSP	Heat-shock protein

L. Gianotti, M.D., Ph.D. (✉) • M. Oldani, M.D. • S. Coppola, M.D. • L. Nespoli, M.D.
Department of Surgery, University of Milano-Bicocca-San Gerardo Hospital, Monza, Italy
e-mail: luca.gianotti@unimib.it

M. Zanello, M.D.
IRCCS Istituto di Science Neurologiche, University Alma Mater of Bologna, Bologna, Italy

M. Braga, M.D.
Department of Surgery, San Raffaele Hospital, Milan, Italy

R. Rajendram et al. (eds.), *Glutamine in Clinical Nutrition*, Nutrition and Health,
DOI 10.1007/978-1-4939-1932-1_12, © Springer Science+Business Media New York 2015

GSH Glutathione
iNOS Inducible nitric oxide synthase
SOFA Sequential organ failure assessment

Introduction

There are clear and sufficient evidences from preclinical and clinical studies showing that glutamine (GLN) plays a key role of in several metabolic pathways. In fact, GLN has been recognized as an essential substrate for the appropriate function of many organs (Table 12.1) and the principal metabolic fuel for rapidly dividing cells, such as macrophages, fibroblasts, lymphocytes, and enterocytes. In general, GLN is essential for cell metabolism because it is able to modulate gluconeogenesis, lipogenesis, and anabolic processes; to preserve mitochondrial ATP levels; and to attenuate the activation of inducible nitric oxide synthase (iNOS) following ischemia, trauma, and sepsis. Although GLN is classified as a nonessential amino acid and is synthesized de novo, for the above reasons it is commonly described as conditionally essential amino acid in critical and catabolic states [1].

Major surgery can be considered as a controlled or a limited trauma and therefore it may induce inflammation and catabolism with a subsequent flux of endogenous glutamine from muscles to other tissues/organs with rapid cell turnover and metabolism. In catabolic states and during hyperinflammation, despite a significant release of GLN from the muscles, its plasma levels decrease during critical illness and this relative deficiency has been recently associated with increased mortality in intensive care units (ICU) [2] (Fig. 12.1). Thus, exogenous glutamine supplementation might be important in such stress to maintain a stable tissue and plasma pool. Theoretically, this should to be associated with a better immune response, an increased protein synthesis, an improved nitrogen balance, a preserved gut barrier structure and function, an enhanced wound healing, a reduced oxidative stress, and a better glucose metabolism.

The core mechanisms of action of GLN are summarized in Table 12.2. For these protective effects on the host metabolism, immune mechanisms and tissue integrity GLN has been considered as one of the most important and essential pharmaconutrients with immunomodulating properties.

Table 12.1 Protective effect of GLN in different organs

Lung:
– Major source of energy for endothelial cells
– May protect epithelial cells against endotoxin/oxidant-related injury
– Enhances heat shock protein expression post-stress
– Preserves cell metabolism following endotoxin injury
Heart:
– Major source of energy (via glutamate) for cardiomyocytes
– Protect cardiomyocyte against ischemia-related injury
– Enhances heat shock protein expression post-stress
Liver:
– Supports hepatocyte glutathione biosynthesis
– Regulator of ammonia metabolism
Gastrointestinal tract:
– Major source of energy for enterocytes
– Supports nucleotide biosynthesis
– May protect epithelial cells against endotoxin/oxidant-related injury
Kidney:
– Regulator of acid/base balance
– Regulator of ammonia metabolism

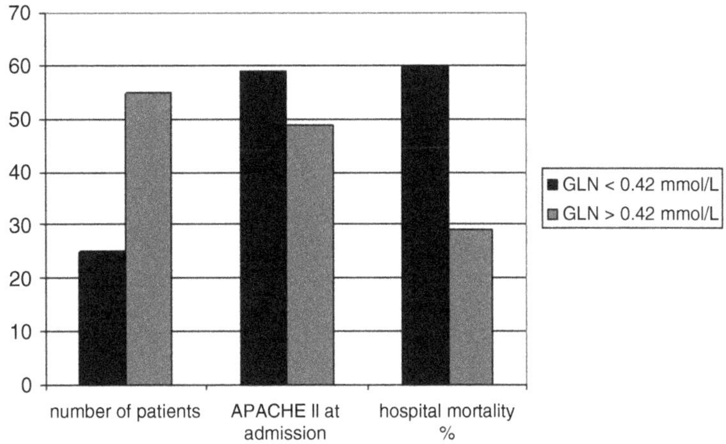

Fig. 12.1 Correlation between GLN plasma levels at ICU admission and outcome. Modified from Oudemans-van Straaten HM, et al. [2]

Table 12.2 The core mechanisms of action of GLN

- Maintenance of intestinal integrity and function with reduced bacterial translocation
- Preservation of the cellular redox state as a precursor of endogenous antioxidants (glutathione), protecting from the harmful effects of free radicals
- Enhancement of the expression of heat-shock proteins reducing cellular apoptosis and inflammation
- Modulation of the synthesis of proinflammatory cytokines
- Enhancement of the monocyte, lymphocyte, and macrophages function
- Reduction of urinary nitrogen loss with improved protein synthesis
- Improvement of wound healing by fibroblast stimulation
- Decrease of hyperglycemia by enhanced tissue insulin sensitivity
- Attenuation of inducible nitric oxide synthase (iNOS) following sepsis and ischemia/reperfusion injury

In critically ill subjects, multiple organ dysfunction syndrome (MODS) is often the ultimate cause of death [3]. MODS may be the result of tissue injury, hypoperfusion and reperfusion, oxidative damage, systemic uncontrolled and excessive inflammation, and hypermetabolism, but severe sepsis is by far the most common trigger and in the USA sepsis-related mortality is similar to the one for acute myocardial infarction [4].

Limited therapeutic options are available to prevent MODS and mortality after the onset of sepsis. Using the body innate stress substrates as a pharmaconutritional intervention to induce endogenous protective pathways may be a promising candidate for the treatment of such conditions. Induction or preservation of these vital stress response pathways via substrates, such as GLN, might be able to prevent MODS and, ultimately, mortality in ICU patients. Thus, GLN has been proposed as a life-saving nutrient in critical conditions as part of an appropriate and optimized nutritional support [5].

Glutamine and Elective Surgery

The pathophysiology of postoperative complications is multifactorial with several well-documented risk factors involved. A preexisting state of malnutrition is only one of the important causes for the development of surgery-related morbidity. In fact, patients with a normal nutritional status may experience frequent and severe complications after major abdominal surgery. Perioperative supplementation of key nutritional substrates, with specific metabolic and immunologic effects, can improve surgical outcome independently from the baseline nutritional status [6, 7]. This suggests that the provision of

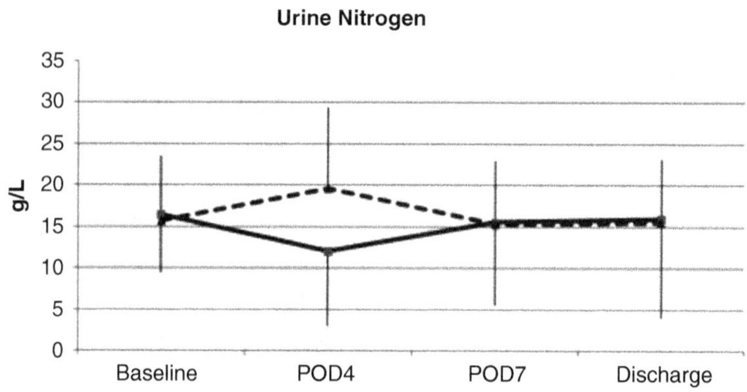

Fig. 12.2 Urinary nitrogen loss in patients receiving parenteral GLN (0.4 g/kg/day) and undergoing major elective abdominal surgery for cancer. Dotted line: control group. Continuous line: GLN group. POD: postoperative day

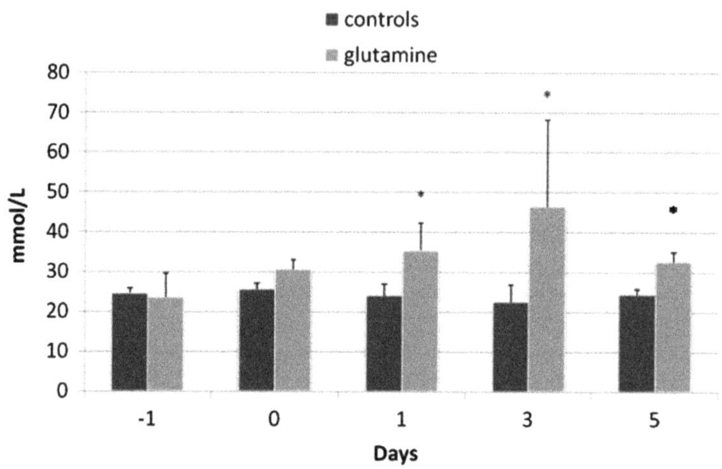

Fig. 12.3 Plasma GLN levels in patients undergoing major elective abdominal surgery for cancer and receiving perioperative GLN supplementation (0.4 g/kg/day). -1 : baseline value. 0: day of surgery. 1–5: days after surgery

such substrates may achieve protective effects that should be ascribed more to pharmacological activity than nutritional repletion.

In elective surgical patients the effects of GLN has been tested as a dipeptide (alanine-glutamine) infused parenterally with a dose ranging from 0.27 to 1 g/kg/day.

1. *Safety profile*
   None of the trials evaluating the safety profile of GLN supplementation in elective surgery [8–14] showed major treatment-related harmful effects except for very few episodes of allergy with cutaneous rush during infusion and moderate alteration of renal and hepatic function with dose exceeding 1 g/kg/day.
2. *Nitrogen balance and glutamine plasma levels*
   Unpublished data from our group showing a reduced but transitory postsurgical urinary nitrogen loss (Fig. 12.2) after GLN supplementation, confirm what reported in several others clinical trials. This effect of protein metabolism was partially associated with an increased GLN plasma levels (Fig. 12.3). The positive nitrogen balance should not be considered exclusively as the result of a higher dose of amino acids because similar findings were obtained when isonitrogenous solutions were compared. These observations confirm GLN as an important nitrogen donor for anabolic processes.
3. *GLN supplementation and immune function/inflammatory response*
   Several randomized controlled trials (RCTs) focused their attention on the potential role of GLN infusion on the alterations of the immune response related to surgery.

Asprer and colleagues [15] evaluated the impact of GLN supplementation, provided exclusively during the preoperative period in a group of malnourished patients undergoing major gastrointestinal surgery. The parenteral administration of GLN for 5 days resulted in a significant increase of lymphocyte, granulocyte, and total white blood cell counts when compared with nonsupplemented patients. This effect rapidly disappeared in the postoperative period when GLN supplementation was stopped.

When given postoperatively, GLN enriched total parenteral nutrition (TPN) was associated with a significant better recovery of total lymphocyte count than after infusion of a standard TPN in both gastrointestinal and vascular surgery [8, 16]. These results were not confirmed measuring the total number of white blood cells [8, 13, 14, 17], suggesting that GLN supplementation predominantly influenced lymphocytes metabolism, through increased T- and B-cell mitogen responses.

Lymphocyte subpopulations were also investigated. The total number and proportion of circulating T-lymphocytes were upregulated in the postoperative period in supplemented patients but no effect was reported in subject undergoing standard treatment [10, 16]. Moreover, O'Riordain and colleagues [18] evaluated T-cell activity by the ex vivo determination of T-cells DNA synthesis in patients candidate to colorectal resection. They observed a significant increase of this parameter in patients who received postoperative GLN-supplemented TPN compared to standard formulas.

A positive impact of GLN supplementation on postoperative CD4, CD8, and NK cells plasma levels and proportion was observed in patients undergoing major vascular surgery [16] but there data were not confirmed by other studies enrolling patients who underwent other types of abdominal operations [13, 19, 20].

The potential immunomodulatory effects of GLN administration on inflammatory cytokine production and release have been also investigated. Most of the trial evaluating cytokine levels did not found a significant difference in postoperative IL-2, IL-6, IL-8, IL-10, and TNF-alpha (Table 12.3). Moreover, also the constitutive expression of the TNF-receptors I and II was not affected by GLN supplementation [19].

Reduced HLA-DR expression on monocytes is considered as a surrogate of postoperative immunosuppression. Two different clinical trials [9, 19] demonstrated that GLN supplementation induced a better preservation of HLA-DR monocyte expression after surgery than in control groups.

The effects of GLN on host defense mechanisms are summarized in Table 12.3.

4. *GLN supplementation and oxidative stress*
   Fan et al. [20] evaluated, in patients undergoing elective abdominal surgery, the impact of GLN supplementation on oxidative stress induced by surgical trauma. They observed in supplemented patients a trend toward a lower reduction of postoperative glutathione levels in plasma and in red blood cells and a significantly higher ratio of glutathione/glutathione disulfide than in control patients. These data suggested that GLN infusion was associated to a better preservation of antioxidant capacity in the postoperative period.
5. *GLN supplementation and intestinal permeability*
   Gut integrity and barrier function are considered crucial in the postoperative period to minimize bacterial translocation and subsequent infections. Jiang and colleagues [17] evaluated GLN supplementation on intestinal permeability in patients candidate to elective gastrointestinal surgery. Permeability was estimated by the lactulose/mannitol ratio. A significant improvement of gut barrier function was observed in patients receiving GLN supplementation than in controls.

Another trial [13] evaluated postoperative D-xylose extraction by the intestine, as a surrogate marker of gut function. This was tested in patients requiring post-surgical intensive care. The 2-h serum D-xylose concentration was found significantly below the normal range in all patients suggesting a dysfunction of the intestinal mucosa. However, the 2-h serum D-xylose concentration was

Table 12.3 Effects of GLN on immune parameters in elective surgical patients

Author	Parameters
O'Riordain [6]	↑ T cells function; = IL-2, IL-6, TNF
Morlion [7]	↑Lymphocyte recovery, ↑generation of cysteinil-leukotrienes from PMNs
Jacobi [8]	↑ HLA-DR-monocytes, = CD3, CD4, CD8, IL-6 reduction, IL-10
Jiang [9]	= WBCs
Mertes [10]	= TNF-alfa, IL-6
Karwowska [11]	↑ WBCs, lymphocytes, CD3, CD4, CD19, CD8, NK, IgA, Ig G
Neri [12]	= lymphocytes
Spittler [13]	↑ HLA-DR-monocytes; =lymhpocytes, CD3, CD4, CD8, CD4/CD8 ratio, activated T- and T-helper cells, CD19, cytotoxic T-cells and NK-cells, TNF-alfa, IL-6, TNF-receptors I and II
Lin [14]	↑ CD3, CD4; = lymphocytes, CD8
Exner [15]	↑ TNF-alfa; =HLA-DR-monocytes
Klek [16]	= lymphocytes
Yao [17]	↑ soluble CD14; = WBCs
Jo [18]	=lymhpocytes
Estevariz [20]	=CD3,CD4,CD8
Asprer [21]	↑WBCs, granulocytes, lymphocytes
Engel [22]	=IL-1, IL-6, IL-8,TNF-alfa
Fan [23]	=lymphocytes, IgA, IgG, IgM, CD4, CD8, CD4/CD8 ratio
Marton [25]	=TNF-alfa, IL-6, IL-8, procalcitonin
Lu [26]	↑ IL-6; = WBCs, lymphocytes, TNF-alfa, IL-10

↑ Increased in GLN-supplemented patients compared to controls
= No differences between groups
WBCs: white blood cells; IL: interleukin; TNF: tumor necrosis factor, Ig: immunoglobulin; PMNs: polymorphonuclear cells

significantly higher in GLN-supplemented patients than in controls suggesting that GLN may be used by enterocytes during acute conditions.

GLN Supplementation and Clinically Relevant Outcomes

In major elective surgery the impact of GLN supplementation on postoperative outcome has been investigated in several RCTs (Table 12.4) and only three of them [9, 26, 27] reported a significant reduction in infectious morbidity in patients receiving GLN supplementation. Two of these trials [9, 26] compared patients candidate to heterogeneous gastrointestinal operations and randomized to receive postoperative GLN-supplemented TPN (GLN-dipeptide 0.4 g/kg/day) or standard TPN. Oguz et al. [27] reported similar results in patients with colorectal cancer who receive an high perioperatively dose of GLN-dipeptide (1 g/kg/day) in combination with enteral nutrition.

Estivariz et al., [13] evaluated the impact of postoperative GLN infusion in patients candidate to quite heterogeneous elective surgical procedures (cardiac, vascular, colonic, and pancreatic surgery) requiring TPN and a postoperative surgical ICU stay. Although no significant difference in postoperative infection rates was observed comparing GLN to control treatment, a reduction in infectious morbidity was detected in the subgroup of patients who underwent non-pancreatic surgical procedures. The other trials evaluating infectious morbidity as an end-point did not showed any significant difference between GLN-supplemented and controls groups, although a trend toward a reduction in infectious rate has been observed in many cases.

A multicenter trial [28] designed to test the effect of parenteral GLN supplementation enrolled subjects with preoperative weight loss less that 10 %. All patients had gastrointestinal cancer and

Table 12.4 Randomized controlled trials in elective surgery

Study	Year	Number of patients	Nutritional status	Type of surgery	GLN dipeptide dose (g/kg/day)	Morbidity (GLN vs. control)	LOS (GLN vs. control)
O'Riordain [18]	1994	22	Undefined	Colorectal	0.27	No difference	NR
Morlion [8]	1998	28	Undefined	Colorectal	0.3	NR	Reduced
Jacobi [9]	1999	34	Undefined	Upper GI	0.4	Reduced	
Jiang [17]	1999	60	Undefined	Mixed GI	0.5	No difference	Reduced
Mertes [21]	2000	50	Undefined	Mixed GI and vascular	0.5	NR	Reduced
Karwowska [16]	2001	30	Well-nourished	Vascular	0.3	NR	Reduced
Neri [22]	2001	33	Undefined	Mixed GI	0.3	NR	Reduced
Spittler [19]	2001	30	Undefined	Mixed GI	0.74	NR	No difference
Lin [10]	2002	48	Undefined	Mixed GI	0.42	No difference	NR
Exner [23]	2003	45	Undefined	Mixed GI	0.5	No difference	No difference
Klek [11]	2005	105	Well-nourished	Gastric	0.4	No difference	Reduced
Yao [12]	2005	40	Well-nourished	Mixed GI	0.5	No difference	Reduced
Jo [24]	2006	60	Well-nourished and malnourished	Pancreatic	0.3	No difference	No difference
Oguz [27]	2007	109	Undefined	Colorectal	1	Reduced	Reduced
Estevariz [13]	2008	63	Undefined	Cardiac, vascular, pancreatic, colonic surgery	0.5	No difference	No difference
Asprer [15]	2009	34	Malnourished	Mixed GI	0.3	No difference	NR
Engel [14]	2009	78	Undefined	Cardiac	0.74	No difference	No difference
Fan [20]	2009	40	Undefined	Mixed GI	0.2	No difference	No difference
Gianotti [28]	2009	428	Well-nourished	Mixed GI	0.4	No difference	No difference
Marton [25]	2010	55	Well-nourished and malnourished	Esophageal	0.5	No difference	No difference
Lu [26]	2011	50	Undefined	Mixed GI	0.45	Reduced	NR

GLN: glutamine; LOS: length of hospital stay; NR: not reported; GI: Gastrointestinal

were candidate to major surgical procedure. Glutamine infusion begun the day before operation and continued postoperatively for at least 5 days with a dose of 0.4 g/kg/day. No postoperative artificial nutrition (AN) was allowed unless patients could not adequately eat by day 7. The results showed that the mean percent of weight loss was 1.4 in controls and GLN group. Overall postoperative complication rate was 34.9 % (74/212) in GLN and 32.9 % (71/216) in control group ($p=0.65$). Infectious morbidity was 19.3 % (41/212) in GLN group and 17.1 % (37/216) in controls ($p=0.55$). The rate of major complications was 7.5 % (16/212) in GLN group and 7.9 % (17/216) in controls ($p=0.90$). The rate of patients requiring postoperative AN was 13.2 % (28/212) in GLN group and 12.0 % (26/216) in controls ($p=0.71$).

In this study it was not used an isonitrogenous regimen in the control group because it was previously shown that intravenous infusion of amino acid solutions (protein sparing therapy) was not superior to conventional fluid therapy in well-nourished patients undergoing major abdominal surgery.

This was the only trial with a statistical adequate power to detect outcome differences between treated and control group and did no show any advantage of GLN supplementation in this type of surgical patients, but it leaves an open issue about glutamine supplementation in patients with severe weight loss and high risk of surgical morbidity. They should represent cohorts with more elevated glutamine demand, increased glutamine metabolism, and/or baseline deficits. Moreover, a possible treatment underdosing could be hypothesized, although the selected dose (0.4 g/kg/day) was chosen on previous publications showing an optimal clinical effect when GLN was given at a dose higher than 0.3 g/kg/day. Another possible explanation for the results is the insufficient preoperative GLN loading to obtain adequate tissue and plasma levels at time of surgical trauma and in the postoperative course.

The impact of GLN supplementation on length of stay (LOS) was evaluated in several trials with contrasting results (Table 12.4). LOS in surgical patient is usually directly correlated with outcome since duration of hospitalization is strongly dependent from morbidity rate. Therefore, LOS should be considered as a secondary or surrogate end-point of clinical studies unless the discharge criteria are well defined and a priori stated. The variability reported across trials on the effect of GLN supplementation on LOS should be attributed to the lack of definition of discharge criteria.

No difference in death rates has been also observed in evaluated trials, but in general mortality should not be an end-point of elective surgery for the very low incidence.

The RCTs published so far evaluating GLN supplementation, with few exceptions, suffer several important methodological limitations such as lack of sample size calculation, blindness, a priori definition of complications, intention-to-treat analysis, subgroup and post hoc analysis, statistical underpower, nonhomogeneous patient cohorts, and use of TPN without recognized indications. The latter, in particular, may have altered the results because it is well documented that the inappropriate use of TPN particularly in well-nourished or mild-undernourished patients is associated with increased postoperative morbidity.

Glutamine and Critical Illness

The Potential Beneficial Effects of GLN

When given enterally GLN should be active mainly on the gut mucosal layer and subsequently on the barrier function which plays a critical role in the host protection since an increase in intestinal permeability may contribute to the occurrence of systemic infections through the process of bacterial translocation [29]. Translocation is a rather complex event and it is regulated by several mechanisms including the balance between cell proliferation and apoptosis, luminal bacterial and toxin load, and ability of the host to clear translocating microorganisms. GLN is the preferential substrate for the enterocytes and intestinal immune cells and is able to decrease cell apoptosis and activate local host defence mechanisms.

When given systemically, GLN is able to enhance immune response, protect tissues against oxidative stress and toxic agents or pathologic insults by increasing glutathione (GSH) production and

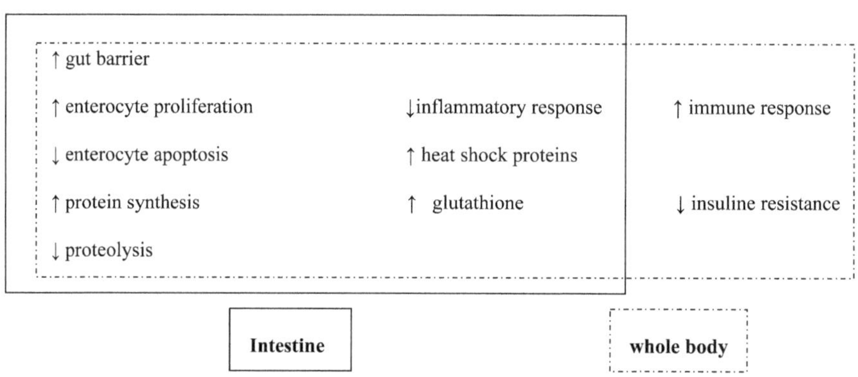

Fig. 12.4 Overlapping protective mechanisms of GLN when given enterally or parenterally

enhancing heat shock protein (HSP) expression. These proteins function as intracellular chaperones for other proteins, mediating functions such as folding and conformation.

Some of the protective mechanisms of GLN given enterally or parenterally have common characteristics (Fig. 12.4).

Mechanisms by Which Glutamine Should Improve Outcome

1. *Tissue protection*
   Wischmeyer et al. [30] tested intravenous GLN (0.75 g/kg/day) in an experimental model of sepsis. They found enhanced lung tissue heat-shock protein HSP-70, HSP 25, and serum HSP-70 expression leading to prevention of ARDS and consequently mortality.
   A double blind RCT conducted by Ziegler and colleagues [31] conducted in ICU patients and requiring TPN for more than 5 days, showed that in the group receiving GLN-dipeptide (0.5 g/kg/day) the serum HSP-70 expression was significantly increased compared to an isonitrogenous control group and ICU stay was decreased. This study demonstrated GLN as the first nontoxic, clinically relevant enhancer of HSP-70 expression in critically ill patients.
2. *Anti-inflammatory effect*
   Despite a large body of evidences from experimental studies, there are quite few data from human trials regarding an active role of GLN in modulation the inflammatory response.
   Andreasen et al. [32] conducted an elegant study in healthy volunteers, injected with *E. coli* endotoxin to test the role of GLN supplementation on immune and inflammatory markers.
   Their findings showed that plasma GLN increased during GLN infusion. Endotoxin reduced plasma GLN, but plasma GLN levels remained above baseline with GLN supplementation. Endotoxin injection was associated with alterations in white blood cell and differential counts, tumour necrosis factor-α, IL-6, cortisol, temperature, and heart rate, but GLN affected neither the endotoxin-induced change in these variables nor the expression of HSP-70 in peripheral circulating monocytes. They concluded that endotoxin reduced plasma GLN independently of GLN infusion, but supplementation allowed plasma levels to be maintained above baseline. GLN altered neither endotoxin-induced systemic inflammation nor early expression of HSP.
3. *Prevention of gut failure*
   De Souza's [33] recent meta-analysis showed an improved gut function in acute patients receiving GLN supplementation. Other investigators [34, 35] demonstrated that GLN prevented the injury-related increase of intestinal permeability. Before starting and after 2 weeks of GLN-enriched TPN vs. standard TPN mucosal biopsy specimens were taken from the second part of the duodenum. The urine concentrations of lactulose/mannitol ratio were used to measure intestinal permeability. After 2 weeks of GLN enriched TPN, intestinal permeability was unchanged, whereas permeability in the standard TPN group increased. This well correlated with a decrease of the intestinal villus height observed in controls.
4. *Preservation of glucose metabolism and insulin sensitivity*
   In vitro and in vivo studies showed that GLN is one of the most effective substrates for gluconeogenesis particularly in the kidney and liver. Infusion of large amounts of GLN (28 g over 4 h) resulted in threefold increased plasma GLN concentrations and a sevenfold increase in glucose formation without changes in plasma insulin and glucagon levels [36]. These results provided evidence in humans that glutamine may act both as a substrate as well as a modulator of glucose metabolism. The glucose-lowering effect of GLN may be in relation to its known effect on fat metabolism such as inhibition of fatty acid oxidation, lipolysis and attenuation of insulin resistance induced by fat.
   Moreover, GLN is known to enhance the release of insulin by the pancreatic beta cells.

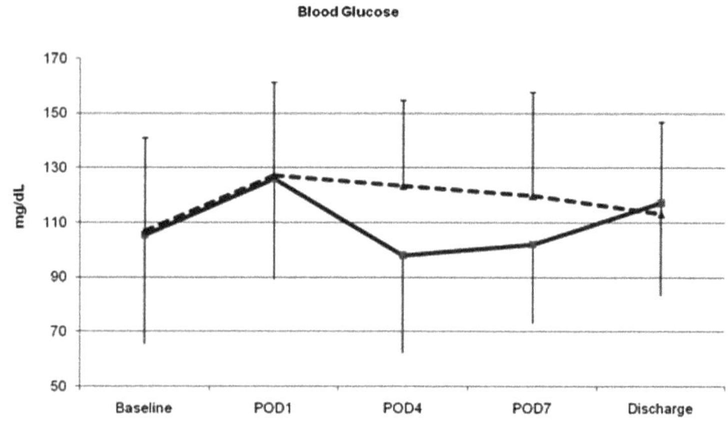

Fig. 12.5 Improved blood glucose control in patients receiving parenteral GLN (0.4 g/kg/day) and undergoing major elective abdominal surgery for cancer. Dotted line: control group. Continuous line: GLN group. POD: postoperative day

Clinical trials in critically ill patients, but also in elective surgery (Fig. 12.5; personal unpublished data) reported a significant better control of hyperglycemia due to an improved insulin sensitivity and signalling in liver and muscle and a reduced insulin resistance in patients receiving GLN supplementation [37, 38].

The key role of prevention of excessive blood glucose levels on survival in ICU patients has been demonstrated in many high quality trials [39] and optimal glucose control by mean of insulin treatment has become a routine practice worldwide.

5. *Antioxidant activity*
   GLN is an important precursor of glutathione, a vital intracellular antioxidant molecule that protects tissues from free radical injury via detoxification of active species and/or repair of injury, and plays an important role in the metabolism of drugs and endogenous substances. GLN appears to be important also for the regeneration of glutathione stores because glutamate is poorly transported into cells and GLN is efficiently transported across the cell membrane and in the mitochondria to produce glutamate and ammonia and to attenuate iNOS expression. Induction of high-output of iNOS usually occurs in an oxidative environment, and thus high levels of nitric oxide have the opportunity to react with superoxide leading to peroxynitrite formation and cell toxicity. These properties may define the role of iNOS in host immunity, enabling its participation in anti-microbial and anti-tumor activities as part of the oxidative burst of macrophages, but on the other hand it may cause self-tissue damage, increased oxygen radical production, and eventually organ dysfunction.

Effect of GLN on Clinically Relevant Outcomes

Novak and colleagues [40] in 2002 performed a comprehensive review of all published trials of GLN therapy. They reported no statistical significant differences between treated and control groups but there were some important trends in subgroup analyses. With respect to mortality, the treatment benefit was observed in studies of parenteral glutamine (RR, 0.71; 95 % CI, 0.51–0.99) compared with trials using enteral glutamine (RR, 1.08; 95 % CI, 0.57–2.01) and with an high-dose of glutamine (RR, 0.73; 95 % CI, 0.53–1.00) versus a low-dose glutamine (RR, 1.02; 95 % CI, 0.52–2.00). A more recent meta-analysis [41] including 40 trials did not confirmed the protective effect of GLN on mortality while a benefit of GLN supplementation was reported for LOS and infection rates.

From these meta-analyses it is difficult to appreciate the relative weight and the value of single studies design and methodology. Therefore, it is essential to highlight the characteristics of the most relevant trials to better understand the potential effect of GLN supplementation in critically ill subjects. The consequence of GLN infusion in trauma patients is described in details in another chapter.

Goeters and al [42]. in 2002 randomized 144 critically ill patients and looked at the effect of parenteral GLN on 6-month outcome in critically ill patients. Ninety-five patients were treated for 5 or more days and 68 patients for 9 or more days under standardized conditions. In the treatment group, plasma glutamine concentrations significantly increased within 6–9 days, resulting in a significant improvement of 6-month survival for patients treated the longer period (66.7 % vs. 40 %, control group).

An effect of GLN in reducing infections was also reported by Griffiths et al. [43]. They randomized 84 ICU patients to receive glutamine-supplemented TPN or standard TPN. Their conclusions were that parenteral nutrition containing glutamine could not reduce the overall incidence of intensive care acquired infections, but it could reduce the risk of dying from acquired infections. Moreover patients receiving GLN showed significantly fewer catheter related infections and developed fewer Candida infections. The improved survival seen at 6 months in the GLN supplemented group appeared mostly related to the reduced mortality in the intensive care unit from multiple organ failure.

More recently, Déchelotte et al. [37] randomized 114 ICU patients admitted for multiple trauma, complicated surgery, or pancreatitis to receive isocaloric isonitrogenous TPN providing 37.5 kcal/kg/day and 1.5 g amino acids/kg/day supplemented with either GLN dipeptide (0.5 g/kg/day, $n=58$) or an isonitrogenous GLN-free dipeptide (control group, $n=56$) over at least 5 days. Their major finding was that TPN supplemented with GLN dipeptide in ICU patients was associated with a significant reduction of the rate of infections and a better glucose tolerance. This study raises again the issue of the potential detrimental effect of overfeeding. The patients were fed parenterally with a very high caloric load. Therefore it is unclear if the beneficial effect on outcome is the results of the true mechanisms of action GLN or in contrast GLN just mitigated the detrimental effect of parenteral overfeeding.

Conejero et al. [44] studied the effect of a GLN enriched enteral diet in a randomized, single blind, multicenter trial including 84 patients with systemic inflammatory response syndrome of any etiology. The number of infected patients was significantly lower in the glutamine group than in the control group, with a relative risk of 0.5 (95 % confidence interval: 0.3–0.9). The most frequent infection was nosocomial pneumonia, with 33 % of patients in the control group and 14 % in the glutamine group. There were no differences with respect to other infections, mortality, or length of stay. The study was interrupted earlier than planned because the infection rate in the control group was significantly higher than in the GLN supplemented group.

Hall et al. [45] in a single-blind, monocenter trial, investigated 363 ICU patients requiring mechanical ventilation and with a median APACHE II score of 14 at admission. One group of patients received 19 g of enteral GLN per day in addition to standard enteral feeding and the controls received no GLN supplementation. The outcomes were similar in the two groups: death within 6 months was 15 % in the glutamine group vs. 16 % in controls; ($p=0.75$; relative risk: 0.95 (95 % confidence interval: 0.71–1.28): Severe sepsis rate was 21 % in the glutamine group vs. 23 % in the control group ($p=0.62$; relative risk: 0.94 (95 % confidence interval: 0.72–1.22). There was also no discernable difference in the secondary outcomes relating to infections, febrile period, antimicrobial therapy, and consumption of inotropes.

Andrews and colleagues [46] investigated in a large multicenter Scottish trial, adult patients admitted in high dependency units for more than 48 h, with gastrointestinal failure and requiring parenteral nutrition. Treatment was parenteral glutamine (20.2 g/day) for up to 7 days. There was no overall effect of glutamine on new infections (134/250 vs. 131/252, odds ratio: 1.07; 95 % confidential interval: 0.75–1.53), even if patients received more than 5 days of supplementation (odds ratio: 0.99; 95 % confidential interval 0.56–1.75). Six-month mortality was not significantly different (115/250 in GLN vs. 106/252 in controls; odds ratio: 1.18; 95 % confidential interval: 0.82–1.70), but there was a nonsignificant trend toward an increased 3-month mortality in the supplemented group (44 %) vs. controls (36 %). Also, length of stay, days of antibiotic use, and modified sequential organ failure assessment (SOFA) score were not significantly affected by glutamine supplementation.

In 413 ICU patients, Wernerman et al. [47] investigated by a multicenter, double-blinded randomized, pragmatic clinical trial the effects of parenteral GLN supplementation on sequential organ failure scores and mortality. Inclusion criteria were the following: ICU patients nourished enterally or parenterally, APACHE score greater than 10. Subjects were included within 72 h after ICU admission. Acute mortality (during ICU stay) was significantly lower in the treatment arm but 6-month mortality was unchanged. The SOFA scores during ICU stay revealed no difference between the two groups.

The results of the most recent multicenter study by Heyland et al. [48] published in April 2013 with the largest randomized series of critically ill patients are somehow surprising given the data from previous large RCTs. Critically ill adults collected in 40 ICUs in Canada, the USA, and Europe who had multiorgan failure and were receiving mechanical ventilation underwent a GLN supplementation ($n=303$) or placebo ($n=302$). GLN dipeptide was given both parenterally (0.5 g/kg/day) and enterally (42.5 g/day) within 24 h after ICU admission. The groups were comparable for demographic data, medical diagnoses, timing and dosage of artificial nutrition, and ICU treatment.

The majority of the patients had septic shock, a very high APACHE score and about on third of them had renal dysfunction at enrolment in the study. A trend toward increased mortality was found at 28 days among patients who received GLN as compared with those who did not receive it (32.4 % vs. 27.2 %; $p=0.05$). In-hospital mortality and mortality at 6 months were significantly higher among those who received glutamine than among those who did not. Glutamine had also no effect on rates of organ failure or infectious complications. The authors concluded that an early provision of glutamine did not improve clinical outcomes, but rather glutamine was associated with an increase in mortality among critically ill patients with multiorgan failure.

Heyland et al. results are persuasive because the trial design overcame many limitations of previous studies such as inappropriate sample size, lack of blindness, intention-to-treat analysis, rigorous definition of morbidity, GLN dosing or delayed start, and the double administration via the enteral and parenteral route which should cover both mechanisms of action and provide maximal protection (Fig. 12.4). Moreover, this study targeted the very severe critically ill patients with MODS, the majority of whom were in shock, whereas previous study typically excluded such patients. This study documented also that the majority of these patients did not have GLN deficiency early in the course of their critical illness in contrast with earlier experiences. This result challenged the prevailing previous concept that GLN is an essential nutrient in critically ill patients and requires immediate supplementation.

The results of this trial place doubts on the potential toxicity of GLN at such high dose and on its metabolic fate in very severe patients. In particular, it was shown in a subgroup analysis that the trend to higher mortality rates in the GLN group was caused by the patients who had renal dysfunction at enrolment in the study. In this subgroup of patients, mortality was significantly increased in the supplemented group, compared with controls. By excluding this subgroup of patients with renal dysfunction the supplemented group and the placebo group had similar 28-day mortality.

Another relevant issue is that glutamine supplementation started earlier than artificial nutrition and therefore in an early phase the nitrogen supply was totally represented by GLN. Also with the later nutrition support, protein requirement was given in a proportion higher than 50 % by GLN alone. This observation cannot exclude that the higher mortality in the GLN supplemented groups may be more related to the deficiency of other important amino acids than to the toxicity of GLN.

It may be suggested that future trials should address more appropriately the dose-finding issue, dose–response kinetics and the fate of both enteral and parenteral GLN given in different subgroups of ICU cohorts.

Table 12.5 summarizes the characteristics of all studies addressing the effects of GLN supplementation in ICU patients.

Table 12.5 Randomized controlled trials in ICU patients

Study	Year	Number of patients	Design	GLN dose/day	Route	Outcome (GLN vs; control)
Heyland [48]	2013	605	DB, multicenter	0.5 g/kg–42.5 g	PN–EN	↑ ICU and 6-month mortality, ↑ LOS, ↑ time of ventilation
Andrews [46]	2011	251	DB, multicenter	20.2 g	PN	= infections, = mortality
Wernerman [47]	2011	413	DB, multicenter	0.283 g/kg	PN	↓ ICU mortality, = 6-month mortality
Schneider [49]	2011	58	SB	30 g	EN	= LOS, = mortality
Grau [38]	2011	127	DB,multicenter	0.5 g/kg	PN	↓ infections; ↑ glucose control; = LOS, = mortality
Cekmen [50]	2011	30	DB	0.5 g/kg	PN	= ICU LOS, = mortality
Fuentes-Orozco [51]	2008	44	DB	0.4 g/kg	PN	= LOS, ↓ infections, = mortality
Perez-Barcena [52]	2008	15	SB	0.35 g/kg	PN	= infections, = ICU LOS, = mortality
Sahin [53]	2007	40	DB	0.3 g/kg	PN	↓ LOS
Déchelotte [37]	2006	114	DB, multicenter	0.5 g/kg	PN	↓ infections; ↑ glucose control, = mortality, = LOS
Ziegler [31]	2005	29	DB	0.5 g/kg	PN	= LOS, = ICU LOS
Xian-Li [54]	2004	69	DB	0.4 g/kg	PN	↓ infections, ↓ LOS, ↓ mortality
Hall [45]	2003	363	SB	20 g	EN	= mortality, = infections
Conejero [44]	2002	84	SB, multicenter	30.5 g	EN	↓ infections
Griffiths [43]	2002	84	DB	18 g	PN	↓ catheter-related infections, = infections, ↓ 6-month mortality
Ockenga [55]	2002	28	DB	0.3 g/kg	PN	↓ LOS
Goeters [42]	2002	144	Open label	0.3 g/kg	PN	↓ mortality
Powell Tuck [56]	1999	168	DB	20 g	PN	= LOS, = infections

DB: double blind; SB: single blind; PN: parenteral; EN: enteral; LOS: length of stay

Conclusions

Despite the strong rational and the robust evidences of an active role of GLN in protecting cell, tissue, and organ functions, the effect of GLN supplementation on primary outcome measures, such as morbidity and mortality in surgical and ICU patients is not persuasive. The most methodologically robust trials evaluating GLN supplementation showed no protective effects or even a trend to harm in specific subgroups. Up to now the available data do not support the routine use of GLN in elective surgical patients and in critically ill patients. Others large ongoing RCTs are enrolling different population subsets. The results will clarify if there is any role for GLN supplementation in specific patient cohorts.

References

1. Lacey JM, Wilmore DW. Is glutamine a conditionally essential amino acid? Nutr Rev. 1990;48(8):297–309.
2. Oudemans-van Straaten HM, Bosman RJ, Treskes M, van der Spoel HJ, Zandstra DF. Plasma glutamine depletion and patient outcome in acute ICU admissions. Intensive Care Med. 2001;27(1):84–90.
3. Rangel-Frausto MS, Pittet D, Costigan M, Hwang T, Davis CS, Wenzel RP. The natural history of the systemic inflammatory response syndrome (SIRS). A prospective study. JAMA. 1995;273(2):117–23.

4. Martin GS, Mannini DM, Eaton S, et al. The epidemiology of sepsis in the United States from 1979 through 2000. N Eng J Med. 2003;348(16):1546–54.
5. Preiser JC, Wernerman J. Glutamine, a life-saving nutrient, but why? Crit Care Med. 2003;31(10):2555–6.
6. Gianotti L, Braga M, Nespoli L, Radaelli G, Beneduce A, Di Carlo V. A randomized controlled trial of preoperative oral supplementation with a specialized diet in patients with gastrointestinal cancer. Gastroenterology. 2002; 122(7):1763–70.
7. Braga M, Gianotti L, Nespoli L, Radaelli G, Di Carlo V. Nutritional approach in malnourished surgical patients: a prospective randomized study. Arch Surg. 2002;137(2):174–80.
8. Morlion BJ, Stehle P, Wachtler P, Siedhoff HP, Köller M, König W, Fürst P, Puchstein C. Total parenteral nutrition with glutamine dipeptide after major abdominal surgery: a randomized, double-blind, controlled study. Ann Surg. 1998;227(2):302–8.
9. Jacobi CA, Ordemann J, Zuckermann H, Döcke W, Volk HD, Müller JM. The influence of alanyl-glutamine on immunologic functions and morbidity in postoperative total parenteral nutrition. Preliminary results of a prospective randomized trial. Zentralbl Chir. 1999;124(3):199–205.
10. Lin MT, Kung SP, Yeh SL, Lin C, Lin TH, Chen KH, Liaw KY, Lee PH, Chang KJ, Chen WJ. The effect of glutamine-supplemented total parenteral nutrition on nitrogen economy depends on severity of diseases in surgical patients. Clin Nutr. 2002;21(3):213–8.
11. Kłek S, Kulig J, Szczepanik AM, Jedrys J, Kołodziejczyk P. The clinical value of parenteral immunonutrition in surgical patients. Acta Chir Belg. 2005;105(2):175–9.
12. Yao GX, Xue XB, Jiang ZM, Yang NF, Wilmore DW. Effects of perioperative parenteral glutamine-dipeptide supplementation on plasma endotoxin level, plasma endotoxin inactivation capacity and clinical outcome. Clin Nutr. 2005;24(4):510–5.
13. Estívariz CF, Griffith DP, Luo M, Szeszycki EE, Bazargan N, Dave N, Daignault NM, Bergman GF, McNally T, Battey CH, Furr CE, Hao L, Ramsay JG, Accardi CR, Cotsonis GA, Jones DP, Galloway JR, Ziegler TR. Efficacy of parenteral nutrition supplemented with glutamine dipeptide to decrease hospital infections in critically ill surgical patients. JPEN J Parenter Enteral Nutr. 2008;32(4):389–402.
14. Engel JM, Pitz S, Mühling J, Menges T, Martens F, Kwapisz M, Hempelmann G. Role of glutamine administration on T-cell derived inflammatory response after cardiopulmonary bypass. Clin Nutr. 2009;28(1):15–20.
15. Asprer JM, Llido LO, Sinamban R, Schlotzer E, Kulkarni H. Effect on immune indices of preoperative intravenous glutamine dipeptide supplementation in malnourished abdominal surgery patients in the preoperative and postoperative periods. Nutrition. 2009;25(9):920–5.
16. Karwowska KA, Dworacki G, Trybus M, Zeromski J, Szulc R. Influence of glutamine-enriched parenteral nutrition on nitrogen balance and immunologic status in patients undergoing elective aortic aneurysm repair. Nutrition. 2001;17(6):475–8.
17. Jiang ZM, Cao JD, Zhu XG, Zhao WX, Yu JC, Ma EL, Wang XR, Zhu MW, Shu H, Liu YW. The impact of alanyl-glutamine on clinical safety, nitrogen balance, intestinal permeability, and clinical outcome in postoperative patients: a randomized, double-blind, controlled study of 120 patients. JPEN J Parenter Enteral Nutr. 1999;23(5 Suppl):S62–6.
18. O'Riordain MG, Fearon KC, Ross JA, Rogers P, Falconer JS, Bartolo DC, Garden OJ, Carter DC. Glutamine-supplemented total parenteral nutrition enhances T-lymphocyte response in surgical patients undergoing colorectal resection. Ann Surg. 1994;220(2):212–21.
19. Spittler A, Sautner T, Gornikiewicz A, Manhart N, Oehler R, Bergmann M, Függer R, Roth E. Postoperative glycyl-glutamine infusion reduces immunosuppression: partial prevention of the surgery induced decrease in HLA-DR expression on monocytes. Clin Nutr. 2001;20(1):37–42.
20. Fan YP, Yu JC, Kang WM, Zhang Q. Effects of glutamine supplementation on patients undergoing abdominal surgery. Chin Med Sci J. 2009;24(1):55–9.
21. Mertes N, Schulzki C, Goeters C, Winde G, Benzing S, Kuhn KS, Van Aken H, Stehle P, Fürst P. Cost containment through L-alanyl-L-glutamine supplemented total parenteral nutrition after major abdominal surgery: a prospective randomized double-blind controlled study. Clin Nutr. 2000;19(6):395–401.
22. Neri A, Mariani F, Piccolomini A, Testa M, Vuolo G, Di Cosmo L. Glutamine-supplemented total parenteral nutrition in major abdominal surgery. Nutrition. 2001;17:968–9.
23. Exner R, Tamandl D, Goetzinger P, Mittlboeck M, Fuegger R, Sautner T, Spittler A, Roth E. Perioperative GLY-GLN infusion diminishes the surgery-induced period of immunosuppression: accelerated restoration of the lipopolysaccharide-stimulated tumor necrosis factor-alpha response. Ann Surg. 2003;237(1):110–5.
24. Jo S, Choi SH, Heo JS, Kim EM, Min MS, Choi DW, Seo JM, Chung JC, Kim YI. Missing effect of glutamine supplementation on the surgical outcome after pancreaticoduodenectomy for periampullary tumors: a prospective, randomized, double-blind, controlled clinical trial. World J Surg. 2006;30(11):1974–82.
25. Marton S, Ghosh S, Papp A, Bogar L, Koszegi T, Juhasz V, Cseke L, Horvath PO. Effect of glutamine in patients with esophagus resection. Dis Esophagus. 2010;23(2):106–11.

26. Lu CY, Shih YL, Sun LC, Chuang JF, Ma CJ, Chen FM, Wu DC, Hsieh JS, Wang JY. The inflammatory modulation effect of glutamine-enriched total parenteral nutrition in postoperative gastrointestinal cancer patients. Am Surg. 2011;77(1):59–64.
27. Oguz M, Kerem M, Bedirli A, Mentes BB, Sakrak O, Salman B, Bostanci H. L-alanin-L-glutamine supplementation improves the outcome after colorectal surgery for cancer. Colorectal Dis. 2007;9(6):515–20.
28. Gianotti L, Braga M, Biffi R, Bozzetti F, Mariani L. Perioperative intravenous glutamine supplemetation in major abdominal surgery for cancer: a randomized multicenter trial. Ann Surg. 2009;250(5):684–90.
29. Gianotti L, Alexander JW, Gennari R, Pyles T, Babcock GF. Oral glutamine decreases bacterial translocation and improves survival in experimental gut-origin sepsis. JPEN J Parenter Enteral Nutr. 1995;19(1):69–74.
30. Wischmeyer PE, Kahana M, Wolfson R, Ren H, Musch MM, Chang EB. Glutamine induces heat shock protein and protects against endotoxin shock in the rat. J Appl Physiol. 2001;90(6):2403–10.
31. Ziegler TR, Ogden LG, Singleton KD, Luo M, Fernandez-Estivariz C, Griffith DP, Galloway JR, Wischmeyer PE. Parenteral glutamine increases serum heat shock protein 70 in critically ill patients. Intensive Care Med. 2005;31(8):1079–86.
32. Andreasen AS, Pedersen-Skovsgaard T, Mortensen OH, van Hall G, Moseley PL, Pedersen BK. The effect of glutamine infusion on the inflammatory response and HSP70 during human experimental endotoxaemia. Crit Care. 2009;13(1):R7. doi:10.1186/cc7696.
33. De-Souza DA, Greene LJ. Intestinal permeability and systemic infections in critically ill patients: effect of glutamine. Crit Care Med. 2005;33(5):1125–35.
34. Van der Hulst RR, van Kreel BK, von Meyenfeldt MF, Brummer RJ, Arends JW, Deutz NE, Soeters PB. Glutamine and the preservation of gut integrity. Lancet. 1993;341(8857):1363–5.
35. Zhou YP, Jiang ZM, Sun YH, Wang XR, Ma EL, Wilmore D. The effect of supplemental enteral glutamine on plasma levels, gut function, and outcome in severe burns: a randomized, double-blind, controlled clinical trial. JPEN J Parenter Enteral Nutr. 2003;27(4):241–5.
36. Bergman E, Heitmann R. Metabolism of amino acids by the gut, liver, kidneys and peripheral tissue. Fed Proc. 1978;37:1228–32.
37. Déchelotte P, Hasselmann M, Cynober L, Allaouchiche B, Coëffier M, Hecketsweiler B, Merle V, Mazerolles M, Samba D, Guillou YM, Petit J, Mansoor O, Colas G, Cohendy R, Barnoud D, Czernichow P, Bleichner G. L-alanyl-L-glutamine dipeptide-supplemented total parenteral nutrition reduces infectious complications and glucose intolerance in critically ill patients: the French controlled, randomized, double-blind, multicenter study. Crit Care Med. 2006;34(3):598–604.
38. Grau T, Bonet A, Miñambres E, Piñeiro L, Irles JA, Robles A, Acosta J, Herrero I, Palacios V, Lopez J, Blesa A, Martínez P, Metabolism, Nutrition Working Group, SEMICYUC, Spain. The effect of L-alanyl-L-glutamine dipeptide supplemented total parenteral nutrition on infectious morbidity and insulin sensitivity in critically ill patients. Crit Care Med. 2011;39(6):1263–8.
39. Lipshutz AK, Gropper MA. Perioperative glycemic control: an evidence-based review. Anesthesiology. 2009;110(2):408–21.
40. Novak F, Heyland DK, Avenell A, Drover JW, Su X. Glutamine supplementation in serious illness: a systematic review of the evidence. Crit Care Med. 2002;30(9):2022–9.
41. Bollhalder L, Pfeil AM, Tomonaga Y, Schwenkglenks M. A systematic literature review and meta-analysis of randomized clinical trials of parenteral glutamine supplementation. Clin Nutr. 2013;32(2):213–23.
42. Goeters C, Wenn A, Mertes N, Wempe C, Van Aken H, Stehle P, Bone HG. Parenteral L-alanyl-L-glutamine improves 6-month outcome in critically ill patients. Crit Care Med. 2002;30(9):2032–7.
43. Griffiths RD, Jones C, Palmer TE. Six-month outcome of critically ill patients given glutamine-supplemented parenteral nutrition. Nutrition. 1997;13(4):295–302.
44. Conejero R, Bonet A, Grau T, Esteban A, Mesejo A, Montejo JC, López J, Acosta JA. Effect of a glutamine-enriched enteral diet on intestinal permeability and infectious morbidity at 28 days in critically ill patients with systemic inflammatory response syndrome: a randomized, single-blind, prospective, multicenter study. Nutrition. 2002;18(9):716–21.
45. Hall JC, Dobb G, Hall J, de Sousa R, Brennan L, McCauley R. A prospective randomized trial of enteral glutamine in critical illness. Intensive Care Med. 2003;29(10):1710–6.
46. Andrews PJ, Avenell A, Noble DW, Campbell MK, Croal BL, Simpson WG, Vale LD, Battison CG, Jenkinson DJ. Cook JA; Randomised trial of glutamine, selenium, or both, to supplement parenteral nutrition for critically ill patients. BMJ. 2011;342:d1542.
47. Wernerman J, Kirketeig T, Andersson B, Berthelson H, Ersson A, Friberg H, Guttormsen AB, Hendrikx S, Pettilä V, Rossi P, Sjöberg F, Winsö O, Scandinavian Critical Care Trials Group. Scandinavian glutamine trial: a pragmatic multi-centre randomised clinical trial of intensive care unit patients. Acta Anaesthesiol Scand. 2011;55(7):812–8.
48. Heyland D, Muscedere J, Wischmeyer PE, Cook D, Jones G, Albert M, Elke G, Berger MM, Day AG. A randomized trial of glutamine and antioxidants in critically ill patients. N Engl J Med. 2013;368(16):1489–97.

49. Schneider A, Markowski A, Momma M, Seipt C, Luettig B, Hadem J, Wilhelmi M, Manns B, Merle V, Mazerolles M, Samba D, Guillou YM, Petit J, Mansoor O, Colas G, Cohendy R, Barnoud D, Czernichow P, Bleichner G. L-alanyl-L-glutamine dipeptide-supplemented total parenteral nutrition reduces infectious complications and glucose intolerance in critically ill patients: the French controlled, randomized, double-blind, multicenter study. Crit Care Med. 2006;34(3):598–604.
50. Cekmen N, Aydin A, Erdemli O. The impact of L-alanyl-L-glutamine dipeptide supplemented total parenteral nutrition on clinical outcome in critically patients. J Clin Nutr Metab. 2011;6(2):e64.
51. Fuentes-Orozco C, Cervantes-Guevara G, Muciño-Hernández I, López-Ortega A, Ambriz-González G, Gutiérrez-de-la-Rosa JL, Gómez-Herrera E, Hermosillo-Sandoval JM, González-Ojeda A. L-alanyl-L-glutamine-supplemented parenteral nutrition decreases infectious morbidity rate in patients with severe acute pancreatitis. JPEN J Parenter Enteral Nutr. 2008;32(4):403–11.
52. Pérez-Bárcena J, Regueiro V, Marsé P, Raurich JM, Rodríguez A, Ibáñez J, de Lorenzo Mateos AG, Bengoechea JA. Glutamine as a modulator of the immune system of critical care patients: effect on Toll-like receptor expression. A preliminary study. Nutrition. 2008;24(6):522–7.
53. Sahin H, Mercanligil SM, Inanç N, Ok E. Effects of glutamine-enriched total parenteral nutrition on acute pancreatitis. Eur J Clin Nutr. 2007;61(12):1429–34.
54. Xian-Li H, Qjing-jiu M, Jian-guo L, Yan-kui C, Xi-lin D. Effect of total parenteral nutrition (TPN) with and without glutamine dipeptide supplementation on outcome in severe acute pancreatitis (SAP). Clin Nutr. 2004; 1(suppl):43–7.
55. Ockenga J, Borchert K, Rifai K, Peter Manns M, Bischoff SC. Effect of glutamine-enriched total parenteral nutrition in patients with acute pancreatitis. Clin Nutr. 2002;21(5):409–16.
56. Powell-Tuck J, Jamieson CP, Bettany GE, Obeid O, Fawcett HV, Archer C, Murphy DL. A double blind, randomised, controlled trial of glutamine supplementation in parenteral nutrition. Gut. 1999;45(1):82–8.

Chapter 13
Enteral Nutrition Supplemented with L-glutamine in Patients with Sepsis

Ana Augusta Monteiro Cavalcante and Paulo Roberto Leitão de Vasconcelos

Key Points

- Glutamine is a conditionally essential nutrient during catabolic stress conditions.
- The effect of parenteral, enteral or oral nutrition supplemented with L-glutamine and dipeptide L-alanyl-L-glutamine on glycolytic parameters, inflammation, immune function, oxidative stress, intestinal permeability, mortality and morbidity in critically and moderately ill intensive care patients with trauma, SIRS, cancer, sepsis, and infection.
- Glutamine metabolism and mechanisms of action.
- Enteral nutrition supplemented with glutamine increases the percentage and count of lymphocytes, enhancing immune function.
- Glutamine is profoundly depleted in plasma and tissues during catabolic stress conditions, such as trauma, surgery, extensive burns, sepsis, and inflammatory processes.
- No adverse effects have been observed which may be attributed to glutamine in diets enriched with L-glutamine or L-alanyl-glutamine.
- Glutamine-enriched enteral diets are well tolerated.

Keywords Glutamine • Sepsis • Metabolism • Immune system • Enteral Nutrition

Abbreviations

ICU	Intensive Care Unit
ATP	Adenosine Triphosphate
GABA	Aminobutyric Acid
ROS	Oxygen-Reactive Species

A.A.M. Cavalcante, M.Sc., Ph.D. (✉)
Nutrimed Industrial Ltda, Fortaleza, Ceará, Brazil
e-mail: monteirocavalcante@yahoo.com.br

P.R.L. de Vasconcelos, D.Phil.
Department of Surgery, Federal University of Ceará, School of Medicine, Fortaleza, Ceará, Brazil

R. Rajendram et al. (eds.), *Glutamine in Clinical Nutrition*, Nutrition and Health,
DOI 10.1007/978-1-4939-1932-1_13,

TBARS Thiobarbituric Acid-Reactive Substances
SIRS Systemic inflammatory response syndrome
GSH Glutathione
APACHE Acute Physiology and Chronic Health Evaluation
DMBA 7,12-Dimethylbenz[*a*]anthracene

Introduction

Glutamine in Sepsis

Glutamine, a conditionally essential amino acid in stress conditions, has been receiving increasing attention from researchers over the past two decades, and several studies [1–7] have demonstrated its benefits.

Critical clinical illness leads to glutamine deficiency, but intravenous glutamine supplementation has been shown to reduce complications and infection associated with mortality in the intensive care unit (ICU) setting [8, 9].

Clinical trials show that glutamine-enriched parenteral nutrition in critically ill patients increases serum heat-shock protein levels [10] and improves antioxidant defense [11]. Likewise, L-alanyl-glutamine-enriched parenteral nutrition is known to augment glucose utilization in critically ill patients [12] and to decrease insulin resistance in severe trauma patients [13]. Thus, by stimulating glycolysis, glutamine supplementation potentially helps control glucose levels [12, 13] (Table 13.1). However, in a recent study, intravenous nutrition supplemented with L-alanyl-glutamine (0.4 g/kg/day) in severe critical patients with Apache II scores from 22 to 26 produced no significant effect on the total number of lymphocytes, B-lymphocytes, T-lymphocytes, and their subgroups (helper T-lymphocytes, cytotoxic T-lymphocytes); thus, no immunomodulatory benefit could be demonstrated [14].

Glutamine supplementation has been extensively studied in both animals and humans, but the most significant results have been observed with total parenteral nutrition [15, 16]. In enteral diets, glutamine supplementation is safe and well tolerated and can help reduce infectious complications, oxidative stress, intestinal permeability, infections, mortality and morbidity rates, and hospitalization cost

Table 13.1 Effects of glutamine-supplemented parenteral nutrition

Author	Design	Population	Glutamine intervention	Time	Results
Dechelotte et al. 2006 [12]	Randomized, double-blind, multicenter study	114 critical patients	0.5 g/kg body weight/day	5 days	Increased glucose utilization and reduced rates of infections complications
Bakalar et al. 2006 [13]	Randomized, prospective, controlled trial	40 multiple-trauma patients	0.4 g/kg body weight/day	7 days	Better insulin sensitivity
Alves et al. 2010 [44]	Case–control study	32 critical limb ischemia patients recruited for surgery	Exogenous preoperative infusion (50 g L-Ala-Gln) 3 h after surgery	1 time	Reduced muscle cell damage and decreased glycemia

The Table 13.1 summarizes studies examining the effects of glutamine-supplemented parenteral nutrition

Table 13.2 Effects of glutamine-supplemented enteral nutrition

Author	Design	Population	Intervention	Time	Results
Houdijk et al. 1998 [18]	Randomized, double blind	72 critical multiple-trauma patients	30.5 g/day	5 days	Decreased frequency of pneumonia
Senkal et al. 2004 [19]	Prospective open clinical trial	20 cancer patients	30 g/day + supplement with antioxidants	1 time—2–3 h after surgery + 3 days continuous infusion pos operative	No adverse effects; well tolerated; conditionally pharmaconutrients delivery
Cavalcante et al. 2012 [20]	Randomized, crossover, double blind	30 moderately ill intensive care patients with sepsis	30 g/day	5 days	Increased lymphocytesand decreased lipid peroxidation

The Table 13.2 summarizes studies examining the effects of glutamine-supplemented enteral nutrition

and time, potentially benefiting patients with severe SIRS [17], polytrauma [18], cancer [19], sepsis, and infection [20] (Table 13.2).

In a experimental study, Lim et al. [21] showed the beneficial effects of glutamine application (both topical and oral) in carcinogenesis. The results showed that glutamine completely inhibited the development of DMBA-induced leukoplakia and epidermoid carcinoma.

In sepsis, glutamine depletion is a prognostic factor of clinical response. The combination of reduced food intake and upregulated metabolism leads to glutamine depletion despite increased endogenous production in skeletal muscle [22]. Glutamine production may also be increased during sepsis, with stores consumed mainly by the liver and immune cells and, to a lesser extent, by the intestine. In this condition, the liver becomes the main consumer of glutamine from skeletal muscle, which is the main source of glutamine endogenous production. In other words, glutamine supplementation allows to restore glutaminemia and reduce infectious complications [22].

In humans, the plasma carries approximately 25 % of the glutamine produced by the organism [23]. Due to its ability to synthesize and release glutamine, especially during moments of increased demand from other organs and tissues, skeletal muscle plays a key metabolic role in the regulation of glutaminemia [24].

Glutamine is primarily synthesized in skeletal muscle. It allows nitrogen to be transferred to the spleen, kidneys and immune system [25]. The discrepancy between the increase in glutamine utilization by the organism and the relative decrease in de novo glutamine synthesis in skeletal muscle lead to systemic glutamine deficiency and therefore to severe disease [25].

In many body tissues, such as the kidneys, liver, bowels, and immune system, glutamine is found in high concentrations. However, under certain clinical conditions, such as trauma, bone marrow transplantation, burns, sepsis and cancer cachexia, and intramuscular and plasma glutamine concentrations are reduced to such an extent that supplementation becomes necessary [26, 27].

Glutamine can be synthesized by the body in large enough amounts to satisfy nutritional needs under normal physiological conditions, in which case it is considered a non-essential amino acid. It is synthesized from glutamate and ammonium, catalyzed by glutamine synthetase in an ATP-dependent reaction [28]. However, despite being the most abundant amino acid in the human body, in stress states, while glutamine synthesis increases in the muscle in response to aggression, the metabolic demand exceeds the body's capacity to synthesize it.

Thus, despite large muscle stores, glutamine is profoundly depleted in plasma and tissues during catabolic stress conditions, such as trauma, surgery, extensive burns, sepsis, and inflammatory processes [29]. Once glutamine stores are depleted and endogenous production falls short of the demand, dietary glutamine supplementation becomes necessary. In this scenario, due to the combination of reduced food intake and upregulated metabolism, leading to depletion despite increased skeletal muscle synthesis, glutamine may be considered a conditionally essential amino acid [23, 29–32].

Severe infection causes considerable disturbances in the flow of glutamine from organ to organ, accompanied by significant changes in regional cell membrane transport and intracellular glutamine metabolism. During infection, skeletal muscle, the most important repository of glutamine, releases twice the usual amount of glutamine, and endogenous glutamine biosynthesis increases significantly. Despite the increased activity of skeletal muscle glutamine synthetase, the intracellular glutamine pool becomes depleted, indicating that release rates exceed rates of synthesis. The fact that no increase is observed in the levels of circulating glutamine suggests that uptake by other organs has increased concurrently [33].

Under conditions of stress, changes occur in the flow of glutamine among organs. In healthy individuals, glutamine is produced mainly by skeletal muscle and the lungs and is consumed by the intestine, immune cells and the liver. During sepsis, glutamine production increases, while most of the uptake occurs in immune cells and liver tissues, rather than in the intestine. In this scenario, the liver becomes the main organ of uptake of glutamine released by skeletal muscle, the principal glutamine supplier [27, 33].

Novak et al. [8] observed that high-dose glutamine supplementation is associated with improved post-surgical outcomes, including fewer infectious complications and shorter hospital permanence, with no adverse effect on mortality. In severe patients, glutamine supplementation has been associated with reductions in complications and mortality rates. However, supplementation yields the best results when administered parenterally. Mondello et al. [16] investigated the effect of total parenteral nutrition supplemented with glutamine on immune system in anorectic patients and observed the benefit of glutamine supplementation on immune response in anorectic patients.

In a prospective, randomized, controlled, double-blind and crossover clinical study evaluating the effect of enteral nutrition supplemented with nutraceutical doses of L-glutamine (30 g/day) on inflammatory markers, glycolytic metabolism, immune function, and oxidative stress in 30 moderately severe adult and elderly ICU patients, Cavalcante et al. [20] observed an increase in the total number and percentage of lymphocytes (Tables 13.3 and 13.4) induced by L-glutamine supplementation and a decrease in lipid peroxidation, with supplementation of either L-glutamine or calcium caseinate (Table 13.5).

Table 13.3 Lymphocyte counts of 30 patients with sepsis before and after enteral diet supplementation with calcium caseinate (CAS) and glutamine (GLN)

	CAS		GLN		
Time	Median	Interval range	Median	Interval range	Significance (intergroup)
T0	1.288	834–2.209	954	785–1.442	0.1042
T1	1.085	805–1.363	1.916	1.301–2.517	$<0.0001^{+++}$
Significance (intragroup)	0.0324*		<0.0001***		

Source: original material of A.A. Monteiro Cavalcante

Statistical Analysis: Wilcoxon test for intergroup and intragroup, variables and expressed as median, maximum and minimum values. $^{*}p=0.020$ (GLN T1<GLN T0), $^{+++}p<0.0001$ (GLN T1>T0), $^{+++}p<0.0001$ (GLN versus CAS, T1 GLN>T1 CAS)

T0 (before enteral diet supplementation); T1 (after enteral diet supplementation)

Table 13.4 Lymphocyte percentage of 30 patients with sepsis before and after enteral diet supplementation with calcium caseinate (CAS) and glutamine (GLN)

	CAS		GLN		
Time	Median	Interval range	Median	Interval range	Significance (intergroup)
T0	9.50	6.00–19.25	7.50	4.75–15.00	0.104
T1	9.00	6.00–12.00	15.00	9.75–23.25	<0.0001^{+++}
Significance (intragroup)	0.0271*		<0.0001***		

Source: Original material of A.A. Monteiro Cavalcante

Statistical Analysis: Wilcoxon test for intergroup and intragroup, variables and expressed as median, maximum and minimum values. *p=0.0271 (CAS T1<CAS T0), ***p<0.0001 (GLN T1>T0), ^{+++}p<0.0001 (GLN versus CAS, T1 GLN>T1 CAS)

T0 (before enteral diet supplementation); T1 (after enteral diet supplementation)

Table 13.5 TBARS concentrations of 30 patients with sepsis before and after enteral diet supplementation with calcium caseinate (CAS) and glutamine (GLN)

	CAS		GLN		
Time	Median	Interval range	Median	Interval range	Significance (intergroup)
T0	20.560	14.210–38.590	17.670	8.155–34.980	0.484
T1	15.080	13.640–20.560	16.520	5.415–21.860	0.781
Significance (intragroup)	0.001**		0.020*		

Source: original material of A.A. Monteiro Cavalcante

Statistical Analysis: Wilcoxon test for intergroup and intragroup, variables and expressed as median, maximum and minimum values. *p=0.020 (GLN T1<GLN T0), **p=0.001 (CAS T1<CAS T0)

T0 (before enteral diet supplementation); T1 (after enteral diet supplementation); TBARS (thiobarbituric acid-reactive substances)

Immune System

Glutamine acts in tissue protection, has antioxidant and anti-inflammatory effects, regulates the immune system, and helps preserve the metabolic functions of tissues under stress.

It is important in cell growth and differentiation, inter-organ carbon transfer and as a preferential substrate for cells with rapid turnover, such as erythrocytes, and immune cells, such as macrophages and lymphocytes [34]. In addition, glutamine is a precursor to mediators like GABA (γ-aminobutyric acid) and glutamate, acting in the synthesis of amino acids, nucleotides, nucleic acids, amino sugars, proteins, and many other biologically important molecules [27, 28].

Glutamine is a key substrate for activated immune cells, increases lymphocytic response to mitogen stimulation, and alleviates bacteremia and endotoxemia, thereby helping prevent sepsis [35]. The high rate of glutamine utilization by lymphocytes and macrophages suggests that glutamine supply plays an important role in the maintenance of immune function [26, 27]. The activation of cells such as T lymphocytes is essential for the maintenance of adequate immune response and contributes to preventing bacterial translocation [36]. Glutamine is also important in gluconeogenesis, urea synthesis, pH homeostasis, neurotransmission, and cell growth and differentiation [27].

Immune cells utilize large amounts of glutamine to sustain lymphocyte proliferation and cytokine production by lymphocytes and macrophages; in other words, the basic functions of these cells, as demonstrated in vitro, are dependent on glutamine supply [26]. Normally and especially during stress, the digestive tract is the main organ of glutamine uptake and utilization since the intestinal mucosa contains immune and neuroendocrine cells in addition to numerous absorptive enterocytes.

In response, the bowel perceives the nutritional and antigenic environment, acts in immunological screening and defense, and produces endocrine responses to the lumen environment [37].

In short, the administration of glutamine or one of its precursors is beneficial to severely ill patients with inflammatory and immune response due to stress, trauma, sepsis, or any condition which increases susceptibility to infection.

Oxidative Stress

Oxidative stress reflects an imbalance between the production of oxygen-reactive species (ROS) and the ability of the body's antioxidant defense mechanisms to detoxify reactive intermediates. ROS play an important role in the regulation of normal cell functions but, when produced in excess, can be harmful and lead to oxidative stress [38].

Excessive ROS production can damage all cell components, including proteins, lipids and nucleic acids. The greater the oxidative stress, the more extensive the cell damage. Eventually, apoptosis (or even cell necrosis) may occur [38].

Among the consequences of oxidative stress, lipid peroxidation is the most extensively investigated. It is measured by detection in plasma or urine of thiobarbituric acid reactive substances (TBARS), a marker of lipid peroxidation. SIRS, a host response to infection and other forms of tissue injury, is often accompanied by oxidative stress in one or more organic systems. In fact, Takeshi et al. [39] observed that TBARS and lipid peroxidation increase in patients with SIRS.

Glutamine is a precursor of glutathione (GSH) which is found in high concentrations in mammalian cells. GSH is considered the most potent antioxidant substance in the human body and is capable of neutralizing the action of ROS [40]. It is the main component of the antioxidant defense system in cells and has a range of effects on the immune system, stimulating or inhibiting immune response in order to control inflammation [41].

Changes in GSH concentrations play an important role in several clinical conditions, especially in those involving inflammatory and immune responses mediated by oxidative stress reactions. In such situations, failure of the antioxidant defense system to maintain the rate of oxidative balance is usually due to the combination of weakened antioxidant defense and increased production of pro-oxidants [41]. Thus, glutamine depletion can lead to decreased GSH levels and may require replacement by exogenous glutamine supply [42].

The Canadian Critical Care Trials Group [43] has shown that glutamine supplementation is likely to have a positive impact upon oxidative stress in critical patients. Likewise, the observation by Cavalcante et al. [20] that patients receiving glutamine supplementation are likely to sustain antioxidant capacity reflects the role of glutamine as a precursor of GSH.

Alves et al. [44] administered L-alanyl-glutamine (50 g) intravenously 3 h prior to surgery in patients subjected to critical limb ischemia and found decreased TBARS levels and increased GSH concentrations in the muscle half an hour after reperfusion following venous grafting. They also reported reduced levels of lactate dehydrogenase (LDH) and lactate indicating increased glucose oxidation in the limb submitted to ischemia/reperfusion, suggesting that glutamine reduced glycemia in the patients. It may therefore be concluded that pretreatment with L-alanyl-glutamine reduces muscle cell damage, promotes a decrease in glycemia and enhances antioxidant capacity in patients with critical limb ischemia [44] (Table 13.1). GSH replacement may be achieved by means of exogenous glutamine supply, thereby maintaining the intracellular glutamate pool and avoiding GSH depletion.

Intestinal Barrier

Intestinal barrier function depends on a balance between epithelial cell (enterocyte) proliferation and apoptosis and between protein synthesis and proteolysis, but also on the maintenance of the junctions between enterocytes, the so-called tight junctions [22].

The intestinal mucosa plays a key role in intestinal barrier function, preventing systematic dissemination of bacteria and intraluminal endotoxins. However, under conditions of severe damage, anatomical and functional integrity may be lost, allowing bacterial translocation and, consequently, sepsis and multiple organ failure [45].

Bacterial translocation implies the transfer of viable endogenous bacteria from the gastrointestinal tract to extra-intestinal sites, such as the mesenteric lymph node complex, the liver, the spleen or the blood. Among the factors implicated in this condition are long-term nutritional deficits during severe disease, changes in gastrointestinal microflora leading to bacterial overgrowth, physical disruption of the intestinal mucosal barrier through direct damage to enterocytes, thereby favoring penetration, reduced intestinal blood flow, and local or systemic response causing deficiencies in the immune defense and increased permeability or damage to the intestinal mucosal barrier [46, 47]. Thus, the inflammatory response to injury and infection, although an essential part of immune function, carries the risk of severe tissue depletion and immunosuppression [47].

Bacterial translocation can occur in both healthy and diseased individuals regardless of disease severity [47], but tends to increase in severe clinical conditions, such as burns, trauma, surgery and heart failure. Intestinal barrier permeability can be reduced to prevent bacterial translocation by different treatment approaches, including enteral nutrition and immunonutrition [22, 46, 47].

Immunonutrition can modulate the immune system, or the consequences of immune system activation, by supplying specific foods and nutrients in amounts exceeding those found in conventional diets [47, 48]. Glutamine is an immunomodulating amino acid capable of maintaining intestinal integrity and stimulating protein synthesis in human intestinal mucosa [22, 45].

Nutritional glutamine depletion has been associated with reduced glutamine levels in plasma and mucosa and with increased intestinal permeability. In a study on glutamine plasma concentrations and nutritional parameters in 26 patients receiving parenteral nutrition, Hulsewé et al. [49] observed that inflammatory activity occurs regardless of the presence or absence of nutritional depletion.

Several studies on enteral, parenteral or oral administration of recommended doses of glutamine before or just after surgery and burns have shown glutamine to have a protective effect preventing or reducing loss of intestinal permeability, maintaining the physiological intestinal barrier and reducing the frequency of infection.

Glycolytic Metabolism

Hyperglycemia is associated with a poor prognosis in clinical or surgical ICU patients. In this setting, hyperglycemia develops mainly due to gluconeogenesis, insulin resistance, upregulation of insulin counterregulatory hormones, cytokine activity, clinical interventions, and glucose intolerance [50].

Hyperglycemia is multifactorial. Common in sepsis (even in nondiabetic patients), it causes or exacerbates oxidative stress, endothelial injury, neutrophil rolling and inflammation and has proinflammatory and immunosuppressive action [51].

As an alternative to therapy with exogenous insulin supply, studies have shown that nutritional glutamine supplementation can attenuate insulin resistance and subsequent hyperglycemia following severe disease. Clinical studies on glutamine supplementation to severe [12] and polytraumatized patients [13] revealed a reduction in infectious complications and improved metabolic tolerance in a group of patients requiring insulin therapy. Based on these studies, it seems reasonable to affirm that glutamine in dipeptide form has beneficial effects on insulin-dependent glucose metabolism.

Enteral Nutrition and Immunonutrients in Intensive Care

Diet can be used as a tool to modulate health outcomes, improving the clinical and biochemical indicators affected by the disease. One such tool, enteral nutrition, is indicated for patients with conditions which preclude normal oral feeding and, consequently, nutrient absorption. It provides necessary calories and substrates and restores metabolic and immune response, improving host defense and accelerating recovery.

Over the past decades, enteral nutrition has become a vital component in intensive care. It is in most cases the recommended strategy for feeding severely ill patients presenting increased nutritional requirements and, not uncommonly, catabolism with risk of organ failure. In addition, ICU patients often experience depletion of specific nutrients, such as arginine, minerals, and glutamine.

Research has shown the benefits of glutamine supplementation in severe conditions [1–7], in both animals and humans, but results have been most significant for total parenteral nutrition [8–13, 15, 16] and, especially, dipeptides such as L-alanyl-glutamine.

Glutamine may act as a pharmaconutrient at nutraceutical doses (10–50 g/day). Under such conditions, it has specific and important metabolic functions, especially in injury related to infection or wounds or in catabolism and sepsis. The rapid depletion of glutamine in the plasma which is commonly observed in severely ill patients appears to justify the need of replacement by way of supplementation [8, 9, 11, 19].

Enteral glutamine supply benefits primarily splanchnic tissues, whereas parenteral supplementation provides glutamine for the entire organism [25].

Conejero et al. [17] investigated the effect of glutamine-enriched enteral nutrition on intestinal permeability, infectious morbidity and mortality in severe patients developing SIRS following an acute event and concluded that glutamine-enriched enteral nutrition reduced nosocomial infections in this population.

García-de-Lorenzo et al. [52] reviewed several studies and found that enteral glutamine supplementation at nutraceutical doses was safe and well tolerated clinically, with no adverse effects regardless of the disease. Thus, no restrictions or contraindications exist for glutamine supplementation at nutraceutical doses [17, 20, 52, 53].

Glutamine-enriched enteral diets are well tolerated and have been shown to improve immune defense in polytraumatized patients and reduce the cost of intensive care [9]. No evidence or reports of adverse or negative effects attributed to glutamine supplementation have been published to date. Likewise, Garcia et al. [52] and Galera et al. [53] found glutamine supplementation at nutraceutical doses to be safe.

Galera et al. [53] evaluated the safety profile of oral administration of L-glutamine at 30 g/day for 14 days in a sample of healthy middle-aged and elderly subjects, but observed no clinically important effects, apart from the need for permanent control of renal function in this population.

Glutamine-enriched diets at recommended nutraceutical doses (20–30 g/day) should be started as early as possible and maintained for at least 5 days [52]. Since the turnover of glutamine is very high, a daily dose of 30 g may be administered with no risk of significant side effects [20, 53].

Macrophages and lymphocytes are the largest cell components of the immune system. The latter are a group of heterogeneous cells involved in immune cell mediation and immunoregulation. In one study, enteral nutrition supplemented with L-glutamine [20] enhanced immune function by increasing the total number and percentage of lymphocytes. In addition, lipid peroxidation decreased with enteral nutrition supplemented with protein (calcium caseinate) and glutamine in both study groups, but had no effect on glycolytic parameters or inflammatory response.

On the other hand, in a study by Cetinbas et al. [14] administering parenteral nutrition supplemented with L-alanyl-glutamine at 0.4 g/kg/day to severe patients with APACHE II scores from 22 to 26, no significant difference was observed with regard to the total number of lymphocytes, B- lymphocytes, and T-lymphocytes or their subgroups (helper T-lymphocytes and cytotoxic T-lymphocytes).

The findings of these last two studies suggest that severe patients do not benefit as much from glutamine supplementation as moderately ill patients. In a study by Cavalcante et al. [20], glutamine, despite being supplied enterally, increased the percentage of lymphocytes, indicating that the amino acid was not retained by the enterocytes. The finding of an increased percentage and total number of lymphocytes [20] (Tables 13.3 and 13.4) indicates significant improvement of the immune system, especially when considered in combination with a significant decrease in the percentage of leukocytes, as observed in both study groups.

Conclusions

The utilization of glutamine by lymphocytes, particularly when these are challenged by adverse conditions such as sepsis, suggests that exogenous glutamine supplementation favors cell function and, consequently, enhances the efficiency of the immune system. Considering the observed benefits and the absence of adverse effects, enteral and parenteral diets enriched with L-glutamine or L-alanyl-glutamine are currently recommended for severe ICU patients in order to modulate the immune system.

References

1. Bastian L, Weimann A. Immunonutrition in patients after multiple trauma. Br J Nutr. 2002;87(suppl):S133–4.
2. Jiang Z, Jiang H, Fürst P. The impact of glutamine dipeptides on outcome of surgical patients: systematic review of randomized controlled trials from Europe and Asia. Clin Nutr Suppl. 2004;1(1):17–23.
3. Fürst P, Alteheld B, Stehle P. Why should a single nutrient—glutamine—improve outcome? The remarkable story of glutamine dipeptides. Clin Nutr Suppl. 2004;1(1):3–15.
4. Hasenboehler E, Wiliams A, Leinhase I, Morgan SJ, Smith W, Moore EE, Stahel PF. Metabolic changes after polytrauma: an imperative for early nutritional support. World J Emerg Surg. 2006;1(29):1–7.
5. Weitzel LRB, Wischmeyer PE. Glutamine in critical illness: the time has come, the time is now. Crit Care Med. 2010;26(3):515–25.
6. Bongers T, Griffiths RD, McArdle A. Exogenous glutamine: the clinical evidence. Crit Care Med. 2007; 35(suppl):S545–52.
7. Kuhn KS, Muscaritoli M, Wischmeyer P, Stehle P. Glutamine as indispensable nutrient in oncology: experimental and clinical evidence. Eur J Clin Nutr. 2010;49(4):197–210.
8. Novak F, Heyland DK, Avenell A, Drover JW, Su X. Glutamine supplementation in serius illness: a systematic review of the evidence. Crit Care Med. 2002;30(9):2022–9.
9. Fuentes-Orozco C, Anaya-Prado R, González-Ojeda A, Arenas-Márquez H, Cabrera-Privaral C, Cervantes-Guevara G, Barrera-Zepeda L. L-alanyl-l-glutamine-supplemented parenteral nutrition improves infectious morbidity in secondary peritonitis. Clin Nutr. 2004;23(1):13–21.
10. Ziegler TR, Ogden LG, Singleton KD, Luo M, Fernandez-Estivariz C, Griffith DP, Galloway JR, Wischmeyer PE. Parenteral glutamine increases serum heat shock protein 70 in critically ill patients. Intensive Care Med. 2005;31(8):1079–86.
11. Abilés J, Moreno-Torres R, Moratalla G, Castaño J, Abúd RP, Mudarra A, Machado MJ, Planells E, De la Cruz AP. Efectos de la suplementación con glutamina sobre el sistema antioxidante y la peroxidación lipídica en pacientes críticos con nutrición parenteral. Nutr Hosp. 2008;23(4):332–9.
12. Dechelotte P, Hasselmann M, Cynober L, Allaouchiche B, Coëffier M, Hecketsweiler B, et al. L-alanyl-L-glutamine dipeptide-supplemented total parenteral nutrition reduces infectious complications and glucose intolerance in critically

ill patients: The French controlled, randomized, double-blind, multicenter study. Crit Care Med. 2006;34(3): 598–604.
13. Bakalar B, Duska F, Pachl J, Fric M, Otahal M, Pazout J, Andel M. Parenterally administered dipeptide alanyl-glutamine prevents worsening of insulin sensitivity in multiple-trauma patients. Crit Care Med. 2006;34(2):381–6.
14. Cetinbas F, Yelken B, Gulbas Z. Role of glutamine administration on cellular immunity after total parenteral nutrition enriched with glutamine in patients with systemic inflammatory response syndrome. J Crit Care. 2010;25(4):661. e1–6.
15. Windle EM. Glutamine supplementation in critical illness: Evidence, recommendations, and implications for clinical practice in burn care. J Burn Care Res. 2006;27(6):764–72.
16. Mondello S, Italiano D, Giacobbe MS, Mondello P, Trimarchi G, Aloisi C, Bramanti P, Spina E. Glutamine-supplemented total parenteral nutrition improves immunological status in anorectic patients. Nutrition. 2010; 26(6):677–81.
17. Conejero R, Bonet A, Grau T, Esteban A, Mesejo A, Montejo JC, López J, Acosta JA. Effect of a glutamine-enriched enteral diet on intestinal permeability and infectious morbidity at 28 days in critically Ill patients with systemic inflammatory response syndrome: a randomized, single-blind, prospective, multicenter study. Nutrition. 2002;18(9):716–21.
18. Houdijk APJ, Rijnsburger ER, Janse J, Wesdorp RI, Weiss JK, McCamish MA, Teerlink T, Meuwissen SG, Haarman HJ, Thijs LG, van Leeuwen PA. Radomised trial of glutamine-enriched enteral nutrition on infeccious morbity in patients with multiple trauma. Lancet. 1998;352:772–6.
19. Senkal M, Haaker R, Deska T, Hummel T, Steinfort C, Zumtobel V, Alteheld B, Stehle P. Early enteral gut feeding with conditionally indispensable pharmaconutrients in metabolically safe and is well tolerated in postoperative cancer patients—a pilot study. Clin Nutr. 2004;23(5):1193–8.
20. Cavalcante AAM, Campelo MWS, Vasconcelos MPP, Ferreira CM, Guimarães SB, Garcia JHP, Vasconcelos PRL. Enteral nutrition supplemented with L-glutamine in patients with systemic inflammatory response syndrome due to pulmonary infection. Nutrition. 2012;28(4):397–402.
21. Lim V, Korourian S, Todorova VK, Kaufmann Y, Klimberg VS. Glutamine prevents DMBA-induced squamous cell cancer. Oral Oncol. 2009;45(2):148–55.
22. Coëffier M, Tamion F, Déchelotte P. Supplémentation parentérale en glutamine en réanimation: preuves cliniques et mecanismes d'action. Réanimation. 2009;18(6):506–10.
23. Newsholme P. Why is L-glutamine metabolism important to cells of the immune system in health, post injury, surgery or infection? J Nutr. 2001;131(suppl):2515S–22.
24. Cruzat VF, Petry ER, Tirapegui J. Glutamina: Aspectos Bioquímicos, Metabólicos, Moleculares e Suplementação. Revista Brasileira de Medicina do Esporte. 2009;15(5):392–7.
25. Biolo G, Zorat F, Antonione R, Ciocchi B. Muscle glutamine depletion in intensive care unit. Int J Biochem Cell Biol. 2005;37(10):2169–79.
26. Calder PC, Yaqoob P. Glutamine and the immune system. Amino Acids. 1999;17:227–41.
27. Newsholme EA, Calder PC. The proposed role of glutamine in some cells of the immune system and speculative consequences for the whole animal. Nutrition. 1997;13(718):728–30.
28. Moskovitz B, Katz Y, Singer P, Nativ O, Rosenberg B. Glutamine metabolism and utilization: relevance to major problems in health care. Pharmacol Res. 1994;30(1):61–71.
29. Wernerman J. Glutamine supplementation. Annals Intensive Care. 2011;1(25):1–6.
30. Griffiths RD, Allen KD, Andrews FJ, Jones C. Infection, multiple organ failure, and survival in the intensive care unit: Influence of glutamine-supplemented parenteral nutrition on acquired infection. Nutrition. 2002;18:546–52.
31. Arruda IS, Aguilar-Nascimento JE. Benefits of early enteral nutrition with glutamine and probiotics in brain injury patients. Clin Sci. 2004;106:287–92.
32. Dupertius YM, Raguso CA, Pichard C. Basics in clinical nutrition: nutrients which influence immunity—clinical and experimental data. Eur e-J Clin Nutr Metabol. 2009;4(1):e7–9.
33. Karinch AM, Pan M, Lin CM, Strange R, Souba WW. Glutamine metabolism in sepsis and infection. J Nutr. 2001;131(suppl):2535S–8.
34. Wilmore DW, Shabert JK. Role of glutamine in immunologic responses. Nutrition. 1998;14:618–26.
35. Cynober L. Médiateurs de línflammation: contrôle par les nutriments azotes. Nutrition Clinique et Métabolisme. 2000;14(3):194–200.
36. Singer P, Smadja P. Diètes immuno-enrichies en protéines. Nutrition Clinique et Métabolisme. 2010;24(2):45–51.
37. Burrin DG, Stoll B, Jiang R, Chang X, Hartmann B, Holst JJ, Greeley Jr GH, Reeds PJ. Minimal enteral nutrient requirements for intestinal growth in neonatal piglets: how much is enough? Am J Clin Nutr. 2000;71(6): 1603–10.
38. Rosenfeldt F, Wilson M, Lee G, Kure C, Ou R, Braun L, Haan J. Oxidative stress in surgery in an ageing population: pathophysiology and therapy. Exp Gerontol. 2013;48:45–54.
39. Takeshi M, Kazufumi O, Ichirou K, Masamichi H, Yoshihiro K, Hisao O. Possible role of increased oxidant stress in multiple organ failure after systemic inflammatory response syndrome. Crit Care Med. 2003;31(4):1048–52.

40. Fläring UB, Rooyackers OE, Wernerman J, Hammarqvist F. Glutamine attenuates post-traumatic glutathione depletion in human muscle. Clin Sci. 2003;104(3):275–82.
41. Perricone C, Carolis C, Perricone R. Glutathione: a key player in autoimmunity. Autoimmun Rev. 2009; 8(8):697–701.
42. Bonet A, Grau T. La glutamina, un aminoácido casi indispensable en el enfermo crítico. Medicine Intensiva. 2007;31(7):402–6.
43. Heyland DK, Dhaliwal R, Day AG, Muscedere J, Drover J, Suchner U, et al. Canadian critical care trials group. Reducing deaths due to oxidative stress (the REDOXS study): rationale and study design for a randomized trial of glutamine and antioxidant supplementation in critically-ill patients. Proc Nutr Soc. 2006;65(3):250–63.
44. Alves WF, Aguiar EE, Guimarães SB, Filho ARS, Pinheiro PMA, Soares DSD, Vasconcelos PRL. L-alanyl-glutamine preoperative infusion in patients with critical limb ischemia subjected to distal revascularization reduces tissue damage and protects from oxidative stress. Ann Vasc Surg. 2010;24(4):461–7.
45. Francis R, Michel H. Avec quoi nourrir l'intestin agressée? Nutrition Clinique et Métabolisme. 2000;14(4):341–9.
46. Wiest R, Rath HC. Bacterial translocation in the gut. Best Pract Res Clin Gastroenterol. 2003;17(3):397–425.
47. Grimble RF. Nutritional modulation of immune function. Proc Nutr Soc. 2001;60(3):389–97.
48. Grimble RF. Basics in clinical nutrition: Immunonutrition—Nutrients which influence immunity: Effect and mechanism of action. Eur e-J Clin Nutr Metabol. 2009;4(1):e10–3.
49. Hulsewé KWE, van der Hulst RWWJ, van Acker BAC, von Meyenfeldt MF, Soeters PB. Inflammation rather than nutritional depletion determines glutamine concentrations and intestinal permeability. Clin Nutr. 2004;23(5): 1209–16.
50. Van den Berghe G, Wilmer A, Hermans G, Meersseman W, Wouters PJ, Milants I, Wijngaerden EV, Bobbaers H, Bouinllon R. Intensive insulin therapy in the medical ICU. N Engl J Med. 2006;354:449–61.
51. Kumar S, Leaper DJ. Basic science of sepsis. Surgery. 2005;23(8):272–7.
52. Garcia-de-Lorenzo A, Zarazaga A, Garcia-Luna PP, Gonzalezhuix F, López-Martínez J, Miján A, Quecedo L, Casimiro C, Usán L, Lano J. Clinical evidence for enteral nutritional support with glutamine: a systematic review. Nutrition. 2003;19(9):805–11.
53. Galera SC, Fechine FV, Teixeira MJ, Coelho ZCB, Vasconcelos RC, Vasconcelos PRL. The safety of oral use of L-glutamine in middle-aged and elderly individuals. Nutrition. 2010;26(4):375–81.

Chapter 14
Glutamine Supplementation in Multiple Trauma Patients

Ruqaiya M. Al Balushi, Jennifer D. Paratz, Jeremy Cohen, and Merrilyn Banks

Key Points

- Multiple trauma is characterised by alteration and depression of the immune response, which is associated with an elevated rate of infectious complications, sepsis, multiple organ failure, and death.
- Glutamine supplementation has demonstrated improved clinical outcomes in patients receiving parenteral nutrition. However, its effects and the best route of administration in patients receiving enteral nutrition are still debated.
- Despite the numerous clinical trials that have investigated the beneficial effects of glutamine supplementation in patients receiving enteral nutrition, the results are conflicting and inconclusive.
- Previous trials of glutamine supplementation in multiple trauma patients had several limitations.
- A future well-designed multi-centre trial is required to investigate the effect of glutamine supplementation in multiple trauma patients on mortality and infectious complication.

Keywords Multiple trauma • Head injury • Glutamine • Alanyl-glutamine • Supplementation • Enteral • Parenteral • Intravenous

Abbreviations

Ala-Gln	Alanyl-glutamine
CARS	Compensatory Anti-inflammatory Response Syndrome
CRP	C-reactive Protein

R.M. Al Balushi, B.Sc., M.Sc., Ph.D. (✉)
Health and Nutrition Department, College of Food and Agriculture, United Arab Emirates University, P.O. Box 15551, Al Ain, United Arab Emirates
e-mail: ruq.balushi@hotmail.com; albalushi.ruqaiya@gmail.com

J.D. Paratz, M.Phty., Ph.D., F.A.C.P. • J. Cohen, M.R.C.P., F.R.C.A., Ph.D.
Department of Intensive Care Medicine, Royal Brisbane & Women's Hospital, Brisbane, QLD, Australia

Trauma & Critical Care Research Centre, The University of Queensland, School of Medicine, Burns, Brisbane, QLD, Australia

M. Banks, B.Sc., M. Hlth. Sc., Ph.D.
Department of Nutrition and Dietetics, Royal Brisbane & Women's Hospital, Brisbane, QLD, Australia

R. Rajendram et al. (eds.), *Glutamine in Clinical Nutrition*, Nutrition and Health,
DOI 10.1007/978-1-4939-1932-1_14, © Springer Science+Business Media New York 2015

DB	Double-blind
EAA	Essential Amino Acid
EN	Enteral Nutrition
FcγRI/CD64	Fc Receptor
GCS	Glasgow Coma Scale
Gln	Glutamine
HSP	Heat-shock protein
HLA-DR	Human Leukocyte Antigen-DR
ICU	Intensive Care Unit
ICU LOS	ICU length of stay
ISS	Injury Severity Score
IV	Intravenous
MODS	Multiple Organ Dysfunction Syndrome
MOF	Multiple Organ Failure
NB	Nitrogen Balance
NS	Not Significant
RCT	Randomised Clinical Trial
SB	Single-blind
SIRS	Systemic Inflammatory Response Syndrome
SOFA	Sequential Organ Failure Assessment
TLR	Toll-like Receptor
TPN	Total Parenteral Nutrition
UUN	Urinary Urea Nitrogen

Introduction

Multiple trauma is defined as "a syndrome of combined injuries with an injury severity score (ISS) > 17 and consequent systemic inflammatory response syndrome (SIRS) for at least 1 day, leading to dysfunction, or failure of remote organs and vital systems, which themselves had not been injured" [1]. In spite of improved road safety, multiple trauma is undoubtedly still considered the most important cause of death among people under 40 years [2, 3]. Although immediate deaths from multiple trauma result from severe brain injury and haemorrhagic shock [2, 4], many later deaths are related to infections, sepsis and multiple organ failure (MOF) [2, 5, 6].

Multiple trauma is life threatening not only from the trauma insult itself, but also from the subsequent massive immunological dysfunctions and metabolic pathway alterations during the following clinical course [7], which occur as defensive and survival mechanisms to confront a life-threatening injury. This altered immune system [8] is associated with an increased rate of infectious complications and mortality [9, 10]. During critical illness, despite vigorous nutrition support and higher protein intake [11], net protein catabolism is elevated [11, 12]. Muscle catabolism that results in massive loss of lean body mass is considered a major clinical feature that prolongs dependency on mechanical ventilation, delays wound healing and recovery from critical illness, and prolongs hospital length of stay [13]. This muscle catabolism is accompanied by a marked depletion of glutamine levels in plasma and muscle, which is considered a major hallmark of critically ill patients [14–16]. Indeed, a low admission plasma glutamine level in critically ill patients is considered a significant independent risk factor of mortality [17]. Despite the fact that muscle tissue increases glutamine production during stress and critical illness, it cannot maintain the intracellular levels of glutamine [18].

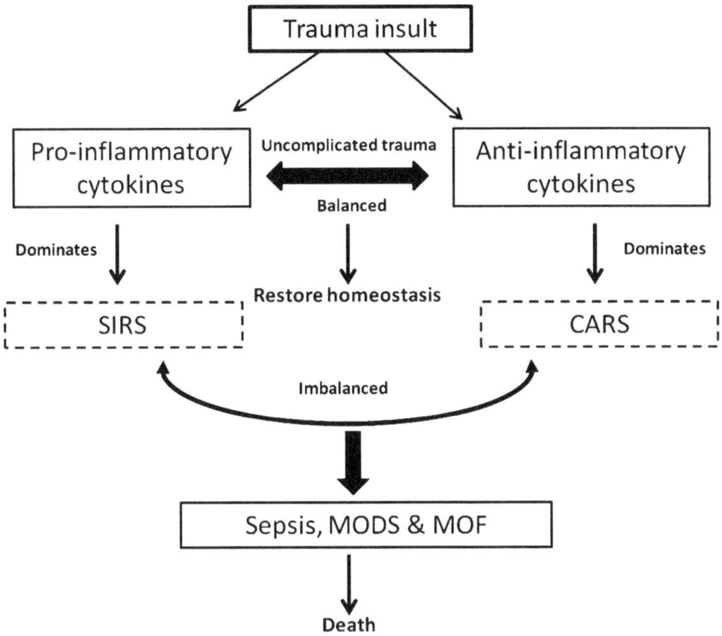

Fig. 14.1 A schematic demonstration of immune response of multiple trauma. SIRS, systemic inflammatory response syndrome; CARS, compensatory anti-inflammatory response syndrome; MODS, multiple organ dysfunction syndrome; MOF, multiple organ failure; modified from Bone [22]

Immune and Metabolic Changes of Multiple Trauma and Critical Illness

Multiple trauma and critical illness trigger an orchestrated cascade of immune and metabolic changes that aim to restore homeostasis and are correlated with the severity and duration of the injury. The traumatic insult stimulates the production of pro-inflammatory cytokines. There is also a subsequent release of anti-inflammatory cytokines [19, 20]. In uncomplicated trauma, there is a balance between the production of pro-inflammatory and anti-inflammatory cytokines, and the body restores homeostasis with no major clinical complications [19, 21]. However, if the trauma is exaggerated and prolonged, cytokine production can become unbalanced and have deleterious consequences. On one hand, if the production of pro-inflammatory cytokines dominates, the patient may develop systemic inflammatory response syndrome (SIRS). On the other hand, if the release of anti-inflammatory cytokines dominates, compensatory anti-inflammatory response syndrome (CARS) occurs [22]. The perturbation between SIRS and CARS may lead to multiple organ dysfunction syndrome (MODS) and MOF, which are associated with high mortality [10, 22–25]. Figure 14.1 demonstrates the immune response to multiple trauma.

The metabolic changes resulting from multiple trauma and injury are triggered by escalated secretion of catabolic and counter-regulatory hormones [19, 26]. These metabolic changes are important for diverting essential substrates from non-essential tasks to more important functions such as activity of the immune system, wound healing and other functions necessary for survival from the trauma. These metabolic changes result in sustained hypermetabolism [27, 28], lipolysis [29, 30] and protein hypercatabolism [27]. This protein hypercatabolism results in a negative nitrogen balance [31] and leads to muscle proteolysis that may reach up to 2 % per day [32]. Muscle proteolysis results in

Fig. 14.2 Metabolic changes after multiple trauma

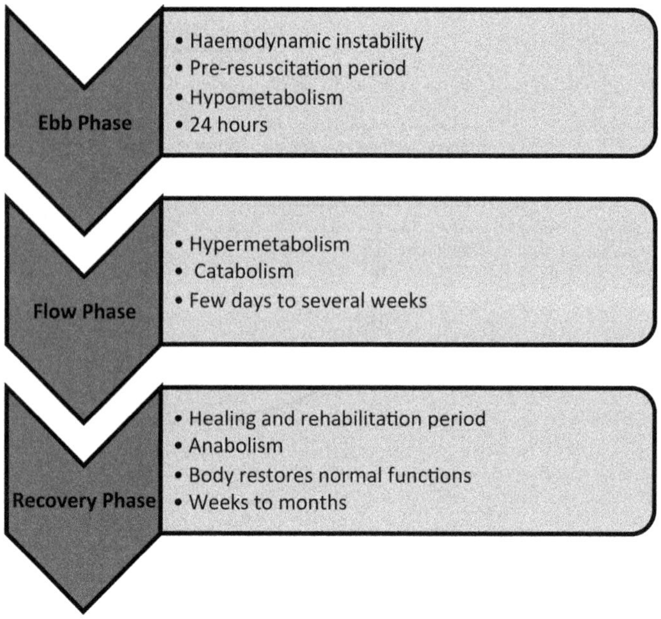

marked and prolonged intracellular and plasma glutamine depletion [12, 32, 33]. Although protein synthesis during trauma and critical illness is increased to some extent, the rate of protein catabolism is much more elevated [34] and this results in muscle degradation and wasting. The metabolic changes of multiple trauma are demonstrated in Fig. 14.2.

Physiological Importance of Glutamine During Multiple Trauma and Critical Illness

Under catabolic conditions such as multiple trauma, burns and sepsis, muscle concentration and plasma levels of glutamine fall dramatically [35–37]. Although glutamine synthesis is not impaired during critical illness, plasma and intramuscular glutamine levels are severely depleted [12, 18] in conditions such as major surgery [38], burn injury [35, 39] and multiple trauma [37, 40, 41] because of increased demand. Therefore, glutamine has been proposed as an essential amino acid during these conditions [42]. Indeed, multiple trauma patients are good candidates for glutamine supplementation. The potential functions and mechanisms of glutamine during multiple trauma and critical illness are summarised in Fig. 14.3.

Safety of Glutamine Supplementation in Trauma and Critical Illness

Glutamine supplementation, either enteral or parenteral, in critically ill patients is considered safe [43]. However, it has been suggested that patients with renal and hepatic impairment should be excluded from such treatment [44]. Specific safety issues have been addressed in a number of studies of intravenous supplementation. In a study of multiple trauma patients received total parenteral nutrition supplemented with high dose of glutamine dipeptide was confirmed to be safe and effective in inducing rise in plasma glutamine levels [45]. Another study reported that the administration of

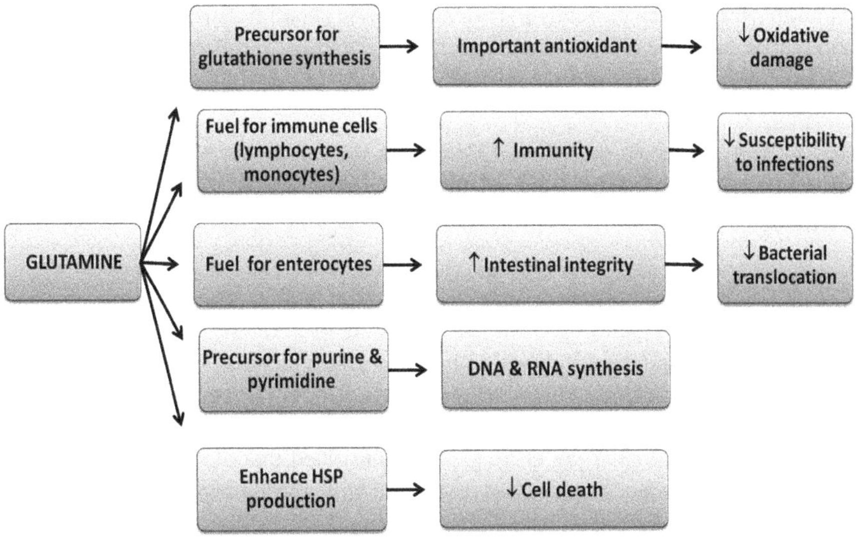

Fig. 14.3 Glutamine functions and mechanisms during stress and critical illness. HSP, heat-shock protien; DNA, deoxyribonucleic acid; RNA, ribonucleic acid, modified from Wischmeyer [84]

undiluted alanyl-glutamine (0.5 g/kg/day) was safe in terms of local vascular tolerance through peripheral vein in critically ill patients [46]. Furthermore, alanyl-glutamine given at a dose of 0.5 g/kg/day was well tolerated in terms of plasma kinetics in critically ill patients and the dipeptide was immediately hydrolysed and cleared in the circulation and there was no detectable glutamine dipeptide in the urine [47].

The safety of parenteral glutamine supplementation in patients with head injury has been addressed in the literature. A pilot study demonstrated that IV Ala-Gln supplementation that increased plasma glutamine levels by 30 % had no effect on plasma glutamate levels or interstitial cerebral glutamate concentrations in patients with head injury, suggesting that parenteral Ala-Gln supplementation is safe in this patient population [48, 49]. Furthermore, a previous trial demonstrated that IV glutamine supplementation that resulted in an increase in plasma glutamine levels in a dose dependent manner had no effect on plasma glutamate levels [50], which indicates that the interstitial cerebral fluid will not be affected. However, both were pilot trials and larger trials are required to confirm the safety of IV Ala-Gln supplementation in patients with head injury. Furthermore, the trials did not investigate the safety of long-term supplementation on levels of glutamate in the interstitial cerebral fluid.

Glutamine Supplementation in Multiple Trauma Patients

Numerous clinical trials have demonstrated the beneficial effects of parenteral glutamine supplementation in critically ill and trauma patients [51–55]. Although many clinical trials have been conducted to investigate the benefits of enteral glutamine supplementation in patients receiving enteral nutrition, the results are conflicting [36, 56–64]. The enteral route of glutamine supplementation is not always practical in critically ill patients as there is a clear difference between the prescribed dose and what can be delivered [60, 65]. In addition, the systemic bioavailability of glutamine through the enteral route is less than the parenteral route [66]. This could be because enteral glutamine is extracted and used mainly by the splanchnic area [67, 68]. Therefore, parenteral glutamine supplementation in patients receiving enteral nutrition is attractive. However, limited trials have investigated the effect this has on multiple trauma and critically ill patients receiving enteral nutrition [65, 69–71]. Tables 14.1 and 14.2 summarise the trials of enteral and parenteral glutamine supplementation in multiple trauma patients.

Glutamine Supplementation and Mortality, SOFA and Infectious Complications

The effect of glutamine supplementation on mortality and infectious complications was reported in a number of trials [36, 71–73]. In one of the largest trials of enteral glutamine supplementation in trauma patients, the in-hospital mortality was higher in the glutamine supplemented patients compared with the control patients [63], but the results were not significant especially after controlling for age and severity of illness. This result suggested that enteral glutamine supplementation might have negative effect [63]. In contrast, Yang et al. [73] demonstrated that alanyl-glutamine supplemented TPN in 46 traumatic brain injury patients was associated with a significant decrease in 2-week mortality rate and alimentary tract haemorrhage. They also reported that this supplementation resulted in a significant decrease in infectious complications. There was a significant decrease in ICU length of stay in the glutamine supplemented patients. However, there are a number of concerns with this trial. Firstly, no stress ulcer prevention was given, which is not an accepted standard management [74]. The main cause of death in the second week (1 patient in the glutamine group versus 6 patients in the control group) was uncontrolled alimentary haemorrhage, which is uncommon in patients with head injury and is potentially related to lack of stress ulcer prevention. This result suggests that glutamine might have a role in prevention of alimentary tract haemorrhage but only if patients are not receiving stress ulcer prevention. Secondly, this was a single centre trial with relatively small number of patients. Therefore, final clear conclusion and recommendations are problematic. Furthermore, the dose used was relatively small (2 mg/kg) compared with other trials that found beneficial effects (0.5 g/kg).

Houdijk et al. [36] demonstrated that glutamine-supplemented enteral feed resulted in a significant decrease in pneumonia, bacteraemia and sepsis. There were no gram-negative bacteraemia cases in the glutamine-supplemented group versus 54 % of the cases in the control group, suggesting that enteral glutamine supplementation might play a role in preventing bacterial translocation form the gut. On the other hand, Schulman and colleagues [72] reported that enteral glutamine supplementation had no significant effect on infectious complications and the use of antibiotics. Eroglu [71] reported that IV glutamine supplementation for 7 days in 40 trauma patients receiving enteral nutrition had no significant effect on infections. However, this was a pilot study with small number of patients and short follow-up duration [71].

As primary outcomes in nutritional intervention trials, infectious complications and mortality require a large number of participants [75–77]. Therefore, critical illness scores that relate to mortality and infectious morbidity endpoints have been considered as an alternative outcome measure [75, 76]. Multiple organ failure is considered as a reliable predictor of mortality in critically ill patients [78]. Sequential organ failure assessment (SOFA) score as a surrogate outcome was reported in two trials [70, 71]. Overall, there was no significant improvement in SOFA score with intravenous glutamine supplementation in both trials.

Nitrogen Balance, Protein Synthesis and Other Biochemical Outcomes

The effect of glutamine supplementation on nitrogen balance, protein synthesis and glutamine plasma and other surrogate biochemical outcomes has been reported in several trials. Long and colleagues [79] reported that enteral glutamine administration for 3 days did not result in significant difference

Table 14.1 Clinical trials of enteral glutamine supplementation in multiple trauma patients

Study	Design	No of patients	Route	Gln dose/day	Commencement and duration	Main outcomes (Gln vs. Control)
Long et al. 1995, 1996 [16, 79]	DB RCT	30	EN (NG)	0.35 g Gln/kg	Approximately 24 h after admission; 3 days	• = NB, protein turnover, synthesis, breakdown • = glucose turnover, oxidation, recycling • = plasma Gln levels • ↑↑ EAA conc. in both groups
Houdijk et al. 1998, 1999 [36, 83]	DB RCT	72 (60 received feeding ≥ 5 days)	EN (NJ)	30.5 g Gln/ 100 g protein	Within 48 h of trauma and until tolerating oral feeding (study period 15 days)	• ↑↑ Gln, ↑↑ citrulline, ↑↑ arginine plasma levels • ↓↓ serum levels of TNF-receptors • ↓↓ pneumonia, ↓↓ bacteraemia 005), ↓↓ sepsis • = ICU LOS, = LOS, = mechanical ventilation days. Glucose levels above normal fasting levels in both groups Plasma levels of stress hormones (cortisol and glucagon) ↑ to high normal levels in both groups (p=NS) • Growth hormone levels in normal range throughout study and = between groups • ↑↑ α_1 – antitrypsin in both groups • ↑↑ CRP in both groups

(continued)

Table 14.1 (continued)

Study	Design	No of patients	Route	Gln dose/day	Commencement and duration	Main outcomes (Gln vs. Control)
Brantley et al. 2000 [61] (Abstract)	RCT unblinded? (not mentioned in abstract) $N=70$	70	EN	0.5 g/kg Gln	7 days	• ↑↑ prealbumin level • ↑ NB (NS) • = infections, = total costs, = ICU LOS, = LOS
Boelenes et al. 2002 [41]	DB RCT	108	EN (NJ)	30.5 g Gln/100 g protein	Within 48 h of trauma and until tolerating oral feeding (pts fed at least 5 days EN were included in results; study period 15 days)	• On day 1 HLA-DR expression much lower in Gln and control groups compared to healthy volunteers group • ↑↑ HLA-DR expression • = FcγRI/CD64 expression in monocytes in Gln and control groups compared to healthy volunteers
Schulman et al. 2005, 2006 [63, 72]	Sequential rotating assignment, unblinded	185 (175 trauma)	EN (NJ or PEG)	0.6 g Gln/kg	EN continued until oral diet is tolerated or TPN was required	• = infections, = antibiotic use • = mechanical ventilation days, = ICU LOS, = LOS • = in-hospital mortality between groups (after controlling for age and severity of illness)
McQuiggan et al. 2008 [64]	Pilot, unblinded RCT	20	EN (NG)	0.5 g Gln/kg/day	Start during the first 24 h of resuscitation; 10 days	• Gln well tolerated during resuscitation, no adverse events • ↓↓ instances of high gastric output, ↓↓ abdominal distension, ↓↓ total instances of intolerance • = CRP on day 4 between groups ↑↑ Total UUN

DB double-blind, *RCT* randomised clinical trial, *Gln* glutamine, *EN* enteral nutrition, *NG* nasogastric, *NJ* nasojejunal, *PEG* percutaneous endoscopic gastrostomy, *TPN* total parenteral nutrition, = no significant difference, ↑↑ significant increase, ↓↓ significant decrease, ↑ increased, *NS* not significant, *NB* nitrogen balance, *EAA* essential amino acid, *NEAA* non-essential amino acid, *UUN* urinary urea nitrogen, *ICU* intensive care unit, *TNF* tumour necrosis factor, *HLA-DR* human leukocyte antigen-DR, *FcγRI/CD64* Fc receptor

Table 14.2 Clinical trials of parenteral glutamine supplementation in multiple trauma patients

Study	Design	No of patients	Route	Gln dose/day	Commencement and duration	Main outcomes (Gln vs. Control)
Bakalar et al. 2006 [70]	Pilot, unblinded RCT	40	PN	0.4 g/kg/day Ala-Gln	Started 24 h after injury for 7 days + EN or PN	• = protein breakdown • = SOFA score • ↓ energy expenditure • ↑↑ insulin-mediated glucose disposal • ↑↑ endogenous insulin secretion in control group • ↑↑ insulin sensitivity
Yang et al. 2007 [73]	RCT	46	PN	Ala-Gln (2 mg Ala-Gln/kg	Started within 24 h for 2 weeks TPN started on day 3 after injury, EN gradually replaced TPN in the first week	• ↓↓ 2-week mortality, ↓↓ICU LOS • = GCS • ↓↓ lung infection, ↓↓ alimentary tract haemorrhage • = urinary tract infection • ↑↑ total serum protein, ↑↑ total lymphocyte count
Eroglu 2009 [71]	DB RCT	40	PN	0.5 g Ala-Gln/kg/day	7 days + EN	• ↑↑ total plasma glutathione levels • = CRP, = prealbumin, = glucose levels • = SOFA score • = Infections, = ICU LOS • = 1- month mortality
Pérez-Bárcena et al. 2010 [81]	SB RCT	43	PN	0.5 g Ala-Gln / kg/day	5 days + TPN	• = TLR4 (glutamine-supplemented TPN doesn't improve expression or functionality of TLRs in peripheral blood monocytes)

RCT randomised clinical trial, *DB* double-blind, *SB* single-blind, *Gln* glutamine, *PN* parenteral nutrition, *TPN* total parenteral nutrition, *EN* enteral nutrition, ↑↑ significant increase, ↓↓ significant decrease, = no significant difference, *GCS* Glasgow Coma Score, *CRP* C-reactive protein, *SOFA* Sequential Organ Failure Assessment, *TLR* toll-like receptor

in nitrogen balance, protein synthesis and breakdown. There was also no significant difference in plasma glutamine levels. Yang et al. reported that IV glutamine supplementation resulted in significant increase in total serum protein. Houdijk et al. [36] demonstrated that glutamine-supplemented enteral nutrition resulted in a significant increase in glutamine, citrulline and arginine plasma levels. McQuiggan et al. [64] investigated the effect of enteral glutamine supplementation during the first 24 h of resuscitation, before starting the enteral feed for 10 days. This was a pilot unblinded trial in 20 patients with severe trauma. The supplementation was given as a bolus two to three times per day. The glutamine supplementation was well tolerated during resuscitation with no adverse events. The glutamine supplemented patients had significantly less instances of high gastric output and abdominal distension, suggesting the safety of enteral glutamine supplementation during active shock resuscitation. Total urinary urea nitrogen was significantly higher in the glutamine group compared with the control group. A larger trial is required to investigate the effect of enteral glutamine supplementation during active shock resuscitation on other clinical outcomes.

The effect of parenteral alanyl-glutamine on insulin resistance was investigated by Bakalar et al. [70], who showed significantly improved insulin sensitivity and insulin-mediated glucose disposal in the glutamine-supplemented patients. The rate of protein breakdown was not different between groups during the study, but hypermetabolism was attenuated in the glutamine group by reducing energy expenditure. It was concluded that glutamine supplementation was associated with significantly better insulin sensitivity in trauma patients, offering a new approach to glycaemic control in this group.

Glutamine Supplementation and Immune Function

The potential role of glutamine supplementation on the immune system and inflammation has been investigated in a number of trials. Boelens et al. [41] reported, as part of Houdijk et al. [36] trial, that glutamine-supplemented enteral nutrition could play a role modulating immune functions. The study investigated the effect of glutamine-supplemented enteral nutrition versus isocaloric, isonitrogenous enteral nutrition, and both groups were compared with healthy volunteers on human leukocyte antigen-DR (HLA-DR) and Fc receptor (FcγRI/CD64) expression in monocytes, which are severely depleted in trauma patients [9, 80]. As expected, HLA-DR expression was much lower in both groups compared to healthy volunteers. However, glutamine supplementation resulted in significantly increased expression of HLA-DR but did not restore normal values. There was no difference in the FcγRI/CD64 expression between both groups and healthy volunteers. It was concluded that glutamine increased HLA-DR expression and thus improved cellular immune function, and this may play a role in reducing infectious complications in trauma patients.

Pérez-Bárcena et al. [81] investigated in a single-blind, randomised trial the effect of glutamine supplemented total parenteral nutrition on toll-like receptors (TLR2 and TLR4), which are key receptors for sensing infections. The expression levels of TLR2 in monocytes were found to be similar between the groups before and after supplementation. There was also no significant difference in TLR4 levels between groups before and after treatment. Although the trial was not powered to investigate the clinical effect of glutamine on reducing infectious complications, there were fewer incidences of infections and shorter hospital length of stay in the glutamine group that did not reach significance. It was concluded that glutamine-supplemented parenteral nutrition in trauma patients had no influence on the expression or functionality of TLRs in monocytes.

In a well-designed large multi-centre trial Heyland et al. [82] investigated the effect of early (within 24 h of ICU admission) enteral and parenteral supplementation in very critically ill patients with oxidative stress and included multiple trauma patients The trial reported a trend towards increased 28-day mortality and a significant increase in 6-month mortality. Furthermore, glutamine supplementation had no significant effect on organ failure and infectious complications. However, these trauma patients had MOF and the dose received was twice the dose of other trials. Contrary to previous reports, in a sub-study of 66 patients around 30 % of patients did not have low admission plasma glutamine level. Although the safety of this high dose of parenteral and enteral glutamine was investigated in a previous dose-finding trial [43], the harmful effect was reported in this multi-centre trial.

Limitations of Glutamine Supplementation Trials

Although many trials have been conducted to investigate the effect of enteral and parenteral glutamine in multiple trauma patients, the results are still controversial and inconclusive. There are a number of limitations in the trials of glutamine supplementation in trauma including random allocation concealment, blinding and no the intention-to-treat analysis of data. Another limitation is the small sample size of many trials and not being sufficiently powered to investigate major clinical outcomes such as infectious complications and mortality. In enteral glutamine supplementation trials receiving the prescribed dose is difficult due to high gastric output and feed intolerance. In addition, the trials were single-centre trials. Therefore, many of these trials should be considered as pilot trials. The intention to include only multiple trauma patients in these trials to obtain a homogenous population might have resulted in reducing the applicability and the generalisability of the results. Investigating surrogate outcomes is another limitation in many trials. Furthermore, the doses used in different trials are not consistent, making clear comparison between the trials problematic. Also, the period of supplementation was short in many trials.

Conclusion

Although there is strong evidence that glutamine supplementation has beneficial effect in improving clinical outcomes in critically ill patients and should be part of nutritional therapeutic approach in multiple trauma and critically ill patients, limitations of these trials make final conclusion problematic. To overcome the challenges and limitations of previous trials, well-designed, adequately powered, multi-centre trials are required to ensure strong clinical evidence. Due to the uncertainty of absorption of enteral glutamine supplementation in patients receiving enteral nutrition and the splanchnic use of enteral glutamine, investigating the effect of intravenous glutamine supplementation in multiple trauma patients receiving enteral nutrition is advocated for future trials. Investigating clinically relevant outcome measures such as mortality and infectious complications rather than short-term surrogate measures is also strongly encouraged. Future trials should also focus on both the clinical outcomes and the underlying mechanisms of glutamine supplementation.

References

1. Keel M, Trentz O. Pathophysiology of polytrauma. Injury. 2005;36(6):691–709.
2. Acosta JA, Yang JC, Winchell RJ, Simons RK, Fortlage DA, Hollingsworth-Fridlund P, et al. Lethal injuries and time to death in a level I trauma center. J Am Coll Surg. 1998;186(5):528–33.
3. Matthes G, Seifert J, Ostermann PA, Wurfel S, Ekkernkamp A, Wich M. Early death of the severly injured patient– A retrospective analysis. Zentralbl Chir. 2001;126(12):995–9.
4. Demetriades D, Murray J, Charalambides K, Alo K, Velmahos G, Rhee P, et al. Trauma fatalities: time and location of hospital deaths. J Am Coll Surg. 2004;198(1):20–6.
5. Osborn TM, Tracy JK, Dunne JR, Pasquale M, Napolitano LM. Epidemiology of sepsis in patients with traumatic injury. Crit Care Med. 2004;32(11):2234–40.

6. Sauaia A, Moore FA, Moore EE, Moser KS, Brennan R, Read RA, et al. Epidemiology of trauma deaths: a reassessment. J Trauma. 1995;38(2):185–93.
7. Napolitano LM, Faist E, Wichmann MW, Coimbra R. Immune dysfunction in trauma. Surg Clin North Am. 1999; 79(6):1385–416.
8. Faist E, Schinkel C, Zimmer S. Update on the mechanisms of immune suppression of injury and immune modulation. World J Surg. 1996;20(4):454–9.
9. Ditschkowski M, Kreuzfelder E, Rebmann V, Ferencik S, Majetschak M, Schmid EN, et al. HLA-DR expression and soluble HLA-DR levels in septic patients after trauma. Ann Surg. 1999;229(2):246–54.
10. Baker CC, Oppenheimer L, Stephens B, Lewis FR, Trunkey DD. Epidemiology of trauma deaths. Am J Surg. 1980;140(1):144–50.
11. Streat SJ, Beddoe AH, Hill GL. Aggressive nutritional support does not prevent protein loss despite fat gain in septic intensive care patients. J Trauma. 1987;27(3):262–6.
12. Jackson NC, Carroll PV, Russell-Jones DL, Sonksen PH, Treacher DF, Umpleby AM. The metabolic consequences of critical illness: acute effects on glutamine and protein metabolism. Am J Physiol. 1999;276(1 Pt 1):E163–70.
13. De Jonghe B, Bastuji-Garin S, Durand MC, Malissin I, Rodrigues P, Cerf C, et al. Respiratory weakness is associated with limb weakness and delayed weaning in critical illness. Crit Care Med. 2007;35(9):2007–15.
14. Liu W, Lopez JM, VanderJagt DJ, Glew RH, Fry DE, Schermer C, et al. Evaluation of aminoaciduria in severely traumatized patients. Clin Chim Acta. 2002;316(1–2):123–8.
15. Gore DC, Wolfe RR. Glutamine supplementation fails to affect muscle protein kinetics in critically ill patients. JPEN J Parenter Enteral Nutr. 2002;26(6):342–9. discussion 49-50.
16. Long CL, Borghesi L, Stahl R, Clark JA, Geiger JW, DiRienzo DB, et al. Impact of enteral feeding of a glutamine-supplemented formula on the hypoaminoacidemic response in trauma patients. J Trauma. 1996;40(1):97–102.
17. Oudemans-van Straaten HM, Bosman RJ, Treskes M, van der Spoel HJ, Zandstra DF. Plasma glutamine depletion and patient outcome in acute ICU admissions. Intensive Care Med. 2001;27(1):84–90.
18. Mittendorfer B, Gore DC, Herndon DN, Wolfe RR. Accelerated glutamine synthesis in critically ill patients cannot maintain normal intramuscular free glutamine concentration. JPEN J Parenter Enteral Nutr. 1999;23(5):243–52.
19. Brochner AC, Toft P. Pathophysiology of the systemic inflammatory response after major accidental trauma. Scand J Trauma Resusc Emerg Med. 2009;17(1):43.
20. Keel M, Ecknauer E, Stocker R, Ungethum U, Steckholzer U, Kenney J, et al. Different pattern of local and systemic release of proinflammatory and anti-inflammatory mediators in severely injured patients with chest trauma. J Trauma. 1996;40(6):907–12. discussion 12-4.
21. Lenz A, Franklin GA, Cheadle WG. Systemic inflammation after trauma. Injury. 2007;38(12):1336–45.
22. Bone RC. Sir Isaac Newton, sepsis, SIRS, and CARS. Crit Care Med. 1996;24(7):1125–8.
23. Napolitano LM, Ferrer T, McCarter Jr RJ, Scalea TM. Systemic inflammatory response syndrome score at admission independently predicts mortality and length of stay in trauma patients. J Trauma. 2000;49(4):647–52. discussion 52-3.
24. Schroder O, Laun RA, Held B, Ekkernkamp A, Schulte KM. Association of interleukin-10 promoter polymorphism with the incidence of multiple organ dysfunction following major trauma: results of a prospective pilot study. Shock. 2004;21(4):306–10.
25. Moore FA, Sauaia A, Moore EE, Haenel JB, Burch JM, Lezotte DC. Postinjury multiple organ failure: a bimodal phenomenon. J Trauma. 1996;40(4):501–10. discussion 10-2.
26. Vermes I, Beishuizen A. The hypothalamic-pituitary-adrenal response to critical illness. Best Pract Res Clin Endocrinol Metab. 2001;15(4):495–511.
27. Monk DN, Plank LD, Franch-Arcas G, Finn PJ, Streat SJ, Hill GL. Sequential changes in the metabolic response in critically injured patients during the first 25 days after blunt trauma. Ann Surg. 1996;223(4):395–405.
28. Uehara M, Plank LD, Hill GL. Components of energy expenditure in patients with severe sepsis and major trauma: a basis for clinical care. Crit Care Med. 1999;27(7):1295–302.
29. Klein S, Peters EJ, Shangraw RE, Wolfe RR. Lipolytic response to metabolic stress in critically ill patients. Crit Care Med. 1991;19(6):776–9.
30. Wolfe RR, Martini WZ. Changes in intermediary metabolism in severe surgical illness. World J Surg. 2000; 24(6):639–47.
31. Frankenfield DC, Smith JS, Cooney RN. Accelerated nitrogen loss after traumatic injury is not attenuated by achievement of energy balance. JPEN J Parenter Enteral Nutr. 1997;21(6):324–9.
32. Gamrin L, Andersson K, Hultman E, Nilsson E, Essen P, Wernerman J. Longitudinal changes of biochemical parameters in muscle during critical illness. Metabolism. 1997;46(7):756–62.
33. Biolo G, Zorat F, Antonione R, Ciocchi B. Muscle glutamine depletion in the intensive care unit. Int J Biochem Cell Biol. 2005;37(10):2169–79.
34. Arnold J, Campbell IT, Samuels TA, Devlin JC, Green CJ, Hipkin LJ, et al. Increased whole body protein breakdown predominates over increased whole body protein synthesis in multiple organ failure. Clin Sci. 1993;84(6): 655–61.

35. Gore DC, Jahoor F. Glutamine kinetics in burn patients. Comparison with hormonally induced stress in volunteers. Arch Surg. 1994;129(12):1318–23.
36. Houdijk AP, Rijnsburger ER, Jansen J, Wesdorp RI, Weiss JK, McCamish MA, et al. Randomised trial of glutamine-enriched enteral nutrition on infectious morbidity in patients with multiple trauma. Lancet. 1998;352(9130): 772–6.
37. Weingartmann G, Oehler R, Derkits S, Oismuller C, Fugger R, Roth E. HSP70 expression in granulocytes and lymphocytes of patients with polytrauma: comparison with plasma glutamine. Clin Nutr. 1999;18(2):121–4.
38. Parry-Billings M, Baigrie RJ, Lamont PM, Morris PJ, Newsholme EA. Effects of major and minor surgery on plasma glutamine and cytokine levels. Arch Surg. 1992;127(10):1237–40.
39. Parry-Billings M, Evans J, Calder PC, Newsholme EA. Does glutamine contribute to immunosuppression after major burns? Lancet. 1990;336(8714):523–5.
40. Askanazi J, Carpentier YA, Michelsen CB, Elwyn DH, Furst P, Kantrowitz LR, et al. Muscle and plasma amino acids following injury. Influence of intercurrent infection. Ann Surg. 1980;192(1):78–85.
41. Boelens PG, Houdijk AP, Fonk JC, Nijveldt RJ, Ferwerda CC, Von Blomberg-Van Der Flier BM, et al. Glutamine-enriched enteral nutrition increases HLA-DR expression on monocytes of trauma patients. J Nutr. 2002;132(9): 2580–6.
42. Lacey JM, Wilmore DW. Is glutamine a conditionally essential amino acid? Nutr Rev. 1990;48(8):297–309.
43. Heyland DK, Dhaliwalm R, Day A, Drover J, Cote H, Wischmeyer P. Optimizing the dose of glutamine dipeptides and antioxidants in critically ill patients: a phase I dose-finding study. JPEN J Parenter Enteral Nutr. 2007; 31(2):109–18.
44. Sacks GS. The data in support of glutamine supplementation. Nutr Clin Pract. 2003;18(5):386–90.
45. Weingartmann G, Fridrich P, Mauritz W, Gotzinger P, Mittlbock M, Germann P, et al. Safety and efficacy of increasing dosages of glycyl-glutamine for total parenteral nutrition in polytrauma patients. Wien Klin Wochenschr. 1996; 108(21):683–8.
46. Berg A, Forsberg E, Wernerman J. The local vascular tolerance to an intravenous infusion of a concentrated glutamine solution in ICU patients. Clin Nutr. 2002;21(2):135–9.
47. Berg A, Rooyackers O, Norberg A, Wernerman J. Elimination kinetics of L-alanyl-L-glutamine in ICU patients. Amino Acids. 2005;29(3):221–8.
48. Berg A, Bellander BM, Wanecek M, Gamrin L, Elving A, Rooyackers O, et al. Intravenous glutamine supplementation to head trauma patients leaves cerebral glutamate concentration unaffected. Intensive Care Med. 2006;32(11):1741–6.
49. Berg A, Bellander BM, Wanecek M, Norberg A, Ungerstedt U, Rooyackers O, et al. The pattern of amino acid exchange across the brain is unaffected by intravenous glutamine supplementation in head trauma patients. Clin Nutr. 2008;27(6):816–21.
50. Tjäder I, Rooyackers O, Forsberg AM, Vesali RF, Garlick PJ, Wernerman J. Effects on skeletal muscle of intravenous glutamine supplementation to ICU patients. Intensive Care Med. 2004;30(2):266–75.
51. Goeters C, Wenn A, Mertes N, Wempe C, Van Aken H, Stehle P, et al. Parenteral L-alanyl-L-glutamine improves 6-month outcome in critically ill patients. Crit Care Med. 2002;30(9):2032–7.
52. Fuentes-Orozco C, Anaya-Prado R, Gonzalez-Ojeda A, Arenas-Marquez H, Cabrera-Pivaral C, Cervantes-Guevara G, et al. L-alanyl-L-glutamine-supplemented parenteral nutrition improves infectious morbidity in secondary peritonitis. Clin Nutr. 2004;23(1):13–21.
53. Zhou Y-P, Jiang Z-M, Sun Y-H, He G-Z, Shu H. The effects of supplemental glutamine dipeptide on gut integrity and clinical outcome after major escharectomy in severe burns: a randomized, double-blind, controlled clinical trial. Clin Nutr Suppl. 2004;1(1):55–60.
54. Dechelotte P, Hasselmann M, Cynober L, Allaouchiche B, Coeffier M, Hecketsweiler B, et al. L-alanyl-L-glutamine dipeptide-supplemented total parenteral nutrition reduces infectious complications and glucose intolerance in critically ill patients: the French controlled, randomized, double-blind, multicenter study. Crit Care Med. 2006; 34(3):598–604.
55. Grau T, Bonet A, Minambres E, Pineiro L, Irles JA, Robles A, et al. The effect of l-alanyl-l-glutamine dipeptide supplemented total parenteral nutrition on infectious morbidity and insulin sensitivity in critically ill patients. Crit Care Med. 2011;39(6):1263–8.
56. Conejero R, Bonet A, Grau T, Esteban A, Mesejo A, Montejo JC, et al. Effect of a glutamine-enriched enteral diet on intestinal permeability and infectious morbidity at 28 days in critically ill patients with systemic inflammatory response syndrome: a randomized, single-blind, prospective, multicenter study. Nutrition. 2002;18(9):716–21.
57. Garrel D, Patenaude J, Nedelec B, Samson L, Dorais J, Champoux J, et al. Decreased mortality and infectious morbidity in adult burn patients given enteral glutamine supplements: a prospective, controlled, randomized clinical trial. Crit Care Med. 2003;31(10):2444–9.
58. Zhou YP, Jiang ZM, Sun YH, Wang XR, Ma EL, Wilmore D. The effect of supplemental enteral glutamine on plasma levels, gut function, and outcome in severe burns: a randomized, double-blind, controlled clinical trial. JPEN J Parenter Enteral Nutr. 2003;27(4):241–5.

59. Peng X, Chen RC, Wang P, You ZY, Wang SL. Effects of enteral supplementation with glutamine on mitochondria respiratory function of intestinal epithelium in burned rats. Zhongguo Wei Zhong Bing Ji Jiu Yi Xue. 2004; 16(2):93–6.
60. Jones C, Palmer TE, Griffiths RD. Randomized clinical outcome study of critically ill patients given glutamine-supplemented enteral nutrition. Nutrition. 1999;15(2):108–15.
61. Brantley S, Pierce J. Effects of enteral glutamine on trauma patients. Nutr Clin Pract. 2000;15:S13.
62. Hall JC, Dobb G, Hall J, de Sousa R, Brennan L, McCauley R. A prospective randomized trial of enteral glutamine in critical illness. Intensive Care Med. 2003;29(10):1710–6.
63. Schulman AS, Willcutts KF, Claridge JA, Evans HL, Radigan AE, O'Donnell KB, et al. Does the addition of glutamine to enteral feeds affect patient mortality? Crit Care Med. 2005;33(11):2501–6.
64. McQuiggan M, Kozar R, Sailors RM, Ahn C, McKinley B, Moore F. Enteral glutamine during active shock resuscitation is safe and enhances tolerance of enteral feeding. JPEN J Parenter Enteral Nutr. 2008;32(1):28–35.
65. Luo M, Bazargan N, Griffith DP, Estivariz CF, Leader LM, Easley KA, et al. Metabolic effects of enteral versus parenteral alanyl-glutamine dipeptide administration in critically ill patients receiving enteral feeding: a pilot study. Clin Nutr. 2008;27(2):297–306.
66. Melis GC, Boelens PG, van der Sijp JR, Popovici T, De Bandt JP, Cynober L, et al. The feeding route (enteral or parenteral) affects the plasma response of the dipetide Ala-Gln and the amino acids glutamine, citrulline and arginine, with the administration of Ala-Gln in preoperative patients. Br J Nutr. 2005;94(1):19–26.
67. Haisch M, Fukagawa NK, Matthews DE. Oxidation of glutamine by the splanchnic bed in humans. Am J Physiol Endocrinol Metab. 2000;278(4):E593–602.
68. Ligthart-Melis GC, van de Poll MC, Dejong CH, Boelens PG, Deutz NE, van Leeuwen PA. The route of administration (enteral or parenteral) affects the conversion of isotopically labeled L-[2-15 N]glutamine into citrulline and arginine in humans. JPEN J Parenter Enteral Nutr. 2007;31(5):343–8. discussion 49-50.
69. Wischmeyer PE, Lynch J, Liedel J, Wolfson R, Riehm J, Gottlieb L, et al. Glutamine administration reduces Gram-negative bacteremia in severely burned patients: a prospective, randomized, double-blind trial versus isonitrogenous control. Crit Care Med. 2001;29(11):2075–80.
70. Bakalar B, Duska F, Pachl J, Fric M, Otahal M, Pazout J, et al. Parenterally administered dipeptide alanyl-glutamine prevents worsening of insulin sensitivity in multiple-trauma patients. Crit Care Med. 2006;34(2):381–6.
71. Eroglu A. The effect of intravenous alanyl-glutamine supplementation on plasma glutathione levels in intensive care unit trauma patients receiving enteral nutrition: the results of a randomized controlled trial. Anesth Analg. 2009;109(2):502–5.
72. Schulman AS, Willcutts KF, Claridge JA, O'Donnell KB, Radigan AE, Evans HL, et al. Does enteral glutamine supplementation decrease infectious morbidity? Surg Infect (Larchmt). 2006;7(1):29–35.
73. Yang DL, Xu JF. Effect of dipeptide of glutamine and alanine on severe traumatic brain injury. Chin J Traumatol. 2007;10(3):145–9.
74. Schirmer CM, Kornbluth J, Heilman CB, Bhardwaj A. Gastrointestinal prophylaxis in neurocritical care. Neurocrit Care. 2012;16(1):184–93.
75. Beale RJ, Sherry T, Lei K, Campbell-Stephen L, McCook J, Smith J, et al. Early enteral supplementation with key pharmaconutrients improves Sequential Organ Failure Assessment score in critically ill patients with sepsis: outcome of a randomized, controlled, double-blind trial. Crit Care Med. 2008;36(1):131–44.
76. Macfie J. European round table: the use of immunonutrients in the critically ill. Clin Nutr. 2004;23(6):1426–9.
77. Wernerman J. Glutamine and acute illness. Curr Opin Crit Care. 2003;9(4):279–85.
78. Marshall JC, Cook DJ, Christou NV, Bernard GR, Sprung CL, Sibbald WJ. Multiple organ dysfunction score: a reliable descriptor of a complex clinical outcome. Crit Care Med. 1995;23(10):1638–52.
79. Long CL, Nelson KM, DiRienzo DB, Weis JK, Stahl RD, Broussard TD, et al. Glutamine supplementation of enteral nutrition: impact on whole body protein kinetics and glucose metabolism in critically ill patients. JPEN J Parenter Enteral Nutr. 1995;19(6):470–6.
80. Hershman MJ, Cheadle WG, Wellhausen SR, Davidson PF, Polk Jr HC. Monocyte HLA-DR antigen expression characterizes clinical outcome in the trauma patient. Br J Surg. 1990;77(2):204–7.
81. Pérez-Bárcena J, Crespí C, Regueiro V, Marsé P, Raurich JM, Ibáñez J, et al. Lack of effect of glutamine administration to boost the innate immune system response in trauma patients in the intensive care unit. Crit Care. 2010; 14(6):R233.
82. Heyland D, Muscedere J, Wischmeyer PE, Cook D, Jones G, Albert M, et al. A randomized trial of glutamine and antioxidants in critically ill patients. N Engl J Med. 2013;368(16):1489–97.
83. Houdijk AP, Nijveldt RJ, van Leeuwen PA. Glutamine-enriched enteral feeding in trauma patients: reduced infectious morbidity is not related to changes in endocrine and metabolic responses. JPEN J Parenter Enteral Nutr. 1999;23(5 Suppl):S52–8.
84. Wischmeyer PE. Clinical applications of L-glutamine: past, present, and future. Nutr Clin Pract. 2003;18(5): 377–85.

Chapter 15
Glutamine Dipeptide and Insulin Sensitivity in Critically Ill Patients

Teodoro Grau-Carmona and Carol Lorencio Cárdenas

Key Points

- Glutamine is a conditional amino acid in critically ill patients that influences glucose metabolism, and particularly it can improve insulin sensitivity in critically ill patients.
- There are several mechanisms that can explain these phenomena: through the glucose-glutamine cycle, increasing insulin secretion, improving insulin sensitivity in muscle, increasing fatty acids oxidation and decreasing the inflammatory response.
- Assess glycaemia variability in critically ill patients is a difficult task. Specialized techniques to assess variability must take in account the changes across time.
- There is enough evidence that support the use of time series analysis as the best statistical method to explain glucose variability.
- Glutamine exerts a beneficial effect controlling hyperglycaemia and decreasing insulin needs in critically ill patients.

Keywords Alanyl-glutamine dipeptide • Glycaemia variability • Insulin sensitivity • Total parenteral nutrition • Critically ill patients

Abbreviations

ARMA	Autoregressive Moving Average Model
DTA	Detrended Fluctuation Analysis
FFA	Free Fatty Acids
GLI	Glycaemic Liability Index
GLUT-4	Glucose Transporter 4
GPI	Glycaemic penalty Index
HGI	Hyperglycaemic Index

T. Grau-Carmona, M.D., Ph.D. (✉)
Intensive Care Department, Hospital Universitario Doce de Octubre, Madrid, Spain
e-mail: teodoro.grau@salud.maadrid.org; teograu@terra.com

C.L. Cárdenas, M.D.
Intensive Care Department, Hospital Josep Trueta, Girona, Spain

R. Rajendram et al. (eds.), *Glutamine in Clinical Nutrition*, Nutrition and Health,
DOI 10.1007/978-1-4939-1932-1_15, © Springer Science+Business Media New York 2015

HoGI	Hypoglycaemic Index
HSF-1	Heat-Shock Factor 1
JkApEn	Jack-knifed Approximate Entropy
MAG	Mean Absolute Glucose
MAGE	Mean Amplitude of Glycaemia Excursions
NF-κβ	Nuclear Factor κβ
RMSE	Root Mean-Square Error
TNF-α	Tumour Necrosis Factor α
TPN	Total Parenteral Nutrition

Introduction

Hyperglycaemia is a landmark metabolic feature associated with the stress response in critically ill patients. The stress response gives an exaggerated production of catecholamines and cortisol that combined with the presence of inflammatory cytokines, results in insulin resistance. Moreover, the use of exogenous catecholamines and nutritional support results in an exaggerated hyperglycaemia. Stress hyperglycaemia has been linked to poor outcomes and until recently, many efforts have been done to control high glucose levels using intensive insulin administration [1]. In the last two decades, intensive insulin administration has been the cornerstone therapy to maintain glycaemia in an acceptable range in order to avoid hyperglycaemia related complications in these patients [2, 3]. Nevertheless, there is also a risk associated to hypoglycaemia and, in fact, the most recent study has not shown beneficial effects of thigh glucose control with insulin therapy [4]. Two subsequent meta-analyses have shown that thigh glycaemic control does not decrease mortality in critically ill patients [5, 6], and some authors suggest that acquired insulin resistance in these patients could be of benefit [7].

When looking at glycaemia control in critical care patients we should consider not only the presence or not of insulin resistance, but the effect of different substrates and the level of inflammation. Dietary restriction improves insulin resistance sensitivity quickly and before substantial weight loss is achieved. During the stress response, different inflammatory mediators play a key roll in intermediate metabolism, increasing the endogenous production of glucose [8]. Amino acids are the main source for gluconeogenesis and oxidation, and glutamine is the main donor of carbon chains for this process. Indeed, glutamine is involved in immune processes that can modulate the inflammatory response during the critical illness. In this chapter we review the potential roll of glutamine to preserve insulin sensitivity in critically ill patients.

Altered Glucose Metabolism After Injury

Hyperglycaemia in critically ill patients is directly related to the level of injury and is due to insulin resistance. Studies using euglycaemic hyperinsulinaemic clamps have demonstrated that the level of insulin resistance in these patients correlates with the severity of the injury [9]. The two classical patterns of the stress response are called the "ebb phase" and the "flow phase". The ebb phase occurs immediately after the injury and correlates with the severity of the disease. The hyperglycaemia seen at this moment is not associated with high levels of plasmatic insulin but it appears during the flow period [10]. At this time there are three landmarks changes of fuel substrate metabolism: increased levels of glycaemia with impaired oxidation, increased levels of plasma-free fatty acids (FFA) with increased oxidation and an increased liberation of amino acids from the skeletal muscle, mainly glutamine, for hepatic gluconeogenesis.

During the flow phase, hepatic gluconeogenesis is elevated and not suppressed by the exogenous administration of glucose. At the same time, glycogen formation is inhibited in the muscle and the liver, and glucose is metabolized to pyruvate and lactate (non-oxidative utilisation of glucose). This phenomenon is named central insulin resistance and represents the failure of insulin to inhibit gluconeogenesis and glycogenolysis in the liver, and it is responsible for the development of hyperglycaemia and persistent stimulation of insulin production. Peripheral insulin resistance results in a diminished insulin-mediated uptake of glucose by skeletal muscle, adipose tissue and other insulin-mediated glucose uptake tissues [11]. The final result of these metabolic processes is the presence of large amounts of glucose that are stored in the form of lipids via the novo lipogenesis. Cortisol and epinephrine are responsible of the impaired insulin mediated glucose uptake. Moreover, cytokines such as TNFα and interleukin inhibit post-receptor insulin signalling and down-regulate glucose transporter 4 (GLUT-4). Hyperglycaemia by itself exacerbates the cytokine production, and the inflammatory response setting up a vicious cycle whereby hyperglycaemia leads to further hyperglycaemia [12].

During the flow phase, there is an enhanced release of Fatty Acids (FFA) from peripheral tissues and enhanced whole-body fat oxidation. This increased flux of Fatty

Acids are not clearly associated to high levels of plasma FFA but glycerol concentrations are increased, reflecting an exaggerated lipolysis. Under conditions of hyperglycaemia and hyperinsulinaemia, hepatic oxidation of FFA and secretion seems to be inhibited, particularly when the amount of released FFA exceeds the energy needs, and triglycerides accumulate in hepatocytes and muscle. FFA overload at mitochondrial level, and high amounts of triglycerides stored in muscle and liver result in more impaired insulin sensitivity in these tissues [13, 14].

Figure 15.1 shows an integrated approach to the development of hyperglycaemia and insulin resistance in critically ill patients. In the first phase (ebb), stress hormones promote glucogenolysis, gluconeogenesis and lipolysis. The inflammatory response mediated by TNF-α results in mitochondrial damage and muscle and liver with the result of insulin resistance. Circulating FFA and hyperglycaemia perpetuates the response during the flow phase [14].

Glutamine Actions on Insulin Sensitivity

Glutamine is the most abundant non-essential amino acid in humans and it is involved in numerous metabolic processes. During critical illness, plasmatic levels of glutamine are usually low and have been correlated with an increased mortality [15]. It seems that glutamine is the main donor of carbon chains for gluconeogenesis in the liver and the kidney. It acts as a substrate but also as a modulator of glucose metabolism, reducing hyperglycaemia and plasmatic levels of insulin. There are several proposed mechanisms that could explain why glutamine improves hyperglycaemia and insulin sensitivity (Table 15.1).

The Glucose Glutamine Cycle

In the post-absorptive state, oral or parenteral glutamine is converted in glucose in the muscle, liver, kidneys and small intestine. The skeletal muscle account for more than 50 % of glutamine uptake from the plasma and, at the same time, is responsible of the 65–75 % of plasmatic glutamine release. Studies in humans during euglycaemic hyperinsulinaemic clamps have shown that skeletal muscle is largely responsible for the increased release of glutamine into plasma, and this may be due to an increased conversion of glucose to glutamine as a part of the glucose-glutamine cycle. But during hypoglycemic hyperinsulinaemic clamps there is a decreased glutamine uptake by skeletal muscle

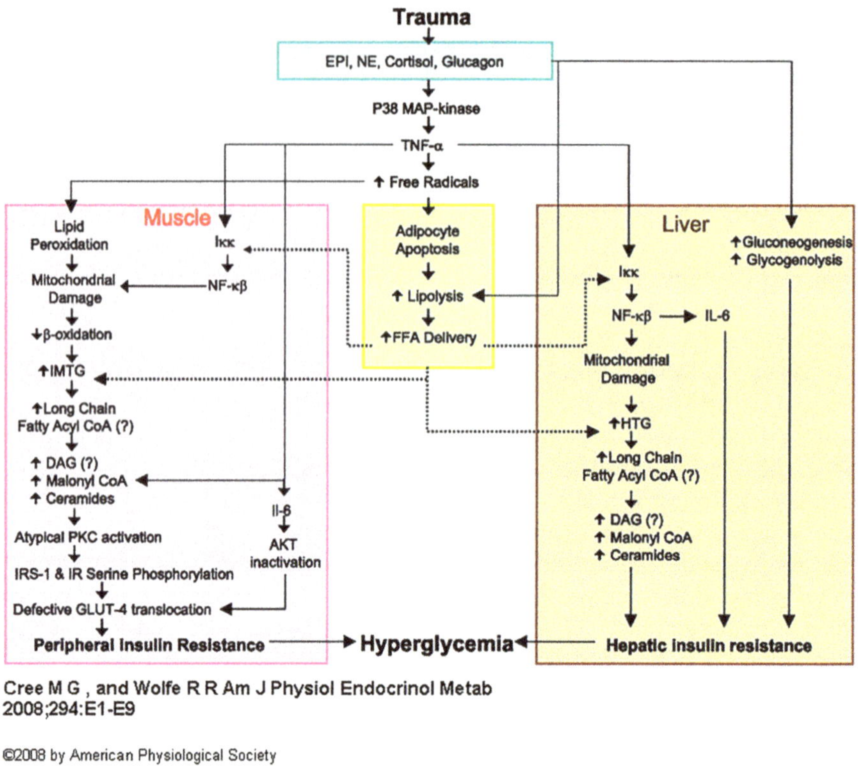

Fig. 15.1 Proposed pathways of insulin resistance in the ebb and flow stages of burn. *Abbreviations*: *DAG* diacylglycerol, *EPI* epinephrine, *FFA* free fatty acids, *GLUT-4* glucose transporter-4, *TG* triglyceride, *HTG* hepatic TG, *IL-6* interleukin-6, *IMTG* intramyocellular TG, *IR* insulin receptor, *IRS-1* insulin receptor substrate-1, *NE* norepinephrine, *TNF-α* tumor necrosis factor- α, *NF-κB* nuclear factor-κB, *PKC* protein kinase C reference [14]

Table 15.1 Proposed mechanisms of how glutamine can improve hyperglycaemia

- The glucose-glutamine cycle
- Increasing insulin secretion
- Improving insulin sensitivity in muscle
- Increasing fatty acid oxidation
- Decreasing the inflammatory response

because it is diverted to the liver for gluconeogenesis [16]. These results suggest that carbon transfer from glucose to glutamine may depend on adequate insulin availability and action. In critically ill patients, administering insulin to maintain tight glycaemic control promotes an increased release of glutamine from skeletal muscle probably due to increased de novo net synthesis of glutamine suggesting a cause–effect relationship [17].

Increasing Insulin Secretion

In vivo, pancreatic β-cells constantly monitor nutrient availability and can generate appropriate secondary stimulus-coupling signals in response to minor changes in the concentration of specific substrates. Exocytose of insulin granules in β-cells is directly related to ATP metabolism in mitochondria in presence of high levels of glucose. Nevertheless, it seems that some amino acids, and particularly glutamine, play also a significant roll to maintain insulin secretion. In vitro and human studies have demonstrated that glutamine is metabolized to glutamate in β-cells through glutamate DH, and it stimulates directly insulin exocytose [18]. It is a well-known phenomenon in children's glutamate DH mutation that present the Hyperinsulinism Hyperammonaemia Syndrome [19]. This effect has not been proven in critically ill patients.

Improving Insulin Sensitivity in Muscle

Experimental studies have shown that glutamine can improve insulin mediated glucose uptake. During euglycaemic hyperinsulinaemic clamps, intravenous glutamine improved whole body glucose utilization without changes in glucagon levels. The higher uptake was observed in the liver and in the muscle, indicating that there is an improved sensitivity to insulin in these tissues [20]. It is unknown if glutamine modifies the insulin sensitivity of the receptor or if it is a post-receptor effect. Human studies have shown that glutamine improves insulin sensitivity in muscle. Using euglycaemic hyperinsulinaemic clamps, there are two studies that have demonstrated that glutamine diminishes insulin resistance. The first one was performed in multiple trauma patients in the first week after the injury, and show that glucose disposal is higher and fasting insulin resistance is lower in patients receiving alanyl-glutamine dipeptide in the first week after the injury. This effect is not due to a reduction in the lean body mass and an increased proteolysis or a change in the inflammatory response, measured with C-reactive protein [21]. The second one explored the combined effect of low dose of alanyl-glutamine and growth hormone on insulin resistance and substrate oxidation. Glucose disposal was higher in the group of patients with glutamine alone when compared with the control group, or the other one that receives simultaneously alanyl-glutamine and growth hormone [22].

Increasing Fatty Acid Oxidation

Related with the changes in insulin sensitivity, one can expect that glutamine can modify fatty acid oxidation. In the study performed in multiple trauma patients mentioned above, glutamine treated group showed higher carbohydrate oxidation rates than lipid oxidation [21]. It could be explained by the named Randle's cycle or glucose-fatty acid cycle. It describes that the release and oxidation of lipids inhibits glucose oxidation in muscles, and conversely glucose inhibit release of lipids fuels and thereby facilitate uptake and oxidation of carbohydrates. Probably, glutamine improves insulin sensitivity of adipose tissue, can blunt lipolysis and lipid oxidation in the liver and can reverse hyperglycaemia related to a lipid infusion [23]. Human studies have shown that glutamine, administered with a mixed meal [24], can regulate glucose and lipid oxidation but this effect has not been deeply studied in critically ill patients.

Decreasing the Inflammatory Response

Decreasing the inflammatory response has a direct effect on glucose and fat metabolism (Fig. 15.1). It has been shown that glutamine attenuate the expression of pro-inflammatory cytokines and decreases systemic inflammation. The mechanism is interfering with the signal transduction of the nuclear factor NF-kB, and protein-kinase pathways [25]. The same group has demonstrated that glutamine exerts a beneficial after a heat-stress injury, because it is able to modify the Heat-Shock Factor 1 (HSF-1) expression and enhances the Heat-Shock Protein response after injury, increasing the resistance to cellular apoptosis can also decrease the inflammatory response [26].

Glycaemic Control and Glutamine

When looking at glycaemic control, it has been demonstrated that the level of glycaemia and insulin needs are dependent of the status of the patient. In the outpatient setting, insulin requirements in physiologic terms are classified as of basal and prandial needs. In the hospital, nutritional intake is not necessarily provided as discrete meals. The insulin dose requirement can be classified as basal and for nutritional needs. Nutritional insulin requirements refer to the amount of insulin necessary to cover intravenous dextrose, TPN, enteral feedings, nutritional supplements administered or discrete meals. When patients eat discrete meals without receiving other nutritional supplementation, the nutritional insulin requirement is the same as the prandial requirement, and it is the amount of exogenous insulin necessary to prevent gluconeogenesis and ketogenesis. An additional variable that determines total insulin needs in the hospital is an increase in insulin requirement related to the acute illness. The net effect of these factors is an increase in insulin requirements, compared with a non-sick population. This proportion of insulin requirement specific to illness is referred to as illness or stress-related insulin and varies across the in one individual and between individuals. In fact, in critically ill patients, the amount of basal insulin needed to obtain glycaemic control is around 50 % of the total amount, artificial nutrition (enteral or parenteral) represent as much as the 40 % of the insulin needs and the disease by itself increase the insulin needs between 20 and 30 %, giving a total amount more than 120 % of the basal needs under a healthy status [27].

There are several studies that support the hypothesis that glutamine can improve glycaemic control and decrease insulin needs in healthy humans [28]. Moreover, glutamine seems to exert better glycaemic control [29]. In this paper, hyperglycaemia was less frequent in glutamine-treated patients, and the need for insulin therapy was also significantly reduced.

Glycaemia Variability and Glycaemia Dynamics

One major concern in glycaemic control is the variability across the time. Classical studies have shown that elevated levels of glycaemia, the episodes f hypoglycaemia and an increased variability correlate with mortality [30]. Glycaemia variability seems to be more toxic that hyperglycaemia by itself. Experimental and clinical studies have shown that variability or oscillating hyperglycaemia increases oxidative stress more than sustained chronic hyperglycaemia in diabetes type 2 patients [31]. In critically ill patients, it has been clearly demonstrated that hyperglycaemia and hypoglycaemia are toxic and increase mortality by itself [4]. Nevertheless, it is not clear if the variability has the same relevance in critically ill patients. A meta-analysis designed to evaluate the results of assessing glycaemia variability found a significant heterogeneity of the 12 studies selected. Thirteen different methods to assess variability were found, and the studies reported a significant association between mortality, but there were a lot of methodological problems. The meta-analysis does not support a clear evidence of the association between glycaemia variability and bad clinical outcomes [32].

The evaluation of the different methods to assess glycaemia variability in critically ill patients is out of the scope of this chapter, but several considerations should be done.

Glucose values are not necessarily normally distributed or even symmetric about the mean, because there are not negative values below a number of standard deviations from the mean. Hyperglycaemia and hypoglycaemia should have a common threshold. Indexes like mean absolute glucose (MAG),

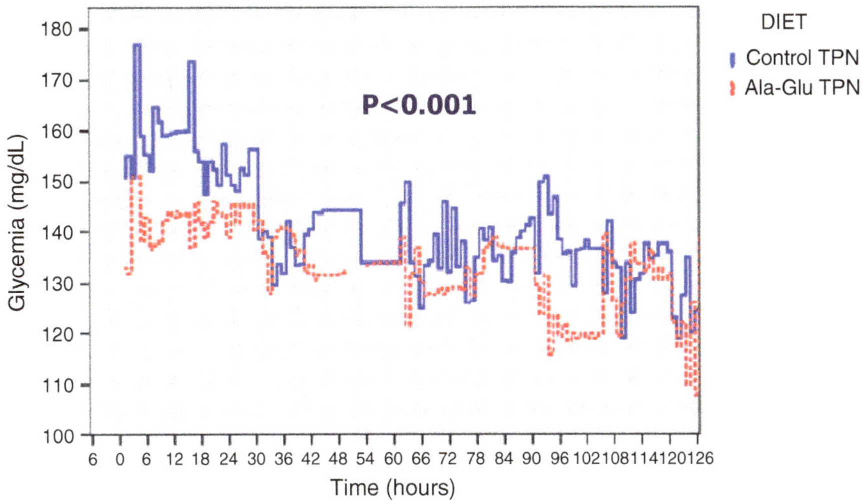

Fig. 15.2 Glycaemia time series in patients treated with alanine dipeptide and control patients

mean amplitude of glycaemic excursions (MAGE) and glycaemic labiality index (GLI) do not assess the direction of changes. Mean and standard deviations values, hypoglycaemia, hyperglycaemia, mean daily blood glycaemia or changes across the time do not take into account the time elapsed between determinations. Caregivers will respond differently to different levels of glycaemia changing the threshold levels or modifying insulin doses. Moreover, race, sex, previous disease, the clinical status of the patient, the severity of the disease and the typical interventions in critically ill patients, like the use of catecholamines or steroids, can blunt the clear effect of glycaemia variability on clinical outcomes.

Analysis of the Oscillatory Patterns of Glycaemia

It is clearly established that glucose stimulates insulin secretion from pancreatic cells. Oscillations in insulin secretion have been measured in vivo and in isolated pancreatic islets. The oscillations have two components: the faster one has a period of tens of seconds, and the slower one period of 4–6 min. This latter component appears to play an important physiological role in insulin action. It seems that the fast oscillations result from electrical mechanisms generated endogenously within the β-cells themselves and, slow oscillations are due to the effects of glycolysis in Ca^{++} channels of the β-cells. This model take in account the variability or time course of the Ca^{++} intracellular levels and other metabolic variables observed in glucose-stimulated pancreatic islets. The oscillatory pattern of intracellular levels of Ca^{++} results in a pulsatile pattern of insulin secretion [33].

There are several clinical studies that have tried to identify this oscillatory pattern. A study in trauma and burn patients assessed the variability of glycaemia and exogenous insulin requirements trying to find a pattern comparing the changes in both data. Hourly blood glucose and insulin dose requirements were matched between subjects for a time of day given. Average blood glucose and insulin requirement for the study population were analyzed with a linear and cosine regression to determine daily and overall trends. Cosine regression confirmed the diurnal glucose and insulin patterns and simple regression of the data identifies the overall trend in mean levels. The average insulin dose to correct hyperglycaemia in the study population was lowest at admission and increased at a constant rate, showing the evidence that insulin activity decreases over time and that there is an increasing insulin resistance [34] (Fig. 15.2).

The second study was done in a mixed population of critically ill patients. The authors analyzed glucose variability assuming that it has a nonlinear dynamics. Glycaemia levels seem to be unpredictable and be random (pseudorandom) as other physiologic processes like cardiac rhythm, or temperature. They use a complexity analysis based on time series calculations. Complexity was assessed with a technique named detrended fluctuation analysis (DFA). DFA estimates the degree of long-range correlations within a signal, analyzing how the time series diverge as the time considered increases. High-complexity series, or series with high variability, show that two consecutive values diverge whereas, in low complexity series, two consecutive values are closer. Low values of DFA represent high complexities and high values indicate low complexity. This analysis correlates one value with the closest values and is linked with them. This kind of analysis can detect small differences between values that traditional statistical methods (median, range, standard deviation) are unable to find. Usually physiological conditions show high levels of complexity and low variability whereas pathological conditions have low complexity and high variability. A nice example is the complexity of the sinus rhythm and the variability of cardiac dysrhythmias. In this study, DFA was significantly lower (higher complexity) in surviving patients than in patients who died and the difference remained when confounding factors as the age and severity score were included in the model [35].

The last study is derived from the Leuven study [2]. They used the large amount of patient included in the study that time series of all blood glucose measurements were available. Several indexes of glucose variability, as markers of variability, were calculated: the hyperglycaemic index (HGI), the hypoglycaemic index (HoGI), and the glycaemic penalty index (GPI). In addition, they calculated jack-knifed approximate entropy (JkApEn) of the blood glucose signal, as a marker of patterns of variation over time. With this statistical technique, large values of entropy correlates high variability and small values correlate with low variability of the value. A physiological system has low levels of entropy and a pathological one has high levels. This study assessed the effect of an intensive insulin treatment on amplitude variation and entropy of glycaemia in a multivariable logistic regression model. It demonstrated that a lower blood glucose amplitude variation and a more regular blood glucose signal with recognizable patterns were independently associated with a lower mortality [36].

Glycaemic Control with Glutamine: Time-Series Analysis

In 2008, our group published the results of a prospective, double-blind, randomized trial was to assess the clinical efficacy of glutamine dipeptide-supplemented TPN, defined by the occurrence of nosocomial infections, or new organ failure as clinical endpoints. A secondary objective was to analyze the effect of glutamine. The aim of this study was to assess the effect of glutamine dipeptide supplemented TPN on tight glycaemic control in critically ill patients compared with a standard TPN using a time series analysis. Entry criteria were the following: adult patients in ICU requiring TPN for 3 or more days and APACHE II score higher than 12. Both groups received isonitrogenous and isocaloric TPN. Nutritional needs were calculated: 0.25 g N kg^{-1} day^{-1} and 25 kcal kg^{-1} day^{-1}. Glutamine-TPN group received 0.5 g kg^{-1} day^{-1} of glutamine dipeptide and the standard TPN group a similar amount of amino acids. A tight glycemic control protocol was placed using a target plasmatic glycaemia of 120 mg/dL. Hourly glycaemia and the hourly dose of insulin were recorded at least 15 times a day. After an exploratory analysis, glycaemia and insulin values were depurated. We apply six different time series models to find the model that better fits using the root mean-square error (RMSE) between patients and individual determinations (Table 15.2). The model that better fits was an autoregressive moving average model ARMA that included the values of insulin 1 and 2 h before the next determination (Table 15.3). Because glycaemia and insulin data were unbalanced, we applied a hierarchical mixed linear model that overcomes the limitations of multivariate analysis of variance. We used two levels of hierarchy, patient and measurement, to identify the effect of insulin dose and the type of diet. A lineal and sinusoidal model was used to assess the circadian rhythm.

Table 15.2 The best model of different time series analysis was the auto-regressive moving average model, ARMA (2,1). Measured and predicted values were the closest obtained from different models

Model	RMSE
AR (1)	27,406
AR (2)	25,496
ARMA (1,1)	26,329
ARMA (2, 1)	24,546
ARMA (1,2)	25,138
ARIMA (1,1,0)	32,561

RMSE: Root mean-square error
Measured Values
N. measurements: 19,782
Glycaemia: 133 mg/dL (CI 95 % 105–171)
Insulin: 5 UI/h (CI 95 %: 3–12)
Predicted Values
N. measurements: 20,017
Glycaemia: 130 mg/dL (CI 95 %: 103–163)
Insulin: 4 UI/h (CI 95 %: 2–6)

Table 15.3 The time series analysis with ARMA (2,1) show that glycaemia is dependent of the insulin dose one before the determination, and the effect of glutamine diet (β) is higher that the control diet with a significant difference

	β	SE(β)	*p*-value
ARIMA (1,2)			
Insulin dose	7.14	0.24	<0.001
Insulin 1 h before	−0.94	0.13	<0.0001
Diet and insulin 1 h			
Control	−0.8	0.1	<0.0001
Glutamine	−1.1	0.2	<0.0001
Difference	−0.5	0.1	<0.0001

The effect of insulin dose on plasmatic glycaemia was best measured using a regression model with autocorrelation (ARMA) with one previous measurement. It has a physiological explanation because insulin action starts 6 min after the administration. When looking to the effect of the different diets, the glutamine treated group TPN group had lower levels of glycaemia and needed lesser insulin than the control TPN group with a 54 % reduction of the amount of insulin for the same levels of plasmatic glycaemia (Fig. 15.3). We were unable to find circadian differences between the doses of insulin in both groups [37].

Conclusions

Hyperglycaemia is a landmark metabolic feature associated with the stress response in critically ill patients mediated by catecholamines and inflammatory metabolites, particularly cytokines and the nuclear factor κβ. The de novo acquired hyperglycaemia in these patients is mainly due to a decreased insulin sensitivity in liver and muscle. The efforts to control these phenomena must be addressed not only to use insulin but to explore the effect of different nutritional substrates on glucose metabolism. It has been suggested that glutamine, a conditionally essential amino acid in critically ill patients, can influence glucose metabolism, and particularly it can improve insulin sensitivity in critically ill patients. There are several mechanisms that can explain these phenomena: through the glucose-glutamine cycle, increasing insulin secretion, improving insulin sensitivity in muscle, increasing fatty acid oxidation and decreasing the inflammatory response.

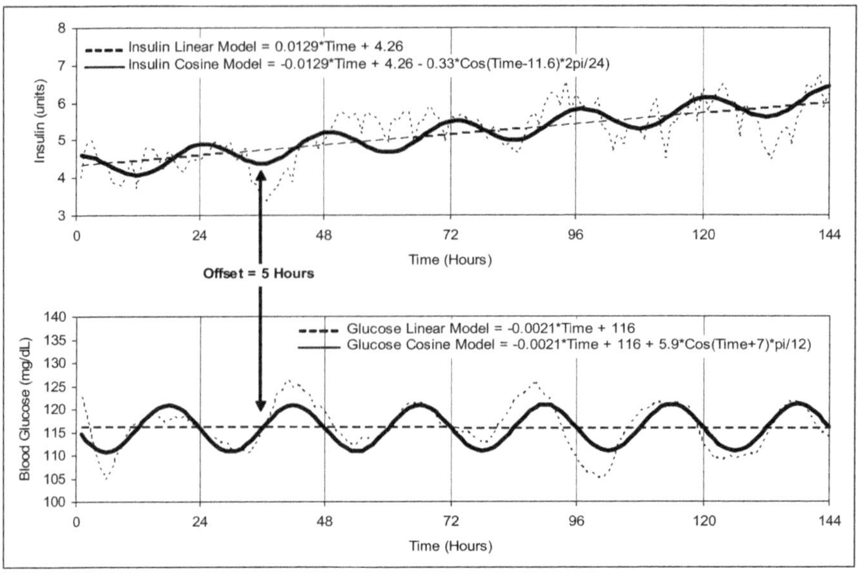

Fig. 15.3 Diurnal patterns over time of insulin requirement (*top*) and blood glucose (*bottom*). Simple regression formula for insulin requirement (*large dash*) demonstrates that the slope increases over time, while that of glucose remains nearly constant. Diurnal peaks and troughs are offset by 5 h reference [34]

Assess glycaemia variability in critically ill patients is a difficult task. It is important to consider the variations across the time using specialized statistical methods due to the characteristic oscillatory pattern of glycaemia levels and insulin secretion. The use of different methods of time series analysis can explain this variability and demonstrate the effectiveness of some interventions like tight glycaemic control with intensive insulin administration. Also, we have demonstrated that assessing glucose variability with different hierarchical models why can explain how a glutamine dipeptide exerts a beneficial effect controlling hyperglycaemia and decreasing insulin needs in critically ill patients.

References

1. Dungan KM, Braithwaite SS, Preiser JC. Stress hyperglycaemia. Lancet. 2009;373:1798–807.
2. Van den Berghe G, Wilmer A, Hermans G, et al. Intensive insulin therapy in the medical ICU. N Engl J Med. 2006;354:449–61.
3. Preiser JC, Devos P, Ruiz-Santana S, et al. A prospective randomised multi-centre controlled trial on tight glucose control by intensive insulin therapy in adult intensive care units: the Glucontrol study. Intensive Care Med. 2009; 35:1738–48.
4. The NICE-SUGAR Study Investigators. Intensive versus conventional glucose control in critically ill patients. N Engl J Med. 2009;360:1283–97.
5. Wiener RS, Wiener DC, Larson RJ. Benefits and risks of tight glucose control in critically ill adults: a meta-analysis. JAMA. 2008;300:933–44.
6. Griesdale DEG, de Souza RJ, van Dam RM, Heyland DK, Cook DJ, Malhotra A, et al. Intensive insulin therapy and mortality among critically ill patients: a meta-analysis including NICE-SUGAR study data. CMAJ. 2009;180: 821–7.
7. Soeters MR, Soeters PB. The evolutionary benefit of insulin resistance. Clin Nutr. 2012;31:1002–7.
8. Frayn KN. Hormonal control of metabolism in trauma and sepsis. Clin Endocrinol. 1986;24:577–99.
9. Saberi F, Heyland D, Lam M, Rapson D, Jeejeebhoy K. Prevalence, incidence, and clinical resolution of insulin resistance in critically ill patients: an observational study. JPEN J Parenter Enteral Nutr. 2008;32:227–35.
10. Wolfe RR. Review: acute versus chronic response to burn injury. Circ Shock. 1981;8:105–15.

11. Biddinger SB, Kahn CR. From mice to men: insights into the insulin resistance syndromes. Annu Rev Physiol. 2006;68:123–58.
12. Ling P, Smith R, Bistrian B. Hyperglycemia enhances the cytokine production and oxidative responses to a low but not high dose of endotoxin in rats. Crit Care Med. 2005;33:1084–9.
13. Schenk S, Saberi M, Olefsky M. Insulin sensitivity: modulation by nutrients and inflammation. J Clin Invest. 2008;118:2992–3002.
14. Cree MG, Wolfe RR. Postburn trauma insulin resistance and fat metabolism. Am J Physiol Endocrinol Metab. 2008;294:E1–9.
15. Oudemans-van Straatcn HM, Bosman RJ, Treskes M, et al. Plasma glutamine depletion and patient outcome in acute ICU admissions. Intensive Care Med. 2001;27:84–90.
16. Meyer C, Woerle HJ, Gerich J. Paradoxical Changes of Muscle Glutamine Release During Hyperinsulinemia Euglycemia and Hypoglycemia in Humans: Further Evidence for the Glucose-Glutamine Cycle. Metabolism. 2004;53:1208–14.
17. Biolo G, De Cicco M, Lorenzon S, et al. Treating hyperglycemia improves skeletal muscle proteína metabolism in cancer patients after major surgery. Crit Carc Med. 2008;36:1768–75.
18. Newsholme P, Brennan L, Bender K. Amino Acid Metabolism, β-Cell Function, and Diabetes. Diabetes. 2006;55 Suppl 2:S39–47.
19. Stanley CA, Lieu YK, Hsu BY, Burlina AB, et al. Hyperinsulinism and hyperammonemia in infants with regulatory mutations of the glutamate dehydrogenase gene. N Engl J Med. 1998;338:1352–7.
20. Borel MJ, Williams PE, Jabbour K, et al. Parenteral glutamine infusion alters insulin-mediated glucose metabolism. JPEN J Parenter Enteral Nutr. 1998;22:280–5.
21. Bakalar B, Duska F, Pachl J, et al. Parenterally administered dipeptide alanyl-glutamine prevents worsening of insulin sensitivity in multiple-trauma patients. Crit Care Med. 2006;34:381–6.
22. Duska F, Fric M, Waldauf P, et al. Frequent intravenous pulses of growth hormone together with glutamine supplementation in prolonged critical illness after multiple trauma: effects on nitrogen balance, insulin resistance, and substrate oxidation. Crit Care Med. 2008;36:1707–13.
23. Ballard TC, Farag A, Branum GD, et al. Effect of L-glutamine supplementation on impaired glucose regulation during intravenous lipid administration. Nutrition. 1996;12:349–54.
24. Iwashita S, Mikus C, Baier S, et al. Glutamine supplementation increases postprandial energy expenditure and fat oxidation in humans. JPEN J Parenter Enteral Nutr. 2006;30:76–80.
25. Singleton KD, Beckey VE, Wischmeyer PE. Glutamine prevents activation of NF-kappa-β and stress kinase pathways, attenuates inflammatory cytokine release, and prevents acute respiratory distress syndrome (ARDS) following sepsis. Shock. 2005;24:583–9.
26. Morrison AL, Dinges M, Singleton KD, et al. Glutamine's protection against cellular injury is dependent on heat shock factor-1. Am J Physiol Cell Physiol. 2006;290:C1625–32.
27. Clement S, Braithwaite SS, Magee MF, et al. Management of diabetes and hyperglycemia in hospitals. Diabetes Care. 2004;27:553–91.
28. Coeffier M, Claeyssens S, Hecketsweiler B, Lavoinne A, Ducrotte P, Dechelotte P. Enteral glutamine stimulates protein synthesis and decreases ubiquitin mRNA level in human gut mucosa. Am J Physiol Gastrointest Liver Physiol. 2003;285:G266–73.
29. Déchelotte P, Hasselmann M, Cynober L, et al. L-alanyl-L-glutamine dipeptide-supplemented total parenteral nutrition reduces infectious complications and glucose intolerance in critically ill patients: the French controlled, randomized, double-blind, multicenter study. Crit Care Med. 2006;34:598–604.
30. Bagshaw SM, Bellomo R, Jacka MJ, et al. The impact of early hypoglycemia and blood glucose variability on outcome in critical illness. Crit Care. 2009;13:R91.
31. Monnier L, Mas E, Ginet C, et al. Activation of oxidative stress by acute glucose fluctuations compared with sustained chronic hyperglycemia in patients with diabetes type 2. JAMA. 2006;295:1681–7.
32. Slami S, Taherzadeh Z, Schultz MJ, et al. Glucose variability measures and their effect on mortality: a systematic review. Intensive Care Med. 2011;37:583–93.
33. Bertram R, Sherman A, Satin LS. Metabolic and elcctrical oscillations: partners in controlling pulsatile insulin secrction. Am J Physiol Endocrinol Metab. 2007;293:E890–900.
34. Pidcoke HF, Salinas J, Wanek SM, et al. Patterns of exogenous insulin requirement reflect insulin sensitivity changes in trauma. Am J Surg. 2007;194:798–803.
35. Lundelin K, Vigil L, Bua S, et al. Differences in complexity of glycemic profile in survivors and nonsurvivors in an intensive care unit: a pilot study. Crit Care Med. 2010;38:849–54.
36. Meyfroidt G, Keenan DM, Wang X, et al. Dynamic characteristics of blood glucose time series during the course of critical illness: effects of intensive insulin therapy and relative association with mortality. Crit Care Med. 2010;38:1021–9.
37. Grau T, Bonet A, Miñambres E, et al. The effect of L-alanyl-L-glutamine dipeptide supplemented total parenteral nutrition on infectious morbidity and insulin sensitivity in critically ill patients. Crit Care Med. 2011;39:1263–8.

Chapter 16
Potential for Glutamine Supplementation in Critically Ill Children

Efrossini Briassouli, Luise Victoria Marino, and George Briassoulis

Key Points

- Glutamine serves as a primary fuel for rapidly dividing cells and is used as a source of nitrogen to refill the citric acid cycle.
- During critical illness, the demand for glutamine may exceed that which can be mobilised from muscle stores.
- No glutamine supplementation recommendations exist for critically ill children.
- The beneficial effect of glutamine, in experimental or animal models of sepsis, appears to be dependent on the heat-shock protein-70 response.
- In order to understand the role of glutamine supplementation in critically ill children and premature infants, future studies should address previous methodological problems within clinical studies, with the aim of investigating interrelationships between glutamine supplementation, stress-induced heat-shock protein and the inflammatory response.

Keywords Glutamine • Enteral • Parenteral • Children • Infants • Premature • Supplementation

Abbreviations

ARDS	Acute respiratory distress syndrome
ATP	Adenosine triphosphate
ASPEN	American Society of Parenteral and Enteral Nutrition
CRP	C-reactive protein

E. Briassouli, M.D.
1st Department of Internal Medicine–Propaedeutic, "Laiko" Hospital, University of Athens, Agiou Thoma Road, Athens, Attiki 115 27, Greece
e-mail: efroelesar@hotmail.com

L.V. Marino, M. Med. Sci. Nutrition, Ph.D.
Department of Paediatrics, Imperial College London, Norfolk Place, St. Mary's Campus, London W2 1PG, UK
e-mail: Luise.marino@uhs.nhs.uk; l.marino@imperial.ac.uk; Marinoluise37@gmail.com

G. Briassoulis, M.D., Ph.D. (✉)
Department of Paediatric Intensive Care, School of Medicine, University of Crete
Voutes area, Heraklion, Crete 71110, Greece
e-mail: ggbriass@otenet.gr

R. Rajendram et al. (eds.), *Glutamine in Clinical Nutrition*, Nutrition and Health,
DOI 10.1007/978-1-4939-1932-1_16,

DAMPS	Damage-associated molecular patterns
DC	Dendritic cells
ESPEN	European Society of Parenteral and Enteral Nutrition
ELBW	Extremely low birth weight
HSF-1	Heat-shock factor 1
HSP	Heat-shock protein
HSP25	Heat-shock protein 25
HSP70	Heat-shock protein 70
HBP	Hexosamine biosynthetic pathway
IL	Interleukin
IEC	Intestinal epithelial cells
IV	Intravenously
IKK	IκB kinase
LOS	Length of stay
LPS	Lipopolysaccharide
mRNA	Messenger ribonucleic acid
MAPK	Mitogen-activated protein kinase pathway
MYD88	Myeloid differentiation primary response 88
NF-κB	Nuclear factor kappa B
PICU	Paediatric intensive care unit
PRISM	Paediatric risk of mortality
PAMPS	Pathogen-associated molecular patterns
PRR	Pattern recognition receptors
RCT	Randomised controlled trial
SIRS	Systemic inflammatory response syndrome
TLR	Toll-like receptors
TNF-α	Tumour necrosis factor alpha
UK	United Kingdom
US	United States of America
VLBW	Very low birth weight

Introduction

Amino acids trigger signalling cascades, which regulate various aspects of protein synthesis and energy metabolism serving as precursors for important substrates. Glutamine is the most abundant extracellular amino acid, with a concentration of between 0.6 and 0.7 mmol/L, which becomes conditionally essential during stress, injury or illness [1]. Conversely, glutamate is usually the most abundant intracellular amino acid with a concentration of 2–20 mmol/L depending on the cell type. Glutamate facilitates de novo amino acid transamination, donating an amino group or ammonia. In some organs, e.g. liver, and cells, e.g. astrocytes, glutamate and ammonia are combined by glutamine synthetase to form glutamine, which is then exported from the cell.

Organs and skeletal muscle are the main source of endogenous glutamine with high intracellular concentrations of 20–25 mmol/L glutamine. Blood glutamine levels reflect the balance between synthesis, release and consumption by all types of cells. Glutamine serves as a metabolic intermediate and precursor, providing carbon and nitrogen for the de novo synthesis of other amino acids, nucleic acids, fatty acids, nucleotides and proteins. During times of stress, skeletal muscle is an active net exporter of free glutamine. Glutamine provides fuel source for rapidly dividing cells such as those of the immune system and gastrointestinal tract, reticulocytes and fibroblasts; it is a precursor for nucleic acid synthesis, hexosamines, nucleotides and precursors for arginine; glutathione and helping to maintain acid–base homeostasis in the kidney and renal regulation of inter-organ glutamine flow in metabolic acidosis [2]. In the acute phase of critical illness, glutamine is released in large amounts from muscle tissue. Glutamine's functions within the cell may be broadly categorised into four main categories: (1) nitrogen transport; (2) maintenance of the cellular redox state through glutathione; (3) a metabolic intermediate and (4) a source of energy.

Nutrition support, especially in children who have limited metabolic reserves, has traditionally been seen as a means to prevent malnutrition by providing substrate e.g. protein, fat and carbohydrate [3]. Recent advances in the field of nutrition research have resulted in the realisation that specific nutrients such as glutamine may be of benefit to critically ill patients with immune modulating effects altering the host response to stress. In critically ill adults, plasma glutamine levels decrease significantly, remaining low for up to 21 days, and are associated with increased morbidity and mortality [4]. Accordingly, the American Society of Parenteral and Enteral Nutrition (ASPEN)/European Society of Enteral and Parenteral Nutrition (ESPEN) recommend that 0.3–0.5 g/kg of glutamine is added to parenteral nutrition in critically ill adults [5]. However, no such recommendations exist for critically ill children. This is because much of the work considering the use of glutamine in critical illness has been completed in adults, with little data available from paediatric critical illness.

Paediatric Sepsis

There is a growing interest into how individual nutrients particularly glutamine could influence morbidity and mortality in critical illness. Globally, sepsis and septic shock remain a leading cause of mortality in adults and children. Mortality from severe sepsis in children is reported to be between 10.3 and 14 %, which is lower than the mortality rates reported in adults of between 27 and 54 %. Recently published data shows that amongst children admitted to a paediatric intensive care unit (PICU) 82 % had evidence of systemic inflammatory response syndrome (SIRS), with 23 % of these meeting the criteria for sepsis, of which 4 % had severe sepsis and 2 % had septic shock [6].

In the USA, paediatric sepsis costs nearly $2 billion per annum and in the UK the estimated total cost of adult care was between £7,000 and £28,000 per patient per admission. The cost of healthcare during acute disease does not account for hidden costs relating to post-discharge rehabilitation following severe sepsis, especially in children and the long-term impact on cognitive abilities, executive functioning and psycho/social difficulties experienced into adulthood [7].

The Inflammatory Response

Young infants and those with underlying medical conditions (e.g. neurodevelopmental delay, chronic lung disease and primary immunodeficiency) are at particular risk of bacterial blood stream infections due to immature mucosal barriers and immune system (including macrophages, neutrophils, immunoglobulin and complement).

Many bloodstream infections in children are caused by colonising pathogenic bacteria, which are present on the skin or mucosal surfaces such as the nasopharynx. Bloodstream infections can arise when there is disruption to the mucosal-epithelia barrier allowing bacterial adherence to occur. The endothelial mucosal layer acts as an early detection system for pathogen invasion, stimulating host defence mechanisms by recruiting leukocytes to the bloodstream entry site. From bloodstream infection to the development of sepsis there is an interplay between the invading organism and the host response; the systemic inflammatory response is the body's organised response to infection promoting the activation of the complement system and innate immune response. These mechanisms are initiated through the recognition of pathogen-associated molecular patterns (PAMPs) by receptors sites on the cell surface such as toll-like receptors (TLR) known as pattern recognition receptors (PRRs). PRRs (such as TLRs) form the first line of cellular defence, recognising and transducing signals via ligand receptors, on the host cell surface, when they come into contact with PAMPs [8].

Pathogens and the subsequent host response results in tissue and cell damage, stimulating the release of intracellular proteins, such as heat-shock protein 70 (HSP70), known as alarmins, which aim to protect tissue or cells from further damage. As alarmins and PAMPs elicit similar innate and adaptive immune responses they are broadly known as damage-associated molecular patterns (DAMPs) acting to promote an inflammatory response to infection. Inflammation, as co-ordinated by the innate immune system, is a necessary response to infection promoting increased blood flow to the injured site. In the absence of an inflammatory response the host would succumb to overwhelming infection, however, an exaggerated host response results in septic shock and increased risk of mortality [8].

During the early phase of sepsis, DAMPs are released in large amounts, both from the invading organism and the host's damaged tissue promoting the release of inflammatory cytokines (TNF-α, IL-1, IL-6, IL-12, IL-8) in addition to free radicals and enzymes in large amounts. HSP70 acts as a DAMP and signal through CD14-TLR4 complex, eliciting rapid signal transduction via MYD88–IKK/NF-κB pathway, activating NF-κB and MAPK pathways and promoting the release pro-inflammatory mediators (TNF-a, IL-1β and IL-6). In addition, the NF-κB family is capable of regulating genes associated with the inflammatory response, immunity and apoptosis, further promoting the release of inflammatory mediators such as TNF-α [9].

Heat-Shock Protein 70 and Glutamine

The beneficial effects of glutamine in critical illness are postulated to be due to increased production of HSP70. The initial response to infection results in a rapid and ubiquitous use of glutamine by immune cells, for a myriad of cell functions including the release of extracellular HSP70 (both via necrotic cell death and passive cell release), promoting high plasma levels of HSP70 [10]. In vitro glutamine supplementation upregulates HSP70 release in lung macrophages and epithelial cells protecting against sepsis related injury. The beneficial effect of glutamine appears to be HSP70 dependent, since when a knockout septic mouse model was used HSP70 (-/-) no benefit was derived from glutamine supplementation. In experimentally induced ARDS, glutamine supplementation improved ATP levels reversing lactate accumulation, by restoring HSP70 levels. HSP70 deficiency led to a decline in lung tissue metabolism, lung injury and organ failure in a rat model of sepsis. In an experimental septic mouse model glutamine administration in combination with antimicrobial significantly decreased morbidity and mortality via HSP70-mediated effects on the inflammatory response [11]. It is thought that glutamine depletion may affect the efficacy and biological activity of heat-shock factor 1 (HSF-1), HSP70, and the half-life of HSP70 mRNA levels limiting functional efficacy and activity of HSP70 during times of stress.

Glutamine Is a Pro-chaperone

A large body of literature has hypothesised a relationship between HSP70 expression and glutamine's protection in both in vitro and in vivo settings [12]. Glutamine has been shown to induce heat shock protein expression and to attenuate lipopolysaccharide (LPS)-mediated cardiovascular dysfunction. Glutamine has also been shown to exert an effect on HSP70 production relative to the upstream influence of glutamine on HSF-1 and HSE [13]. Glutamine is metabolised via the hexosamine biosynthetic pathway (HBP), which appears to be part of an early cellular protective response to stress and is a key substrate required for optimal activity of the HBP. It has been shown that a single dose of intravenous glutamine enhances phosphorylation of nuclear HSF-1, a vital step in its transcriptional activation, causing a rapid and significant increase in HSP25 and HSP70 expression in unstressed Sprague–Dawley rat [14]. In vitro models showed that glutamine supplementation attenuated lethal heat and oxidant injury and delayed spontaneous apoptosis in neutrophils, protecting activated T cells via glutathione upregulation [15]. Recently, by inducing HSP70 in an experimental model, glutamine was also shown to attenuate LPS-induced cardiomyocyte damage [16].

Marked attenuation of tissue metabolic dysfunction was observed after glutamine administration as measured by lung tissue adenosine 5′-triphosphate/adenosine 5′-diphosphate ratio and the oxidised form of nicotinamide adenine dinucleotide. Glutamine supplementation has been shown to enhance HSP70 release, protecting intestinal epithelial cells in a dose-dependent fashion against heat stress and oxidant injury, decreasing lung injury, and improving survival [14]. Recent results demonstrated for the first time that orally administered glutamine can enhance tissue HSP70 expression [4] and improve survival following lethal hyperthermia injury [17]. In cardiac disease, oral glutamine taken for 3 days prior to coronary artery bypass graft (with a final dose given 2 h prior to surgery), promoted HSP70 release decreasing myocardial ischaemic reperfusion injury and post-operative complications [18]. It was hypothesised that glutamine may act as an HSF-1 activator and increase the entire family of HSPs after stress or injury since in HSF-1 knockout cells, glutamine's ability to generate an HSP response is lost and the protection conferred by glutamine is also completely abrogated.

Glutamine Depletion During Critical Illness

During critical illness, glutamine is released into the system to provide fuel for the accelerated metabolic functions such as RNA synthesis and perhaps as a cell primer against further injury, making it a conditionally essential amino acid during periods of severe stress [4]. The benefit of intravenous compared to enteral administration is that glutamine is available for systemic circulation benefitting immune cells in addition to those within the gut. Glutamine given intravenously (IV) mimics endogenously produced glutamine as shown by its even uptake across the splanchnic area [19]. On the other hand, enteral glutamine is rapidly metabolised within the upper part of the small bowel (jejunum) leaving little available for the remainder of the bowel. Portal circulation studies also show that little glutamine makes it across the "first-pass elimination" to the liver and for subsequent systemic circulation. Enteral administration of glutamine is not as effective at restoring plasma glutamine levels to within normal range when compared to parenteral glutamine [20].

During times of stress there is a net export of glutamine from muscle stores, which become rapidly depleted. Protein flux and turnover in rapidly growing children is considerably higher than in adults and as such the need for amino acids such as glutamine is considerably more, suggesting a preferential use by rapidly dividing cells such as enterocytes and immune cells. Protein kinetic studies using leucine isotopes have shown glutamine supplementation attenuates protein breakdown. However, glutamine supplementation is not able to increase the rate of protein synthesis, but does exert a protein-sparing effect, in very-low-birth weight infants and in surgical neonates. Increased amino acid delivery in stressed, very-low-birth-weight infants, resulted in an increase in de novo glutamine synthesis [21].

Muscle glutamine depletion occurs within hours of severe illness by up to 72 %. Griffiths et al. have shown that in adults there is a precipitous drop in plasma glutamine levels by up to 58 % with the onset of catabolism, which can last for up to 21 days, increasing mortality [22]. Up to 14 g of free glutamine is reported as being depleted from skeletal muscle, in uncomplicated critically ill adults. Furthermore, during the first few days of acute illness, nutrition support is often suboptimal which is of concern as up to 40 % of children are malnourished on admission to PICU [23]. Plasma glutamine levels of ≤0.43 mmol are associated with increased mortality and non-surviving adult septic patients lost up to 90 % of their skeletal muscle glutamine mass [24].

Although plasma concentrations do not accurately reflect the intracellular glutamine concentration, which varies dependent on the type of cell, is currently the best proxy for glutamine depletion [25]. Low plasma glutamine levels are not necessarily due to glutamine shortage, but can be reflective of intra- and extravascular fluid redistribution in parallel with disease severity, thereby explaining controversial results in adult studies [26, 27].

One study considering glutamine levels in critically ill children, found they have early significantly glutamine depletion (glutamine 0.31 mmol/L; ±SD 0.13; range 0.05–0.64) ($p<0.001$) compared to convalescent levels (0.40 mmol/L; ±SD 0.14; range 0.07–0.64) [28]. Glutamine levels were 52 % below the lower limit of the normal reference range (i.e. 0.6 mmol/L) during the acute phase of illness, whilst in the convalescent samples levels were 26 % below, suggesting depletion rather than on going consequence of fluid shifts [22]. Importantly, HSP70 levels in critically ill children [29] were higher (26.7 ng/mL; ±SD 79.95; range 0.09–600.5) [28] than those described in adult critical illness (median 1.75 ng/mL), assuming a more rapid protective response to stress among young people.

Glutamine Supplementation in Children

In children, the use of glutamine remains largely undefined with paucity of data regarding the benefits of glutamine as a pharmacological agent in paediatric critical illness. Conflicting results with respect to the benefits of glutamine supplementation was found in preterm infants [30] infants with gastrointestinal disease and surgery, burns and malnutrition [31]. Reasons for the lack of consistent results, following glutamine supplementation in children may be as a result of the different individual study designs, heterogeneity of the populations studied [32, 33], route of enteral administration chosen, e.g. enteral or IV, dosage g/kg given (Fig. 16.1) and duration of glutamine supplementation [34].

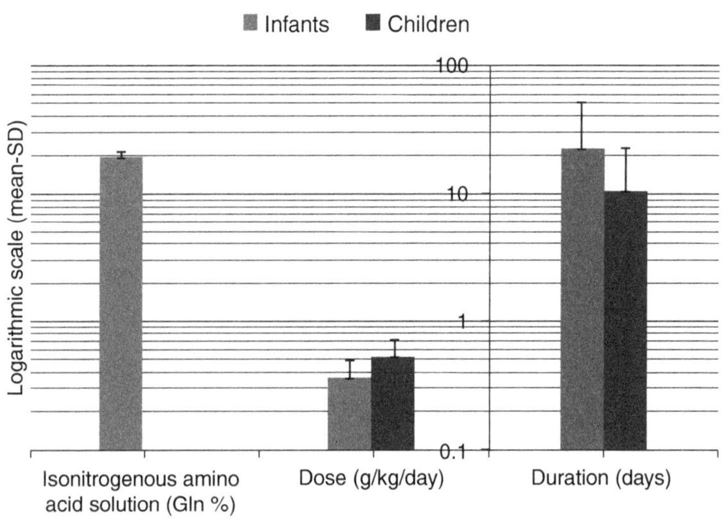

Fig. 16.1 Glutamine-dosing regimens in randomised control clinical studies in infants and children

However, beneficial effects of glutamine have been reported in children, which include decreased duration of acute diarrhoea, reduced severity of mucositis post-bone marrow transplant, decreased muscle catabolism in Duchene muscular dystrophy and improved growth in sickle cell anaemia [35].

Parenteral Supplementation of Glutamine in Preterm and Extremely Low-Birth Weight (ELBW) Infants

Glutamine is conditionally essential and safe for use in extremely low birth weight infants (ELBW) with supplementation increasing levels of plasma glutamine. In ELBW parental glutamine, given for a 2 weeks, was associated with fewer days on parenteral nutrition and length of stay in hospital, in addition to decreased hospital acquired infection episodes in premature infants [36]. Glutamine had an acute protein-sparing effect, as it suppressed leucine oxidation and protein breakdown, in parenterally fed very low birth weight infants [37], and was associated with lower whole-body protein breakdown and protein accretion in low birth weight (LBW) infants. Glutamine supplementation also improved hepatic tolerance in very low birth weight infants (VLBW) infants, suggesting a hepatoprotective effect. Although parenteral glutamine was well tolerated in ill preterm neonates, reducing the time to achieving enteral nutrition, nosocomial culture-positive sepsis or age at discharge was not reduced.

In a large multicentre, randomised clinical trial, the safety and efficacy of early parenteral nutrition (PN) supplemented with glutamine in decreasing the risk of death or late-onset sepsis were assessed in extremely low-birth weight infants. Although there were significant beneficial effects with glutamine supplementation, similar studies considering surgical neonates did not show any benefit [38]. Importantly, glutamine-enriched enteral nutrition in VLBW infants had neither beneficial nor detrimental effects on long-term cognitive, motor and behavioural outcomes of very preterm and/or VLBW children at school age, although visuomotor abilities were poorer in children that received glutamine [39].

Enteral Supplementation of Glutamine in Preterm and Extremely Low-Birth Weight (ELBW) Infants

In blinded randomised trials in VLBW infants, enteral glutamine supplementation did not decrease morbidity or mortality [40]. Preliminary results in VLBW suggest glutamine supplementation results in lower sepsis rates and a blunting of the inflammatory process [41]. Importantly, examining the effect of enteral glutamine on whole-body kinetics of glutamine in growing preterm infants, enterally administered glutamine was shown to be entirely metabolised in the gut and to have not a discernible effect on whole-body protein and nitrogen kinetics [42]. Similarly no differences between groups for plasma concentrations of glutamine, glucose or ammonia were shown during the glutamine enteral supplementation period [43].

Furthermore, the beneficial effects of glutamine supplementation especially in pre-term population may only be seen beyond the neonatal period. Follow-up studies of VLBW infants having received enteral preterm formula or breast milk supplemented with glutamine showed a lower risk of atopic dermatitis. However, there were no differences in incidence of bronchial hyperactivity, infections of upper respiratory, lower respiratory, urinary or gastrointestinal tracts [44], of intestinal microbiota, neurodevelopmental impairment or cerebral palsy. At 1 year of age intestinal (faecal) microbiota did not differ between the two groups. There was also no difference in Th1 and Th2 cytokine profiles either during the days of supplementation or at 1 year of age following in vitro whole-blood stimulation [45].

A Cochrane review concluded that glutamine supplementation confers no benefits to preterm infants and as such glutamine should not be an active research stream [30]. However, other groups argue the mode, timing, duration and type of analogue used in the randomised controlled trials included in the Cochrane review influenced the outcome measures. The use of glutamine in preterm infants has received considerable attention, with some results showing benefit with respect to infectious complications and time to full enteral feeds, and others showing no difference [46]. There are, however, inherent difficulties with trying to interpret the data from these studies as outlined below.

- Heterogeneous groups, e.g. sick versus relatively well versus surgical neonates.
- Isonitrogenous—many of the preterm studies compared the use of total parental nutrition enriched with glutamine to isonitrogenous control, the issue with this is that it potentially leads to suboptimal delivery of other essential amino acids, especially tyrosine and phenyl alanine.
- Time taken to get to goal rate—due to the delivery method some of the studies took up to 10 days to reach the goal rate of delivery, e.g. 0.3 g/kg.

Supplementation of Glutamine (Immunonutrition) in Critically Ill Children

Glutamine supplementation of 0.3–0.5 g/kg is recommended in critically ill adults [5], although no such recommendations exist for critically ill children. In critically ill children the amount of glutamine delivered enterally is often suboptimal providing only 28 % of the recommended adult intake [28], in addition to a low total protein intake of 0.88 g/kg (range 0.62–3.76 g/kg) [47]. Protein-rich feeds in critically ill children are reported to be of benefit as such protein intake should aim for the ASPEN recommendations [48].

In a multicentre randomised, double-blinded, comparative effectiveness trial, enteral zinc, selenium, glutamine and intravenous metoclopramide conferred no advantage in the immune-competent population of children requiring long-term intensive care compared with whey protein supplementation [49]. Further evaluation of these constituents' supplementation was thought to be warranted only in the immunocompromised long-term paediatric intensive care unit patient.

In another blinded, prospective, randomised, controlled clinical trial in critically ill children given an immune-enhancing formula supplemented with glutamine, nutritional indices and antioxidant catalysts showed a higher increasing trend but also higher osmolality, sodium and urea [50]. Similarly to the control group, gastrointestinal complications (diarrhoea and gastric distention) were the most frequently recorded in the immunonutrition group. Length of stay or mortality did not differ between groups, however there was a trend for fewer nosocomial infections in those receiving immunonutrition compared to conventional group. In another single-centre, randomised, blinded controlled trial in children with septic shock who received 5 days of early enteral feeding of immunonutrition, there was a decrease in pro-inflammatory cytokine IL-6 [32]. The differences in cytokines were independently correlated with PRISM, however, mortality and other paediatric intensive care unit outcome endpoints did not differ between the two groups. In two randomised studies in trauma patients (adults and children) there were no significant differences in mortality, LOS, lung infection or immunologic or biochemical parameters between the glutamine supplemented groups (enteral or parenteral) and controls [51] (Table 16.1).

Conclusions

Studies in critically ill children and in premature neonates remain inconsistent, partly because of the different effects of enteral and parenteral glutamine supplementation, different dosing and timing regimens, co-administered multi-immune-enhancing constituents, heterogeneity and pathways

Table 16.1 Outcome effect of glutamine in clinical randomised control studies in infants and children

Population	Number of studies/ patients	Mortality	Hospital-acquired infections	Length of stay	Inflammation
Extremely low-birth weight infants	1/1,433	No effect	No effect	No effect	NA
Premature or very-low-birth weight infants	12/1,359	No effect (8 studies)	3 studies (25 %) showed reduced infections/ hospital-acquired sepsis	1 (8 %) study showed reduced los	Higher lymphocyte count, blunted the rise in HLA-DR+and CD16/CD56 subsets (1 study each)
Post-surgery infants	2/215	No effect (1 study)	No effect	No effect	No effect
Ill preterm neonates, critically ill infants	2/44	No effect	No effect	No effect	No effect
Critically ill children	4/421	No effect	2 studies (50 %) showed reduced infections	No effect	Decreased IL-6, or IL-6, or Increased NB (1 study)

triggered in different stress states. Especially, findings of a number of RCTs are rather diverse and it remains unclear whether this variability is a consequence of inadequacy of innate immune heat-shock protein-response to stress or of true heterogeneity across individual trials or of the low power of many of these trials and the resulting chance effects. Since these studies are scarce and insufficient to allow safe recommendations to be made regarding immune-competent infants and children, additional large-scale, high-quality RCTs are needed.

Acknowledgements This research has been cofinanced by the European Union (European Social Fund (ESF)) and Greek national funds through the Operational Program "Education and Lifelong Learning" of the National Strategic Reference Framework (NSRF)-Research Funding Program: THALES.

Conflict of Interests The authors declare that there have no conflicts of interests.

References

1. Wischmeyer PE. Can glutamine turn off the motor that drives systemic inflammation? Crit Care Med. 2005;33:1175–8.
2. Gong J, Jing L. Glutamine induces heat shock protein 70 expression via O-GlcNAc modification and subsequent increased expression and transcriptional activity of heat shock factor-1. Minerva Anestesiol. 2011;77:488–95.
3. Briassoulis G, Zavras N, Hatzis T. Malnutrition, nutritional indices, and early enteral feeding in critically ill children. Nutrition. 2001;17:548–57.
4. Wischmeyer PE. Glutamine: role in critical illness and ongoing clinical trials. Curr Opin Gastroenterol. 2008;24:190–7.
5. Singer P, Berger MM, Van den Berghe G, Biolo G, Calder P, Forbes A, et al. ESPEN guidelines on parenteral nutrition: intensive care. Clin Nutr. 2009;28:387–400.
6. Proulx F, Fayon M, Farrell CA, Lacroix J, Gauthier M. Epidemiology of sepsis and multiple organ dysfunction syndrome in children. Chest. 1996;109:1033–7.
7. Vermunt LC, Buysse CM, Joosten KF, Duivenvoorden HJ, Hazelzet JA, Verhulst FC, et al. Survivors of septic shock caused by Neisseria meningitidis in childhood: psychosocial outcomes in young adulthood. Pediatr Crit Care Med. 2011;12:e302–9.

8. Cinel I, Opal SM. Molecular biology of inflammation and sepsis: a primer. Crit Care Med. 2009;37:291–304.
9. Guha M, Mackman N. LPS induction of gene expression in human monocytes. Cell Signal. 2001;13:85–94.
10. Roth E. Nonnutritive effects of glutamine. J Nutr. 2008;138:2025S–31.
11. Mazloomi E, Jazani NH, Sohrabpour M, Ilkhanizadeh B, Shahabi S. Synergistic effects of glutamine and ciprofloxacin in reduction of Pseudomonas aeruginosa-induced septic shock severity. Int Immunopharmacol. 2011;11:2214–9.
12. Briassouli E, Briassoulis G. Glutamine randomized studies in early life: the unsolved riddle of experimental and clinical studies. Clin Dev Immunol. 2012;2012:749189.
13. Morrison AL, Dinges M, Singleton KD, Odoms K, Wong HR, Wischmeyer PE. Glutamine's protection against cellular injury is dependent on heat shock factor-1. Am J Physiol Cell Physiol. 2006;290:C1625–32.
14. Wischmeyer PE, Kahana M, Wolfson R, Ren H, Musch MM, Chang EB. Glutamine induces heat shock protein and protects against endotoxin shock in the rat. J Appl Physiol. 2001;90:2403–10.
15. Pithon-Curi TC, Schumacher RI, Freitas JJ, Lagranha C, Newsholme P, Palanch AC, Doi SQ, Curi R. Glutamine delays spontaneous apoptosis in neutrophils. Am J Physiol Cell Physiol. 2003;284:C1355–61.
16. Singleton KD, Beckey VE, Wischmeyer PE. Glutamine prevents activation of NF-kappaB and stress kinase pathways, attenuates inflammatory cytokine release, and prevents acute respiratory distress syndrome (ARDS) following sepsis. Shock. 2005;24:583–9.
17. Singleton KD, Wischmeyer PE. Oral glutamine enhances heat shock protein expression and improves survival following hyperthermia. Shock. 2006;25:295–9.
18. Sufit A, Weitzel LB, Hamiel C, Queensland K, Dauber I, Rooyackers O, et al. Pharmacologically dosed oral glutamine reduces myocardial injury in patients undergoing cardiac surgery: a randomized pilot feasibility trial. J Parenter Enteral Nutr. 2012;36:556–61.
19. Berg A, Rooyackers O, Norberg A, Wernerman J. Elimination kinetics of L-alanyl-L-glutamine in ICU patients. Amino Acids. 2005;29:221–8.
20. Houdijk AP, Rijnsburger ER, Jansen J, Wesdorp RI, Weiss JK, McCamish MA, et al. Randomised trial of glutamine-enriched enteral nutrition on infectious morbidity in patients with multiple trauma. Lancet. 1998;352:772–6.
21. Kadrofske MM, Parimi PS, Gruca LL, Kalhan SC. Effect of intravenous amino acids on glutamine and protein kinetics in low-birth-weight preterm infants during the immediate neonatal period. Am J Physiol Endocrinol Metab. 2006;290:E622–30.
22. Griffiths RD. Outcome of critically ill patients after supplementation with glutamine. Nutrition. 1997;13:752–4.
23. Joosten KF, Hulst JM. Malnutrition in pediatric hospital patients: current issues. Nutrition. 2011;27:133–7.
24. Roth E, Funovics J, Muhlbacher F, Schemper M, Mauritz W, Sporn P, et al. Metabolic disorders in severe abdominal sepsis: glutamine deficiency in skeletal muscle. Clin Nutr. 1982;1:25–41.
25. Wernerman J. Glutamine supplementation. Ann Intens Care. 2011;1:25.
26. Heyland DK, Dhaliwal R. Role of glutamine supplementation in critical illness given the results of the REDOXS study. J Parenter Enteral Nutr. 2013;37:44.
27. Heyland D, Muscedere J, Wischmeyer PE, Cook D, Jones G, Albert M, Elke G, Berger MM, Day AG, Canadian Critical Care Trials Group. A randomized trial of glutamine and antioxidants in critically ill patients. N Engl J Med. 2013;368:1489–97.
28. Marino LV, Pathan N, Meyer R, Wright V, Habibi P. Glutamine depletion and heat shock protein 70 (HSP70) in children with meningococcal disease Clin Nutr. 2014;33(5):915-21. http://www.ncbi.nlm.nih.gov/pubmed/?term=Marino+LV+and+glutamine.
29. Wheeler DS, Fisher Jr LE, Catravas JD, Jacobs BR, Carcillo JA, Wong HR. Extracellular hsp70 levels in children with septic shock. Pediatr Crit Care Med. 2005;6:308–3011.
30. Tubman TR, Thompson SW, McGuire W. Glutamine supplementation to prevent morbidity and mortality in preterm infants. Cochrane Database Syst Rev. 2012;3:CD001457.
31. Lima AA, Brito LF, Ribeiro HB, Martins MC, Lustosa AP, Rocha EM, et al. Intestinal barrier function and weight gain in malnourished children taking glutamine supplemented enteral formula. J Pediatr Gastroenterol Nutr. 2005;40:28–35.
32. Briassoulis G, Filippou O, Kanariou M, Hatzis T. Comparative effects of early randomized immune or non-immune-enhancing enteral nutrition on cytokine production in children with septic shock. Intensive Care Med. 2005; 31:851–8.
33. Briassoulis G, Filippou O, Kanariou M, Papassotiriou I, Hatzis T. Temporal nutritional and inflammatory changes in children with severe head injury fed a regular or an immune-enhancing diet: a randomized, controlled trial. Pediatr Crit Care Med. 2006;7:56–62.
34. Neu J. Glutamine supplements in premature infants: why and how. J Pediatr Gastroenterol Nutr. 2003;37:533–5.
35. Yalcin SS, Yurdakok K, Tezcan I, Oner L. Effect of glutamine supplementation on diarrhea, interleukin-8 and secretory immunoglobulin A in children with acute diarrhea. J Pediatr Gastroenterol Nutr. 2004;38:494–501.

36. Li ZH, Wang DH, Dong M. Effect of parenteral glutamine supplementation in premature infants. Chin Med J (Engl). 2007;120:140–4.
37. des Robert C, Le Bacquer O, Piloquet H, Rozé JC, Darmaun D. Acute effects of intravenous glutamine supplementation on protein metabolism in very low birth weight infants: a stable isotope study. Pediatr Res. 2002;51:87–93.
38. Ong EG, Eaton S, Wade AM, Horn V, Losty PD, Curry JI, Sugarman ID, Klein NJ, Pierro A, SIGN Trial Group. Randomized clinical trial of glutamine-supplemented versus standard parenteral nutrition in infants with surgical gastrointestinal disease. Br J Surg. 2012;99:929–38.
39. de Kieviet JF, Oosterlaan J, van Zwol A, Boehm G, Lafeber HN, van Elburg RM. Effects of neonatal enteral glutamine supplementation on cognitive, motor and behavioural outcomes in very preterm and/or very low birth weight children at school age. Br J Nutr. 2012;108:2215–20.
40. Vaughn P, Thomas P, Clark R, Neu J. Enteral glutamine supplementation and morbidity in low birth weight infants. J Pediatr. 2003;142:662–8.
41. Neu J, Roig JC, Meetze WH, Veerman M, Carter C, Millsaps M, Bowling D, Dallas MJ, Sleasman J, Knight T, Auestad N. Enteral glutamine supplementation for very low birth weight infants decreases morbidity. J Pediatr. 1997;131:691–9.
42. Parimi PS, Devapatla S, Gruca LL, Amini SB, Hanson RW, Kalhan SC. Effect of enteral glutamine or glycine on whole-body nitrogen kinetics in very-low-birth-weight infants. Am J Clin Nutr. 2004;79:402–9.
43. Roig JC, Meetze WH, Auestad N, Jasionowski T, Veerman M, McMurray CA, Neu J. Enteral glutamine supplementation for the very low birthweight infant: plasma amino acid concentrations. J Nutr. 1996;126(Suppl):1115S–20.
44 van Zwol A, Moll HA, Fetter WP, van Elburg RM. Glutamine-enriched enteral nutrition in very low birthweight infants and allergic and infectious diseases at 6 years of age. Paediatr Perinat Epidemiol. 2011;25:60–6.
45. van Zwol A, van den Berg A, Nieuwenhuis EE, Twisk JW, Fetter WP, van Elburg RM. Cytokine profiles in 1-yr-old very low-birth-weight infants after enteral glutamine supplementation in the neonatal period. Pediatr Allergy Immunol. 2009;20:467–70.
46. Poindexter BB, Langer JC, Dusick AM, Ehrenkranz RA, National Institute of Child H, Human Development Neonatal Research N. Early provision of parenteral amino acids in extremely low birth weight infants: relation to growth and neurodevelopmental outcome. J Pediatr. 2006;148:300–5.
47. Botran M, Lopez-Herce J, Mencia S, Urbano J, Solana MJ, Garcia A. Enteral nutrition in the critically ill child: comparison of standard and protein-enriched diets. J Pediatr. 2011;159:27–32.
48. Mehta NM, Compher C. A.S.P.E.N. Clinical Guidelines: nutrition support of the critically ill child. J Parenter Enteral Nutr. 2009;33:260–76.
49. Carcillo JA, Dean JM, Holubkov R, Berger J, Meert KL, Anand KJ, Zimmerman J, Newth CJ, Harrison R, Burr J, Willson DF, Nicholson C, Eunice Kennedy Shriver National Institute of Child Health and Human Development (NICHD) Collaborative Pediatric Critical Care Research Network (CPCCRN). The randomized comparative pediatric critical illness stress-induced immune suppression (CRISIS) prevention trial. Pediatr Crit Care Med. 2012;13:165–73.
50. Briassoulis G, Filippou O, Hatzi E, Papassotiriou I, Hatzis T. Early enteral administration of immunonutrition in critically ill children: results of a blinded randomized controlled clinical trial. Nutrition. 2005;21:799–807.
51. Yang DL, Xu JF. Effect of dipeptide of glutamine and alanine on severe traumatic brain injury. Chin J Traumatol. 2007;10:145–9.

Chapter 17
Glutamine and Ammonia in Hepatic Encephalopathy

Sherry Dadsetan, Helle S. Waagepetersen, Arne Schousboe, and Lasse K. Bak

Key Points

- During hyperammonemia, ammonia is fixated into glutamate and glutamine by the enzymes glutamate dehydrogenase and glutamine synthetase, respectively.
- Whereas glutamate dehydrogenase is present in neurons and astrocytes, glutamine synthetase is present in astrocytes only.
- Hyperammonemia leads to an elevated production of glutamine in astrocytes, which is believed to be one cause among several of the pathological changes observed in hepatic encephalopathy.
- Inhibition of glutamine synthetase with the drug methionine sulfoximine leads to lower glutamine levels but is not without side effects.
- Inhibition of glutamine synthetase in vitro and in vivo leads to synthesis of alanine, a process that might serve as an alternative ammonia scavenger pathway in the brain.
- It is concluded that partial inhibition of glutamine synthetase may represent a viable pharmacotherapeutic approach.

Keywords Hepatic encephalopathy • Glutamine • Neuron • Astrocyte • Alanine

Abbreviations

AAT	Aspartate aminotransferase
ALAT	Alanine aminotransferase
BAPTA	1,2-Bis(o-aminophenoxy)ethane-*N*,*N*,*N*′,*N*′-tetraacetic acid
GABA	γ-Aminobutyric acid
GDH	Glutamate dehydrogenase
HE	Hepatic encephalopathy
mPT	Mitochondrial permeability transition
MSO	Methionine sulfoximine
PAG	Phosphate-activated glutaminase

S. Dadsetan • H.S. Waagepetersen • A. Schousboe • L.K. Bak (✉)
Department of Drug Design and Pharmacology, Faculty of Health and Medical Sciences,
University of Copenhagen, 2 Universitetsparken, Copenhagen 2100, Denmark
e-mail: sdadsetan@hotmail.com; helle.waagepetersen@sund.ku.dk;
arne.schousboe@sund.ku.dk; laba@sund.ku.dk

R. Rajendram et al. (eds.), *Glutamine in Clinical Nutrition*, Nutrition and Health,
DOI 10.1007/978-1-4939-1932-1_17, © Springer Science+Business Media New York 2015

Introduction

The amino acid glutamine is present in all tissues and it serves several purposes depending on the tissue in question. This chapter is devoted to a discussion of its role in relation to the elevated ammonia levels found in the brain in the context of hepatic encephalopathy (HE), a disturbance of the central nervous system due to liver failure [1] characterized by cognitive, psychiatric, and motor deficits. Early symptoms include reversal of sleep pattern, apathy, hypersomnia, irritability, and personal neglect and HE can progressively lead to coma and death [2]. Brain ammonia homeostasis is functionally associated with metabolism in the liver since this organ is responsible for removal of excess ammonia from the bloodstream. Thus, this chapter is intended to focus on glutamine metabolism in these two organs.

In the brain glutamine plays an important role in the maintenance of amino acid mediated neurotransmission that involves the two metabolically closely related amino acids glutamate and GABA in addition to glycine. The latter amino acid will not be dealt with, as its metabolism is not directly related to glutamine. Glutamine is the precursor for glutamate, which subsequently can be α-decarboxylated to form GABA. This means that the excitatory transmitter glutamate can be converted to the inhibitory neurotransmitter GABA and since these neurotransmission systems account for the vast majority of synapses in the brain [3], the common precursor glutamine is at center stage regarding the availability of these transmitters having opposite effects on neurons.

Glutamine Metabolism in the Brain

Interconversion of glutamine and glutamate is catalyzed by two different enzymes, glutaminase and glutamine synthetase (GS). As the former enzyme is activated by phosphate [4] it is normally referred to as phosphate-activated glutaminase (PAG). The enzyme catalyzes a hydrolysis of the amide group in glutamine resulting in the production of glutamate and ammonia. This ammonia, which is primarily produced in glutamatergic neurons due to a large demand for transmitter production [5], needs subsequently to be transferred to surrounding astrocytes and this aspect will be dealt with below. The expression level of PAG is high in glutamatergic neurons but it does not serve as a marker enzyme as it is present in other types of neurons including GABAergic cells as well as in astrocytes [5].

The reaction in the opposite direction, i.e., conversion of glutamate to glutamine catalyzed by GS, is energy dependent and requires ATP in addition to the co-substrate ammonia to occur [6]. The K_m values for the three substrates [6] are within the range of their cellular concentrations but it is unlikely that the enzyme will be saturated, which means that its activity will fluctuate with changes in the cellular level of the substrates [5]. This enzyme has been shown to be irreversibly inhibited by the compound methionine sulfoximine (MSO) and this inhibitor is of importance for the assessment of the functional significance of GS [7].

It is important to note that while PAG is ubiquitously expressed, albeit with a higher level in neurons compared to astrocytes [8], GS is exclusively expressed in astrocytes [9]. As mentioned above this means that ammonia produced in neurons by the action of PAG must be transferred to the astrocytes to function as a substrate in the GS catalyzed formation of glutamine. This requires a mechanism responsible for transfer of ammonia from neurons to astrocytes and different shuttle mechanisms based on transfer of the amino acids alanine or one of the branched chain amino acids have been proposed [10]. A detailed discussion about this is beyond the scope of this chapter. The different cellular location of PAG and GS requires that glutamine can be shuttled between astrocytes and neurons with a concomitant opposite flux of glutamate. This constitutes the glutamate-glutamine cycle (Fig. 17.1) which was formulated several decades ago based on fundamental studies of glutamate and glutamine metabolism in brain tissue [11].

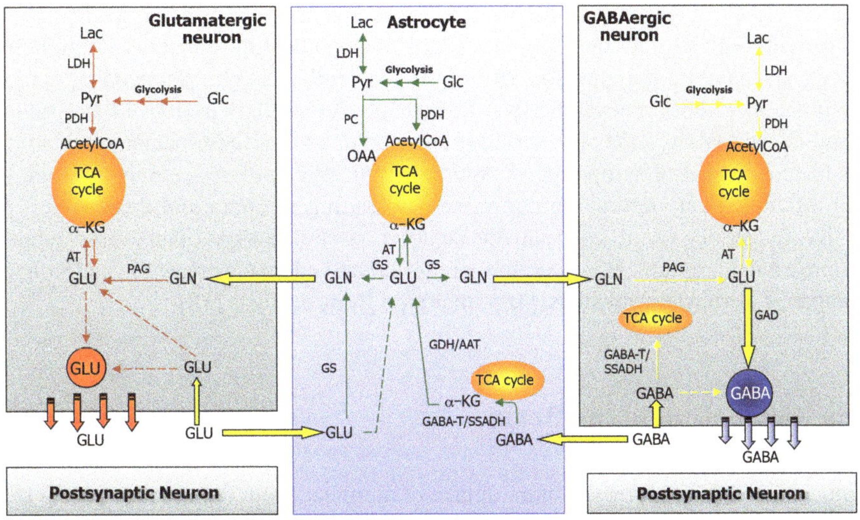

Fig. 17.1 Cartoon depicting the metabolic interactions between a glutamatergic neuron, a GABAergic neuron and an astrocyte. In all cell types, glucose (Glc) is metabolized to pyruvate (Pyr) via the multi-step process of glycolysis and either reduced to lactate (Lac; by lactate dehydrogenase, LDH) or oxidized to acetylCoA (by pyruvate dehydrogenase complex, PDH) that will subsequently be oxidized in the tricarboxylic acid (TCA) cycle. In astrocytes, pyruvate may also undergo carboxylation to form oxaloacetate (OAA), an anaplerotic reaction catalyzed by pyruvate carboxylase (PC). At the glutamatergic synapse, glutamate (GLU) released as neurotransmitter will be taken up by nearby astrocytes and amidated to glutamine (GLN) by glutamine synthetase (GS) and returned to the neuron for reuse as neurotransmitter, thus concluding the so-called glutamate-glutamine cycle. In neurons, glutamate is re-formed from glutamine by the mitochondrial enzyme phosphate-activated glutaminase (PAG). A similar cycle exists at the GABAergic synapse; however, the carbon skeleton of GABA enters the TCA cycle as indicated. GABA is transformed to the TCA cycle intermediate succinate via two reactions catalyzed by GABA-transaminase (GABA-T) and succinic semialdehyde dehydrogenase (SSADH). The GABA-T catalyzed reaction produces glutamate from α-ketoglutarate (α-KG) that may then be used as precursor for glutamine synthesis and eventual synthesis of GABA in the neuron. This process is known as the GABA shunt since it bypasses two reactions of the (astrocytic) TCA cycle. In GABAergic neurons, GABA is synthesized from glutamate by the enzyme glutamate decarboxylase (GAD). Notice that in all cell types, glutamate is in transamination equilibrium (catalyzed by aminotransferases, AT) with α-ketoglutarate linking TCA cycle metabolism with glutamate and GABA homeostasis. Also notice that reuptake of released glutamate and GABA takes place to some extent as well and that the GABA shunt works in GABAergic neurons when GABA is taken up into the presynaptic terminal

Ammonia Metabolism in the Liver

In the liver glutamine metabolism is in principle identical to that described above for the brain involving the same set of enzymes albeit the liver seems to primarily express a glutaminase isozyme different from the major isoform in the brain [12]. It is important to note that contrary to the brain, the liver has the capacity to dispose of ammonia by producing urea. However, if this pathway is disturbed during liver failure, the result will be a large increase in the blood level of ammonia, which will lead to uptake of ammonia into the brain [13] that may progress to HE. The liver is responsible for metabolism of exogenous and endogenous substances, mainly into hydrophilic excretable compounds and it is the only tissue expressing a complete urea cycle. Ammonia generated in the gastrointestinal tract, due to breakdown of proteins, is released into the portal blood and transported to the liver. In the hepatocytes ammonia is detoxified by incorporation in urea, which is subsequently excreted in the urine and accordingly providing low ammonia levels in the circulatory system of healthy subjects. During liver failure a diminished capacity for hepatic urea synthesis and increased portosystemic shunting results in an impaired ability to detoxify ammonia. Consequently, arterial ammonia levels may rise up to 400 μM in patients with liver failure from the 30 μM found in healthy subjects with highest increases found in acute liver failure patients [14–16]. Acute liver failure is characterized by a rapid loss of hepatocyte function without preexisting liver disease most commonly as a result of viral hepatitis or drug-induced hepatotoxicity [17]. The onset of encephalopathy in these patients typically occurs in 1–2 weeks from the onset of symptoms. A common clinical feature of acute liver failure is cerebral edema and intracranial hypertension consequently leading to coma and death if left untreated. In chronic liver failure due to cirrhosis, patients do not show clinical signs of an overt cerebral edema or increased intracranial pressure. However, low-grade cerebral edema is present in addition to morphological changes of astrocytes known as Alzheimer type II astrocytosis [18].

Ammonia Metabolism in the Brain

Hyperammonemia leads to increased brain uptake of ammonia from the blood [13, 19]. In the brain, blood-borne ammonia is primarily metabolized by GS, which as stated above is exclusively located in the astrocytes and catalyzes the incorporation of ammonia in glutamate to form glutamine. Glutamine is released from the astrocytes and may subsequently be either released from the brain into the circulatory system or taken up by the neurons. In neurons, glutamine will be hydrolyzed by the mitochondrial enzyme PAG deamidating glutamine, thus forming glutamate while liberating ammonia. In glutamatergic neurons the excitatory neurotransmitter glutamate is released upon depolarization from the presynaptic neuron. The released glutamate is for the major part transported into surrounding astrocytes equipped with extremely efficient glutamate transporters [20]. Altogether these processes constitute the glutamate-glutamine cycle (Fig. 17.1) also mentioned above. In both neurons and astrocytes the mitochondrial enzyme glutamate dehydrogenase (GDH) upholds a link between neurotransmission and energy metabolism and it catalyzes the reversible conversion of tricarboxylic acid cycle intermediate α-ketoglutarate to glutamate during fixation of ammonia while using NADH as a co-factor. The amino group of glutamate may subsequently be transferred to keto acids through aminotransferase reactions. The aminotransferases aspartate aminotransferase (AAT) and alanine aminotransferase (ALAT), which exist in both a cytosolic and a mitochondrial isoform, transfer the amino group of glutamate to either oxaloacetate or pyruvate forming aspartate or alanine, respectively (Fig. 17.2).

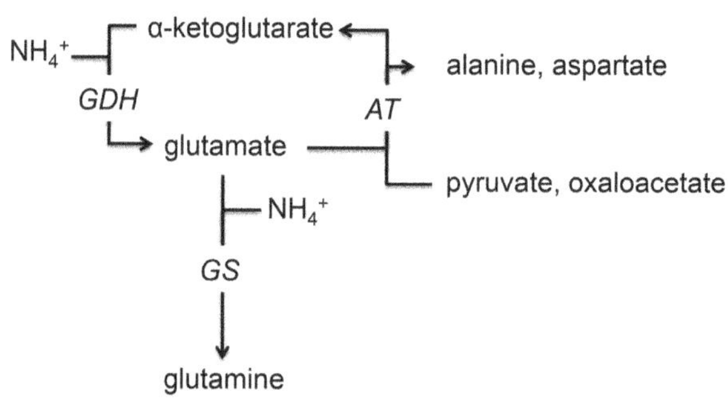

Fig. 17.2 Depiction of the enzymatically catalyzed chemical reactions involving fixation of ammonia into glutamate and glutamine by glutamate dehydrogenase (GDH) and glutamine synthetase (GS), respectively. The associated transamination reactions producing alanine and aspartate from pyruvate and oxaloacetate, respectively, are also shown. These reactions are catalyzed by designated aminotransferases (ATs). It should be noted that GS is only expressed in astrocytes whereas GDH is expressed in both neurons and astrocytes

The most pivotal reaction in brain ammonia detoxification is through glutamine synthesis via GS and studies reveal that up to 85 % of blood-borne ammonia is incorporated in glutamine [21–23]. Consequently, hyperammonemia is associated with elevated brain glutamine levels. Alternative mechanisms for removal of excess ammonia are discussed below.

Effects of Hyperammonemia on Brain Cells

The pathological mechanisms leading to HE remains poorly understood. However, there is a consensus that hyperammonia plays a pivotal role in the etiology of this condition. In HE the astrocytes are the principal cells affected by ammonia. The astrocytic end-feet completely cover the CNS capillaries ensuring that any ammonia entering the brain is immediately metabolized, thus protecting the neurons from immediate ammonia toxicity.

Studies in vivo and in astrocyte cultures have shown that elevated ammonia levels induce oxidative stress through a mechanism that remains incompletely understood [18, 24]. However, oxidative stress has multiple effects on astrocytes and seems to play an important role in the pathogenesis of HE [18, 24]. Exposure of ammonia to astrocyte cultures causes an intracellular rise in Ca^{2+} resulting in free radical production leading to oxidative stress [24]. Furthermore, ammonia induced activation of the Ca^{2+}-dependent enzymes constitutive nitric oxide synthase, NADPH oxidase and phospholipase A2 which generate nitric oxide and superoxide was diminished by the Ca^{2+} chelator BAPTA (1,2-bis(o-aminophenoxy)ethane-*N*,*N*,*N*′,*N*′-tetraacetic acid) as well as by specific inhibitors of the enzymes, indicating a role of these enzymes in mediating oxidative stress during hyperammonemia [25]. Oxidative stress and intracellular Ca^{2+} increases can lead to induction of the mitochondrial permeability transition (mPT) pore characterized by an increased permeability of the inner mitochondrial membrane to small molecules. The mPT is mediated through a large increase in mitochondrial Ca^{2+} levels leading to a collapse of the mitochondrial inner membrane potential which consequently results in osmotic swelling of the mitochondrial matrix, uncoupling of oxidative phosphorylation, interruption of ATP synthesis, and generation of reactive oxygen species. In astrocyte cultures ammonia exposure was demonstrated to lead to induction of the mPT and this effect as well as free radical production was blocked by addition of the GS inhibitor, methionine sulfoximine (MSO) implying that glutamine rather than ammonia per se is responsible for these events [26, 27]. This effect of glutamine in astrocyte mitochondria has been coined the 'Trojan Horse' hypothesis (see Fig. 17.3) and is based on the observation that exposure of astrocytes to glutamine results in free radical generation, which could be prevented by inhibition of PAG [28, 29]. It was also found that glutamine had no such effect in neurons. This is likely due to a difference between neuronal and astrocytic PAG with regard to inhibition by ammonia since only the neuronal enzyme exhibits this inhibitory pattern [29]. This together with a similar result in cultured cortical neurons treated with ammonia showing that this was not associated with induction of mPT [26] indicate a vital role for the increased glutamine synthesis in astrocytes in mediating the mPT.

Glutamine synthesis is the main mechanism for removal of ammonia in brain and the glutamine level is increased during hyperammonemia. In 1964 it was demonstrated by Warren and Schenker [30] how addition of MSO protected mice from ammonia toxicity implying a pathogenic role for glutamine in the development of HE. Decades later Brusilow and Traystman [31] put forward the hypothesis that glutamine formation in astrocytes was a key mechanism for astrocyte swelling in hyperammonemia, with elevated glutamine levels acting as an osmolyte leading to influx of water into the cell. Although numerous studies have demonstrated that MSO ameliorates astrocyte swelling and increases survival of mice it remains controversial that glutamine acts through an osmotic effect [32].

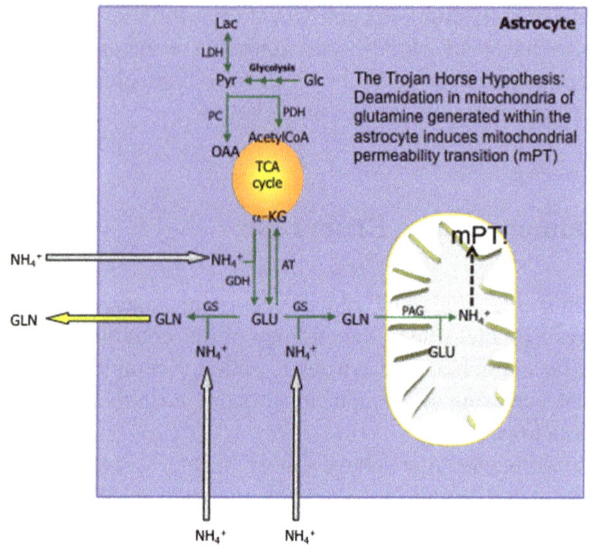

Fig. 17.3 Cartoon depicting the ammonia fixating pathways active during hyperammonemic conditions in astrocytes, and the putative induction of mitochondrial membrane permeability transition (MPT) by deamidation of glutamine (GLN) by phosphate-activated glutaminase (PAG) in mitochondria; the latter is known as the Trojan Horse Hypothesis. Ammonia fixation is catalyzed by glutamate dehydrogenase (GDH) and glutamine synthetase (GS). Please see text and legends to Figs. 17.1 and 17.2 for details. *AT* aminotransferase, *Glc* glucose, *GLU* glutamate, *α-KG* α-ketoglutarate, *Lac* lactate, *LDH* lactate dehydrogenase, *OAA* oxaloacetate, *PDH* pyruvate dehydrogenase, *PC* pyruvate carboxylase, *Pyr* pyruvate, *TCA* tricarboxylic acid

Alternative Processes for Ammonia Fixation in the Brain

While glutamine synthesis is pivotal for brain ammonia detoxification during hyperammonemia studies in co-cultures of neurons and astrocytes have demonstrated significantly increased incorporation of ammonia in alanine during hyperammonemic conditions [33]. This suggests that transamination into alanine following reductive amination by GDH may constitute an important pathway for ammonia detoxification (Fig. 17.2). Since the blood–brain barrier expresses transport systems that could facilitate alanine efflux [34] it would be plausible that alanine synthesis, release into the extracellular space and further on into the bloodstream could serve as a detoxification pathway distinct from cerebral synthesis of glutamine and subsequent brain efflux. Ammonia incorporation in aspartate is augmented during hyperammonemic conditions in co-cultures [33, 35] suggesting that transamination reactions of both ALAT and AAT display enhanced activity during hyperammonemia. However, since aspartate is an excitatory amino acid, thus only present in the extracellular space at very low levels, synthesis of aspartate cannot be considered an alternative ammonia-scavenging pathway. In support of this, aspartate is not released from healthy astrocytes due to glutamate transporters generating an inward gradient of glutamate and aspartate. In vivo studies demonstrated that during inhibition of GS with MSO rats infused with $^{15}NH_4^+$ exhibited increased incorporation of ^{15}N in cerebral alanine, suggesting that inhibiting GS leads to an additional enhancement of alanine formation for ammonia detoxification during hyperammonemia. In co-culture experiments, the de novo synthesis of alanine was mediated through the concerted action of GDH and ALAT [35, 36]. It may be noted that while the ammonia-induced increased glutamine production was associated with an enhanced pyruvate carboxylase dependent anaplerosis (for further explanation, see Fig. 17.4) the augmented alanine production seen in the presence of the GS inhibitor MSO was associated with an increased glycolysis [36]. This means that the astrocytic pyruvate metabolism is regulated by the demand for alanine production or oxaloacetate production to compensate for removal of α-ketoglutarate used for

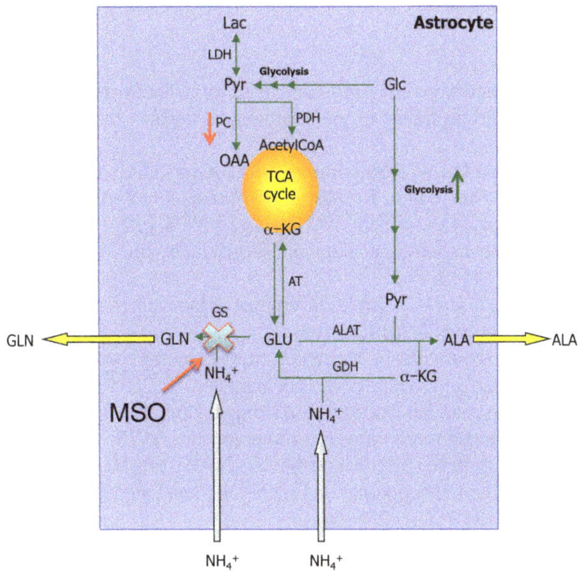

Fig. 17.4 Cartoon showing the putative effects on de novo synthesis and release of alanine (ALA) when glutamine synthetase (GS) is inhibited by methionine sulfoximine (MSO) or a similar drug, as indicated. Under conditions with decreased activity of GS, glycolysis and subsequent de novo synthesis and release of alanine may operate as an alternative ammonia-scavenging pathway. This will decrease pyruvate carboxylase (PC) activity and increase glycolytic activity, as indicated by *red* and *green arrows*, respectively. See text and legends to Figs. 17.1, 17.2, and 17.3 for further details. *ALAT* alanine aminotransferase, *AT* aminotransferase, *GDH* glutamate dehydrogenase, *Glc* glucose, *GLN* glutamine, *GLU* glutamate, *α-KG* α-ketoglutarate, *Lac* lactate, *LDH* lactate dehydrogenase, *OAA* oxaloacetate, *PDH* pyruvate dehydrogenase, *PC* pyruvate carboxylase, *Pyr* pyruvate, *TCA* tricarboxylic acid

glutamine synthesis (Fig. 17.4). Hence, it may be possible that decreasing cerebral GS activity can function as a therapeutic avenue in hyperammonemia alleviating the detrimental effects of glutamine accumulation. The alanine-synthesizing pathway was not sufficient in alleviating the increased ammonia level arisen from whole-body GS inhibition [35]. However, in vivo studies in bile duct-ligated rats infused with $^{15}NH_4^+$ showed that an augmented [^{15}N]ammonia incorporation in alanine is specific to brain and not observed in the peripheral tissues, indicating that alanine as an ammonia scavenging function may still be relevant for cerebral ammonia detoxification [37]. Treatment with a glutamine synthetase inhibitor would indeed be relevant for amelioration of brain edema and intracranial hypertension in acute liver failure patients.

Concluding Remarks

As discussed, fixation of ammonia into glutamine in the brain during hyperammonia is probably causing a number of the symptoms related to HE. Thus, inhibition of glutamine synthesis in conjunction with measures to lower blood ammonia might represent a viable therapeutic avenue, especially if the brain is able to increase synthesis and export of alanine as an alternative ammonia scavenger. However, a number of challenges remain. In particular, to avoid detrimental effects of increased ammonia levels in the circulatory system a full systemic inhibition of glutamine synthesis is not desirable. Ideally, one should aim to develop a pharmacological treatment that is selectively able to partially block the synthesis of glutamine in the brain, although this will be a major challenge. Future work is needed to prove if this is indeed a viable solution, and if it is at all possible.

References

1. Blei AT, Cordoba J. Hepatic encephalopathy. Am J Gastroenterol. 2001;96:1968–76.
2. Al Sibae MR, Mcguire BM. Current trends in the treatment of hepatic encephalopathy. Ther Clin Risk Manag. 2009;5:617–26.
3. Madsen KM, Larsson OM, Schousboe A. Regulation of excitation by GABA neurotransmission: focus on metabolism and transport. In: Darlison MG, editor. Results and problems in cell differentiation. Inhibitory regulation of excitatory neurotransmission, vol. 44. New York, NY: Springer; 2008. p. 201–21.
4. Errera M, Greenstein JP. Phosphate-activated glutaminase in kidney and other tissues. J Biol Chem. 1949;178: 495–501.
5. Schousboe A, Bak LK, Waagepetersen HS. Astrocytic control of biosynthesis and turnover of the neurotransmitters glutamate and GABA. Front Endocrinol. 2013;15:102.
6. Pamiljans V, Krishnaswamy PR, Dumville G, Meister A. Studies on the mechanism of glutamine synthesis; isolation and properties of the enzyme from sheep brain. Biochemistry. 1962;1:153–8.
7. Brusilow SW, Koehler RC, Traystman RJ, Cooper AJ. Astrocyte glutamine synthetase: importance in hyperammonemic syndromes and potential target for therapy. Neurotherapeutics. 2010;7:452–70.
8. Lovatt D, Sonnewald U, Waagepetersen HS, Schousboe A, He W, Lin JH, Han X, Takano T, Wang S, Sim FJ, Goldman SA, Nedergaard M. The transcriptome and metabolic gene signature of protoplasmic astrocytes in the adult murine cortex. J Neurosci. 2007;27:12255–66.
9. Norenberg MD, Martinez-Hernandez A. Fine structural localization of glutamine synthetase in astrocytes of rat brain. Brain Res. 1979;161:303–10.
10. Bak LK, Schousboe A, Waagepetersen HS. Brain energy and ammonia metabolism. In: Keiding S, Sorensen M, editors. Functional molecular imaging in hepatology. Aarhus Denmark: Bentham Books; 2012. p. 129–44.
11. Schousboe A. Studies of brain metabolism: a historical perspective. In: Choi I-Y, Gruetter R, editors. Advances in neurobiology. Neural metabolism in vivo, vol. 4. New York, NY: Springer; 2012. p. 909–20.
12. Marquez J, Tosina M, de la Rosa V, Segura JA, Alonso FJ, Mates JM, Campos-Sandoval JA. New insights into brain glutaminases: beyond their role on glutamatergic transmission. Neurochem Int. 2009;55:64–70.
13. Keiding S, Sorensen M, Bender D, Munk OL, Ott P, Vilstrup H. Brain metabolism of 13N-ammonia during acute hepatic encephalopathy in cirrhosis measured by positron emission tomography. Hepatology. 2006;43:42–50.
14. Butterworth RF. Pathophysiology of hepatic encephalopathy: a new look at ammonia. Metab Brain Dis. 2002;17:221–7.
15. Olde Damink SW, Deutz NE, Dejong CH, Soeters PB, Jalan R. Interorgan ammonia metabolism in liver failure. Neurochem Int. 2002;41:177–88.
16. Wright G, Noiret L, Olde Damink SW, Jalan R. Interorgan ammonia metabolism in liver failure: the basis of current and future therapies. Liver Int. 2011;31:163–75.
17. Lee WM. Acute liver failure. Semin Respir Crit Care Med. 2012;33:36–45.
18. Haussinger D, Schliess F. Pathogenetic mechanisms of hepatic encephalopathy. Gut. 2008;57:1156–65.
19. Dam G, Keiding S, Munk OL, Ott P, Vilstrup H, Bak LK, Waageptersen HS, Schousboe A, Sorensen M. Hepatic encephalopathy is associated with decreased cerebral oxygen metabolism and blood flow, not increased ammonia uptake. Hepatology. 2013;57:258–65.
20. Danbolt NC. Glutamate uptake. Prog Neurobiol. 2001;65:1–105.
21. Cooper AJ, McDonald JM, Gelbard AS, Gledhill RF, Duffy TE. The metabolic fate of 13N-labeled ammonia in rat brain. J Biol Chem. 1979;254:4982–92.
22. Yudkoff M, Nissim I, Pleasure D. Astrocyte metabolism of [15N]glutamine: implications for the for the glutamine-glutamate cycle. J Neurochem. 1988;51:843–50.
23. Sonnewald U, Westergaard N, Jones P, Taylor A, Bachelard HS, Scousboe A. Metabolism of [U-13C5]glutamine in cultured astrocytes studied by NMR spectroscopy: first evidence of astrocytic pyruvate recycling. J Neurochem. 1996;67:2566–72.
24. Norenberg MD, Rama Rao KV, Jayakumar AR. Signaling factors in the mechanism of ammonia neurotoxicity. Metab Bran Dis. 2009;24:103–17.
25. Jayakumar AR, Rama Rao KV, Tong XY, Norenberg MD. Calcium in the mechanism of ammonia-induced astrocyte swelling. J Neurochem. 2009;109 suppl 1:252–7.
26. Bai G, Rama Rao KV, Murthy CR, Panickar KS, Jayakumar AR, Norenberg MD. Ammonia induces the mitochondrial permeability transition in primary cultures of rat astrocytes. J Neurosci Res. 2001;66:981–91.
27. Murthy CR, Rama Rao KV, Bai G, Norenberg MD. Ammonia-induced production of free radicals in primary cultures of rat astrocytes. J Neurosci Res. 2001;66:282–8.
28. Albrecht J, Norenberg MD. Glutamine: a Trojan horse in ammonia neurotoxicity. Hepatology. 2006;44:788–94.
29. Jayakumar AR, Rama Rao KV, Schousboe A, Norenberg MD. Glutamine-induced free radical production in cultured astrocytes. Glia. 2004;46:296–301.

30. Warren KS, Schenker S. Effect of inhibitor of glutamine synthesis (methionine sulfoximine) on ammonia toxicity and metabolism. J Lab Clin Med. 1964;64:442–9.
31. Brusilow SW, Traystman R. Hepatic encephalopathy. New Engl J Med. 1986;314:786–7.
32. Rama Rao KV, Norenberg MD. Glutamine in the pathogenesis of hepatic encephalopathy: the trojan horse revisited. Neurochem Res. 2014;39:593.
33. Leke R, Bak LK, Anker M, Melø TM, Sorensen M, Keiding S, Vilstrup H, Ott P, Portela LV, Sonnewald U, Schousboe A, Waagepetersen HS. Detoxification of ammonia in mouse cortical GABAergic cell cultures increases neuronal oxidative metabolism and reveals an emerging role for release of glucose-derived alanine. Neurotox Res. 2011;19:496–510.
34. Hawkins RA, O'Kane RL, Simpson IA, Vina JR. Structure of the blood-brain barrier and its role in the transport of amino acids. J Nutr. 2006;136 suppl 1:s218–26.
35. Dadsetan S, Kukolj E, Bak LK, Sorensen M, Ott P, Vilstrup A, Schousboe A, Keiding S, Waagepetersen HS. Brain alanine formation as an ammonia-scavenging pathway during hyperammonemia: effects of glutamine synthetase inhibition in rats and astrocyte-neuron co-cultures. J Cereb Blood Flow Metab. 2013;33:1235–41.
36. Dadsetan S, Bak LK, Sorensen M, Keiding S, Vilstrup H, Ott P, Leke R, Schousboe A, Waagepetersen HS. Inhibition of glutamine synthesis induces glutamate dehydrogenase-dependent ammonia fixation into alanine in co-cultures of astrocytes and neurons. Neurochem Int. 2011;59:482–8.
37. Fries A, Dadsetan S, Keiding S, Bak LK, Schousboe A, Waagepetersen HS, Simonsen M, Ott P, Vilstrup H, Sorensen M. Effect of glutamine synthetase inhibition on brain and interorgan ammonia metabolism in bile duct ligated rats. J Cereb Blood Flow Metab. 2014;34(3):460–6.

Chapter 18
The Oral Glutamine Challenge in Liver Cirrhosis

Javier Ampuero and Manuel Romero-Gómez

Key Points

- Glutamine is an essential amino acid in catabolic states.
- Glutamine is metabolized to glutamate and ammonia by the enzyme glutaminase.
- Glutaminase plays a crucial role in the cause of hepatic encephalopathy.
- Oral glutamine challenge is a test which increases blood ammonia after glutamine intake.
- Oral glutamine challenge is easy to perform and is comfortable and safe for patients.
- Oral glutamine challenge predicts minimal hepatic encephalopathy and is related to poor survival

Keywords Oral glutamine challenge • Glutaminase • Ammonia • Cirrhosis • Hepatic encephalopathy

Abbreviations

GA	Glutaminase
GS	Glutamine synthetase
HE	Hepatic encephalopathy
KGA	Kidney-type glutaminase
LGA	Liver-type glutaminase
LOLA	L-Ornithine-L-aspartate
MHE	Minimal hepatic encephalopathy
OGC	Oral glutamine challenge
OHE	Overt hepatic encephalopathy
T2DM	Type 2 diabetes mellitus

J. Ampuero, M.D.
Unit for Clinical Management of Digestive Diseases, Valme University Hospital, Sevilla, Spain,
Jose María Pemán Street, number 8, 3°2, Córdoba, Andalucía 14004, Spain
e-mail: javi.ampuero@gmail.com

M. Romero-Gómez, M.D., Ph.D. (✉)
Unit for Clinical Management of Digestive Diseases, Valme University Hospital, Sevilla, Spain,
Avenida de Bellavista s/n, Sevilla, Andalucía 41014, Spain
e-mail: mromerogomez@us.es

R. Rajendram et al. (eds.), *Glutamine in Clinical Nutrition*, Nutrition and Health,
DOI 10.1007/978-1-4939-1932-1_18, © Springer Science+Business Media New York 2015

Introduction

Glutamine is one of the 20 amino acids (a nonessential neutral amino acid) encoded by the genetic code. When it is enterally administered, glutamine is absorbed from the jejunum. Then, it is metabolized to glutamate and ammonia by the enzyme glutaminase (GA). It has been described that there are three forms of mitochondrial glutaminase in the body: liver-type glutaminase (LGA), kidney-type glutaminase (KGA), and C-type glutaminase (CGA) (found in peripheral mononuclear cells). The LGA is mainly restricted to the liver whereas the KGA is widely distributed in most glutamine-using tissues [1]. The liver plays an essential role in glutamine metabolism (especially regulation), since the liver takes up large amounts of glutamine derived from the gut; it has been documented that at least 50–60 % of total gut ammonia is derived from uptake of glutamine [2]. Ultimately, the enzyme glutamine synthetase (GS) plays a pivotal role in ammonia detoxification; its function is effectively to remove ammonia during the process of conversion of glutamate to glutamine.

The Test

Oral Glutamine Challenge

Oral glutamine challenge (OGC) is a test which aims to measure increase in blood ammonia after glutamine intake, what is similar to the situation that occurs after a protein meal. The test is performed in the morning following an overnight fast. A venous cannula is inserted and maintained patent with saline solution. Then, patients are given either 10 or 20 g of glutamine in a solution of 100 ml of water. Twenty grams of glutamine contains 3.8 g of nitrogen, which approximates to 24 g of protein. Blood samples are taken at time 0, 30, 60 and 90 min post-glutamine load to measure blood ammonia (Fig. 18.1).

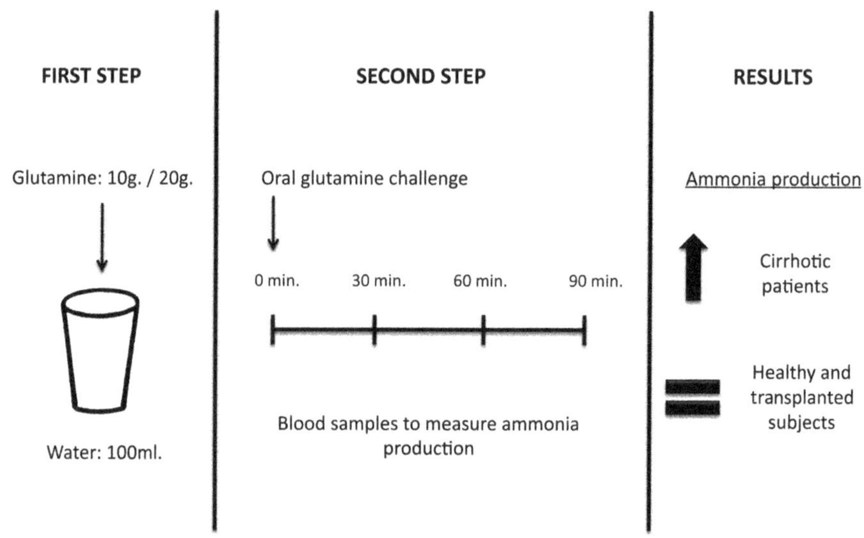

Fig. 18.1 (a) Oral glutamine challenge: steps and interpretation; (b) 10 or 20 g of glutamine is dissolved in 100 ml of water. After that, blood samples are taken at time 0, 30, 60 and 90 min post-glutamine load to measure blood ammonia. OGC induces an increase in blood ammonia in patients with cirrhosis but not in healthy control

Interpretation of the Test

OGC induces an increase in blood ammonia in patients with cirrhosis but not in healthy controls or transplanted subjects [3]. Ammonia response is defined as the ammonia concentration at 1 h following the oral glutamine load. The ammonia concentration reaches the peak between 30 and 60 min after the load; this period of time suggests that the increase in blood ammonia is due to the metabolism of glutamine in the small intestine. Normal venous blood ammonia values in healthy adults are less than 75 mg/dl. A pathological response curve for glutamine tolerance is defined as an ammonia rise to 128 mg/dl at 60 min after the glutamine ingestion.

Adverse Effects

No serious adverse effects have been described in the different published studies, especially with 10 g of glutamine. Typical symptoms described are nausea, vomiting, or dizziness.

Glutamine in Cirrhosis

Glutamine deamidation by intestinal GA seems to be the main source of ammonia in patients with cirrhosis. Thus, blood ammonia levels increase and get to the central nervous system where ammonia may promote toxic effects. Similar effects have been described in rats [4]. Consequently, hepatic encephalopathy (HE) can be triggered without the participation of gut bacteria. When glutamine entries in astrocyte, it causes cell swelling, which leads to a cascade of events resulting in HE. Thus, glutaminase activity has been linked to ammonia production and HE, especially type C (Table 18.1). However, patients with cirrhosis and the same liver dysfunction, which show the same precipitating factor, not always develop overt hepatic encephalopathy (OHE). These data support the hypothesis that a genetic factor is implicated in the development of HE. In fact, Romero-Gómez et al. identified two different haplotypes, related to glutaminase gene, which were linked to the risk of overt HE. Furthermore, they identified a microsatellite in the promoter region of glutaminase gene that, depending on the lenght of alleles, increased the risk of overt HE. The study included 286 cirrhotic patients (109 in estimation cohort and 177 in validation cohort) and 107 healthy control subjects. Patients having two long alleles of the microsatellite in estimation cohort (H.R. 3.12 (95 % CI 1.39–7.02)) and validation cohort (H.R. 2.1 (95 % CI 1.17–3.79)) showed an increased risk of HE (Fig. 18.2). These data was supported by functional studies: higher luciferase activity was observed in cells transfected with the long form of the microsatellite, which suggested that the long microsatellite enhances glutaminase transcriptional activity [5].

Table 18.1 Classification of hepatic encephalopathy

Type	Definition
A	Acute and hyperacute liver failure
B	Portosystemic bypass without intrinsic hepatocellular disease
C	Cirrhosis and portal hypertension with portosystemic shunts

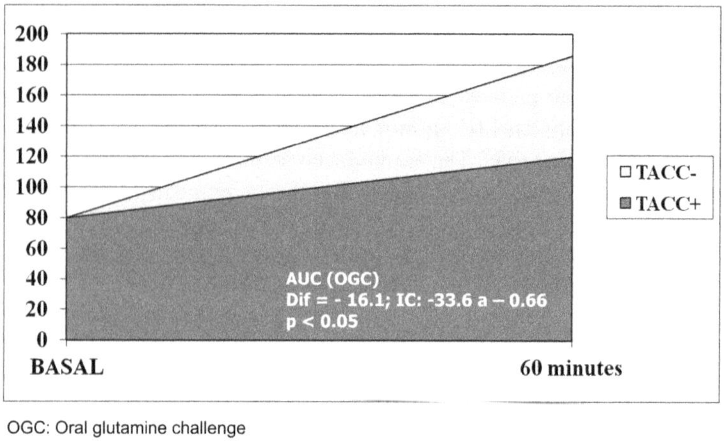

Fig. 18.2 (a) Intestinal ammonia production according to TACC haplotype after OGC; (b) TACC haplotype decreases ammonia production and, consequently, shows a decreased risk of HE

Table 18.2 Mental status according to West Haven criteria

	Conscious	Neuropsyquiatric symptoms	Neurological symptoms
Grade 0 (MHE)	Normal	Impairments detectable by psychometric tests	None
Grade 1	Slight mental impairment	Dysphoria, irritability, anxiety	Psychomotor slowing
Grade 2	Fatigue, apathy, letarghy	Subtle personality changes, slight disorientation, inappropriate behavior	Flapping tremor, ataxia
Grade 3	Somnolence to stupor	Gross disorientation	Clonus, asterixis
Grade 4	Coma	None	Increased intracranial pressure

MHE Minimal hepatic encephalopathy

OGC as a Prognostic Tool

Many studies have used OGC like prognostic tool to predict the development of minimal hepatic encephalopathy (MHE), HE, and survival (Table 18.2). In 2002, Romero-Gómez et al. assessed the usefulness of OGC and MHE (diagnosed by neuro-psychological tests) in evaluating risk of OHE in 70 cirrhotic patients and 10 healthy control subjects. A threshold of 128 mg/dl was established as a pathological value for OGC. Patients with altered OGC and MHE showed higher risk of OHE during follow-up than those without MHE and normal OGC. This result suggests that an abnormal response to OGC could operate as a prognostic factor for the development of OHE in patients with MHE [6]. However, 20 of the 56 patients without MHE had abnormal OGC, so it appeared not to be useful as a diagnostic tool for MHE. Later, the same researching group carried out a prospective study in 49 cirrhotic patients and 36 control subjects to assess the intestinal activity of GA (Fig. 18.3). Intestinal GA was found to be higher in cirrhotic patients than control subjects (four times higher) and it was also increased in patients with MHE. The highest glutaminase activity was observed in patients showing altered OGC and MHE, compared to patients without MHE or normal OGC. Additionally, it was increased in cirrhotic patients and correlated with MHE. Consequently, they found glutaminase activity to be strongly related to MHE and to correlate with the psychometric diagnosis [7]. These data suggest that glutaminase activity in the enterocyte is increased in cirrhotic patients.

Ditisheim et al. looked for improving the performance of blood ammonia for the diagnosis of MHE and explored the value of ammonia in capillary blood. They included 57 cirrhotic patients (19 of them with previous HE) and 13 healthy control subjects in the study. They concluded that determination of

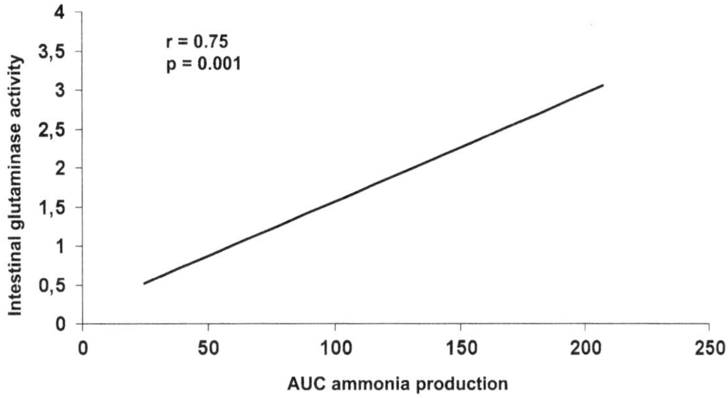

Fig. 18.3 (a) Ammonia production after OGC according to intestinal glutaminase activity; (b) Ammonia production is increased proportionally to intestinal activity glutaminase

capillary blood ammonia after OGC is superior to basal levels (raising the AUROC value from 0.541 at baseline to 0.727 at 60 min after the oral glutamine challenge) for the diagnosis of MHE. However, OGC did not show as a valid tool for the diagnosis of HE and was a poor predictor of future clinical episodes of HE [8].

Romero-Gómez et al. assessed the survival prognosis of patients with cirrhosis who have altered OGC and MHE. Survival among patients who developed overt HE was 59 % at 1 year and 38 % at 3 years; in patients without HE, survival was 96 and 86 % at 1 and 3 years; and an altered OGC response in patients with MHE was associated with a decreased survival rate (80 % at 1 year and 39 % at 3 years). Patients with MHE and abnormal OGC had elevated mortality risk (HR 5.5; 95 % CI, 1.81–16.6). They concluded that a pathological OGC response in patients with MHE appears to be associated with lower survival rate [9]. Enhanced glutaminase activity, portal-systemic shunts and an impaired ammonia detoxification capacity (by liver dysfunction) were proposed to explain these results.

Influence of Portosystemic Shunts on OGC

Portosystemic shunt is an abnormality connection between the portal vein and systemic circulation; most of them are congenital. This means that toxins absorbed by the intestine bypasses the liver and is shunted directly into the systemic circulation. Thus, ammonia is able to reach astrocytes, resulting in deleterious effects. Córdoba et al. investigated this effect and observed the findings in magnetic resonance spectroscopy, after OGC. Three patients with congenital portosystemic shunts and six cirrhotic patients were included. Ammonia production was measured in capillary blood of the ear lobe, following the method previously published [10]. Patients with congenital portosystemic shunts showed impairments in neuropsychological tests, magnetic resonance spectroscopy and in response to the OGC, similar to observed in patients with cirrhosis. Therefore, neurological manifestations of patients with congenital portosystemic shunts show similar mechanisms and risk factors than cirrhotic patients to develop HE [11]. These results have been also observed in animals. In fact, a significant delay in ammonia plasmatic clearance after OGC was obtained in CCl4-induced cirrhotic rats [12].

On the other hand, portal thrombosis is related to portosystemic shunts in non-cirrhotic patients, which can cause HE in absence of cirrhosis. Mínguez et al. performed a study to investigate the neurological consequences of portal vein thrombosis in patients without cirrhosis and no clinical signs of encephalopathy. Ten cirrhotic patients and ten healthy control subjects were included. In this study, patients with non-cirrhotic portal vein thrombosis developed subclinical neurological abnormalities compatible with MHE, such as impairment of neuropsychological tests, higher levels of ammonia after OGC and most marked abnormalities in magnetic resonance similar to cirrhotic patients with HE [13].

Drugs Tested with OGC and Glutaminase Activity

Many drugs have been tested to observe if the glutaminase activity is decreased and, consequently, to decrease the risk of HE. Masini et al. performed a study in which tested if non-absorbable disaccharides (lactulose and lactitol) reduced the small intestine ammonia generation. All cirrhotic patients underwent to two OGC; the ammonia production was lower when OGC was carried out after lactitol use. Their hypothesis was that non-absorbable disaccharides could shorten the transit time of intestinal contents and increase fecal fat excretion cathartic effect) [14].

L-Ornithine-L-aspartate (LOLA) has been shown to reduce ammonia in patients with HE [15]. LOLA stimulates the urea cycle and glutamine synthesis which are important mechanisms in ammonia detoxification. Rees et al. assessed the effect of LOLA in 15 cirrhotic patients without prior HE (7 with TIPS), after OGC. They underwent to OGC on one occasion and placebo on the other in random order. In non-TIPS patients, ammonia increased to 36 μmol/l when LOLA was administered and to 62 μmol/l with placebo. Thus, LOLA ameliorated the deleterious psychometric effects of glutamine in cirrhotic patients without TIPS [16].

Sodium benzoate (SB) is used as a food preservative and has been used to reduce ammonia toxicity in patients born with genetic defects in the urea cycle and to treat cirrhotic patients with HE [17]. The supposed mechanism of action of SB is the elimination of nitrogen as hippurate. Efrati et al. aimed the effect of SB on ammonia production in cirrhotic patients without HE. However, SB increased both the basal and post-OGC ammonia levels [18].

On the other hand, it has been described mersalyl, *N*-ethyl maleimide, 5-oxo-6-norleucine (DON) as a glutaminase inhibitor. DON has been used in the inhibition of glutaminase in cell cultures of astrocytes. The product THDP-17 reduces 42 % of the initial glutaminase activity in Caco-2 cells, while DON reduces 46 % of the initial activity.

Metformin has been the last drug tested in this field. Ampuero et al. included 82 type 2 diabetes mellitus (T2DM) cirrhotic patients and 41 were classified as insulin sensitizers experienced (metformin) and 41 as controls (cirrhotic patients with type 2 diabetes mellitus without metformin treatment). HE was diagnosed during follow-up in 4.9 % in patients receiving metformin and 41.5 % in patients without metformin treatment (H.R. 11.4; $p=0.034$). Patients with MHE and altered OGC showed an increased risk of HE (H.R. 21.3; $p=0.003$). Furthermore, in vitro analysis was performed. In chemical assay, 17.5 % of glutaminase activity inhibition was obtained with a metformin concentration of 10 mM, and up to 68 % inhibition was reached using 100 mM. Additionally, glutaminase activity was decreased up to 24 % at 72 h post-treatment with metformin (20 mM) in Caco2 cells (Fig. 18.4). Therefore, metformin could be useful to reduce ammonia production [19].

Conclusions

Glutamine is an essential amino acid in catabolic states such as injury or illness. However, glutaminase plays a crucial role in the cause of hepatic encephalopathy, as glutaminase activity is increased in cirrhotic patients. Oral glutamine challenge is easy to perform and is comfortable and safe for patients. It is able to predict minimal hepatic encephalopathy and is associated with a poor survival. On the other hand, glutaminase enzyme is an excellent target to develop new drugs that reduce its activity.

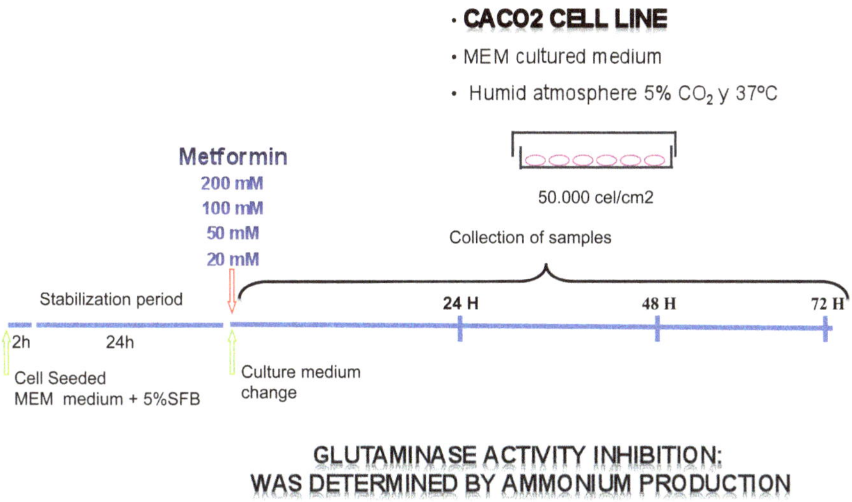

Fig. 18.4 (a) Process to measure ammonia production in Caco-2 cells. (b) In vitro analysis in Caco-2 cells to measure ammonia production after different metformin doses administration at 24, 48, and 72 h posttreatment

Many drugs have been investigated (non-absorbable disaccharides, L-ornithine-L-aspartate, sodium benzoate, THDP-17, or metformin) but the results and/or the study design have been inconclusive. Prospective and randomized studies are needed to evaluate the usefulness of different therapies to normalize this alteration and to improve survival in cirrhotic patients.

References

1. Kovacevic Z, McGivan JD. Mitochondrial metabolism of glutamine and glutamate and its physiological significance. Physiol Rev. 1983;63(2):547–605.
2. Olde Damink SW, Jalan R, Redhead DN, Hayes PC, Deutz NE, Soeters PB. Interorgan ammonia and amino acid metabolism in metabolically stable patients with cirrhosis and a TIPS. Hepatology. 2002;36(5):1163–71.
3. Oppong KN, Al-Mardini H, Thick M, Record CO. Oral glutamine challenge in cirrhotics pre- and post-liver transplantation: a psychometric and analyzed EEG study. Hepatology. 1997;26(4):870–6.
4. Romero-Gomez M, Jover M, Diaz-Gomez D, de Teran LC, Rodrigo R, Camacho I, et al. Phosphate-activated glutaminase activity is enhanced in brain, intestine and kidneys of rats following portacaval anastomosis. World J Gastroenterol. 2006;12(15):2406–11.
5. Romero-Gómez M, Jover M, Del Campo JA, Royo JL, Hoyas E, Galán JJ, et al. Variations in the promoter region of the glutaminase gene and the development of hepatic encephalopathy in patients with cirrhosis: a cohort study. Ann Intern Med. 2010;153(5):281–8.
6. Romero-Gómez M, Grande L, Camacho I, Benitez S, Irles JA, Castro M. Altered response to oral glutamine challenge as prognostic factor for overt episodes in patients with minimal hepatic encephalopathy. J Hepatol. 2002;37(6):781–7.
7. Romero-Gómez M, Ramos-Guerrero R, Grande L, de Terán LC, Corpas R, Camacho I, et al. Intestinal glutaminase activity is increased in liver cirrhosis and correlates with minimal hepatic encephalopathy. J Hepatol. 2004;41(1):49–54.
8. Ditisheim S, Giostra E, Burkhard PR, Goossens N, Mentha G, Hadengue A, et al. A capillary blood ammonia bedside test following glutamine load to improve the diagnosis of hepatic encephalopathy in cirrhosis. BMC Gastroenterol. 2011;11:134.
9. Romero-Gómez M, Grande L, Camacho I. Prognostic value of altered oral glutamine challenge in patients with minimal hepatic encephalopathy. Hepatology. 2004;39(4):939–43.
10. Huizenga JR, Gips CH, Conn HO, Jansen PL. Determination of ammonia in ear-lobe capillary blood is an alternative to arterial blood ammonia. Clin Chim Acta. 1995;239(1):65–70.

11. Ortiz M, Córdoba J, Alonso J, Rovira A, Quiroga S, Jacas C, et al. Oral glutamine challenge and magnetic resonance spectroscopy in three patients with congenital portosystemic shunts. J Hepatol. 2004;40(3):552–7.
12. Miquel M, Bartolí R, Odena G, Serafín A, Cabré E, Galan A, et al. Rat CCl(4)-induced cirrhosis plus total portal vein ligation: a new model for the study of hyperammonaemia and brain oedema. Liver Int. 2010;30(7):979–87.
13. Mínguez B, García-Pagán JC, Bosch J, Turnes J, Alonso J, Rovira A, et al. Noncirrhotic portal vein thrombosis exhibits neuropsychological and MR changes consistent with minimal hepatic encephalopathy. Hepatology. 2006;43(4):707–14.
14. Masini A, Efrati C, Merli M, Attili AF, Amodio P, Ceccanti M, et al. Effect of lactitol on blood ammonia response to oral glutamine challenge in cirrhotic patients: evidence for an effect of nonabsorbable disaccharides on small intestine ammonia generation. Am J Gastroenterol. 1999;94(11):3323–7.
15. Rose C, Michalak A, Pannunzio P, Therrien G, Quack G, Kircheis G, et al. L-ornithine-L-aspartate in experimental portal-systemic encephalopathy: therapeutic efficacy and mechanism of action. Metab Brain Dis. 1998;13(2):147–57.
16. Rees CJ, Oppong K, Al Mardini H, Hudson M, Record CO. Effect of L-ornithine-L-aspartate on patients with and without TIPS undergoing glutamine challenge: a double blind, placebo controlled trial. Gut. 2000;47(4):571–4.
17. Sushma S, Dasarathy S, Tandon RK, Jain S, Gupta S, Bhist MS. Sodium benzoate in the treatment of acute hepatic encephalopathy: a double-blind randomized trial. Hepatology. 1992;16(1):138–44.
18. Efrati C, Masini A, Merli M, Valeriano V, Riggio O. Effect of sodium benzoate on blood ammonia response to oral glutamine challenge in cirrhotic patients: a note of caution. Am J Gastroenterol. 2000;95(12):3574–8.
19. Ampuero J, Ranchal I, Nuñez D, Díaz-Herrero Mdel M, Maraver M, del Campo JA, et al. Metformin inhibits glutaminase activity and protects against hepatic encephalopathy. PLoS One. 2012;7(11):e49279. doi:10.1371/journal.pone.0049279.

Part III
Glutamine in Normal Metabolism and Under Surgical Stress

Chapter 19
Insulin Secretion and the Glutamine-Glutamate-Alpha-Ketoglutarate Axis

Changhong Li

Key Points

- Protein-sensitive hypoglycemia in children with congenital hyperinsulinism (HI) highlights the important role of amino acids in pancreatic β-cell insulin secretion.
- The mechanism of amino acid-stimulated insulin secretion in HI with a glutamate dehydrogenase (GDH) gain of function mutations is due to increased amino acid oxidation via glutamine (Q)-glutamate (E)-alpha-ketoglutarate (αKG) axis.
- Short-chain 3-hydroxyacyl-CoA dehydrogenase (SCHAD) inhibits GDH via protein-protein interaction; HI due to SCHAD deficiency shares a similar mechanism with GDH gain of function.
- Loss of function mutations of ATP-dependent potassium channels are sensitive to glutamine but not to leucine-stimulated insulin secretion.
- The signaling role of glutamine in insulin secretion may be mediated by cAMP-dependent steps of amplification.
- GABA shunt, a branch of the Q-E-αKG axis, mediates glucose suppression of glucagon secretion via production of γ-hydroxybutyrate.
- The key enzymes in the Q-E-αKG axis, including glutaminase, GDH, and glutamine synthetase, serve as intracellular energy sensors which can determine the sensitivity of amino acid stimulation of insulin secretion.

Keywords Insulin secretion • Leucine • Glutamine • Glutamate dehydrogenase • Glutaminase • Glutamine synthetase • Hyperinsulinism

Abbreviations

ECG	Epicatechin gallate
EGCG	Epigallocatechin gallate
GABA-T	GABA transaminase
GAD	Glutamate decarboxylase
GDH	Glutamate dehydrogenase

C. Li, M.D., Ph.D. (✉)
Division of Endocrinology, The Children's Hospital of Philadelphia, Perelman School of Medicine, University of Pennsylvania, 3615 Civic Center Blvd., Philadelphia, PA 19104, USA
e-mail: li@email.chop.edu; Lichanghong2011@gmail.com

R. Rajendram et al. (eds.), *Glutamine in Clinical Nutrition*, Nutrition and Health,
DOI 10.1007/978-1-4939-1932-1_19, © Springer Science+Business Media New York 2015

GHB	γ-hydroxybutyrate
GS	Glutamine synthetase
GSIS	Glucose-stimulated insulin secretion
HI	Hyperinsulinism
K_{ATP}	ATP-dependent potassium channels
LSIS	Leucine stimulated insulin secretion
MSO	Methionine-sulfoximine
PDG	Phosphate-dependent glutaminase
SCHAD	Short-chain 3-hydroxyacyl-CoA dehydrogenase
SSA	Succinate semialdehyde
SUR1	Sulfonylurea receptor 1
αKG	Alpha-ketoglutarate

Introduction

The study of genetic disorders of insulin secretion expands our understanding of interaction between fuel metabolism and secretion coupling in pancreatic β-cells [1]. The glucokinase diseases, including congenital hyperinsulinism (HI) and diabetes (maturity onset diabetes of the young, MODY 2) caused either by a gain of function mutations or a loss of function mutations of glucokinase, have confirmed the basic theories of this enzyme as the sensor and key player for glucose-stimulated insulin secretion (GSIS) [2]. Similarly, protein-induced hypoglycemia in patients with HI due to a gain-of-function mutation of glutamate dehydrogenase (GDH) highlights the important role of amino acid metabolism in the regulation of insulin secretion. Patients with the GDH gain of function are sensitive to leucine and protein challenges; after receiving oral protein or intravenous infusion of leucine, patients showed a rapid increase in insulin secretion and a decline of blood glucose levels [3, 4]. Leucine, the essential amino acid, stimulates insulin release via allosteric activation of GDH, which by causing oxidation of glutamate to produce ATP and resulting in the closure of the ATP-dependent potassium (K_{ATP}) channel, β-cell depolarization, and subsequent calcium influx leads to insulin granule exocytosis [5, 6]. In contrast of leucine and protein hypersensitivity in GDH-HI, HI caused by inactivating mutations of the β-cell K_{ATP} channel (K_{ATP}-HI) is also protein-sensitive but not leucine sensitive [7, 8]. The protein hypersensitivity in K_{ATP}-HI is mainly caused by glutamine-stimulated insulin secretion via a signaling pathway [7]. These discoveries of the role of GDH and glutamine in HI insulin secretion have suggested that the glutamine-glutamate-α-ketoglutarate (Q-E-αKG) is a critical axis for mediating the effects of amino acids in the regulation of insulin secretion. The goal of this chapter is to describe how glutamine-glutamate-α-ketoglutarate axis regulates amino acid and glucose-stimulated insulin secretion based on studies of mouse models of congenital hyperinsulinism and studies on human islets.

Glutaminolysis and Insulin Secretion

Glutaminolysis has been recognized as a pathway to stimulate insulin secretion since the 1980s [5], and as an allosteric activator of GDH, leucine or its non-metabolizable analog, 2-aminobicyclo[2, 2, 1]heptane-2-carboxylic acid, which stimulates insulin secretion by increasing glutamine oxidation. The key steps of glutaminolysis, including phosphate-dependent glutaminase (PDG) and GDH, both serve as intracellular energy sensors in β-cells, play their function by switching on or off of glutamine oxidation in response to the changes of fuel supply, mainly glucose. When glucose supply is limited such as by prolonged fasting, intracellular phosphate potential (ATP and GTP) falls, while free phosphate and ADP increase. Those changes lead to "on" switch of PDG and GDH, which results to the increase of glutamine oxidation. Therefore, β-cell fuel-sensing switches from glucose to amino acids under this circumstance. In contrast, after a meal, glucose oxidation becomes the predominant fuel supplier in the β-cell. Glucose oxidation increases ATP and GTP production; following a drop in phosphate and ADP, as results of these changes, both PDG and GDH are inhibited and glutamine oxidation is turned off. This "Ying and Yang" relationship between glucose oxidation and glutaminolysis is supported by the following evidences.

"Run-Down" Phenomenon

When leucine-stimulated insulin secretion (LSIS) in perifused rat islets were performed, the islets failed to respond to leucine stimulation of insulin secretion after 50 min of "run-down," i.e., fuel depletion by glucose-free perifusion in islets which have been cultured in 10 mM glucose for 3 days. In contrast, a prolonged "run-down" of 120 min caused islets to become leucine sensitive (Fig. 19.1a) [6]. This leucine

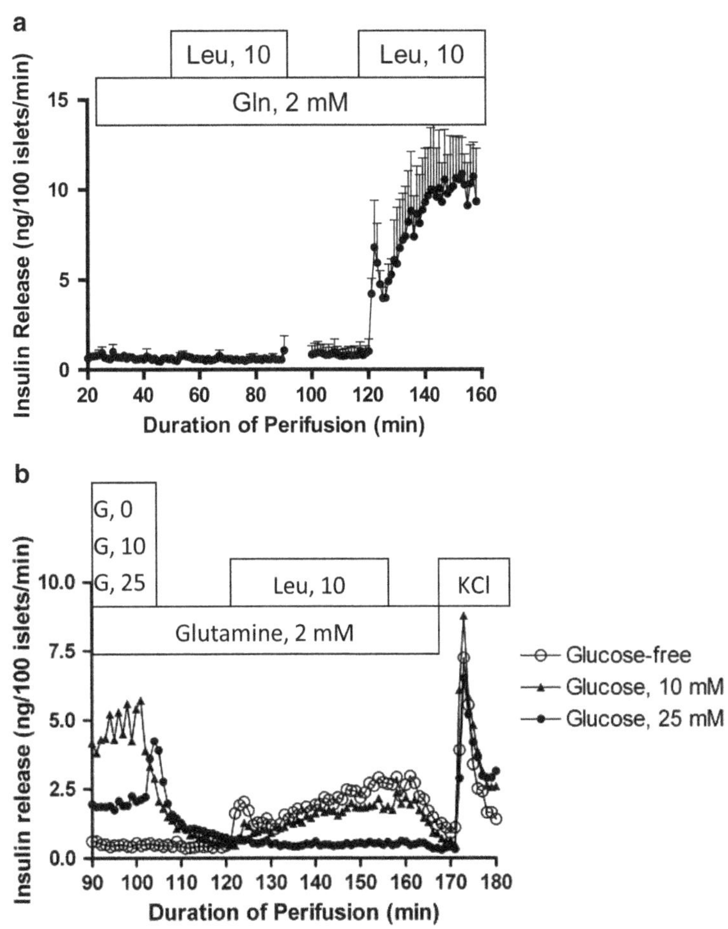

Fig. 19.1 Leucine stimulated insulin secretion in rat islets. After 3 days of culturing in 10 mM glucose, 100 rat islets were perifused with glucose-free Krebs ringer bicarbonate buffer for 50 or 120 min, and then exposed to 10 mM leucine in the presence of 2 mM glutamine (panel **a**, data: mean ± S.E., $n=3$). Leucine-stimulated insulin secretion only occurred in islets with a 120-min "run-down." Panel (**b**) shows that islets were perifused with 0, 10, or 25 mM glucose for 100 min; after withdrawing from glucose for 20 min, islets were then stimulated by 10 mM leucine and finally exposed to 30 mM potassium chloride (KCl). Leucine-stimulated insulin secretion was inhibited by preexposure to high glucose

sensitivity can be completely blocked by preexposure to high glucose (Fig. 19.1b). This "run-down" phenomenon also occurred in mouse islets. After preexposure to high glucose, mouse islets were also no longer sensitive to LSIS [9]. This "run-down" phenomenon supports the notion that GDH serves as an intracellular energy sensor. When intracellular phosphate potential is high, GDH is inhibited by GTP or ATP; in contrast, after a "run-down," the intracellular energy is depleted and GDH gains the sensitivity to leucine activation.

Regulation of PDG in Mouse and Rat Islets

The first step of glutamine oxidation is PDG. PDG is a phosphate-dependent enzyme that can be activated by free phosphate with half-maximally stimulation of 40 mM in rat islets [10]. Previous study of PDG in islets was limited since it was only focused on enzyme kinetics [10]. Recent studies using ^{15}N stable isotope tracing and the GC/MS technique advanced the understanding of regulation of PDG in isolated islets. This technology allows us to calculate the flux of PDG in intact islets [6, 11]. Mouse or rat islets were incubated with 10 mM [2-^{15}N]glutamine as a basal condition, and then incubated with an additional 10 mM leucine, 25 mM glucose or both. The PDG fluxes were calculated based on ^{15}N incorporation into glutamate/aspartate and into ammonia. As showed in Fig. 19.2, leucine stimulates PDG flux in both mouse (panel A) and rat islets (panel B), which may result from direct activation of PDG by leucine [10] or secondary of GDH activation by removing glutamate [12]. High glucose not only inhibits basal PDG fluxes, but also eliminates leucine-stimulated PDG fluxes. The enzyme flux data suggest that glucose oxidation has strong inhibitory effects on PDG. Glucose oxidation and/or "phosphate flush" [13–15] lower intracellular inorganic phosphate in the processes of phosphorylation and ATP production, and therefore, islets will have less phosphate available for PDG activation.

GDH Gain of Function and Insulin Secretion

GDH catalyzes the reversible oxidative deamination of L-glutamate to αKG using NAD(P)$^+$ as coenzyme. GDH can be allosterically activated by ADP and leucine, and inhibited by GTP and ATP [16]. In 1998, mutations of GDH were identified in children with hyperinsulinism and hyperammonemia

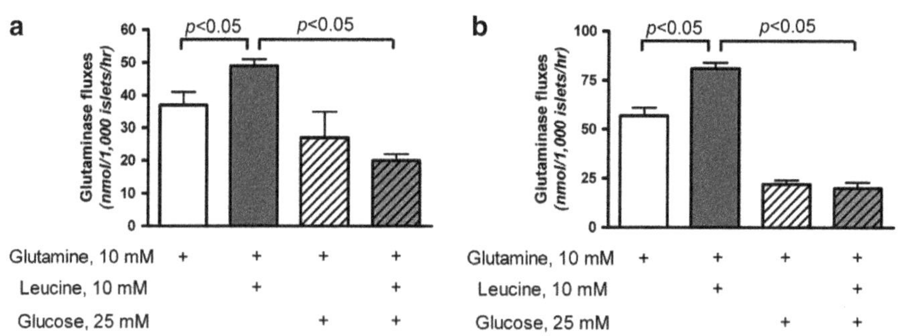

Fig. 19.2 Flux rate of phosphate-dependent glutaminase (PGD) in mouse or rat islets. 1,000 cultured mouse (panel **a**) or rat (panel **b**) islets were incubated with 10 mM [2-^{15}N]glutamine as basal, or with an additional 10 mM leucine, 25 mM glucose or leucine plus glucose for 120 min. PDG flux rate was calculated based on the ^{15}N incorporation into glutamate/aspartate and ammonia. Data: mean ± S.E., $n = 3$. Leucine stimulates PDG fluxes in both mouse and rat islets, while high glucose inhibits basal and leucine-stimulated PDG fluxes

syndrome [17]. GDH enzyme kinetics in the patients with GDH gain-of-function mutations showed a lack of sensitivity to GTP allosteric inhibition [17, 18]. The clinical phenotype is interesting: GDH-HI patients are sensitive to protein feeding and hyperinsulinemic hypoglycemia occurred after a protein-rich meal or a mixture of an amino acid load. GDH-HI also has exaggerated acute insulin responses to intravenous leucine stimulation [3, 4]; this leucine response can be blocked by rising blood glucose levels [4]. We hypothesize that the elevated amino acid oxidation augments ATP production by increasing flux through GDH, which leads to closure of the K_{ATP} channel and subsequently β-cell depolarization and calcium influx, which finally activates the "triggering" pathway for insulin release, similar to GSIS [6, 19].

To further examine the hypothesis of which GDH gain of function mutations is responsible for hyperinsulinism, we generated a transgenic mouse model to express one severe form of GDH mutation (H454Y), specifically in β-cells following a rat insulin promoter. GDH-transgenic mice (GDH-TG) showed a consistent hypoglycemia phenotype [11] which is similar to the GDH-HI patient [3, 17]. An oral amino acids tolerance test showed that GDH-TG mice are sensitive to stimulation by a physiological amino acid mixture and react with rapid falls of blood glucose and increases of insulin secretion [20], also similar to GDH-HI patients [3]. GDH enzyme kinetics in isolated islets from GDH-TG mice showed a right shift of the GTP inhibition curve, confirming the H454Y expression in islet [11, 18]. Dynamic insulin secretion in perifused islets isolated from GDH-TG mice was also sensitive to the amino acid mixture and leucine stimulation and even responded to glutamine alone, whereas control islets were unresponsive to either glutamine or a mixture of amino acids [11]. This study confirms that the GDH gain of function mutation is disease-causing in GDH-HI.

GDH Flux, Measured by ^{15}N Tracing

To directly examine the effects of the H454Y GDH mutation on flux through the GDH, a metabolomic approach was applied in isolated islets by using a stable isotope-tracing technique to trace ^{15} flux from [2-^{15}N]glutamine to [2-^{15}N]glutamate and subsequently to [^{15}N]ammonia, which can help us to determine the specific flux via GDH reaction. Compared to wild-type control littermates, H454Y transgenic islets have greater insulin secretion, ammonia production, [^{15}N]ammonia enrichment, and GDH fluxes in response to 10 mM [2-^{15}N]glutamine. As shown in Fig. 19.3, activation of GDH in control

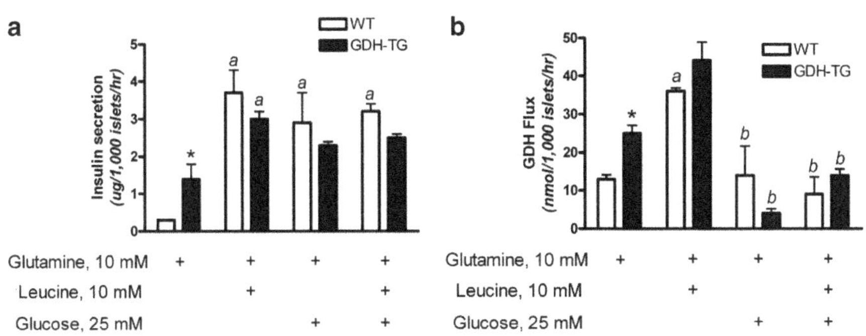

Fig. 19.3 Insulin secretion and GDH flux in GDH transgenic and wild-type islets. 1,000 cultured islets isolated from GDH H454Y transgenic or wild-type mice were incubated with 10 mM [2-^{15}N]glutamine as basal, or with an additional 10 mM leucine, 25 mM glucose or leucine plus glucose for 120 min. GDH flux rate was calculated based on ^{15}N-ammonia production. Insulin secretion (panel **a**) and GDH flux (panel **b**) are shown. Data: mean ± S.E., $n = 3$. vs. WT, *:$p < 0.05$, vs. glutamine alone, *a*: $p < 0.05$, vs. glutamine/leucine, *b*: $p < 0.05$. GDH fluxes in GDH-TG islets are similar to leucine-stimulated GDH fluxes in wild-type islets, while glucose strongly inhibits GDH fluxes, and leucine is unable to overcome this inhibition

islets with 10 mM leucine leads to an increase of insulin release (panel A), accompanied by increased rates of ammonia production and a threefold stimulation of fluxes through GDH (panel B). The effect of leucine on GDH flux in control islets were similar to the rates seen in transgenic islets in absence of leucine, suggesting that GDH flux in TG islets were close to maximal even without leucine activation [11]. The elevated GDH flux in transgenic islets results in increased production of ATP, which is responsible for activation of the triggering pathway of insulin release. Glucose inhibition of LSIS observed in GDH-HI patients [4] can be explained by the high glucose inhibition of GDH flux in normal and transgenic islets; leucine was unable to override this inhibitory effect of glucose [4, 11], which is similar to PDG regulation as shown in Fig. 19.2. High phosphate potential produced from glucose oxidation results in a strong inhibition of GDH activity. This study provides convincing evidence that GDH serves as intracellular energy sensor. In response to the changes of phosphate potential driven by glucose metabolism, the "on and off" switch of GDH will lead to an increase or decrease of amino acid oxidation. Functional expression in islets is the changes of sensitivity to leucine or amino acid stimulation of insulin release.

SCHAD-GDH Interaction, a Novel Mechanism of GDH Regulation

Recently, a new form of HI has been described which is associated with deficiency of the mitochondrial fatty acid β-oxidation enzyme, short-chain 3-hydroxyacyl-CoA dehydrogenase (SCHAD) [21, 22]. SCHAD catalyzes the β-oxidation cycle for medium and short-chain 3-hydroxy fatty acyl-CoAs (C4 to C10). Children with SCHAD deficiency have hypoglycemia and accumulations of fatty acid metabolites, such as plasma 3-hydroxy-butyrylcarnitine and urinary 3-hydroxyglutaric acid [21, 22]. Unlike ketotic hypoglycemia, which occurs in the other forms of genetic defects of fatty acid oxidation, hypoglycemia in SCHAD deficiency results from hyperinsulinism [23]. In order to investigate the mechanisms responsible for hypoglycemia in SCHAD deficiency, SCHAD knockout mice were generated [24]. SCHAD-KO mice have lower plasma glucose levels than controls in both fed and fasting states. Plasma acylcarnitine profiles in SCHAD-KO mice showed a fourfold elevation of plasma 3-hydroxy-butyrylcarnitine compared with controls and had similar values to those reported in children with SCHAD deficiency. SCHAD-KO mice also had an increased accumulation of medium-chain 3-OH-fatty acids, which confirmed the complete knockout of this gene. Compared to wild-type mice, SCHAD-KO mice showed a rapid decline of blood glucose after receiving oral amino acids, which is due to stimulation of insulin release in response to an amino acid challenge. This is similar to the protein-induced hypoglycemia seen in patients with SCHAD deficiency [25]. SCHAD-KO mice have similar glucose tolerance test as compared to the control littermates. Studies in isolated islets confirmed the in vivo findings. SCHAD-KO islets were very sensitive to stimulation to a physiological mixture of amino acids, similar to islets from GDH-TG mice, but had a higher threshold of amino acid-stimulated insulin secretion. When glutamine and leucine were removed from the amino acid mixture, KO islets were completely unresponsive to the other 17 amino acids, indicating that GDH activation was essential for abnormal insulin release in KO islets. KO islets were also more sensitive to leucine stimulation (Fig. 19.4a), but, unlike islets from GDH-TG, failed to respond to glutamine alone. The results of insulin secretion from isolated islets indicated an activation of GDH in SCHAD-KO islets as evidenced by increased [U-^{14}C]glutamine oxidation (Fig. 19.4b) in KO islets, but this was not as active as the GDH gain-of-function mutation observed in GDH-TG mice. GSIS was similar between KO and wild-type islets, suggested that hyperinsulinism in SCHAD-KO is not likely due to increased GSIS as initially hypothesized [26]. Measurement of GDH enzyme kinetics indicates that while KO islets have a normal response to GTP inhibition, they also have a reduced affinity of GDH for α-KG and an increased enzyme efficiency (Fig. 19.4c), suggesting

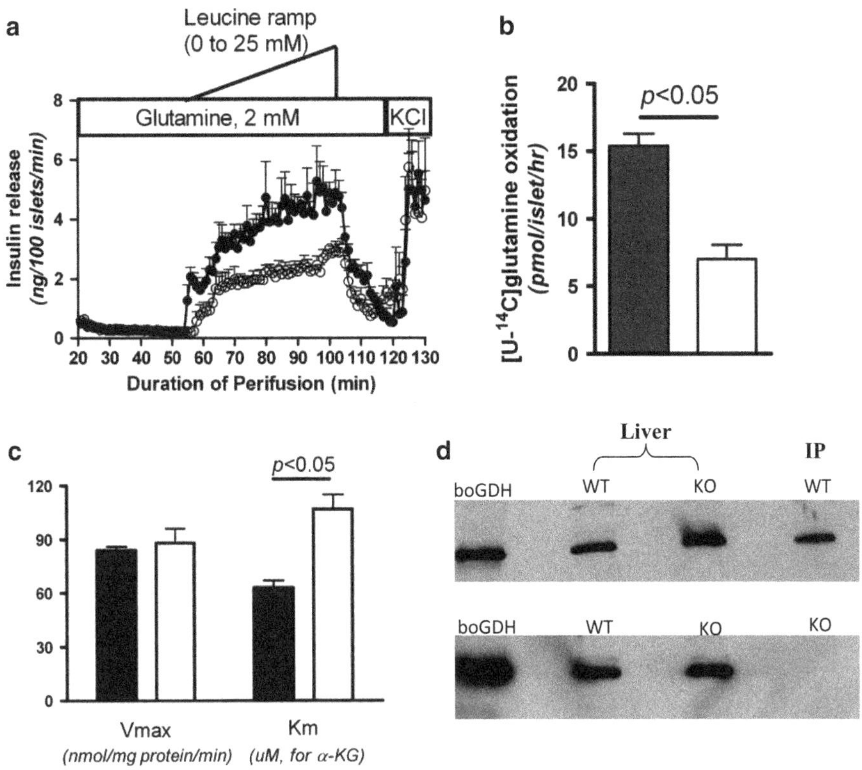

Fig. 19.4 Insulin secretion, glutamine oxidation, GDH enzyme activity and GDH-SCHAD interaction in SCHAD knockout and wild-type mice. Panel (**a**) shows islet perifusion in response to a leucine ramp (0–25 mM) stimulation in the presence of 2 mM glutamine, *filled circles*: SCHAD-knockout islets, *open circles*: wild-type islets; data: mean ± S.E., $n=3$. Panel (**b**) shows [U-^{14}]glutamine oxidation in isolated islets from SCHAD knockout (*filled bar*) or wildtype (*open bar*) mice. 100 cultured islets were incubated with 2 mM glutamine in the presence of 2 μCi [U-^{14}C]glutamine; glutamine oxidation was calculated based on $^{14}CO_2$ production. Data: mean ± S.E., $n=5$. Panel (**c**) shows Vmax and Km for α-ketoglutarate of GDH enzyme activity, *filled bar*: SCHAD knockout, *open bar*: wild-type, $n=4$. Panel (**d**) shows GDH-SCHAD interaction by immunoprecipitation using an anti-SCHAD antibody as bait; GDH in pull-down products was detected by an anti-GDH antibody in isolated liver mitochondria; GDH was co-precipitated with SCHAD in wild-type liver mitochondria, but not in the SCHAD knockout

that the presence of SCHAD protein affects binding of the substrate in the catalytic site of GDH. The effect was limited to islet GDH, perhaps reflecting the high levels of SCHAD and high ratio of SCHAD to GDH in islet tissue [24, 27]. We further examined the possibility of protein-protein interactions between the two enzymes. When the anti-SCHAD antibody was used as bait, GDH was co-precipitated with SCHAD in wild-type mouse liver mitochondria, but not in KO mice, which is consistent with a GDH-SCHAD protein complex in WT liver mitochondria (Fig. 19.4d). Our findings suggest that GDH activation in SCHAD deficiency is due to the loss of a direct protein-protein interaction between the two enzymes. It is interesting to speculate that the inhibitory effect of SCHAD on GDH might be part of a mechanism for reciprocal controlling of fatty acid and amino acid oxidation. GDH may be the center regulatory step in the metabolic interaction, including glucose, fatty acid, and amino acid. Further studies found that SCHAD not only binds to GDH, it also associates with other proteins, for example, carbamoyl phosphate synthase 1, citrate synthase, glutamine syntheses, pyruvate dehydrogenase, and ATP synthase [28]. This involves ureagenesis, metabolism of glucose and amino acid, and ATP production and highlights the complexity of SCHAD interaction.

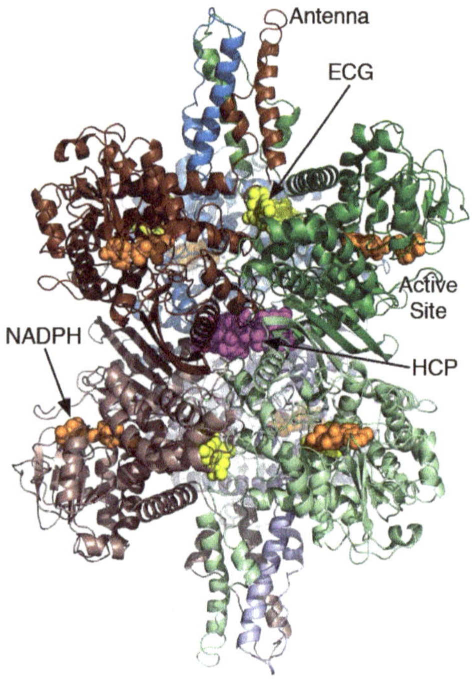

Fig. 19.5 Structure of the GDH-ECG complex. This is a ribbon diagram of bovine glutamate dehydrogenase hexamer complexed with NADPH (*orange*), ECG (*yellow*), and HCP (*purple*)

EGCG Allosterically Inhibits GDH

Green tea is often emphasized as a rich source of polyphenols. Among the four major polyphenols in green tea epigallocatechin gallate (EGCG), epigallocatechin, epicatechin gallate (ECG), and epicatechin, EGCG and ECG have a strong inhibitory effect on GDH activity with nanomolar ED_{50} [23]. Co-crystallization of GDH protein with ECG showed that ECG binds to the ADP activation site (Fig. 19.5), pre-occupying the activation site with ECG and resulting in the inhibition of GDH enzyme activity [20]. Mutations of the ADP binding site (R90S, D123A, and S397I) disrupt the ADP bindings as well as the EGCG inhibition, which strongly supports that EGCG binds to the same site as ADP. Interestingly, EGCG also inhibits several disease-causing GTP-insensitive GDH mutations, including H454Y, simply because EGCG binds to the ADP site, not to the GTP site. This special feature of the EGCG inhibition of GTP-insensitive GDH mutations provides a therapeutic potential to treat GDH-HI by EGCG. The experiments in GDH-TG mice indeed showed that pre-exposure to oral EGCG (100 mg/Kg of body weight) diminished amino acid-induced hypoglycemia in GDH-TG mice. In vitro study showed that EGCG also blocked glutamine-stimulated calcium influx and insulin secretion in GDH-TG islets, which suggests that the action of EGCG in GDH-TG mice is on β-cell insulin secretion [20]. This study provides the "proof of concept" that GDH inhibition by small molecules will lead to novel treatment of GDH-HI, since current treatment only targets dysregulated insulin secretion by diazoxide, an insulin secretion inhibitor. The hyperammonemia and neurological abnormalities are neglected and it certainly requires attention from clinical management [17, 29]. Early attempts already identified several GDH inhibitors by high-throughput compound screening, including hexachlorophene (HCP) of which the binding site also showed in Fig. 19.5 [30].

Signaling Role of Glutamine in Insulin Secretion

In the entire process of insulin secretion, K_{ATP} channels serve as the "gate-keeper" to control insulin release; they are the key components of the triggering and application pathway of insulin secretion [19]. Inactivating mutations in β-cell K_{ATP} channels cause the most common and severe form of HI (K_{ATP}-HI). K_{ATP}-HI is characterized by severe fasting hypoglycemia [8] and impaired GSIS [31]; it often requires pancreatectomy to control hypoglycemia [1]. The absence of K_{ATP} channels in β-cells induces persistent plasma membrane depolarization and elevation of cytosolic calcium, resulting in constant insulin secretion regardless of blood glucose levels [32]. The defective GSIS paradoxically impairs both the turning off and turning on of insulin secretion in response to glucose, which leads to hypoglycemia early in life and a risk of diabetes later [33, 34]. Interestingly, K_{ATP}-HI also has protein-sensitive hypoglycemia, but, unlike GDH-HI, is not leucine sensitive [8]. The fact that amino acid- but not leucine-stimulated insulin secretion occurred without functional K_{ATP}-channels suggests that oxidation of amino acids via the flux of the Q→E→αKG axis is unlikely the cause. The studies of sulfonylurea receptor 1 (SUR1) knockout mice suggests an alternative mechanism of amino acid stimulation of insulin secretion, in which glutamine plays a signaling role in insulin secretion.

SUR1 Knockout and Glutamine-Stimulated Insulin Secretion

To investigate the mechanism of protein-induced hypoglycemia in K_{ATP}-HI, we examined insulin secretion in islets from SUR1 knockout mice [7, 35]. SUR1-KO islets had elevated basal intracellular calcium and basal insulin secretion, which are characteristic features of dysfunctional K_{ATP} channels. Unlike wild-type islets, SUR1-KO islets have no response to leucine or to glucose-stimulated insulin release, but they do release insulin in response to a mixture of amino acids and glutamine (Fig. 19.6). The paradoxical effect of glutamine and leucine on insulin secretion was unlikely to be caused by glutamine oxidation via GDH as we described previously, since activation of GDH by leucine failed to stimulate insulin secretion and the sensitivity to glutamine cannot be inhibited by the PDG inhibitor 6-Diazo-5-oxo-L-norleucine. Therefore, we hypothesized that glutamine may have specific effects on the downstream amplification pathways for insulin release, distal to the elevation of cytosolic calcium.

cAMP and Glutamine Signaling

Recent studies suggest that the signaling effect of glutamine may involve cAMP-dependent pathways [36]. As shown in Fig. 19.7A, amino acids stimulated cAMP production while simultaneously stimulating insulin secretion in SUR1-KO mouse islets; a similar effect can be obtained by glutamine alone. Additional evidence also supported this hypothesis. Inhibition of the GLP-1 receptor by its antagonist, Exendin-(9-39), decreased baseline intracellular cAMP and also blocked the stimulatory effect of amino acids on both cAMP production and insulin secretion (Fig. 19.7, panel A and B). The same phenomenon can be reproduced in control islets during GSIS, suggesting that amino acid amplification of insulin secretion is an important pathway during GSIS [7, 36]. This study suggests that blockage of cAMP production by the GLP-1 receptor antagonist inhibits amino acid-stimulated insulin secretion in K_{ATP}-HI, of which concept may provide a novel therapeutic target to treat K_{ATP}-HI. In vitro experiments in SUR1-KO mice strongly support this hypothesis; fasting hypoglycemia in SUR1-KO

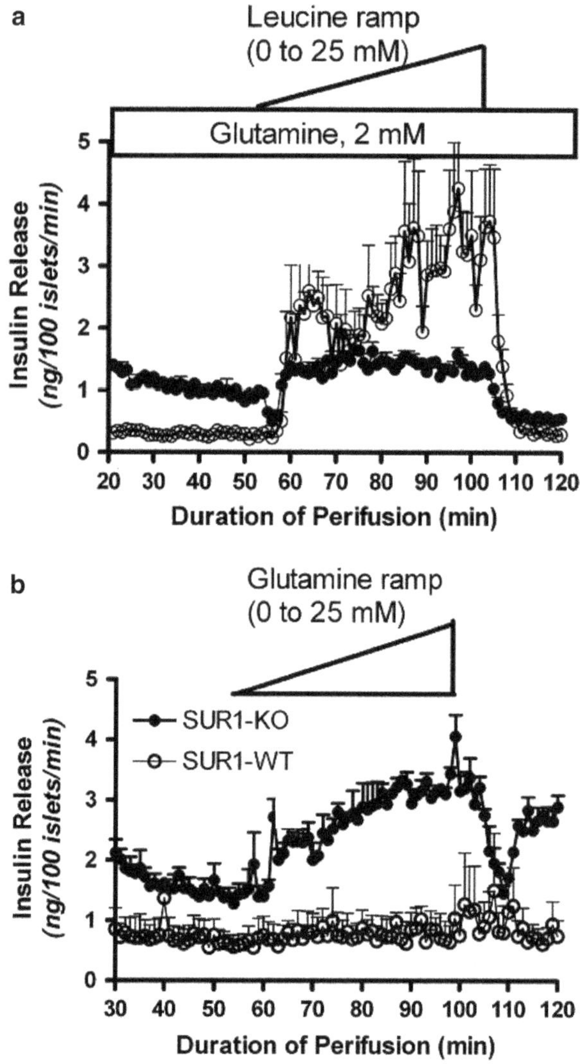

Fig. 19.6 Leucine and glutamine-stimulated insulin secretion in SUR1 knockout and wildtype islets. After 3 days of culturing in 10 mM glucose, isolated islets from the SUR1 knockout (*filled circles*) and wild-type (*open circles*) mice were perifused with a ramp of leucine (0–25 mM) in the presence of 2 mM glutamine (panel **a**), or perifused with a ramp of glutamine (0–25 mM) (panel **b**), data: mean ± S.E., $n=3$. Glutamine, not leucine, stimulates insulin secretion in SUR1 knockout islets

mice can be prevented by prolonged subcutaneous infusions of Exendin-(9-39) [36]. A pilot clinical study in K_{ATP}-HI patients confirmed the findings that observed in mouse models, Exendin-(9-39) administration significantly increased fasting glucose levels in K_{ATP}-HI patients [37]. Studies in islets isolated from surgical specimens after pancreatectomy in K_{ATP}-HI patients suggested that human islets with loss of function mutations of K_{ATP}-channel are indeed supersensitive to amino acid stimulation and that Exendin-(9-39) blocked such effects [37]. Those results suggest that amino acid-sensitive hypoglycemia or amino acid-stimulated insulin secretion play important roles in pathophysiology of K_{ATP}-HI patients. Thus, this approach can serve as a novel target for drug development to control hypoglycemia in K_{ATP}-HI. Although the precise mechanism by which glutamine or amino acid exert their effects on the amplification pathways of insulin secretion remains to be determined, it seems to be of major importance clinically in children with K_{ATP}-HI disorders and may also be important as a major pathway in amplifying the stimulation of insulin secretion in normal individuals in response to glucose and other metabolic fuels.

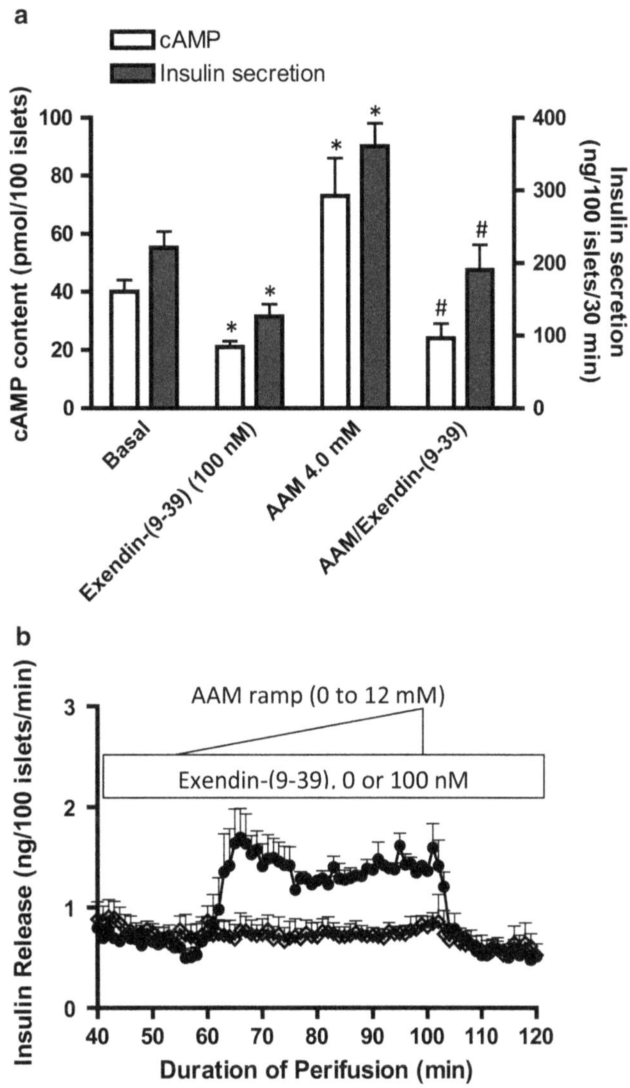

Fig. 19.7 Exendin-(9-39) inhibits cAMP production and insulin secretion in SUR1 knockout islets. As shown in panel (**a**), basal and amino acid mixture stimulated insulin secretion and cAMP production in batch-incubated SUR1 knockout islets. Exendin-(9-39), an inhibitor of the GLP-1 receptor, inhibits amino acid-induced increase of cAMP production and insulin secretion (vs. basal, *: $p<0.05$; vs. amino acid stimulation, #: $p<0.05$, data: mean ± S.E., $n=4$–8). Panel (**b**) shows the inhibitory effects of Exendin-(9-39) on an amino acid mixture ramp (0–12 mM) which stimulated insulin secretion in SUR1 knockout islets ($n=3$)

Glutamine Synthesis Pathway

The amplifying effect of glutamine on insulin secretion in SUR1-KO islets was also observed in normal control islets under conditions where the cytosolic calcium had been elevated by exposure to glyburide or glucose stimulation [7]. As shown in Table 19.1, islet content and release of glutamine was increased twofold during exposure to 25 mM glucose. When islets were stimulated with 25 mM [U-^{13}C]glucose, over 50 % of the glutamine carbon came from glucose. Inhibition of glutamine synthetase (GS) by methionine-sulfoximine (MSO), but not by its inactive analog buthionine sulfoximine, abolished the carbon flux from glutamate to glutamine and also reduced the response to GSIS. These results indicate that the metabolic flux from αKG → E → Q (αKG → E via transaminases) might play an important role in normal mouse islets during the process of GSIS [35]. The inhibitory effect of MSO on GSIS was reversed by the addition of exogenous glutamine in a dose-dependent manner, and could also be reversed by the addition of 6-Diazo-5-oxo-L-norleucine, which is a

Table 19.1 Insulin secretion and glutamine production in normal mouse islets

	Insulin secretion (μg/1,000 islets/h)	Glutamine (nmol/1,000 islets)		^{13}C enrichment (APE, sum of M +2, +3, +4, +5)
		Content	Release	
G, 0	0.2±0.03	0.2±0.02	4.1±0.5	
G, 25	5.4±0.7[a]	0.4±0.04[b]	7.4±0.7[b]	
G, 25/MSO, 1 mM	3.5±0.2[c]	NA	NA	
AAM, 4 mM	0.2±0.0	0.8±0.1		
[U-^{13}C]G, 5/AAM, 4 mM	0.5±0.0[d]	1.3±0.0[e]		34±1.2
[U-^{13}C]G, 25/AAM,4 mM	4.5±0.2[df]	1.3±0.1[e]		57±1.0[f]
[U-^{13}C]G, 25/AAM, 4 mM/MSO, 1 mM	4.7±0.4[df]	NA		ND

Cultured islets were incubated with different concentrations of [U-^{13}C]glucose in presence of 4 mM amino acid mixture, glutamine was determined by HPLC, ^{13}C enrichment was measured by GC/MS
Compare with G, 0, *a*: $p<0.01$, *b*: $p<0.05$; compare with G, 25, *c*: $p<0.05$
Compare with AAM, 4 mM, *d*: $p<0.01$, *e*: $p<0.05$
Compare with G, 5/AAM 4.0, *f*: $p<0.01$
Data: mean±S.E, $n=3$; NA: data not determined, ND: undetectable

non-metabolizable analog of glutamine. These data support the hypothesis in which glutamine generated during glucose oxidation via reversed Q-E-αKG axis amplifies insulin secretion, similar to the other metabolic amplifiers, i.e., glutamate, NADPH, long-chain acyl-CoA, and diacylglycerol [38].

GABA Shunt: A Branch of Q-E-αKG Axis

As a branch of Q-E-αKG axis, the pathway of GABA shunt operates specifically in β-cells, but not in α-cells [39]. The three steps of the GABA shunt include production of GABA via glutamate decarboxylase (GAD) using glutamate as substrate, conversion of GABA to succinate semialdehyde (SSA) by GABA transaminase (GABA-T) while converting αKG to glutamate, and finally entry into the tricarboxylic acid (TCA) cycle as succinate following oxidation by SSA dehydrogenase (SSADH) [39].

GABA Shunt and GDH Interaction: Metabolic Oscillation Hypothesis

During glucose oxidation, glucose carbon flows from αKG to glutamate and then to GABA, and finally re-enters TCA cycle via succinate. Thus, the GABA shunt pathway bypasses the GTP generating step in TCA cycle (succinate CoA synthetase). We can postulate that the operation of GABA shunt in β-cells will lead to less production of GTP and result in the release of the GDH inhibition by GTP, which will ensure the anaplerosis supply of αKG from glutamate. As we discussed in previous sections, production of GTP and ATP during glucose oxidation inhibits GDH. The operation of GABA shunt pathway to bypass GTP production suggests that such inhibition may function in an oscillated pattern. As we expected, inhibition of GDH leads to less production of αKG from glutamate, resulting in an accumulation of glutamate which facilitates the production of GABA via GAD. Once GDH inhibition has been released by increasing flux of GABA shunt, increased GDH flux will have less glutamate available for GAD, which will produce less GABA; slower GABA shunt in turn leads to more GTP production and an inhibition of GDH. Such metabolic oscillation may result in insulin secretion in an oscillated pattern as well.

GABA Shunt in SUR1-KO Mice

Chronic activation of the β-cell K_{ATP} channel by sulfonylureas in normal mice results in "glucose blindness" [40], similar to the lack of GSIS in islets from SUR1-KO islets [7, 41]. Based on those data, we can postulate that the consequence of chronic β-cell depolarization and elevation of cytosolic calcium will affect glucose metabolism in general and result in impaired GSIS. In order to test this hypothesis, a metabolomic approach was used to trace ^{13}C flux from [U-^{13}C]glucose to amino acid in islets isolated from SUR1-KO and wild-type mice. In the presence of a 4 mM physiological amino acid mixture, ^{13}C enrichments of amino acid in islets were detected in alanine, aspartate, glutamate, GABA, and glutamine, which indicate the incorporation of glucose carbon into those amino acids. Serving as metabolic indicators, those amino acids can be used to calculate carbon fluxes from glucose. The results showed that mouse islets operate the GABA shunt pathway and that glucose lowers GABA levels and increases it ^{13}C enrichment, which suggests increased GABA shunt flux during glucose oxidation. Compared to wild-type islets, SUR1-KO islets have a 75 % reduction of GABA shunt. Impaired GABA shunt in SUR1-KO islets can be explained by downregulated GAD gene expression [35]. Glyburide-treated wild-type islets showed similar changes of GABA shunt compared to SUR1-KO. This alteration of metabolic pathways in SUR1-KO islets may be part of the mechanisms of decreased glucose sensing and increased amino acid sensing.

GABA Shunt in Type 2 Diabetic Human Islets

Resent study in both normal human and type 2 diabetic human islets using [U-^{13}C]glucose tracing showed that similar results occurred in mouse islets [35, 42]. In normal human islets, glucose stimulates insulin release while inhibiting glucagon secretion. Type 2 diabetic human islets have impaired insulin secretion in response to glucose stimulation. A subgroup of type 2 diabetic human islets failed to response to glucose-mediated suppression of glucagon secretion. This group of type 2 diabetic human islets also showed the impairment of GABA shunt, which is due to downregulated GAD gene expression [42], similar to SUR1-KO mouse islets. This result suggests that GABA shunt may be responsible for metabolic control of glucagon secretion from β-cells. Further study showed that blockage of GABA shunt by GABA-T inhibitor, vigabatrin, leads to loss of glucose-mediated suppression of α-cell function [42].

γ-Hydroxybutyrate Loop and Glucagon Suppression

The association of impaired glucose-mediated suppression of glucagon release with impaired GABA shunt activity in this subgroup of type 2 diabetic human islets suggested the possibility of a causal link between these two phenomena, such as a deficiency of GABA per se or a deficiency of some downstream metabolite of GABA mediating glucose suppression of glucagon secretion. In consequence of GABA metabolism, SSA produced via GABA shunt enters the TCA cycle through SSADH. In the central nervous system, a fraction of SSA is diverted to γ-hydroxybutyrate (GHB) via the NADPH-dependent SSA reductase [43]. GHB, a potent inhibitory neurotransmitter, is then converted back to SSA via the NAD-dependent GHB dehydrogenase to form the "GHB loop" [44–46]. The expression of key enzymes of the GHB loop and production of GHB in human islets confirmed that the GHB loop, as an extension of GABA shunt, is an active pathway in the β-cell. We hypothesize that production of GHB from GABA shunt in β-cells mediates glucose suppression of glucagon secretion in α-cells via receptor-based mechanism [42]. The pathways are described in Fig. 19.8.

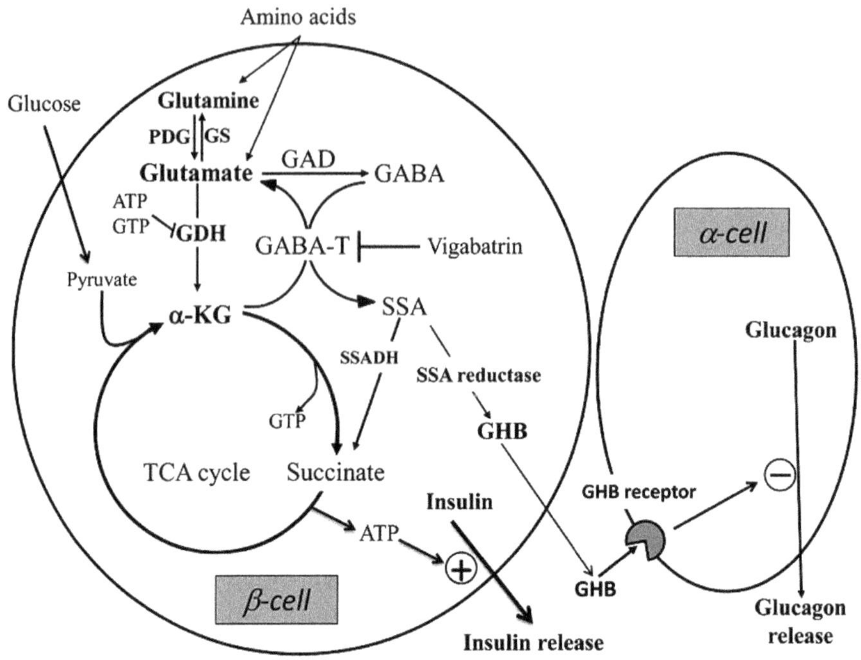

Fig. 19.8 The Q-E-αKG axis, GABA shunt, insulin secretion, and β-α-cell interaction: The Q-E-αKG axis involves three key enzymes: glutamate dehydrogenase (GDH), phosphate-dependent glutaminase (PDG), and glutamine synthetase (GS). The activities of all three enzymes are regulated by changes in the β-cell phosphate potential. During glucose stimulation of insulin secretion, increased generation of αKG from the tricarboxylic acid (TCA) cycle supports enhanced flux through the GABA shunt, which leads to increased production of GHB. GHB is generated from succinate semialdehyde (SSA) via SSA reductase, inhibiting glucagon secretion from α-cell via its receptor. GABA is produced via glutamate decarboxylase (GAD). Vigabatrin acts as a GABA transaminase (GABA-T) inhibitor

Conclusions

The importance of amino acid-stimulated insulin secretion is emphasized in three forms of HI. Amino acid sensitivity in GDH-HI and SCHAD-HI are due to GDH gain of function by either GDH mutation or lack of inhibition by SCHAD via protein-protein interaction. GDH gain of function leads to elevation of amino acid oxidation via Q → E → αKG axis and more ATP production, which triggers insulin secretion. However, glucose oxidation increases intracellular phosphate potential, leading to β-cell depolarization, inhibition of GDH and activation of glutamine synthesis. Under high-energy conditions and β-cell depolarization, glutamine serves as a signaling molecule to amplify insulin release; similar phenomena also occurred in SUR1-KO islets. Therefore, the sensitivity of amino acid stimulation of insulin secretion reflects the changes of intracellular phosphate potential in pancreatic islets; when intracellular phosphate potential is low, islets become sensitive to leucine stimulation due to a release of GDH inhibition. In contrast, glucose oxidation increases phosphate potential, which results in inhibition of GDH but activates glutamine synthesis via α-KG → E → Q axis, leading to amplification of GSIS. As branch of Q-E-αKG axis, GABA shunt activity is closely related to the operation of Q-E-αKG axis. Production of GABA and GHB from GABA shunt may mediate glucose suppression of glucagon secretion in α-cells. GABA shunt may play an important role in the process of β- and α-cell communication. Understanding the mechanisms of amino acid hypersensitivity in HI will not only help us to identify disease-causing metabolic pathways, but also will provide new targets for drug development for both HI and diabetes treatment.

Acknowledgment I gratefully acknowledge the important contributions to this work by colleagues including Charles A. Stanley, Michael J. Bennett, Diva D. De León (The Children's Hospital of Philadelphia, Philadelphia, PA), Franz M. Matschinsky (Perelman School of Medicine, University of Pennsylvania, Philadelphia, PA) and Thomas J. Smith (Donald Danforth Plant Science Center, St Louis, MO). These studies were supported in part by NIH grants, U01DK089529, DK53012, DK22122, and a pilot grant from the Institute of Diabetes, Obesity and Metabolism (University of Pennsylvania, DK19525). Additional support was provided by the Radioimmunoassay and Islet Cores of the Diabetes Research Center of the University of Pennsylvania, Perelman School of Medicine (DK19525).

References

1. De Leon DD, Stanley CA. Mechanisms of Disease: advances in diagnosis and treatment of hyperinsulinism in neonates. Nat Clin Pract Endocrinol Metab. 2007;3(1):57–68.
2. Zelent D, Najafi H, Odili S, et al. Glucokinase and glucose homeostasis: proven concepts and new ideas. Biochem Soc Trans. 2005;33(Pt 1):306–10.
3. Hsu BY, Kelly A, Thornton PS, Greenberg CR, Dilling LA, Stanley CA. Protein-sensitive and fasting hypoglycemia in children with the hyperinsulinism/hyperammonemia syndrome. J Pediatr. 2001;138(3):383–9.
4. Kelly A, Ng D, Ferry Jr RJ, et al. Acute insulin responses to leucine in children with the hyperinsulinism/hyperammonemia syndrome. J Clin Endocrinol Metab. 2001;86(8):3724–8.
5. Sener A, Malaisse WJ. L-leucine and a nonmetabolized analogue activate pancreatic islet glutamate dehydrogenase. Nature. 1980;288(5787):187–9.
6. Li C, Najafi H, Daikhin Y, et al. Regulation of leucine-stimulated insulin secretion and glutamine metabolism in isolated rat islets. J Biol Chem. 2003;278(5):2853–8.
7. Li C, Buettger C, Kwagh J, et al. A signaling role of glutamine in insulin secretion. J Biol Chem. 2004;279(14):13393–401.
8. Fourtner SH, Stanley CA, Kelly A. Protein-sensitive hypoglycemia without leucine sensitivity in hyperinsulinism caused by K(ATP) channel mutations. J Pediatr. 2006;149(1):47–52.
9. Gao ZY, Li G, Najafi H, Wolf BA, Matschinsky FM. Glucose regulation of glutaminolysis and its role in insulin secretion. Diabetes. 1999;48(8):1535–42.
10. Michalik M, Nelson J, Erecinska M. Glutamate production in islets of Langerhans: properties of phosphate-activated glutaminase. Metabolism. 1992;41(12):1319–26.
11. Li C, Matter A, Kelly A, et al. Effects of a GTP-insensitive mutation of glutamate dehydrogenase on insulin secretion in transgenic mice. J Biol Chem. 2006;281(22):15064–72.
12. Zaleski J, Wilson DF, Erecinska M. beta-2-Aminobicyclo-(2.2.1)-heptane-2-carboxylic acid. A new activator of glutaminase in intact rat liver mitochondria. J Biol Chem. 1986;261(30):14091–4.
13. Freinkel N, el Younsi C, Bonnar J, Dawson RM. The "phosphate flush": a new index of secretory stimulation in pancreatic islets. Trans Assoc Am Physicians. 1974;87:306–14.
14. Freinkel N, Younsi CE, Bonnar J, Dawson RM. Rapid transient efflux of phosphate ions from pancreatic islets as an early action of insulin secretagogues. J Clin Invest. 1974;54(5):1179–89.
15. Doliba NM, Vatamaniuk MZ, Buettger CW, et al. Differential effects of glucose and glyburide on energetics and Na+ levels of betaHC9 cells: nuclear magnetic resonance spectroscopy and respirometry studies. Diabetes. 2003; 52(2):394–402.
16. Li M, Li C, Allen A, Stanley CA, Smith TJ. The structure and allosteric regulation of glutamate dehydrogenase. Neurochem Int. 2011;59(4):445–55.
17. Stanley CA, Lieu YK, Hsu BY, et al. Hyperinsulinism and hyperammonemia in infants with regulatory mutations of the glutamate dehydrogenase gene. N Engl J Med. 1998;338(19):1352–7.
18. Fang J, Hsu BY, MacMullen CM, Poncz M, Smith TJ, Stanley CA. Expression, purification and characterization of human glutamate dehydrogenase (GDH) allosteric regulatory mutations. Biochem J. 2002;363(Pt 1):81–7.
19. Henquin JC. Triggering and amplifying pathways of regulation of insulin secretion by glucose. Diabetes. 2000;49(11):1751–60.
20. Li C, Li M, Chen P, et al. Green tea polyphenols control dysregulated glutamate dehydrogenase in transgenic mice by hijacking the ADP activation site. J Biol Chem. 2011;286(39):34164–74.
21. Hussain K, Clayton PT, Krywawych S, et al. Hyperinsulinism of infancy associated with a novel splice site mutation in the SCHAD gene. J Pediatr. 2005;146(5):706–8.
22. Molven A, Matre GE, Duran M, et al. Familial hyperinsulinemic hypoglycemia caused by a defect in the SCHAD enzyme of mitochondrial fatty acid oxidation. Diabetes. 2004;53(1):221–7.
23. Li C, Allen A, Kwagh J, et al. Green tea polyphenols modulate insulin secretion by inhibiting glutamate dehydrogenase. J Biol Chem. 2006;281(15):10214–21.

24. Li C, Chen P, Palladino A, et al. Mechanism of hyperinsulinism in short-chain 3-hydroxyacyl-CoA dehydrogenase deficiency involves activation of glutamate dehydrogenase. J Biol Chem. 2010;285(41):31806–18.
25. Kapoor RR, James C, Flanagan SE, Ellard S, Eaton S, Hussain K. 3-Hydroxyacyl-coenzyme A dehydrogenase deficiency and hyperinsulinemic hypoglycemia: characterization of a novel mutation and severe dietary protein sensitivity. J Clin Endocrinol Metab. 2009;94(7):2221–5.
26. Eaton S, Chatziandreou I, Krywawych S, Pen S, Clayton PT, Hussain K. Short-chain 3-hydroxyacyl-CoA dehydrogenase deficiency associated with hyperinsulinism: a novel glucose-fatty acid cycle? Biochem Soc Trans. 2003; 31(Pt 6):1137–9.
27. Martens GA, Vervoort A, Van de Casteele M, et al. Specificity in beta cell expression of L-3-hydroxyacyl-CoA dehydrogenase, short chain, and potential role in down-regulating insulin release. J Biol Chem. 2007;282(29): 21134–44.
28. Narayan SB, Master SR, Sireci AN, et al. Short-chain 3-hydroxyacyl-coenzyme A dehydrogenase associates with a protein super-complex integrating multiple metabolic pathways. PLoS One. 2012;7(4):e35048.
29. Bahi-Buisson N, Roze E, Dionisi C, et al. Neurological aspects of hyperinsulinism-hyperammonaemia syndrome. Dev Med Child Neurol. 2008;50(12):945–9.
30. Li M, Smith CJ, Walker MT, Smith TJ. Novel inhibitors complexed with glutamate dehydrogenase: allosteric regulation by control of protein dynamics. J Biol Chem. 2009;284(34):22988–3000.
31. Grimberg A, Ferry Jr RJ, Kelly A, et al. Dysregulation of insulin secretion in children with congenital hyperinsulinism due to sulfonylurea receptor mutations. Diabetes. 2001;50(2):322–8.
32. Remedi MS, Koster JC. K(ATP) channelopathies in the pancreas. Pflugers Arch. 2010;460(2):307–20.
33. Huopio H, Reimann F, Ashfield R, et al. Dominantly inherited hyperinsulinism caused by a mutation in the sulfonylurea receptor type 1. J Clin Invest. 2000;106(7):897–906.
34. Leibowitz G, Glaser B, Higazi AA, Salameh M, Cerasi E, Landau H. Hyperinsulinemic hypoglycemia of infancy (nesidioblastosis) in clinical remission: high incidence of diabetes mellitus and persistent beta-cell dysfunction at long-term follow-up. J Clin Endocrinol Metab. 1995;80(2):386–92.
35. Li C, Nissim I, Chen P, et al. Elimination of KATP channels in mouse islets results in elevated [U-13C]glucose metabolism, glutaminolysis, and pyruvate cycling but a decreased gamma-aminobutyric acid shunt. J Biol Chem. 2008;283(25):17238–49.
36. De Leon DD, Li C, Delson MI, Matschinsky FM, Stanley CA, Stoffers DA. Exendin-(9-39) corrects fasting hypoglycemia in SUR-1-/- mice by lowering cAMP in pancreatic beta-cells and inhibiting insulin secretion. J Biol Chem. 2008;283(38):25786–93.
37. Calabria AC, Li C, Gallagher PR, Stanley CA, De Leon DD. GLP-1 receptor antagonist exendin-(9-39) elevates fasting blood glucose levels in congenital hyperinsulinism owing to inactivating mutations in the ATP-sensitive K+ channel. Diabetes. 2012;61(10):2585–91.
38. Newsholme P, Gaudel C, McClenaghan NH. Nutrient regulation of insulin secretion and beta-cell functional integrity. Adv Exp Med Biol. 2010;654:91–114.
39. Sorenson RL, Garry DG, Brelje TC. Structural and functional considerations of GABA in islets of Langerhans. Beta-cells and nerves. Diabetes. 1991;40(11):1365–74.
40. Remedi MS, Nichols CG. Chronic antidiabetic sulfonylureas in vivo: reversible effects on mouse pancreatic beta-cells. PLoS Med. 2008;5(10):e206.
41. Doliba NM, Qin W, Vatamaniuk MZ, et al. Restitution of defective glucose-stimulated insulin release of sulfonylurea type 1 receptor knockout mice by acetylcholine. Am J Physiol Endocrinol Metab. 2004;286(5):E834–43.
42. Li C, Liu C, Nissim I, et al. Regulation of glucagon secretion in normal and diabetic human islets by gamma-hydroxybutyrate and glycine. J Biol Chem. 2013;288(6):3938–51.
43. Kaufman EE, Nelson T, Goochee C, Sokoloff L. Purification and characterization of an NADP+-linked alcohol oxido-reductase which catalyzes the interconversion of gamma-hydroxybutyrate and succinic semialdehyde. J Neurochem. 1979;32(3):699–712.
44. Bessman SP, Fishbein WN. Gamma-hydroxybutyrate, a normal brain metabolite. Nature. 1963;200:1207–8.
45. Gibson KM, Hoffmann GF, Hodson AK, Bottiglieri T, Jakobs C. 4-Hydroxybutyric acid and the clinical phenotype of succinic semialdehyde dehydrogenase deficiency, an inborn error of GABA metabolism. Neuropediatrics. 1998;29(1):14–22.
46. Kaufman EE, Relkin N, Nelson T. Regulation and properties of an NADP+ oxidoreductase which functions as a gamma-hydroxybutyrate dehydrogenase. J Neurochem. 1983;40(6):1639–46.

Chapter 20
Glutamine-Cycling Pathway in Metabolic Syndrome: Systems Biology-Based Characterization of the Glutamate-Related Metabolotype and Advances for Diagnosis and Treatment in Translational Medicine

Silvia Sookoian and Carlos J. Pirola

Key Points

- The metabolic syndrome (MS) is a cluster of strongly related intermediate phenotypes, such as central obesity, glucose intolerance, dyslipidemias, hypertension, and fatty liver, with a common underlying metabolic derangement characterized by insulin resistance (IR).
- The glutamine-cycling pathway participates in the pathogenesis of MS and might be prominently involved in the development of systemic underlying metabolic derangement. High-throughput metabolomic profiling in patients with MS showed a distinctive metabolic signature associated with branched-chain amino acids (BCCA). In fact, circulating levels of glutamic acid and other BCAA have prognostic value in the risk prediction of MS-related complications. The hyperamino-acidemia observed in patients with MS might be involved in the modulation of insulin signaling, and BCAA are potent modulators of the mTOR/p70 S6 kinase pathway.
- The reactions of transaminations mediated by the enzymes ALT and AST regulate the levels of major Krebs cycle-intermediate metabolites and reprogram their activity according to the cellular metabolic environment. Hence, circulating levels of liver transaminases ALT and AST might be regarded as sensors of the systemic metabolic derangement occurring in patients with MS, and a change in the paradigm that ALT and AST are just markers of liver injury is proposed. Mechanisms behind the transcriptional and posttranscriptional regulation of the liver transaminases are explored by systems biology approaches.
- Gene variants in glutaminase 2 (*GLS2*) or glutamine synthase (glutamate-ammonia ligase, GLUL) might provide a molecular explanation to connect genomic variation with enzymatic defects in patients with MS, and may explain the rise in glutamic acid levels observed in these patients, suggesting a "genotype-dependent glutamate-metabolotype." In addition, glutamate dehydrogenase (GLUD1), a mitochondrial matrix enzyme that catalyzes the oxidative deamination of glutamate to alpha-ketoglutarate and ammonia, may have an important role in incorporating ammonia to the

S. Sookoian, M.D., Ph.D. (✉)
Department of Clinical and Molecular Hepatology, Institute of Medical Research A Lanari-IDIM, University of Buenos Aires-National Scientific and Technical Research Council,
Av. Combatiente de Malvinas 3150, Ciudad Autónoma de Buenos Aires 1427, Argentina
e-mail: sookoian.silvia@lanari.fmed.uba.ar

C.J. Pirola, M.D., Ph.D.
Department of Molecular Genetics and Biology of Complex Diseases, Institute of Medical Research A Lanari-IDIM, University of Buenos Aires-National Scientific and Technical Research Council,
Av. Combatiente de Malvinas 3150, Ciudad Autónoma de Buenos Aires 1427, Argentina
e-mail: pirola.carlos@lanari.fmed.uba.ar

R. Rajendram et al. (eds.), *Glutamine in Clinical Nutrition*, Nutrition and Health,
DOI 10.1007/978-1-4939-1932-1_20, © Springer Science+Business Media New York 2015

amino acid metabolism and regulating amino acid-induced insulin secretion, because activating mutations in this gene are a common cause of congenital hyperinsulinism.
- Glutamate might be involved in the fetal metabolic programming of MS-related phenotypes by regulating the hypothalamic signaling cascade of appetite control.

Keywords Diabetes • Insulin resistance • Cardiovascular risk • Fatty liver • ALT • AST • Metabolomics • Biomarkers • Glutamic acid • Branched-chain amino acid • Fetal metabolic programming • Liver cancer • GWAS • GLS2

Abbreviations

ALT	Alanine aminotransferase
AST	Aspartate aminotransferase
BCAA	Branched-chain amino acid
CAD	Coronary artery disease
CVD	Cardiovascular disease
GOT	Glutamic-oxaloacetic transaminase
GPT	Glutamic-pyruvate transaminase
IR	Insulin resistance
MS	Metabolic syndrome
NAFLD	Nonalcoholic fatty liver disease
SHR	Spontaneously hypertensive rats
TCA cycle	Tricarboxylic acid cycle

Introduction

The metabolic syndrome (MS) is a complex disorder that encompasses a cluster of highly related diseases, such as type 2 diabetes (T2D), dyslipidemias, central obesity, arterial hypertension, and some other clinical phenotypes recently included, such as nonalcoholic fatty liver disease (NAFLD), prothrombotic and proinflammatory states, and ovarian polycystosis. Altogether, these disorders constitute a combination of underlying risk factors for an adverse outcome, which is cardiovascular disease (CVD) [1].

The pathogenesis of MS is linked to insulin resistance (IR). In fact, in its original description MS was regarded as "insulin resistance syndrome" or "Syndrome X" [2]. Hence, it is biologically plausible to speculate that MS is a cluster of strongly related intermediate phenotypes with a common underlying metabolic derangement. Nevertheless, there is still debate on whether MS is a "syndrome" or just a cluster of specific diseases that have their own pathogenic mechanism [3].

Regardless of this dilemma, it is obvious that in clinical practice all the intermediate phenotypes of MS often coexist, and all the clustered conditions of MS converge in a common phenotype that, from the clinical point of view, depicts a patient at higher risk of CVD morbidity and mortality.

In this chapter, we introduce the hypothesis that the glutamine-cycling pathway participates in the pathogenesis of MS and might be prominently involved in the development of the systemic underlying metabolic derangement. In addition, we postulate the critical role that some enzymatic reactions occurring in the liver tissue, such as the transamination reactions, play in the pathogenesis of MS.

For simplicity, we refer to the natural L form of the amino acids except where mentioned otherwise.

Evidence from Clinical Studies and Insights from Metabolite Profiling by Emerging Technologies of High-Throughput Metabolomics

Recent studies on the entire set of metabolites of a cell, tissue or biofluid, also called "metabolome" by high-throughput technologies (metabolomics), such as chromatography coupled to mass spectrometry techniques, have elucidated interesting pathways in the pathophysiology of MS-intermediate phenotypes. For example, the identification of human plasma metabolites in obese patients compared with non-obese individuals suggested a distinctive metabolic signature associated with branched-chain amino acid (BCAA) catabolism in obese subjects [4]. Actually, several essential (leucine, isoleucine, valine, and phenylalanine) and nonessential amino acids (alanine, tyrosine, glutamate/glutamine, aspartate/asparagine, and arginine) were significantly elevated in obese versus lean participants, whereas glycine levels were lower in obese subjects [4]. Interestingly, glutamate levels in obese patients (118.4 μM) were significantly higher compared with lean subjects (81.2 μM) [4]. In this scenario, Newgard and colleagues speculated that the accumulation of glutamate and changes in the rate of BCAA metabolism may be associated with an increase of transamination of pyruvate to alanine [4]. Thus, according to the authors' hypothesis, this increase in alanine contributes to the development of IR in obesity-associated states, because alanine is a gluconeogenic amino acid.

On the other hand, Thomas Wang and coworkers explored the plasma metabolic profiling of 189 subjects of the Framingham Offspring Study who developed T2D during the follow-up and 189 matched controls who did not develop diabetes. They observed that a panel of amino acids (isoleucine, leucine, valine, tyrosine, and phenylalanine) predicted the future development of diabetes in healthy, normoglycemic individuals [5]. Similar findings were reported by Huffman et al. in overweight patients with IR [6].

Another study, which examined the plasma concentrations of >350 metabolites in fasted obese T2DM vs. obese non-diabetic African-American women, observed that leucine and valine concentrations rose with increasing HbA1c [7].

A large study exploring the metabolic signatures of IR in 7,098 young adults confirmed that abnormalities in BCAA extend beyond obesity and lipid abnormalities and reflect the degree of IR [8].

Finally, Cheng and coworkers observed that all the intermediate phenotypes of MS, including obesity, IR, high blood pressure, and dyslipidemia, were associated with an abnormal metabolite profile that included BCAA, other hydrophobic amino acids, tryptophan breakdown products, and nucleotide metabolites [9]. Interestingly, the authors were able to predict the risk of incident diabetes by changes in the glutamine-glutamate ratio in a very accurate fashion [9].

Surprisingly, this metabolic pattern of altered amino acids was also observed in patients with CVD. In fact, mass spectrometry-based profiling of 69 metabolites in subjects from "The CATHGEN" biorepository, which includes subjects recruited sequentially through the cardiac catheterization laboratories at Duke University Medical Center (Durham, NC), confirmed that levels of several amino acids, including leucine, isoleucine, valine, proline, methionine, and glutamate/glutamine, were significantly different between cases and controls, and were able to discriminate subjects with coronary artery disease [10].

Table 20.1 summarizes recent results of metabolic profiling explored by technologies of high-throughput metabolomics in patients with MS.

Overall, these clinical reports show that abnormal circulating concentrations of BCAA and glutamate are commonly observed in patients with MS-related phenotypes, and this metabolic profile might be regarded as a novel predictor of long-term impairment of insulin sensitivity. Thus, these findings depict a common underlying metabolic derangement of MS.

Is this a novel finding? Probably not, because changes in plasma amino acid levels and insulin secretion in patients with obesity were initially described in 1969 by Philip Felig, who reported that among 20 plasma amino acids measured, valine, leucine, isoleucine, tyrosine, and phenylalanine

Table 20.1 Summary of recent publications of metabolic profiling explored by technologies of high-throughput metabolomics in patients with MS

First author	Phenotype characteristics	Study design, number of participants	Metabolite quantification	Altered metabolite
Newgard, C.B	Obesity: Obese individuals enrolled from weight loss programs	Hospital-based *N*: 141	Capillary gas chromatography/mass spectrometry (GC/MS)	BCAA
Wang T	IR/T2D: Nested case–control study in the Framingham Offspring Study	Population-based cohort study *N*: 189 selected from 2,422 normoglycemic individuals followed for 12 years	Liquid chromatography-tandem mass spectrometry	BCAA
Huffman, K.M	IR/T2D: 73 subjects who enrolled in studies of targeted risk reduction interventions through exercise	Hospital-based *N*: 73	Mass spectrometry-based platform	BCAA
Fiehn, O	T2D	Population-based *N*: 56	Capillary gas chromatography/mass spectrometry (GC/MS)	BCAA
Wurtz, P	IR/T2D	Population-based The Northern Finland Birth Cohort 1966 (NFBC) and the Cardiovascular Risk in Young Finns Study (YFS) *N*: 1,873	High-throughput nuclear magnetic resonance (NMR) spectroscopy platform	BCAA
Cheng, S	MS	Population-based cohort study Framingham Heart Study (*N*=1,015) and Malmo Diet and Cancer Study (*N*=746)	Liquid chromatography/mass spectrometry	Glutamic acid Glutamine-glutamate ratio
Shah, S.H	CAD Subjects recruited sequentially through the cardiac catheterization	Hospital-based 174 CAD cases and 174 sex/race-matched controls Replication: 140 CAD cases and 140 CAD- controls	Mass spectroscopy	BCAA

BCAA branched-chain amino acid, IR insulin resistance, T2D type 2 diabetes, CAD coronary artery disease

increased, and glycine decreased, in obese subjects compared with age- and sex-matched controls [11]. Felig suggested that hyperaminoacidemia modulates insulin signaling given the ability of most amino acids to stimulate pancreatic beta cell output [11].

Moreover, previous in vitro studies demonstrated that BCAA and their metabolites, such as leucine, isoleucine, valine, and ketoisocaproic acid, the product of leucine transamination, exert effects on insulin signal transduction and glucose transport, including decreased insulin-stimulated tyrosine phosphorylation of IRS-1 (insulin receptor substrate 1) and IRS-2 and a marked inhibition of insulin-stimulated phosphatidylinositol 3-kinase [12].

On the other hand, human studies have demonstrated that glutamine and alanine stimulate secretion of insulin and glucagon with a marked increase in gluconeogenesis [13, 14].

The Liver, the Glutamine-Cycling Pathway, and MS: The Reactions of Transamination and a Change in the Paradigm of the Meaning of Biomarkers of Liver Injury in the Context of MS

The family of enzymes called "transaminases" is involved in the transference of an amine group of one amino acid to a ketone group of another acid, and this reaction is known as transamination. All these enzymes need pyridoxal phosphate as a cofactor. This conversion of the *amino acids* into *keto acids* normally feeds the citric acid cycle, also known as the tricarboxylic acid (TCA) cycle or the Krebs cycle.

In the context of this chapter, we will illustrate that the transaminases are significantly involved in glutamine-cycling as glutamic and pyruvic acids as a result of the transamination of alanine. In fact, it is know from previous experimental studies that the main route of glutamine and glutamate entrance into the TCA cycle via 2-oxoglutarate is transamination by aspartate aminotransferase (AST) [15].

The cytoplasmatic enzyme glutamic-pyruvate transaminase (GPT) or glutamate-pyruvate transaminase 1, also known as alanine aminotransferase (ALT), catalyzes the reversible transamination between alanine and 2-oxoglutarate to generate pyruvate and glutamate (Fig. 20.1). Thus, by mediating the conversion of four major intermediate metabolites, ALT activity modulates their levels in different metabolic scenarios from fasting to excess of dietary nutrients. Transcript variants encoding two different isoforms have been found for the GPT genes; GPT1 is mostly related to hepatocytes, renal tubular epithelial cells, and salivary gland epithelial cells, while GPT2 is expressed in the adrenal gland cortex, neuronal cell bodies, cardiac myocytes, skeletal muscle fibers, and endocrine pancreas. GPT1 represents the major contributor of circulating levels and ALT activity [16].

The glutamic-oxaloacetic transaminase (GOT) or AST exists in two forms, cytoplasmic and mitochondrial: GOT1 and GOT2, respectively. The two enzymes are homodimeric and show close homology. AST catalyzes the reversible transamination between aspartate and 2-oxoglutarate to generate oxaloacetate and glutamate (Fig. 20.1).

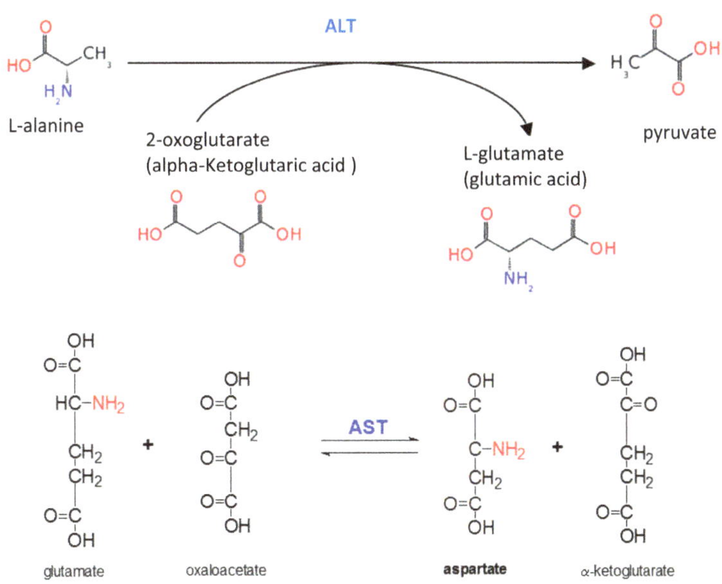

Fig. 20.1 Schematic representation of the transamination reactions: ALT (alanine aminotransferase) and AST (aspartate aminotransferase). ALT catalyzes the reversible transamination between alanine and 2-oxoglutarate to form pyruvate and glutamate, and AST catalyzes the reversible transamination between glutamate and oxaloacetate to form aspartate and alpha ketoglutarate. Transamination reactions are reversible and can be used for both amino acid degradation and synthesis; the coenzyme for the reaction is pyridoxal phosphate

Are ALT and AST Important Players in the Regulation of the Metabolic Cell Environment?

Certainly, they are. In fact, ALT has an important role in the intermediary metabolism of glucose and amino acids, and AST plays a central role in amino acid metabolism and the TCA, and also facilitates the metabolite uptake of long-chain free fatty acids. Actually, AST is important for the metabolite exchange between mitochondria and cytosol.

Likewise, the reactions of transamination that most often occur in the liver mediate the synthesis of glucose from amino acids such as aspartate, asparagine, glutamate, and glutamine under fasting conditions. ALT and AST balance the levels of pyruvate and alpha ketoglutarate, which are precursors to glucose via gluconeogenesis. In addition, if there are excess proteins in the diet, those amino acids converted into pyruvic acid and acetyl CoA can be converted into lipids by the lipogenesis process. Hence, transamination reactions are strong modifiers of the pathogenesis of IR and MS-associated phenotypes.

The serum activity levels of ALT and AST are widely and almost exclusively used in clinical practice as routine biomarkers of liver injury of different etiologies. Surprisingly, however, they are not regarded as sensors of the metabolic derangements occurring in patients with IR and MS. Nonetheless, in large and well-characterized epidemiological studies, ALT (or GPT) and AST (or GOT) are strongly and reproducibly associated with MS-related phenotypes. For instance, in the Framingham Offspring Heart Study that included 2,812 participants (mean age, 44 years; 56 % women) followed up for the development of MS, T2D, CVD, and all-cause mortality, both normal and increased levels of ALT were associated with the long-term development of multiple metabolic disorders [17]. Aminotransferase levels were also correlated with multiple cardiometabolic risk factors above and beyond visceral adipose tissue and IR in the same cohort, as recently demonstrated [18].

On the other hand, in a large population-based community cohort of 1,532 adults from the Cameron County Hispanic Cohort, the epidemiologist tried to identify the most likely cause of elevated ALT and found that the risk factors most strongly associated with elevated ALT in this population were the components of MS [19].

A multiethnic epidemiological study encompassing 633 African-American, Hispanic, and non-Hispanic white subjects aged 40–69 years showed that ALT and the AST-to-ALT ratio predict MS independently of potential confounding variables, including directly measured insulin sensitivity and acute insulin response [20].

A population-based study that included the healthy British South Asian population showed that raised ALT was significantly associated with an adverse metabolic and atherothrombotic risk profile [21]. Likewise, in 1,439 subjects of the Hoorn Study, a population-based cohort of Caucasian men and women 50–75 years of age, which assessed the incidence of CVD and coronary heart disease events, the predictive value of ALT for coronary events seems independent of traditional risk factors and the features of MS [22].

Elevated liver function enzymes were also associated with the development of pre-diabetes and T2D in young adults from the Bogalusa Heart Study, a retrospective cohort study that included adults aged 26–50 years followed up over an average period of 16 years since their young adulthood [23].

In addition, in an Australian population (3,719 subjects, 1,544 men and 2,175 women, aged 25–84 years), ALT was significantly associated with MS, and each of its five components and the association with MS remained significant after adjustment for IR [24].

Among subjects enrolled in the Firenze Bagno a Ripoli (FIBAR) study, elevated AST levels were independent predictors of CVD and the incident diabetes [25]. Higher ALT levels were also associated with obesity, and peripheral and hepatic IR in Pima Indians [26].

Finally, and even more surprising, the findings of the Framingham Heart Study Original and Offspring cohorts, which included a total of 3,744 participants, recently demonstrated that both ALT and AST levels might be associated with the incident of atrial fibrillation [27].

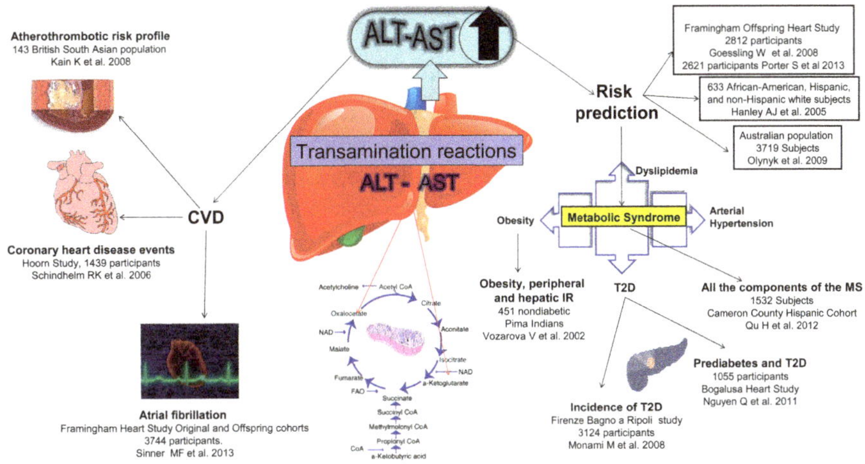

Fig. 20.2 Summary of the epidemiological and clinical data about the role of liver transaminases ALT and AST in the risk prediction of the metabolic syndrome and cardiovascular disease. Transamination reactions mediated by ALT and AST most often occur in the liver tissue and have a significant role in the intermediary metabolism of glucose and amino acids. As ALT and AST feed some components of the TCA cycle, like oxaloacetate and alpha ketoglutarate, both also sense the metabolic cellular environment. These enzymes also mediate metabolite exchange between mitochondria and cytosol. Elevated circulating levels of ALT and AST were reported in patients with MS-associated phenotypes, and they have been useful for predicting MS-associated disease risk, like the development of future CVD complications or diabetes development. In fact, in well-characterized epidemiological cohort studies, ALT better predicts the risk of complications than IR or visceral adipose tissue.

Figure 20.2 shows a picture summarizing the epidemiological and clinical data regarding the role of liver transaminases in the intermediate phenotypes of MS and CVD risk.

Thus, while the evidence from observational and cohort studies is overwhelming in terms of risk prediction and association with the diseases that integrate MS, none of the studies have elucidated the pathophysiological mechanisms behind these observations. Conversely, almost all the epidemiological studies have regarded the elevation of circulating transaminase levels as indicators of liver injury associated with MS and IR, and have speculated that ALT levels just mirror the presence of NAFLD. Surprisingly, none of these studies have ever considered the possibility that high levels of ALT or AST are indicators of high levels of tissue enzymic activities or gene activation.

Is There Any Evidence That Serum ALT or AST Might Reflect the Metabolic Derangement Occurring in the Liver of MS Independent of the Presence of a Liver Disease?

In a rodent study, we observed that spontaneously hypertensive rats (SHR), a strain with genetic CVD and all the metabolic traits related with MS, including high blood pressure, dyslipidemia, and IR, show hepatomegaly, increased ALT levels, and liver upregulation of hypoxia-inducible factor 1 alpha (*Hif1α*) [28]. In this study we showed that the liver seems to be a target for cardiovascular organ damage and that CVD may predispose to an increased susceptibility of the liver to undergo pathological changes, including liver inflammation after exposure to a nutritional insult [28]. We also observed that in the disease model the behavior of liver transcripts involved in the regulation of metabolic functions, such as peroxisome-proliferator-activated receptors α and γ, the nuclear receptor Nr1d1 and Sirtuin 1 (*Sirt1*), showed a singular programming of the liver metabolism associated with a stress response [28].

Not surprisingly, *gpt* and *got* transcripts were elevated in the liver of the SHR rats regardless of the diet insult (unpublished data).

Furthermore, the metabolomic data from recent human studies also suggest that MS is associated with a profound metabolic derangement in which the reactions of transamination are critical modulators [4, 9]. Actually, we postulated the hypothesis that serum levels of the transaminases ALT and AST are associated with a deregulation of normal amino acid metabolism in the liver, and in patients with MS the levels of transaminases are not necessarily markers of liver injury [29]. On the contrary, changes in the level of transaminases in patients with MS might provide a molecular explanation of the altered glutamate-related metabolotype and may suggest a dramatic change in the paradigm of the role of ALT and AST as biomarkers of metabolic derangement. Hence, we suggest that circulating levels of transaminases in patients with MS mirror the liver metabolic reprogramming reflecting high levels of hepatic transamination of amino acids in the liver [29]. We thus postulate that circulating levels of ALT represent a good indicator of protein utilization being a "barometer" of the metabolic state of the body.

Unfortunately, human research around liver transaminases is confined to liver diseases that involve some degree of liver damage. Nevertheless, research in other species has shown interesting findings regarding the physiological regulation of liver transaminases. For example, a high degree of correlation was shown between food ration size and the activity of the enzyme ALT (EC 2.6.1.2) in fish, indicating that long-term limited feeding decreased ALT activity [30].

It would be exciting to better understand the regulation of ALT transcriptional activity. Some previous work indicates that Kruppel-like factor 15 (KLF15), which is regulated by insulin and plays an important role in the regulation of gluconeogenesis, might regulate the enzymatic activity of ALT [31]. Actually, Gray and coworkers demonstrated a decrease in liver ALT activity in mice lacking KLF15. In addition, it was shown that peroxisome proliferator-activated receptor α might act as transcriptional regulator of the liver ALT gene by a direct action on a response element in its proximal promoter [32].

On the other hand, experimental data suggest that the cytosolic but not mitochondrial AST gene is regulated by cAMP under a high-protein diet [33]. Horio and colleagues suggest that the metabolic function of cytosolic AST physiologically increases the supply of oxaloacetate for liver gluconeogenesis [33].

Glutamine-Cycling Pathway and MS: Systems Biology Reveals Clues for Future Research and Deciphers Putative Disease Molecular Mechanisms Underlying This Association

In this section, we propose the use of systems biology approaches to reveal and decipher the putative disease pathways or molecular mechanisms underlying the role of the glutamate in the pathogenesis of MS.

Why Systems Biology to Answer This Question?

Systems biology approaches often combine OMIC (genomics, proteomics, or metabolomics) data, including expression array analysis, the measurement of transcript levels, gene–gene and protein–protein interactions, the relation between transcript levels and clinical traits, etc., which allow scientists to identify hidden connections among known genes, proteins, or molecular targets, and thus integrate the knowledge to predict novel functional implications.

Hence, our first approach was to use data-mining approaches to collect the available published evidence from biomedical literature. Therefore, by text mining we were able to retrieve meaningful biological information that might be hidden in the classic search by key words in the repositories of biomedical literature. Thus, we used the PESCADOR platform (*P*latform for *E*xploration of *S*ignificant *C*oncepts *A*ssociate*D* to co-*O*ccurrence *R*elationships) [34] with the query "metabolic syndrome AND (glutamine OR glutamate OR glutamic acid)"; after abstract tagging, 375 gene/protein terms were identified in 265 published abstracts.

Therefore, we explored the interactions among the gene/proteins tagged by PESCADOR under the above-mentioned terms or key words, and we displayed them in a graphic that depicts a hierarchical hub centered on one gene/protein, GAD1 (glutamate decarboxylase 1), the gene of which encodes for a intracellular widely expressed protein involved in the conversion of the amino acid and excitatory neurotransmitter glutamate to the inhibitory neurotransmitter gamma-aminobutyric acid (GABA) (Fig. 20.3).

Furthermore, this enzyme has been identified as an autoantigen in insulin-dependent diabetes. Moreover, the immediate downstream terms were INS (insulin), PDIA3 (protein disulfide isomerase family A, member 3), ADIPOQ (adiponectin), ERP20 (reticuloplasmin), TXNDC5, GLUD1 (glutamate dehydrogenase 1), GAD2 (glutamate decarboxylase 2), and GLYAT (glycine-*N*-acyltransferase) (Fig. 20.3). Interestingly, gene variants in *GAD2* were associated with the susceptibility for morbid obesity in some [35] but not all the candidate gene studies [35]. Nevertheless, other studies support the role of variants in the promoter of GAD2 as putative risk factors for obesity in children [36] and suggest that they are associated with eating behaviors and weight gain [37].

Based on the list of genes/proteins identified as explained earlier (Table 20.2 shows the term list), we performed a functional association analysis using the bioinformatic resource GenMANIA [38].

Thus, the analysis of the genetic interactions, pathways, protein co-expression, co-localization, and protein domain similarity of our query list showed a network of predicted genes (Fig. 20.4) that

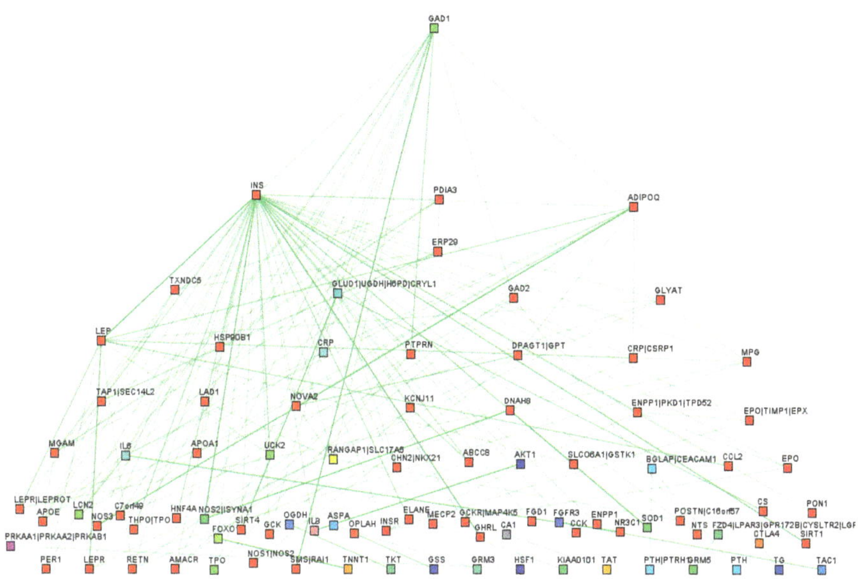

Fig. 20.3 Graphic illustration of gene/protein co-occurrence and its relatedness to biological concepts with the query "metabolic syndrome AND glutamine OR glutamate OR glutamic acid". Prediction was performed by PESCADOR (available at http://cbdm.mdc-berlin.de/tools/pescador/). The graph was constructed using the free available program MEDUSA, which is a Java application for visualizing and manipulating graphs of interaction (www.bork.embl.de/medusa)

Table 20.2 Genes terms identified in 265 published abstracts by the PESCADOR platform with the query "metabolic syndrome AND glutamine OR glutamate OR glutamic acid"

Human symbol	Gene ID
OPLAH	26873
AACS	65985
GAA	2548
OGDH	4967
APOA1	335
APOE	348
CRP	1401
CCK	885
EPOR	2057
GHRL	51738
NR3C1	2908
GCKR	2646
GSS	2937
HSF1	3297
IL8	3576
INS	3630
INSR	3643
LEP	3952
LEPR	3953
GRM3	2913
PAF1	54623
PTH	5741
PCSK1	5122
RETN	56729
TAC1	6863
TG	7038
TPO	7173
TKT	7086
FGFR3	2261
ADIPOQ	9370
AKT1	207
PRKAA2	5563
NOVA2	4858
ASPA	443
CA1	759
CS	1431
CTLA4	1493
NOS3	4846
ENPP1	5167
EPO	2056
ERP29	10961
TXNDC5	81567
FOXO1	2308
GAD1	2571
GAD2	2572
GLUD1	2746
GPBAR1	151306
GPT	2875
HSP90B1	7184

(continued)

Table 20.2 (continued)

Human symbol	Gene ID
GSTK1	373156
ELANE	1991
PTPRN	5798
IL6	3569
KCNJ11	3767
LAD1	3898
LCN2	3934
CCL2	6347
MECP2	4204
GRM5	2915
HNF4A	3172
C7orf49	78996
NOS1	4842
NTS	4922
PER1	5187
USB1	79650
PON1	5444
AMACR	23600
B4GALNT2	124872
SIRT1	23411
SIRT4	23409
SMS	6611
SOD1	6647
ABCC8	6833
TAP1	6890
TAT	6898
TNNT1	7138
UCK2	7371

include, among others, *GPT* and *SIRT1* as newly predicted genes. In addition, there was a marked redundancy of pathways associated with the regulation of glucose metabolism (Table 20.3). Interestingly, if we restrict the functional analysis to genes/proteins associated with transaminases and glucose control, we can see expected and obvious genes, such as insulin, insulin receptor, and glucokinase, and among the newly predicted genes, we can see *GPT* and *SIRT1* (Fig. 20.5) as predicted to have a potential role in the glucose metabolic process and insulin secretion, respectively.

Moreover, *GPT* was predicted to have interactions with *GLUD1* (glutamate dehydrogenase 1). The glutamate dehydrogenase, which is allosterically activated by ADP and inhibited by GTP and ATP and regulated in a complex manner by a number of negative (palmitoyl-coenzyme A) and positive (leucine) allosteric regulators, has an important tissue-specific role. For example, in beta cells glutamate dehydrogenase regulates the amino acid-stimulated insulin secretion; in hepatocytes, it participates in the modulation of amino acid catabolism and ammoniagenesis; and in brain neurons, it participates in the maintenance of glutamate neurotransmitter concentrations, which is relevant to feeding behavior, as discussed later. Furthermore, activating mutations in the *GLUD* gene are a common cause of congenital hyperinsulinism and hyperammonemia syndrome.

GPT also has interactions with *PON1* (paraoxonase 1), *SLC16A10* (solute carrier family 16, member 10), *PTPRN* (protein tyrosine phosphatase, receptor type, N), *APOA1* (apolipoprotein A-I), *GSTK1* (glutathione S-transferase kappa 1), *ACSS2* (acyl-CoA synthetase short-chain family member 2), and *SIRT4* (sirtuin 4). Table 20.4 summarizes these interactions.

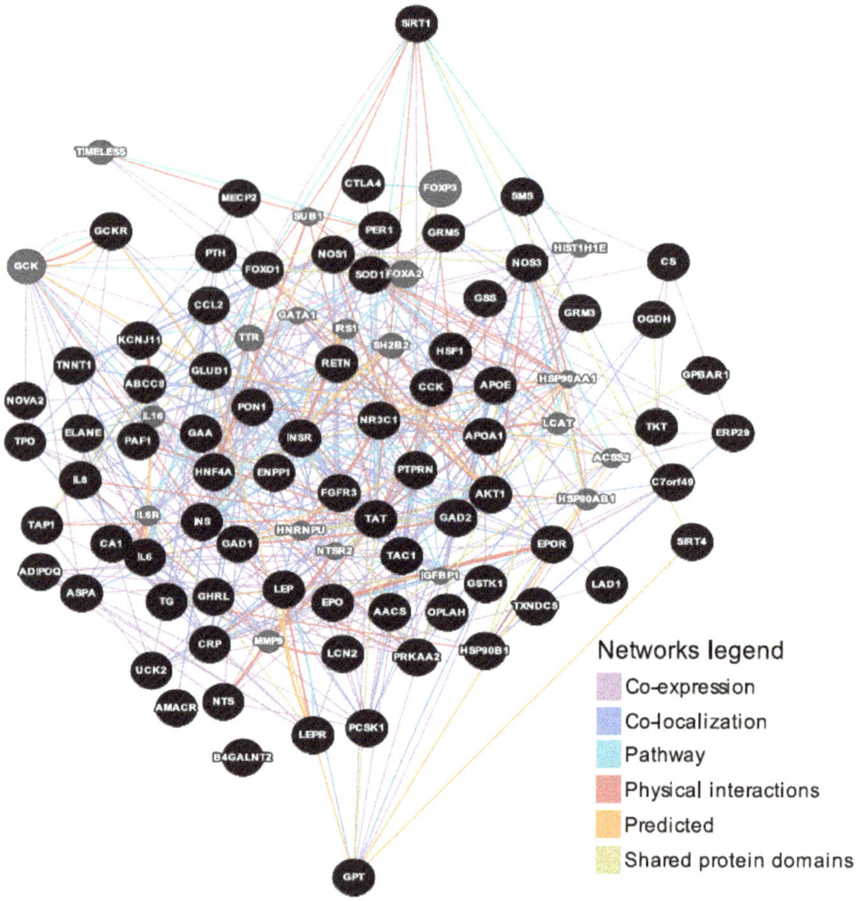

Fig. 20.4 Results of functional association analysis performed by the bioinformatics resource GenMANIA (available at http://www.genemania.org/, Toronto, Canada). Illustration includes molecular functions summarized in GO terms (the gene ontology pathway GO) based on a set of input genes identified by the text-mining tool PESCADOR (Table 20.2)

Table 20.3 Gene ontology (GO) annotation of predicted biological process, in which the candidate genes listed in Table 20.2 are involved by functional enrichment analysis using the GeneMANIA tool (genemania.org)

Molecular functions summarized in GO terms	FDR	Genes in network	Genes in genome
Glucose metabolic process	2.50E−15	17	134
Regulation of glucose metabolic process	2.33E−14	12	47
Hexose metabolic process	2.33E−14	17	162
Monosaccharide metabolic process	2.33E−14	18	196
Regulation of carbohydrate metabolic process	1.26E−13	12	55
Regulation of cellular carbohydrate metabolic process	1.26E−13	12	55
Small molecule catabolic process	3.26E−12	17	228
Energy reserve metabolic process	1.88E−11	14	140
Peptide transport	5.06E−11	13	119
Peptide hormone secretion	5.45E−10	12	111
Peptide secretion	5.52E−10	12	112
Energy derivation by oxidation of organic compounds	6.06E−10	16	276
Signal release	6.06E−10	14	186

(continued)

Table 20.3 (continued)

Molecular functions summarized in GO terms	FDR	Genes in network	Genes in genome
Generation of a signal involved in cell–cell signaling	6.06E−10	14	186
Cellular response to hormone stimulus	8.31E−10	16	283
Regulation of insulin secretion	1.00E−09	11	91
Regulation of carbohydrate biosynthetic process	1.57E−09	8	30
Regulation of response to external stimulus	1.57E−09	14	204
Hormone secretion	1.68E−09	12	129
Regulation of peptide hormone secretion	1.68E−09	11	97
Regulation of peptide transport	1.68E−09	11	98
Regulation of peptide secretion	1.68E−09	11	98
Insulin secretion	1.80E−09	11	99
Regulation of glycogen biosynthetic process	2.01E−09	7	19
Regulation of glucan biosynthetic process	2.01E−09	7	19
Hormone transport	2.01E−09	12	133
Regulation of polysaccharide biosynthetic process	2.01E−09	7	19
Regulation of polysaccharide metabolic process	2.73E−09	7	20
Cellular response to peptide hormone stimulus	2.73E−09	14	220
Regulation of glycogen metabolic process	2.73E−09	7	20
Glucose homeostasis	2.73E−09	9	53
Carbohydrate homeostasis	2.73E−09	9	53
Endocrine pancreas development	3.32E−09	8	35
Carboxylic acid catabolic process	4.10E−09	12	146
Organic acid catabolic process	4.10E−09	12	146
Response to peptide hormone stimulus	4.10E−09	14	230
Regulation of hormone levels	4.77E−09	14	234
Positive regulation of glucose metabolic process	4.77E−09	7	22
Positive regulation of glycogen biosynthetic process	5.49E−09	6	12
Regulation of hormone secretion	5.49E−09	11	115
Regulation of generation of precursor metabolites and energy	6.87E−09	8	39
Positive regulation of glycogen metabolic process	9.53E−09	6	13
Regulation of secretion	9.53E−09	14	249
Pancreas development	9.53E−09	8	41
Endocrine system development	9.53E−09	9	63
Regulation of glucose transport	9.53E−09	9	63
Cellular response to insulin stimulus	9.53E−09	12	160
Positive regulation of carbohydrate metabolic process	1.03E−08	7	25
Positive regulation of cellular carbohydrate metabolic process	1.03E−08	7	25

The list includes the top 50 records with significant results. The analysis was performed by the bioinformatic resource GenMANIA [38], and association data include protein and genetic interactions, pathways, co-expression, co-localization, and protein domain similarity. Genes are linked in a pathway if they participate in the same reaction within a pathway

The GO categories and Q-values from a FDR corrected hypergeometric test for enrichment are shown, along with coverage ratios for the number of annotated genes in the displayed network versus the number of genes with that annotation in the genome. The estimation of *Q*-values was corrected for multiple testing by Benjamini-Hochberg procedure [38]

Furthermore, we performed an additional functional enrichment analysis (Table 20.5) using the bioinformatics resource *ToppGene Suite* (http://toppgene.cchmc.org, Cincinnati, OH, USA). Among the highly predicted pathways, the FOXA2 and FOXA3 transcription factor network was ranked along with the top five. These genes encode members of the forkead class of DNA-binding proteins. *FOXOA2* is also known as hepatocyte nuclear factor 3, beta, and FOXOA3 as hepatocyte nuclear factor 3, gamma, which are transcriptional activators of liver-specific genes that interact with chromatin, opening the compacted chromatin for other proteins through interactions with nucleosomal core histones and

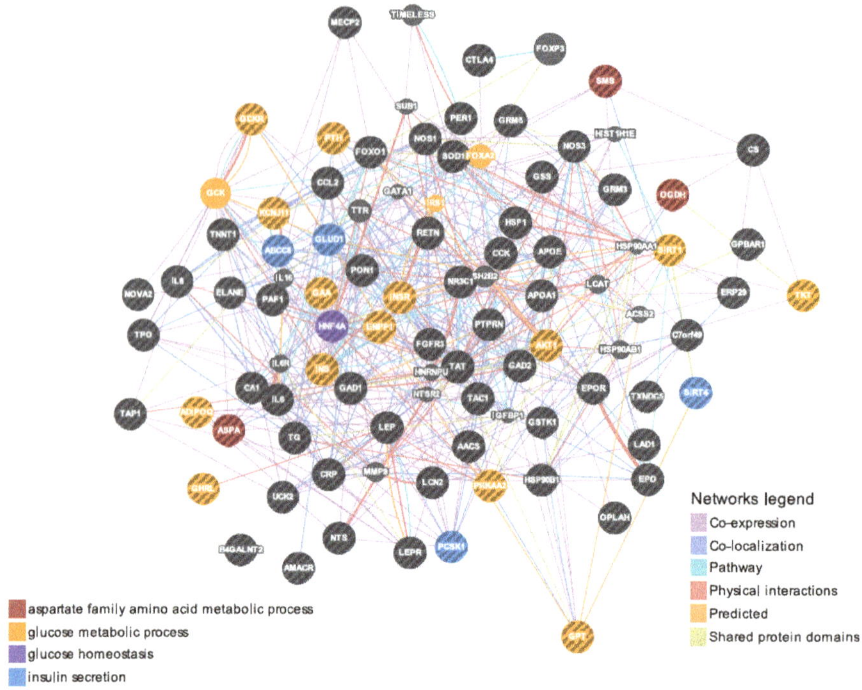

Fig. 20.5 Results of functional association analysis restricted to GO terms: aspartate family, glucose metabolic process and homeostasis and insulin secretion performed by the bioinformatics resource GenMANIA. Illustration includes molecular functions summarized in GO terms (the gene ontology pathway GO) based on a set of input genes identified by the text-mining tool PESCADOR (Table 20.2)

Table 20.4 Interactions of GPT (glutamic-pyruvate transaminase or alanine aminotransferase) gene predicted by the bioinformatic resource GenMANIA [38] based on genomic and proteomic data

Gene 1	Gene 2	Weight	Network group
PTPRN	GPT	0.01880419	Co-expression
PER1	GPT	0.01072104	Co-expression
APOA1	GPT	0.00810353	Co-expression
GSTK1	GPT	0.00674771	Co-expression
GSTK1	GPT	0.01971637	Co-localization
PON1	GPT	0.00952473	Co-localization
GPT	SIRT4	0.02041759	Predicted
ACSS2	GPT	0.00622299	Predicted
GLUD1	GPT	0.00580657	Predicted
TAT	GPT	0.08657161	Shared protein domains

The interaction analysis supposes that two genes are functionally associated if the effects of perturbing one gene were found to be modified by perturbations to a second gene. These data are collected from primary studies and BioGRID [38]

Each interaction is represented as a weighted interaction network where each pair of genes is assigned an association weight, which is either zero indicating no interaction, or a positive value that reflects the strength of interaction or the reliability the observation that they interact. The more the genes are co-expressed, the higher the weight they are linked by, ranging up to 1.0, meaning perfectly correlated expression [38]

thereby replacing linker histones at target enhancer and/or promoter sites. Related family members of FOXOA2 and FOXOA3 in rodents have roles in the differentiation of the liver and pancreas.

Finally, the text mining of glutaminase 2 (*GLS2*), the gene that encodes a mitochondrial phosphate-activated glutaminase that catalyzes the hydrolysis of glutamine to stoichiometric amounts of

Table 20.5 Functional annotations and protein interaction networks of candidate genes and proteins associated with the term list of Table 20.2

ID	Name/source	*p*-Value	Term in query	Term in genome
GO: Molecular function				
GO:0005102	Receptor binding	1.309E−8	25	1304
GO:0005179	Hormone activity	1.415E−8	10	113
GO:0048037	Cofactor binding	8.148E−8	13	293
GO:0042802	Identical protein binding	1.289E−6	20	1016
GO:0016597	Amino acid binding	8.139E−5	7	101
GO: Biological process				
GO:0006082	Organic acid metabolic process	1.768E−18	32	963
GO:0006066	Alcohol metabolic process	4.864E−18	27	611
GO:0006006	Glucose metabolic process	8.350E−18	20	241
GO:0043436	Oxoacid metabolic process	1.417E−17	31	945
GO:0019752	Carboxylic acid metabolic process	1.417E−17	31	945
GO: Cellular component				
GO:0005615	Extracellular space	1.401E−9	22	927
GO:0044421	Extracellular region part	5.886E−9	24	1216
GO:0031410	Cytoplasmic vesicle	5.082E−5	17	978
GO:0016023	Cytoplasmic membrane-bounded vesicle	8.311E−5	16	894
GO:0031982	Vesicle	1.053E−4	17	1030
Human phenotype				
HP:0000855	Insulin resistance	1.261E−4	8	44
HP:0005978	Noninsulin-dependent diabetes mellitus	5.300E−4	7	36
HP:0000818	Abnormality of the endocrine system	1.991E−3	20	477
HP:0000825	Hyperinsulinemic hypoglycemia	2.812E−3	4	8
HP:0003584	Late onset diabetes	4.088E−3	8	68
HP:0006476	Abnormality of the pancreatic islet cells	1.906E−2	4	12
HP:0001952	Abnormal glucose tolerance	3.047E−2	9	116
HP:0003192	Small, short nose	3.054E−2	3	5
HP:0006279	Beta-cell dysfunction	3.054E−2	3	5
HP:0005487	Prominent metopic suture	3.054E−2	3	5
Mouse phenotype				
MP:0005291	Abnormal glucose tolerance	1.830E−11	21	270
MP:0005293	Impaired glucose tolerance	9.948E−11	17	164
MP:0002078	Abnormal glucose homeostasis	1.869E−9	26	573
MP:0000187	Abnormal triglyceride level	2.925E−9	19	270
MP:0005375	Adipose tissue phenotype	7.628E−9	24	505
Pathway				
WP1533	Vitamin B12 metabolism	6.045E−6	8	51
PW:0000208	Diabetes type 2	1.496E−5	4	5
PW:0000027	Glutamate metabolic	3.038E−5	5	13
hnf3bpathway	FOXA2 and FOXA3 transcription factor networks	4.819E−5	7	44
MAP00251_Glutamate_ metabolism	MAP00251 glutamate metabolism	3.489E−4	5	20
Interaction				
int:LEP	LEP interactions	1.469E−6	5	11
int:MEP1A	MEP1A interactions	3.873E−3	4	21
int:NOSIP	NOSIP interactions	4.973E−3	3	7
int:IDE	IDE interactions	3.070E−2	3	12
int:DNAJB1	DNAJB1 interactions	3.602E−2	4	36
Drugs				
D005632	Fructose	6.408E−19	18	125

(continued)

Table 20.5 (continued)

ID	Name/source	*p*-Value	Term in query	Term in genome
CID000005300	Streptozotocin	8.563E–18	27	540
CID000000946	Nitrite	1.708E–17	21	253
CID000004091	Metformin	2.830E–15	19	235
CID000000702	EtOH	4.618E–15	29	837
Disease				
D003924	Diabetes mellitus, type 2	4.841E–6	9	59
20081125:Ridker	C-reactive protein	7.500E–5	4	6
D006946	Hyperinsulinism	1.735E–4	4	7
125853	Diabetes mellitus, noninsulin-dependent; NIDDM	3.377E–4	6	31
D024821	Metabolic syndrome X	3.440E–4	4	8

The analysis was done based on transcriptome, proteome, regulome (TFBS and miRNA), ontologies (the gene ontology (GO) pathway), phenotype (human disease and mouse phenotype), pharmacome (drug–gene associations), literature co-citation, and other features by the bioinformatics resource *ToppGene Suite* (http://toppgene.cchmc.org). The default parameter used was "Bonferroni" for multiple correction method and 0.05 for significance cut-off level

Table 20.6 Disease-gene associations mined from literature for the gene: GLS2 (Glutaminase 2, liver, mitochondrial, ENSP00000310447)

Name of the disease	*z*-Score
Diabetes mellitus	3.8
L-2-hydroxyglutaric aciduria	3.6
Hypoglycemia	3.4
Stomach carcinoma in situ	3.1
Hepatic encephalopathy	3.0
Hypertension	2.8
D-2-hydroxyglutaric aciduria	2.6
Newborn respiratory distress syndrome	2.6
Hereditary hyperbilirubinemia	2.5
Hyperglycemia	2.5

The analysis was performed by the resource DISEASES (http://diseases.jensenlab.org/) Each disease-gene association is based on a text-mining score, which is proportional to (1) the absolute number of conditionings and (2) the ratio of observed to expect conditionings (i.e., the enrichment). These scores are normalized to z-scores by comparing them to a random background

glutamate and ammonia, showed that diabetes mellitus is the first ranked disease (Table 20.6). Likewise, other loci might be interesting targets to explore in the context of human DNA sequence variation and its role in the modulation of glutamic acid in patients with MS, such as *GLUL* (glutamate-ammonia ligase; the protein encoded by this gene catalyzes the synthesis of glutamine from glutamate and ammonia in a ATP-dependent manner as the reaction is energy demanding), *GLS* (or glutaminase; the encoded protein is a phosphate-activated amidohydrolase that catalyzes the hydrolysis of glutamine to glutamate and ammonia), and *GLUD2* (glutamate dehydrogenase 2; the encoded enzyme catalyzes the reversible oxidative deamination of glutamate to alpha-ketoglutarate), as already described. This reaction, which is dependent on NAD+/NADP+ and their reduced forms, is among the most important for ammonia incorporation to amino acids. Interestingly, *GLS*, *GLUD2*, and *GLUL* are predicted to interact with a *GOT2* and subunits of AMPK (AMP-dependent kinase) (Fig. 20.6) that serve as a major sensor of the energy state of the cell modifying gene expression through *SIRT1* [39]. In fact, the observed glutamine decrease observed in MS may be similar to glutamine starvation that induces a cell stress response via AMPK induction [40].

Advances in genotyping technology and information generated by genome-wide association studies (GWAS) have enormously increased our knowledge about gene variants associated with MS-associated phenotypes [41]. Thus, it is tempting to speculate that genomic variation might explain some of the enzymatic defects presented in the previous sections of this chapter.

Surprisingly, few human reports show an association between genetic risk variants for hyperglycemia or T2D with amino acid levels. In fact, Stancakova and coworkers demonstrated that the rs780094 of the *GCKR* gene (glucokinase or hexokinase 4 regulator) was significantly associated with the levels of several amino acids, including alanine, isoleucine, and glutamine [42]. Again, *GLS*, *GLUD2*, and *GLUL* are predicted to interact with *GCKR* (Fig. 20.6).

The lack of information about this topic might be because most of the metabolomic profiling and GWAS studies on the susceptibility of MS-related phenotypes are not performed in concert, and the major disease traits (T2D, obesity, CVD disease) and the major metabolic derangements (dysglucemia and dyslipidemia) are investigated either for gene variants or for metabolomic characterization in an unintegrated fashion.

Perhaps the most representative example of an integrated analysis was recently published, in which in a large collaborative study the authors performed a comprehensive analysis of genotype-dependent

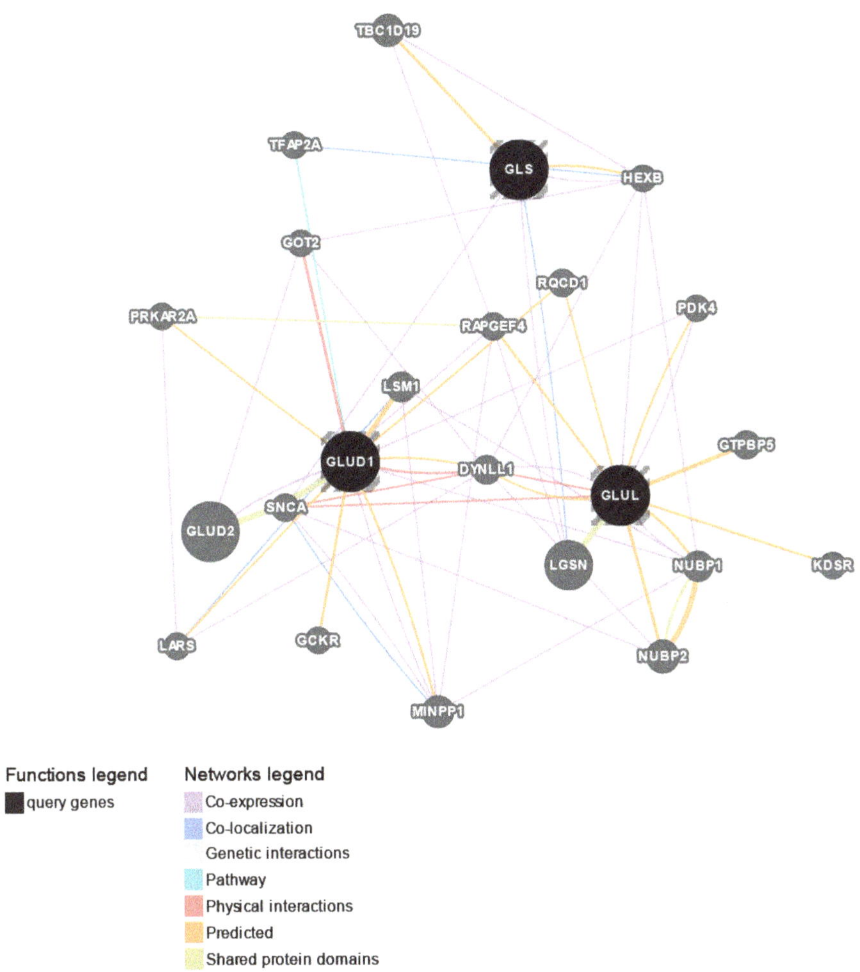

Fig. 20.6 Results of functional association analysis performed by the bioinformatics resource GenMANIA based on a set of input genes identified by the bigger black spheres

metabolic phenotypes using a GWAS with non-targeted metabolomics [43]. Interestingly, the rs780094 in the *GCKR* locus was associated with the mannose/glucose ratio and circulating levels of lactate [43], the rs2216405 in the *CPS1* (carbamoyl-phosphate synthase 1, mitochondrial) gene was associated with ammonia metabolism and glycine levels, the rs477992 in the *PHGDH* (phosphoglycerate ehydrogenase) gene was associated with serine levels, the rs7760535 in *SLC16A10* was associated with isoleucine/tyrosine levels, and finally the rs2657879 in *GLS2* was associated with glutamine levels [43].

Another example of this integrative approach for linking high-throughput metabolomics and genotyping datasets was recently published [44].

Certainly, metabolomic platforms for GWAS that link the genome to the metabolome are promising in terms of understanding the molecular mechanisms behind the connection between the glutamine-cycling pathway and MS [45].

Glutamate and Fetal Metabolic Programming: Glutamine-Cycling Pathway and the Connection Between MS and the Hypothalamic Signaling Cascade of Appetite Control

The worldwide prevalence of MS is alarming. In fact, figures of prevalence of MS from countries that instrument global and periodical epidemiological surveys, such as the National Health and Nutrition Examination Survey (NHANES), a program of studies designed to assess the health and nutritional status of adults and children in the United States, show a significant rise since their inception in 1960 (around 10 %) to the last NHANES 1999–2002 (35 %) [46]. A matter of significant concern is that the prevalence of MS has also reached pandemic proportions in children and adolescents [47], and nearly one-third (31.2 %) of overweight/obese adolescents in the United States have MS, according to the last report [48].

Plenty of experimental and epidemiological data support the hypothesis that MS-associated conditions, such as coronary heart disease and stroke, hypertension, and T2D, may originate through impaired growth and development during fetal life and infancy, as originally described by Barker [49]. This hypothesis is also known as “The thrifty phenotype hypothesis proposes” [50] and originally focused on the development of T2D and MS as resulting from the effects of poor nutrition in early life [50]. Nowadays, the hypothesis of early nutritional programming or metabolic programming has been extended also to a fetal environment of maternal over-nutrition [51, 52]. Interestingly, in the context of observation that fetal over-nutrition plays a critical role in the development of the MS, Hermanussen M and colleagues have suggested that a thrifty phenotype might be the consequence of fetal hyperglutamatemia [53]. This concept was formulated based on the idea that dietary excess of maternal glutamate reaches the fetal circulation by the materno-fetal glutamine-glutamate exchange [53]. As a consequence, glutamate produces a profound remodeling of the hypothalamic leptin-signaling cascade, resulting in a phenotype characterized by a permanent elevation of plasma leptin levels that fail to adequately counter-regulate food intake [53]. It is worth noting that in the above-mentioned abnormal physiological circuit, both the liver and the placenta are key players because there are important inter-organ cycles for amino acids between fetal liver and placenta [54]. Actually, the fetal liver has been shown to be the primary site for glutamate production and release, and the entry of glutamine from the placenta accounts for approximately 60 % of the total glutamine entry rate in fetal plasma [55].

Furthermore, Battaglia and coworkers demonstrated an interesting point about the high rate of transamination of the BCAA to their respective keto acids occurring in the placenta, which modulates the placental production of glutamic acid from oxoglutarate [54]. Hence, the clinical observations derived from the metabolic profiling studies mentioned earlier once again reinforce the biological plausibility of the fetal origin of adult MS.

Based on the idea that high intake of the amino acid glutamate in the periconceptional period determines the propensity of obesity, Hermanussen and colleagues administered monosodium glutamate to pregnant rats and showed that the resulting phenotype was characterized by obesity, voracity, and short stature, suggesting that the neural toxicity of glutamic acid significantly impacts on the animals' behavior and hormonal regulation of appetite [56].

Conclusions

Old concepts from quantitative biology and new evidence from modern laboratory techniques both confirm the significant role of the glutamine-cycling pathway in the modulation of the global metabolic derangement in MS. Actually, changes in the circulating profile of BCCA observed in patients with MS, including glutamic acid or the ratio glutamate/glutamine, may be used in clinical practice as robust and noninvasive biomarkers for both risk prediction and disease complications. The plasma metabolic profiling along with changes in the levels of key enzymes that feed the TCC cycle might suggest a genotype-dependent glutamate metabolotype. Furthermore, high levels of circulating ALT and AST in patients with MS might reflect high levels of hepatic transamination of amino acids in the liver instead of just liver necrosis, and long-term liver metabolic programming might predispose to oncogenic transformation.

Funding Support This study was partially supported by grants PICT 2008-1521 and 2010-0441 (Agencia Nacional de Promoción Científica y Tecnológica), and UBACYT CM04 (Universidad de Buenos Aires). SS and CJP belong to CONICET.

Potential competing interests The authors have no conflict of interest to declare.

References

1. Grundy SM, Cleeman JI, Daniels SR, et al. Diagnosis and management of the metabolic syndrome: an American Heart Association/National Heart, Lung, and Blood Institute Scientific Statement. Circulation. 2005;112:2735–52.
2. Reaven GM. Banting lecture 1988. Role of insulin resistance in human disease. Diabetes. 1988;37:1595–607.
3. Reaven GM. The metabolic syndrome: is this diagnosis necessary? Am J Clin Nutr. 2006;83:1237–47.
4. Newgard CB, An J, Bain JR, et al. A branched-chain amino acid-related metabolic signature that differentiates obese and lean humans and contributes to insulin resistance. Cell Metab. 2009;9:311–26.
5. Wang TJ, Larson MG, Vasan RS, et al. Metabolite profiles and the risk of developing diabetes. Nat Med. 2011;17:448–53.
6. Huffman KM, Shah SH, Stevens RD, et al. Relationships between circulating metabolic intermediates and insulin action in overweight to obese, inactive men and women. Diabetes Care. 2009;32:1678–83.
7. Fiehn O, Garvey WT, Newman JW, Lok KH, Hoppel CL, Adams SH. Plasma metabolomic profiles reflective of glucose homeostasis in non-diabetic and type 2 diabetic obese African-American women. PLoS One. 2010;5:e15234.
8. Wurtz P, Makinen VP, Soininen P, et al. Metabolic signatures of insulin resistance in 7,098 young adults. Diabetes. 2012;61:1372–80.
9. Cheng S, Rhee EP, Larson MG, et al. Metabolite profiling identifies pathways associated with metabolic risk in humans. Circulation. 2012;125:2222–31.
10. Shah SH, Bain JR, Muehlbauer MJ, et al. Association of a peripheral blood metabolic profile with coronary artery disease and risk of subsequent cardiovascular events. Circ Cardiovasc Genet. 2010;3:207–14.
11. Felig P, Marliss E, Cahill Jr GF. Plasma amino acid levels and insulin secretion in obesity. N Engl J Med. 1969;281:811–6.
12. Patti ME, Brambilla E, Luzi L, Landaker EJ, Kahn CR. Bidirectional modulation of insulin action by amino acids. J Clin Invest. 1998;101:1519–29.
13. Krebs M, Brehm A, Krssak M, et al. Direct and indirect effects of amino acids on hepatic glucose metabolism in humans. Diabetologia. 2003;46:917–25.

14. van Loon LJ, Kruijshoop M, Menheere PP, Wagenmakers AJ, Saris WH, Keizer HA. Amino acid ingestion strongly enhances insulin secretion in patients with long-term type 2 diabetes. Diabetes Care. 2003;26:625–30.
15. Brand K, Von HJ, Langer K, Fekl W. Pathways of glutamine and glutamate metabolism in resting and proliferating rat thymocytes: comparison between free and peptide-bound glutamine. J Cell Physiol. 1987;132:559–64.
16. Lindblom P, Rafter I, Copley C, et al. Isoforms of alanine aminotransferases in human tissues and serum—differential tissue expression using novel antibodies. Arch Biochem Biophys. 2007;466:66–77.
17. Goessling W, Massaro JM, Vasan RS, D'Agostino Sr RB, Ellison RC, Fox CS. Aminotransferase levels and 20-year risk of metabolic syndrome, diabetes, and cardiovascular disease. Gastroenterology. 2008;135:1935–44.
18. Porter SA, Pedley A, Massaro JM, Vasan RS, Hoffmann U, Fox CS. Aminotransferase levels are associated with cardiometabolic risk above and beyond visceral fat and insulin resistance: the framingham heart study. Arterioscler Thromb Vasc Biol. 2013;33:139–46.
19. Qu HQ, Li Q, Grove ML, et al. Population-based risk factors for elevated alanine aminotransferase in a South Texas Mexican-American population. Arch Med Res. 2012;43:482–8.
20. Hanley AJ, Williams K, Festa A, Wagenknecht LE, D'Agostino Jr RB, Haffner SM. Liver markers and development of the metabolic syndrome: the insulin resistance atherosclerosis study. Diabetes. 2005;54:3140–7.
21. Kain K, Carter AM, Grant PJ, Scott EM. Alanine aminotransferase is associated with atherothrombotic risk factors in a British South Asian population. J Thromb Haemost. 2008;6:737–41.
22. Schindhelm RK, Diamant M, Dekker JM, Tushuizen ME, Teerlink T, Heine RJ. Alanine aminotransferase as a marker of non-alcoholic fatty liver disease in relation to type 2 diabetes mellitus and cardiovascular disease. Diabetes Metab Res Rev. 2006;22:437–43.
23. Nguyen QM, Srinivasan SR, Xu JH, et al. Elevated liver function enzymes are related to the development of prediabetes and type 2 diabetes in younger adults: the bogalusa heart study. Diabetes Care. 2011;34:2603–7.
24. Olynyk JK, Knuiman MW, Divitini ML, Davis TM, Beilby J, Hung J. Serum alanine aminotransferase, metabolic syndrome, and cardiovascular disease in an Australian population. Am J Gastroenterol. 2009;104:1715–22.
25. Monami M, Bardini G, Lamanna C, et al. Liver enzymes and risk of diabetes and cardiovascular disease: results of the Firenze Bagno a Ripoli (FIBAR) study. Metabolism. 2008;57:387–92.
26. Vozarova B, Stefan N, Lindsay RS, et al. High alanine aminotransferase is associated with decreased hepatic insulin sensitivity and predicts the development of type 2 diabetes. Diabetes. 2002;51:1889–95.
27. Sinner MF, Wang N, Fox CS, et al. Relation of circulating liver transaminase concentrations to risk of new-onset atrial fibrillation. Am J Cardiol. 2013;111:219–24.
28. Burgueno AL, Gianotti TF, Mansilla NG, Pirola CJ, Sookoian S. Cardiovascular disease is associated with high-fat-diet-induced liver damage and up-regulation of the hepatic expression of hypoxia-inducible factor 1alpha in a rat model. Clin Sci (Lond). 2013;124:53–63.
29. Sookoian S, Pirola CJ. Alanine and aspartate aminotransferase and glutamine-cycling pathway: their roles in pathogenesis of metabolic syndrome. World J Gastroenterol. 2012;18:3775–81.
30. Meton I, Mediavilla D, Caseras A, Canto E, Fernandez F, Baanante IV. Effect of diet composition and ration size on key enzyme activities of glycolysis-gluconeogenesis, the pentose phosphate pathway and amino acid metabolism in liver of gilthead sea bream (Sparus aurata). Br J Nutr. 1999;82:223–32.
31. Gray S, Wang B, Orihuela Y, et al. Regulation of gluconeogenesis by Kruppel-like factor 15. Cell Metab. 2007;5:305–12.
32. Thulin P, Rafter I, Stockling K, et al. PPARalpha regulates the hepatotoxic biomarker alanine aminotransferase (ALT1) gene expression in human hepatocytes. Toxicol Appl Pharmacol. 2008;231:1–9.
33. Horio Y, Tanaka T, Taketoshi M, Uno T, Wada H. Rat cytosolic aspartate aminotransferase: regulation of its mRNA and contribution to gluconeogenesis. J Biochem. 1988;103:805–8.
34. Barbosa-Silva A, Fontaine JF, Donnard ER, Stussi F, Ortega JM, Andrade-Navarro MA. PESCADOR, a web-based tool to assist text-mining of biointeractions extracted from PubMed queries. BMC Bioinformatics. 2011;12:435.
35. Boutin P, Dina C, Vasseur F, et al. GAD2 on chromosome 10p12 is a candidate gene for human obesity. PLoS Biol. 2003;1:E68.
36. Meyre D, Boutin P, Tounian A, et al. Is glutamate decarboxylase 2 (GAD2) a genetic link between low birth weight and subsequent development of obesity in children? J Clin Endocrinol Metab. 2005;90:2384–90.
37. Choquette AC, Lemieux S, Tremblay A, et al. GAD2 gene sequence variations are associated with eating behaviors and weight gain in women from the Quebec family study. Physiol Behav. 2009;98:505–10.
38. Warde-Farley D, Donaldson SL, Comes O, et al. The GeneMANIA prediction server: biological network integration for gene prioritization and predicting gene function. Nucleic Acids Res. 2010;38:W214–20.
39. Ruderman NB, Xu XJ, Nelson L, et al. AMPK and SIRT1: a long-standing partnership? Am J Physiol Endocrinol Metab. 2010;298:E751–60.
40. Oehler R, Roth E. Regulative capacity of glutamine. Curr Opin Clin Nutr Metab Care. 2003;6:277–82.
41. Sookoian S, Pirola CJ. Metabolic syndrome: from the genetics to the pathophysiology. Curr Hypertens Rep. 2011;13:149–57.
42. Stancakova A, Civelek M, Saleem NK, et al. Hyperglycemia and a common variant of GCKR are associated with the levels of eight amino acids in 9,369 Finnish men. Diabetes. 2012;61(7):1895–902.

43. Suhre K, Shin SY, Petersen AK, et al. Human metabolic individuality in biomedical and pharmaceutical research. Nature. 2011;477:54–60.
44. Krumsiek J, Suhre K, Evans AM, et al. Mining the unknown: a systems approach to metabolite identification combining genetic and metabolic information. PLoS Genet. 2012;8:e1003005.
45. Adamski J, Suhre K. Metabolomics platforms for genome wide association studies-linking the genome to the metabolome. Curr Opin Biotechnol. 2013;24:39–47.
46. Ford ES, Giles WH, Dietz WH. Prevalence of the metabolic syndrome among US adults: findings from the third National Health and Nutrition Examination Survey. JAMA. 2002;287:356–9.
47. Johnson WD, Kroon JJ, Greenway FL, Bouchard C, Ryan D, Katzmarzyk PT. Prevalence of risk factors for metabolic syndrome in adolescents: National Health and Nutrition Examination Survey (NHANES), 2001–2006. Arch Pediatr Adolesc Med. 2009;163:371–7.
48. de Ferranti SD, Gauvreau K, Ludwig DS, Neufeld EJ, Newburger JW, Rifai N. Prevalence of the metabolic syndrome in American adolescents: findings from the Third National Health and Nutrition Examination Survey. Circulation. 2004;110:2494–7.
49. Barker DJ, Clark PM. Fetal undernutrition and disease in later life. Rev Reprod. 1997;2:105–12.
50. Hales CN, Barker DJ. The thrifty phenotype hypothesis. Br Med Bull. 2001;60:5–20.
51. Poston L. Gestational weight gain: influences on the long-term health of the child. Curr Opin Clin Nutr Metab Care. 2012;15:252–7.
52. Sookoian S, Fernandez GT, Burgueno A, Pirola CJ. Fetal metabolic programming and epigenetic modifications: a systems biology approach. Pediatr Res. 2013;73:531–42.
53. Hermanussen M, Tresguerres JA. Does the thrifty phenotype result from chronic glutamate intoxication? A hypothesis. J Perinat Med. 2003;31:489–95.
54. Battaglia FC. Glutamine and glutamate exchange between the fetal liver and the placenta. J Nutr. 2000; 130:974S–7S.
55. Vaughn PR, Lobo C, Battaglia FC, Fennessey PV, Wilkening RB, Meschia G. Glutamine-glutamate exchange between placenta and fetal liver. Am J Physiol. 1995;268:E705–11.
56. Hermanussen M, Garcia AP, Sunder M, Voigt M, Salazar V, Tresguerres JA. Obesity, voracity, and short stature: the impact of glutamate on the regulation of appetite. Eur J Clin Nutr. 2006;60:25–31.

Chapter 21
Glutamine and Glucagon-Like Peptide-1 Response

Jerry R. Greenfield and Dorit Samocha-Bonet

Key Points

- L-glutamine is a potent secretagogue of glucagon-like peptide-1 from the L-cells model GLUTag cell line and primary intestinal cells in vitro.
- Oral ingestion of L-glutamine increases plasma concentrations of glucagon-like peptide-1 and gastric inhibitory polypeptide (also known as glucose-dependent insulinotropic polypeptide) in healthy and type 2 diabetes patients.
- Oral ingestion of L-glutamine with a meal decreases glycemia in type 2 diabetes patients.
- Decreased postprandial glycemia after glutamine ingestion is likely due to delayed gastric emptying induced by glutamine itself and/or glucagon-like peptide-1.

Keywords Glutamine • Insulin secretion • Glucagon-like peptide-1 • Incretins • Entero-endocrine L-cells

Abbreviations

DPP-IV	Dipeptidyl peptidase-IV
GABA	γ-Aminobutyric acid
GIP	Gastric inhibitory polypeptide also known as glucose-dependent insulinotropic polypeptide
GLP	Glucagon-like peptide
PYY	Peptide YY

J.R. Greenfield, M.B.B.S (Hons 1), Ph.D., F.R.A.C.P. (✉)
Diabetes and Obesity Program, Garvan Institute of Medical Research,
Faculty of Medicine, University of New South Wales, Sydney, NSW, Australia

Department of Endocrinology, St Vincent's Hospital, Sydney, NSW, Australia
e-mail: j.greenfield@garvan.org.au

D. Samocha-Bonet, Ph.D., M.Sc., B.Sc.
Diabetes and Obesity Program, Garvan Institute of Medical Research,
Faculty of Medicine, University of New South Wales, Sydney, NSW, Australia

R. Rajendram et al. (eds.), *Glutamine in Clinical Nutrition*, Nutrition and Health,
DOI 10.1007/978-1-4939-1932-1_21, © Springer Science+Business Media New York 2015

Introduction

Diabetes and hyperglycemia are important causes of morbidity and mortality worldwide. Type 2 diabetes (approximately 90 % of diabetes cases) results from impaired insulin action on target tissues, termed insulin resistance, and is associated with excess body weight and physical inactivity [1, 2]. Defective insulin secretion is a key impairment in type 2 diabetes, contributing to hyperglycemia [3, 4]. Current research is focused on developing treatments that could potentially increase insulin secretion and improve glycemia in response to a meal in type 2 diabetes.

Entero-Endocrine Secretion of and Response to Incretins in Type 2 Diabetes

In healthy humans, plasma insulin excursion is greater in response to iso-glycemic oral compared with intravenous glucose administration [5] (Fig. 21.1). This effect is attributed to one or more humoral or neural factors secreted from the gut following enteral nutrient ingestion, termed incretins.

The first incretin to be purified and characterized in the 1970s was glucose-dependent insulinotropic polypeptide (also known as gastric inhibitory polypeptide, GIP) [6]. Over a decade later, glucagon-like peptide-1 (GLP-1), a peptide co-encoded carboxyterminal to glucagon in the proglucagon gene, was identified [7–9]. Both GIP and GLP-1 play a major role in mediating physiological insulin release following a meal [10, 11]. Previously, it has been suggested that GLP-1 secretion is defective in type 2 diabetes [4, 12–14], developing as a consequence of, rather than cause, the hyperglycemic state [4, 12, 15]. A comprehensive meta-analysis of clinical studies in type 2 diabetes patients and non-diabetic controls suggested that well-controlled type 2 diabetes patients exhibit GLP-1 secretion pattern comparable to non-diabetic individuals [16]. Furthermore, insulin release from the beta cell in response to endogenous GLP-1 is preserved in well-controlled type 2 diabetes [17]. However, the potency of GLP-1 to enhance insulin secretion may be decreased in more advanced disease [18]. GIP secretion is intact in type 2 diabetes, but the insulinotropic response to this incretin hormone is impaired [19]. Interestingly, the blunted insulin response to both GIP and GLP-1 in poorly controlled type 2 diabetes may be restored when glycemic control is improved [18].

Incretin Synthesis and Secretion

GIP is a 42 amino acid peptide produced predominantly in duodenal K-cells in the proximal small intestine. Fasting plasma levels of GIP are low and rise within minutes of food intake. Intact GIP(1–42) is rapidly truncated to bio-inactive GIP(3–42) within minutes of secretion from the gut K-cells by the enzyme dipeptidyl peptidase-4 (DPP-IV) [20]. GLP-1 is produced and secreted from L-cells located in the distal small bowel and colon. Plasma levels of GLP-1 are also low in the fasted state and rise rapidly after food ingestion, well before direct contact between the digested food and the entero-endocrine L-cells. This suggests that both neural and/or endocrine factors promote GLP-1 secretion from L-cells. Bioactive GLP-1 is generated from GLP-1(1–37) and exists as two equipotent circulating molecular forms, GLP-1(7–37) and GLP-1(7–36)amide. The latter form represents the majority of circulating active GLP-1 in human plasma [21]. Bioactive GLP-1 (7–37) and (7–36) are rapidly degraded by DPP-IV to GLP-1(9–37)amide or GLP-1(9–36)amide following release from L-cells.

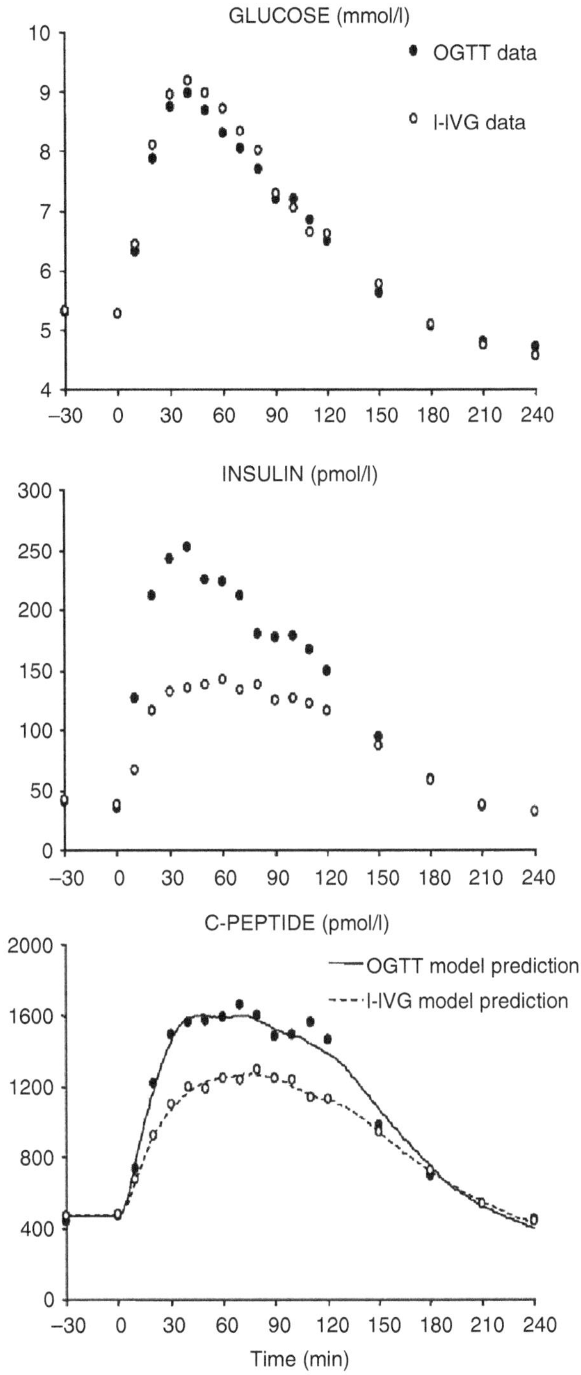

Fig. 21.1 The incretin effect. Mean plasma glucose (*top*), insulin (*middle*), and C-peptide (*bottom*) concentrations during oral glucose tolerance test (OGTT) and isoglycemic intravenous glucose infusion (I-IVG) in 10 healthy normal weight men and women. The extra insulinemic and C-peptide responses observed when glucose is administered orally rather than intravenously is attributed to the incretin effect. Reproduced with permission from Campioni et al. [5]

Stimulating GLP-1 Secretion to Treat Type 2 Diabetes

There has been much recent interest in developing methods by which GLP-1 action can be enhanced in diabetes. GLP-1-based glucose-lowering medications for type 2 diabetes have been in use since 2005. These agents induce significant improvement in glycemic control, albeit with rare, but potentially serious, safety concerns, which are still being evaluated [22, 23]. An alternative approach to the use of

GLP-1 receptor agonists and DPP-IV inhibitors is the direct stimulation of GLP-1 secretion from intestinal L-cells. This approach has the additional benefit of stimulating other entero-endocrine peptides, including peptide YY (PYY) and oxyntomodulin, which suppress appetite and reduce food intake [24, 25], and GLP-2, which stimulates regeneration and repair of intestinal epithelium [26]. Moreover, stimulation of L-cell secretion increases GLP-1(9–36) concentration, the cleaved product of DPP-IV, which is a weak insulinotropic agonist that suppresses hepatic glucose production and possibly exerts antioxidant actions in the heart and vasculature [27].

Low Levels of Circulating L-Glutamine Predict Type 2 Diabetes

Low glutamine concentrations in the circulation have been documented in individuals with impaired fasting glucose and impaired glucose tolerance [28] and in overt type 2 diabetes patients [29]. Recently, large cohort studies have reported that low circulating glutamine levels predict type 2 diabetes incidence [28, 30]. These findings suggest that glutamine may play an important role in glucose homeostasis in humans. In support, in vitro data gathered from the entero-endocrine L-cells model cell line and primary colonic cell line treated with L-glutamine suggested that L-glutamine is a potent GLP-1 secretagogue.

L-Glutamine Is a GLP-1 Secretagogue in GLUTag and Primary Colonic Cells

Some of the earliest evidence implementing glutamine as a potent stimulator of GLP-1 comes from an elegant study by Reimann et al. [31] that examined GLP-1 release from GLUTag, the GLP-1-secreting cells line. The investigators incubated GLUTag cells with a variety of amino acids or glucose (each at 10 mmol/L) for 2 h. As the authors had previously shown [32], GLP-1 secretion was increased 3-fold by glucose (Fig. 21.2a) [31]. However, glutamine was more potent, leading to a 7-fold increase in GLP-1 secretion (Fig. 21.2a). The effect was dose-dependent (Fig. 21.2b) and fairly rapid, occurring within a few minutes, with a continued slow increase in secretion over the 2-h experimental period (Fig. 21.2c). Whilst most other amino acids also increased GLP-1 secretion (Fig. 21.2a), their effect was significantly less than that seen after glutamine. The estimated medium effective concentration was 0.1–1.0 mmol/L, similar to the normal plasma glutamine concentration.

In the same paper, the authors examined the potential mechanism of GLP-1 secretion from GLUTag cells. Glutamine was found to induce a sodium-dependent inward current, triggering depolarization of the membrane and an increase in intracellular calcium. Interestingly, these changes were similar, or even greater, after incubation with other amino acids, including asparagine and alanine, but these amino acids were less effective at inducing GLP-1 secretion (Fig. 21.2a). The authors demonstrate that glutamine perpetuates secretion downstream of the calcium signal.

In a later study, the same group generated a transgenic mouse model, in which they were able to label cells expressing proglucagon with a yellow fluorescent protein [33]. This model allowed Reimann et al. to examine the secretory characteristics of primary L-cells using electrophysiological, fluorescent calcium imaging and expression analysis techniques. Using this model to interrogate glutamine's mode of action, Tolhurst et al. reported a number of novel findings [34]. First, they demonstrated that glutamine dose-dependently stimulates GLP-1 release from primary murine colonic cultures, with a similar EC_{50} to that reported previously in GLUTag cells [34]. Relative GLP-1 secretion by glutamine was again significantly greater than that observed with other amino acids, with only asparagine and phenylalanine significantly affecting GLP-1 release [34]. Second, glutamine increased intracellular calcium, predominately due to calcium entry across the plasma membrane.

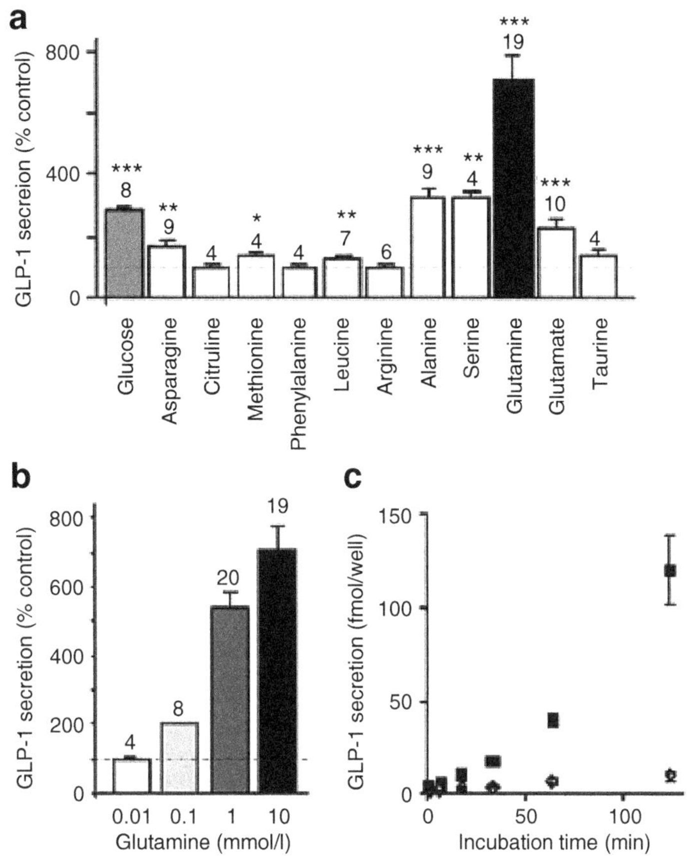

Fig. 21.2 Secretory responses of GLUTag cells to glutamine. GLP-1 secretion from GLUTag cells cultured with 10 mmol/L glucose or the amino acid indicated (**a**). The number of wells is indicated above each bar. Statistical significance was assessed relative to secretion in the absence of nutrients using Student's one-sample *t* test: $^{***}P<0.001$, $^{**}P<0.01$, $^{*}P<0.05$. Concentration dependence of glutamine-induced secretion (**b**). Time course of GLP-1 release in the absence (*open diamonds*) or presence (*closed squares*) of 10 mmol/L glutamine (**c**, $n=4$ per point). Secretion in **a** and **b** was normalized to baseline secretion in the absence of nutrients, measured in parallel on the same day. In **a** and **b** the 10 mmol/L glutamine data are the same. Reproduced with permission from Reimann et al. [31]

Third, when the membrane was "clamped" using diazoxide, a K_{ATP} channel activator, in contrast to asparagine and phenylalanine, glutamine further enhanced GLP-1 secretion, suggesting that it activates a non-electrogenic pathway, as well as stimulating an electrogenic pathway as described above. Fourth, glutamine increased intracellular cAMP to 36 % of that produced by maximal stimulus. Interestingly, phenylalanine led to no increase in intracellular cAMP and asparagine only increased intracellular cAMP by 24 %. The authors conclude that the ability of glutamine to stimulate GLP-1 release from primary murine L-cells occurs via an initial step whereby glutamine stimulates cell excitability, followed by amplification via increased cAMP [34].

These data demonstrate that glutamine may induce GLP-1 secretion by increasing cytosolic calcium and cAMP in L-cells. These synergistic mechanisms are likely to account for the effectiveness of glutamine on GLP-1 secretion. As discussed in the following sections, these data, particularly the results from GLUTag cells, led to an interest in the possibility that glutamine may stimulate GLP-1 secretion in humans, including those with type 2 diabetes, potentially enhancing insulin secretion and improving glycemic control.

Glutamine Ingestion Increases Circulating GLP-1 and Insulin in Healthy Individuals and Type 2 Diabetes Patients

Greenfield and colleagues recruited healthy normal weight and obese individuals and obese individuals with type 2 diabetes or glucose intolerance and studied the effect of ingestion of 30 g glutamine, 75 g glucose or water on circulating glucose, insulin, GLP-1, GIP and glucagon in a randomized study

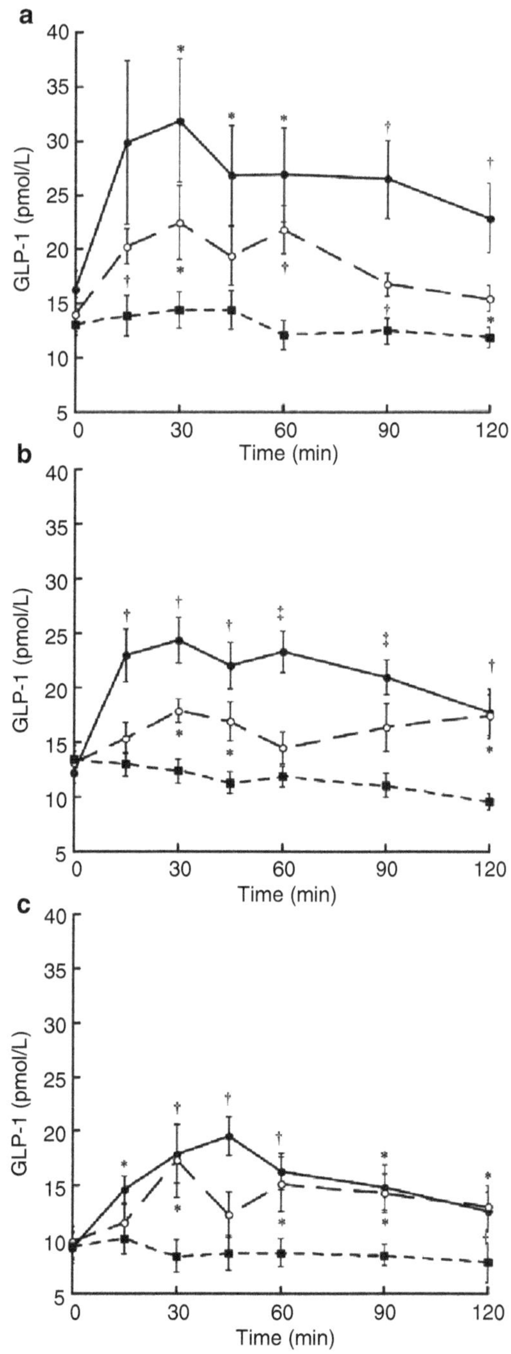

Fig. 21.3 The effect of oral ingestion of L-glutamine on plasma GLP-1 concentrations in healthy lean and obese individuals and obese individuals with type 2 diabetes or impaired glucose tolerance. Plasma GLP-1 concentrations after the ingestion of glucose (*black circles*), glutamine (*white circles*), and water (*black squares*) in 8 lean individuals (**a**), 8 obese non-diabetic control individuals (**b**) and 8 obese individuals with type 2 diabetes or impaired glucose tolerance (**c**). Data represent the mean and SE. $^{*}P<0.05$, $^{\dagger}P<0.01$, $^{\ddagger}P<0.001$ compared with water (paired *t* test). There were no differences in baseline GLP-1 concentrations within each group between visits. Reproduced with permission from Greenfield et al. [35]

with a crossover design [35]. Administration of 30 g of L-glutamine increased circulating GLP-1 concentrations in all study groups, including type 2 diabetes patients (Fig. 21.3) [35], suggesting that glutamine ingestion may have an insulinotropic potential in type 2 diabetes patients. The response to glutamine ingestion was biphasic, with a GLP-1 peak at 30 min and a second at 60–90 min, a pattern observed in all study groups (Fig. 21.3). Glutamine effect was not confined to the L-cell secreting

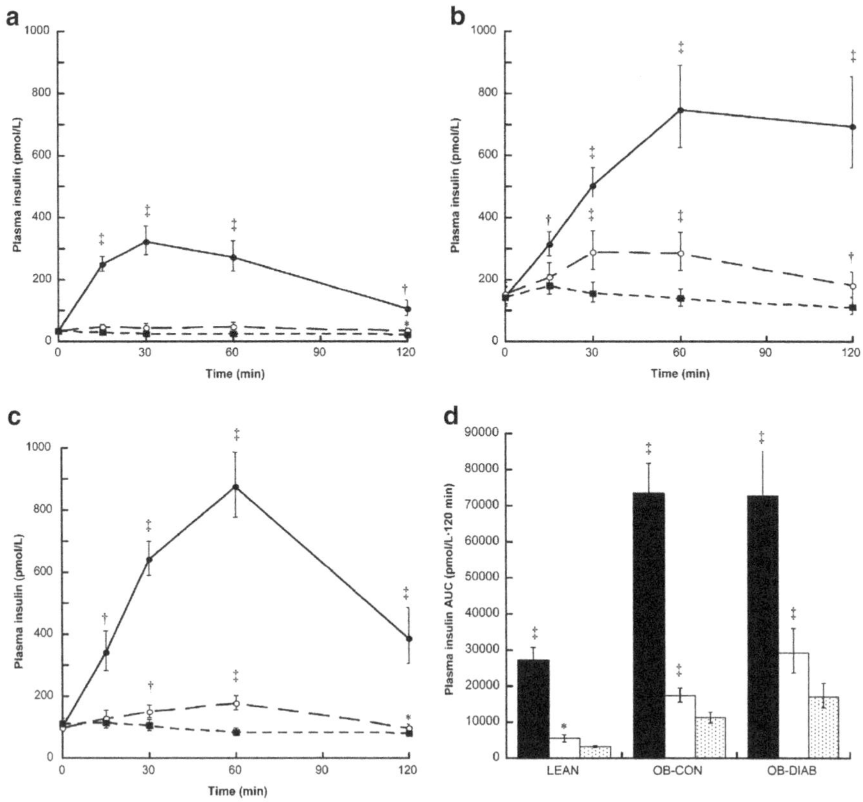

Fig. 21.4 The effect of oral ingestion of L-glutamine on plasma insulin concentrations in healthy lean and obese individuals and obese individuals with type 2 diabetes or impaired glucose tolerance. Plasma insulin concentrations after the ingestion of glucose (*black circles*), glutamine (*white circles*), and water (*black squares*) in 8 lean individuals (**a**), 8 obese non-diabetic control individuals (**b**) and 8 obese individuals with type 2 diabetes or impaired glucose tolerance (**c**). Insulin area under the curve (AUC) after the ingestion of glucose (*black bars*), glutamine (*white bars*), and water (*grey bars*) in the 3 study groups (**d**). Data represent the geometric mean (1 SE range). $^{*}P<0.05$, $^{\dagger}P<0.01$, $^{\ddagger}P<0.001$ compared with water (paired *t* test). There were no differences in baseline insulin concentrations within each group between visits. Reproduced with permission from Greenfield et al. [35]

GLP-1, but also triggered the K-cell-associated GIP in the circulation [35]. Despite augmentation of circulating insulin in response to glutamine ingestion (Fig. 21.4) [35], circulating glucose did not drop significantly (Fig. 21.5) [35], possibly due to a parallel induction of glucagon in the circulation (Fig. 21.6) [35].

Samocha-Bonet and colleagues extended these findings to evaluate the effect of glutamine on postprandial glucose, insulin, C-peptide, total and active GLP-1 and glucagon in well controlled type 2 diabetes patients with short disease duration (mean 2.4 ± SD 1.2 years) [36]. Glutamine was given alone (either 15 or 30 g) or in combination with the DPP-IV inhibitor sitagliptin (15 g glutamine + 100 sitagliptin mg). Control treatments were water and sitagliptin (100 mg) and the study was randomized with a crossover design. Both glutamine 30 g and the combined glutamine 15 g and sitagliptin treatment decreased postprandial glucose excursions significantly compared with water (Table 21.1 and Fig. 21.7a) [36], an effect confined to the first 60 min post meal (Table 21.1). Glutamine 15 g and 30 g increased insulin concentrations significantly (Fig. 21.7b and Table 21.1), but the effect was predominantly observed at 60–120 min post meal (Table 21.1). Relative to glucose, all glutamine treatments

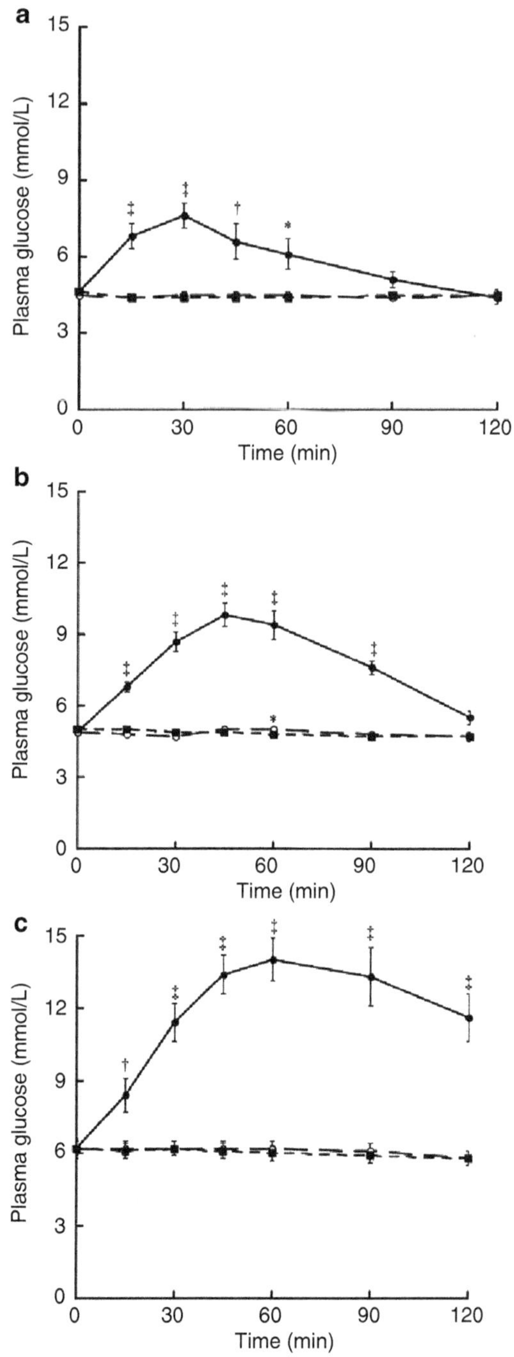

Fig. 21.5 The effect of oral ingestion of L-glutamine on plasma glucose concentrations in healthy lean and obese individuals and obese individuals with type 2 diabetes or impaired glucose tolerance. Plasma glucose concentrations after the ingestion of glucose (*black circles*), glutamine (*white circles*), and water (*black squares*) in 8 lean individuals (**a**), 8 obese non-diabetic control individuals (**b**) and 8 obese individuals with type 2 diabetes or impaired glucose tolerance (**c**). Data represent the mean and SE. $^{*}P<0.05$, $^{\dagger}P<0.01$, $^{\ddagger}P<0.001$ compared with water (paired *t* test). There were no differences in baseline glucose concentrations within each group between visits. Reproduced with permission from Greenfield et al. [35]

significantly augmented insulinemia and glutamine 15 g alone or in combination with sitagliptin had significant effects on both the early (0–60 min) and late (60–180 min) phases post meal ingestion (Fig. 21.7c and Table 21.1). C-peptide was not increased by any treatment (Fig. 21.7d and Table 21.1), but relative to glucose, C-peptide increased in response to glutamine 15 g and glutamine 15 g with

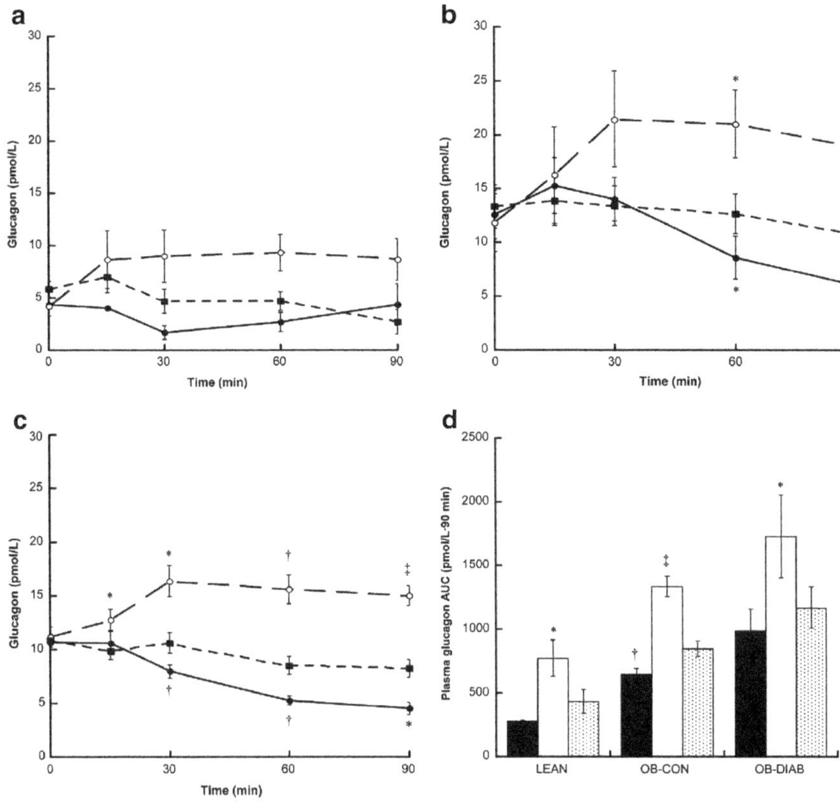

Fig. 21.6 The effect of oral ingestion of L-glutamine on plasma glucagon concentrations in healthy lean and obese individuals and obese individuals with type 2 diabetes or impaired glucose tolerance. Plasma glucagon concentrations after the ingestion of glucose (*black circles*), glutamine (*white circles*), and water (*black squares*) in 8 lean individuals (**a**), 8 obese non-diabetic control individuals (**b**) and 8 obese individuals with type 2 diabetes or impaired glucose tolerance (**c**). Data represent the mean and SE. $^*P<0.05$, $^{\dagger}P<0.01$, $^{\ddagger}P<0.001$ compared with water (paired *t* test). There were no differences in baseline glucagon concentrations within each group between visits. Reproduced with permission from Greenfield et al. [35]

sitagliptin in the first 60 min post meal (Fig. 21.7e and Table 21.1). Total GLP-1 was increased in response to the combined glutamine and sitagliptin treatment and sitagliptin alone (Fig. 21.7h and Table 21.1). Active GLP-1 was increased by glutamine 30 g, similarly to the response to sitagliptin (Fig. 21.7i and Table 21.1). All the glutamine treatments increased glucagon excursions in the circulation (Fig. 21.7f and Table 21.1), but relative to insulin, only the higher glutamine dose had a significant effect in the first 60 min after meal (Fig. 21.7g and Table 21.1).

Glutamine Improves Glycemia via GLP-1-Mediated Slowing of Gastric Emptying

A critical question is whether glutamine-induced increases in GLP-1 reduce glycemia by increasing insulin secretion or slowing of gastric emptying, or both. The study by Samocha-Bonet et al. [36] suggests that the latter is likely to be more important. Firstly, the reduction in postprandial glycemia

Table 21.1 The effect of glutamine (30 or 15 g) or glutamine with the DPP-IV inhibitor sitagliptin (glutamine 15 g + sitagliptin 100 mg) or sitagliptin (100 mg) relative to water on postprandial circulating glucose, insulin, C-peptide and GLP-1 in well controlled type 2 diabetes patients

		Glutamine 30 g	Glutamine 15 g	Glutamine 15 g + sitagliptin 100 mg	Sitagliptin 100 mg
Glucose	Total AUC (0–180 min)	↓		↓	
	AUC 0–60 min	↓		↓	
	AUC 60–180 min				
Insulin	Total AUC (0–180 min)	↑	↑		
	AUC 0–60 min				
	AUC 60–180 min	↑	↑	↑	
Insulin:glucose ratio	Total AUC (0–180 min)	↑	↑	↑	
	AUC 0–60 min		↑	↑	
	AUC 60–180 min	↑	↑	↑	
C-peptide	Total AUC (0–180 min)				
	AUC 0–60 min				
	AUC 60–180 min				
C-peptide:glucose ratio	Total AUC (0–180 min)				↑
	AUC 0–60 min		↑	↑	
	AUC 60–180 min				↑
GLP-1 total	Total AUC (0–180 min)			↑	↑
	AUC 0–60 min				
	AUC 60–180 min				
GLP-1 active	Total AUC (0–180 min)	↑			↑
	AUC 0–60 min	↑			↑
	AUC 60–180 min				
Glucagon	Total AUC (0–180 min)	↑	↑		
	AUC 0–60 min	↑	↑		
	AUC 60–180 min	↑			
Insulin:glucagon ratio	Total AUC (0–180 min)				
	AUC 0–60 min	↑			
	AUC 60–180 min				

↓ or ↑ = decreased or increased relative to water treatment. Areas under the curve (AUC) were calculated using the trapezoidal rule. Treatments were compared with the control (water) using paired *t* test and significance was calculated using the Dunn-Bonferroni correction for the 4 control vs. treatment pairs at an overall significance threshold of 0.05 Participants ($n = 15$) attended the clinic on 5 occasions separated by 1–2 weeks in a random order. Sitagliptin was administered 25 min prior to the meal. L-glutamine powder was consumed in 300 mL of ice-cold water over 2 min immediately prior to the meal which was consumed over 10 min. Meal comprised of 33 g Wheat-Bix and 250 mL low fat milk. Adapted with permission from Samocha-Bonet et al. [36]

preceded any increase in insulinemia. Secondly, although glutamine increased the postprandial insulin response, there was no corresponding increase in C-peptide, suggesting that glutamine may affect insulin clearance, rather than secretion. Although not measured directly in that study, these findings indicate that the effect of glutamine on glycemia is predominantly mediated through slowing of gastric emptying. Indeed, a study in healthy humans has demonstrated that a glutamine and carbohydrate mixed solution prolonged gastric emptying compared to carbohydrate alone [37].

In support of these findings, Chang and colleagues [38] reported that bypassing the stomach by intraduodenal infusion of glutamine prior to glucose infusion did not significantly lower glycemia in healthy individuals and type 2 diabetes patients, despite increases in GLP-1, GIP and insulin (Fig. 21.8) [38]. Glutamine had a significant effect on pyloric stimulation in both study groups, suggesting that

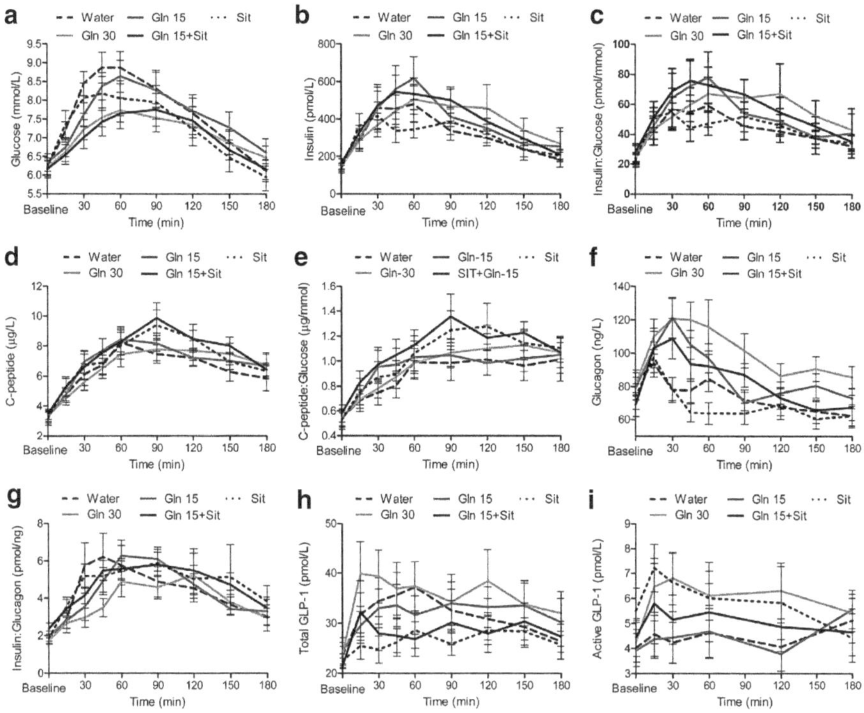

Fig. 21.7 The effect of oral ingestion of L-glutamine alone or in combination with the DPP-IV inhibitor sitagliptin on circulating glucose, insulin, C-peptide, total and active GLP-1 and glucagon in response to a meal in type 2 diabetes patients. Blood glucose (**a**), serum insulin (**b**), the insulin:glucose ratio (**c**), serum C-peptide (**d**) the C-peptide:glucose ratio (**e**), plasma glucagon (**f**), the insulin:glucagon ratio (**g**), plasma total and active GLP-1 (H and I respectively) concentrations in well controlled type 2 diabetes patients in response to a high carbohydrate low fat meal following ingestion of water, 30 g or 15 g glutamine (Gln 30 and Gln 15, respectively), sitagliptin (100 mg) and glutamine (15 g; SIT+Gln) or sitagliptin (100 mg; SIT). Data represent mean and SEM. Reproduced with permission from Samocha-Bonet et al. [36]

delayed gastric emptying may mediate the metabolic effects of glutamine. Notably, slowed gastric emptying in response to glutamine may be indirect due to increased GLP-1. In support, blocking endogenous GLP-1 effect by the GLP-1 receptor antagonist exendin (9–39) amide with a meal accelerates gastric emptying and abolishes the reducing effect on glycemia compared with placebo in healthy individuals [39]. Further, in vitro studies suggest that glutamine is not likely to have a direct insulinotropic effect on pancreatic beta cells, as demonstrated in primary islets or the clonal pancreatic BRIN-BD beta cell lines. Specifically, L-glutamine is rapidly taken up and metabolized by islets and does not stimulate insulin secretion or enhance glucose-induced insulin secretion [40]. This is explained by the conversion of glutamine to γ-aminobutyric acid (GABA) [40, 41].

On the other hand, glucagon secreted from the pancreatic α-cells is induced in response to glutamine ingestion in healthy lean or obese individuals and type 2 diabetes patients (Figs. 21.6 and 21.7f) [35, 36]. Increased glucagonemia is expected to counteract a potential benefit of glutamine on glycemia via enhanced hepatic glucose production. In the fasting state, glucagon maintains normal blood glucose concentration and is maximally active when glucose and insulin concentrations are low. However, postprandial increases in glucagon in parallel with increases in insulin concentration following glutamine ingestion would not be expected to affect hepatic glucose production, which is predominantly relevant in the fasting state.

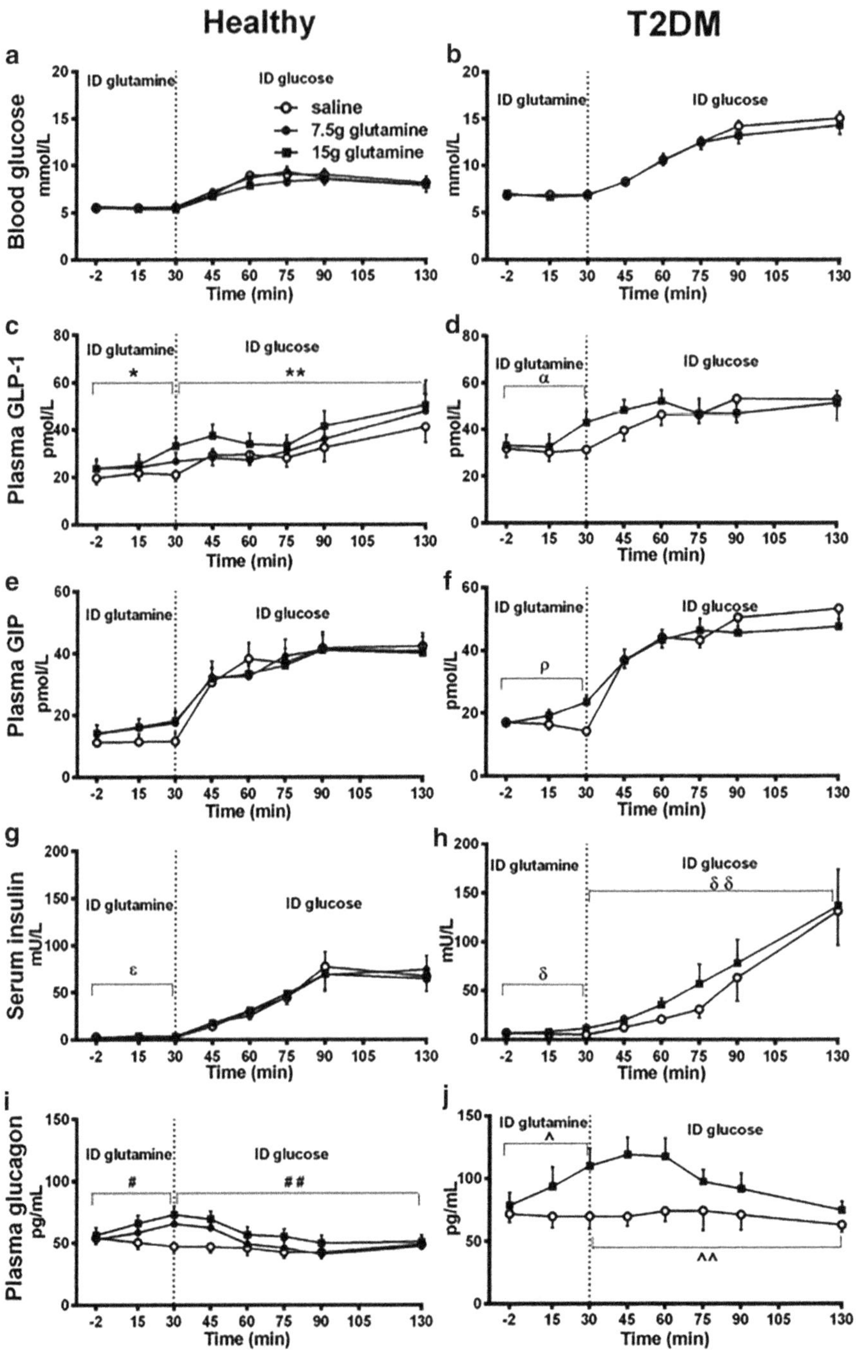

Fig. 21.8 The effect of intraduodenal administration of glutamine on glucose, GLP-1, GIP, insulin and glucagon excursions in response to glucose infusion. Effects of intraduodenal (ID) saline (control) and 7.5 or 15 g glutamine infusions on blood glucose (**a** and **b**), plasma GLP-1 (**c** and **d**), plasma GIP (**e** and **f**), serum insulin (**g** and **h**), and plasma glucagon (**i** and **j**) concentrations in 10 healthy subjects and 9 patients with type 2 diabetes, before (t=0–30 min) and during (t=30–130 min) ID glucose infusion. Healthy subjects received an ID infusion containing 15 or 7.5 glutamine in 350 mL aqueous solution, or 350 mL of 0.9 % saline control, over 30 min (t=0–30 min) in randomized, single blinded order. This was followed by an ID glucose infusion at 3 kcal/min over 100 min (t=30–130 min) with frequent blood sampling. Patients with type 2 diabetes were studied twice (15 g glutamine or saline). Reproduced with permission from Chang et al. [38]

Oral Glutamine Supplementation in Healthy and Type 2 Diabetic Adults: Safety and Tolerance Data

Oral glutamine doses of 0.35–0.65 g/kg result in peak concentrations in the circulation at 30–60 min [35, 42], with similar concentrations attained in individuals with and without diabetes [35]. Oral glutamine intake of up to 0.5 g/kg is relatively palatable [42], but has been shown to induce minor gastrointestinal symptoms [35, 36]. Over 14 days, glutamine ingestion of 0.5 g/kg daily was shown to be safe, with no adverse effects on liver and renal function in middle-aged and elderly individuals [43].

Conclusions

Glutamine ingestion with meals decreases glucose excursions in parallel with increases in insulin and GLP-1 in the circulation and provides a safe approach to enhance glycemic control in well controlled type 2 diabetes patients. The long-term effects of glutamine on glycemic control in type 2 diabetes require further studies.

References

1. Danaei G, Finucane MM, Lu Y, Singh GM, Cowan MJ, Paciorek CJ, et al. National, regional, and global trends in fasting plasma glucose and diabetes prevalence since 1980: systematic analysis of health examination surveys and epidemiological studies with 370 country-years and 2.7 million participants. Lancet. 2011;378:31–40.
2. Global health risks (2009) Mortality and burden of disease attributable to selected major risks. World Health Organization: Geneva, 2009
3. Bonadonna RC, Stumvoll M, Fritsche A, Muggeo M, Haring H, Bonora E, et al. Altered homeostatic adaptation of first- and second-phase beta-cell secretion in the offspring of patients with type 2 diabetes: studies with a minimal model to assess beta-cell function. Diabetes. 2003;52:470–80.
4. Laakso M, Zilinskaite J, Hansen T, Boesgaard TW, Vanttinen M, Stancakova A, et al. Insulin sensitivity, insulin release and glucagon-like peptide-1 levels in persons with impaired fasting glucose and/or impaired glucose tolerance in the EUGENE2 study. Diabetologia. 2008;51:502–11.
5. Campioni M, Toffolo G, Shuster LT, Service FJ, Rizza RA, Cobelli C. Incretin effect potentiates beta-cell responsivity to glucose as well as to its rate of change: OGTT and matched intravenous study. Am J Physiol Endocrinol Metab. 2007;292:E54–60.
6. Brown JC, Dryburgh JR. A gastric inhibitory polypeptide. II. The complete amino acid sequence. Can J Biochem. 1971;49:867–72.
7. Bell GI, Sanchez-Pescador R, Laybourn PJ, Najarian RC. Exon duplication and divergence in the human preproglucagon gene. Nature. 1983;304:368–71.
8. George SK, Uttenthal LO, Ghiglione M, Bloom SR. Molecular forms of glucagon-like peptides in man. FEBS Lett. 1985;192:275–8.
9. Orskov C, Bersani M, Johnsen AH, Højrup P, Holst JJ. Complete sequences of glucagon-like peptide-1 from human and pig small intestine. J Biol Chem. 1989;264:12826–9.
10. Drucker DJ. The biology of incretin hormones. Cell Metab. 2006;3:153–65.
11. Holst JJ. The physiology of glucagon-like peptide 1. Physiol Rev. 2007;87:1409–39.
12. Vollmer K, Gardiwal H, Menge BA, Goetze O, Deacon CF, Schmidt WE, et al. Hyperglycemia Acutely Lowers the Postprandial Excursions of Glucagon-Like Peptide-1 and Gastric Inhibitory Polypeptide in Humans. J Clin Endocrinol Metab. 2009;94:1379–85.
13. Toft-Nielsen MB, Damholt MB, Madsbad S, Hilsted LM, Hughes TE, Michelsen BK, et al. Determinants of the impaired secretion of glucagon-like peptide-1 in type 2 diabetic patients. J Clin Endocrinol Metab. 2001;86: 3717–23.
14. Vilsboll T, Krarup T, Deacon CF, Madsbad S, Holst JJ. Reduced postprandial concentrations of intact biologically active gluccagon-like peptide 1 in type 2 diabetic patients. Diabetes. 2001;50:609–13.

15. Vollmer K, Holst JJ, Baher B, Ellrichmann M, Nauck MA, Schmidt WE, et al. Predictors of incretin concentrations in subjects with normal, impaired, and diabetic glucose tolerance. Diabetes. 2008;57:678–87.
16. Calanna S, Christensen M, Holst JJ, Laferrere B, Gluud LL, Vilsboll T, et al. Secretion of glucagon-like peptide-1 in patients with type 2 diabetes mellitus: systematic review and meta-analyses of clinical studies. Diabetologia. 2013;56:965–72.
17. Salehi M, Prigeon RL, Aulinger B, D'Alessio DA. Effect of endogenous GLP-1 on insulin secretion in type 2 diabetes. Diabetes. 2010;59:1330–7.
18. Hojberg PV, Vilsboll T, Rabol R, Knop FK, Bache M, Krarup T, et al. Four weeks of near-normalisation of blood glucose improves the insulin response to glucagon-like peptide-1 and glucose-dependent insulinotropic polypeptide in patients with type 2 diabetes. Diabetologia. 2009;52:199–207.
19. Nauck MA, Baller B, Meier JJ. Gastric inhibitory polypeptide and glucagon-like peptide-1 in the pathogenesis of type 2 diabetes. Diabetes. 2004;53 Suppl 3:S190–6.
20. Kieffer TJ, McIntosh CH, Pederson RA. Degradation of glucose-dependent insulinotropic polypeptide and truncated glucagon-like peptide 1 in vitro and in vivo by dipeptidyl peptidase IV. Endocrinology. 1995; 136:3585–96.
21. Orskov C, Rabenhoj L, Wettergren A, Kofod H, Holst JJ. Tissue and plasma concentrations of amidated and glycine-extended glucagon-like peptide I in humans. Diabetes. 1994;43:535–9.
22. Butler PC, Elashoff M, Elashoff R, Gale EA. A Critical Analysis of the Clinical Use of Incretin-Based Therapies: Are the GLP-1 therapies safe? Diabetes Care. 2013;36(7):2118–25.
23. Nauck MA. A Critical Analysis of the Clinical Use of Incretin-Based Therapies: The benefits by far outweigh the potential risks. Diabetes Care. 2013;36(7):2126–32.
24. Batterham RL, Cowley MA, Small CJ, Herzog H, Cohen MA, Dakin CL, et al. Gut hormone PYY(3-36) physiologically inhibits food intake. Nature. 2002;418:650–4.
25. Wynne K, Bloom SR. The role of oxyntomodulin and peptide tyrosine-tyrosine (PYY) in appetite control. Nat Clin Pract Endocrinol Metab. 2006;2:612–20.
26. Estall JL, Drucker DJ. Glucagon-like peptide-2. Ann Rev Nutr. 2006;26:391–411.
27. Thomas E, Habener JF. Insulin-like actions of glucagon-like peptide-1: a dual receptor hypothesis. Trends Endocrinol Metab. 2010;21:59–68.
28. Stancakova A, Civelek M, Saleem NK, Soininen P, Kangas AJ, Cederberg H, et al. Hyperglycemia and a common variant of GCKR are associated with the levels of eight amino acids in 9,369 Finnish men. Diabetes. 2012;61:1895–902.
29. Menge BA, Schrader H, Ritter PR, Ellrichmann M, Uhl W, Schmidt WE, et al. Selective amino acid deficiency in patients with impaired glucose tolerance and type 2 diabetes. Regul Pept. 2010;160:75–80.
30. Cheng S, Rhee EP, Larson MG, Lewis GD, McCabe EL, Shen D, et al. Metabolite Profiling Identifies Pathways Associated With Metabolic Risk in Humans. Circulation. 2012;125:2222–31.
31. Reimann F, Williams L, da Silva XG, Rutter GA, Gribble FM. Glutamine potently stimulates glucagon-like peptide-1 secretion from GLUTag cells. Diabetologia. 2004;47:1592–601.
32. Reimann F, Gribble FM. Glucose-sensing in glucagon-like peptide-1-secreting cells. Diabetes. 2002;51:2757–63.
33. Reimann F, Habib AM, Tolhurst G, Parker HE, Rogers GJ, Gribble FM. Glucose sensing in L cells: a primary cell study. Cell Metab. 2008;8:532–9.
34. Tolhurst G, Zheng Y, Parker HE, Habib AM, Reimann F, Gribble FM. Glutamine triggers and potentiates glucagon-like peptide-1 secretion by raising cytosolic Ca2+ and cAMP. Endocrinology. 2011;152:405–13.
35. Greenfield JR, Farooqi IS, Keogh JM, Henning E, Habib AM, Blackwood A, et al. Oral glutamine increases circulating glucagon-like peptide 1, glucagon, and insulin concentrations in lean, obese, and type 2 diabetic subjects. Am J Clin Nutr. 2009;89:106–13.
36. Samocha-Bonet D, Wong O, Synnott EL, Piyaratna N, Douglas A, Gribble FM, et al. Glutamine reduces postprandial glycemia and augments the glucagon-like peptide-1 response in type 2 diabetes patients. J Nutr. 2011; 141:1233–8.
37. Lobo DN, Hendry PO, Rodrigues G, Marciani L, Totman JJ, Wright JW, et al. Gastric emptying of three liquid oral preoperative metabolic preconditioning regimens measured by magnetic resonance imaging in healthy adult volunteers: a randomised double-blind, crossover study. Clin Nutr. 2009;28:636–41.
38. Chang J, Wu T, Greenfield JR, Samocha-Bonet D, Horowitz M, Rayner CK. Effects of Intraduodenal Glutamine on Incretin Hormone and Insulin Release, the Glycemic Response to an Intraduodenal Glucose Infusion, and Antropyloroduodenal Motility in Health and Type 2 Diabetes. Diabetes Care. 2013;36(8):2262–5.
39. Deane AM, Nguyen NQ, Stevens JE, Fraser RJ, Holloway RH, Besanko LK, et al. Endogenous glucagon-like peptide-1 slows gastric emptying in healthy subjects, attenuating postprandial glycemia. J Clin Endocrinol Metab. 2010;95:215–21.
40. Newsholme P, Krause M. Nutritional regulation of insulin secretion: implications for diabetes. Clin Biochem Rev. 2012;33:35–47.

41. Fernandez-Pascual S, Mukala-Nsengu-Tshibangu A, Martin Del Rio R, Tamarit-Rodriguez J. Conversion into GABA (gamma-aminobutyric acid) may reduce the capacity of L-glutamine as an insulin secretagogue. Biochem J. 2004;379:721–9.
42. Ward E, Picton S, Reid U, Thomas D, Gardener C, Smith M, et al. Oral glutamine in paediatric oncology patients: a dose finding study. Eur J Clin Nutr. 2003;57:31–6.
43. Galera SC, Fechine F, Teixeira MJ, Branco Coelho ZC, de Vasconcelos RC, de Vasconcelos PR. The safety of oral use of l-glutamine in middle-aged and elderly individuals. Nutrition. 2010;26:375–81.

Chapter 22
Glutamine Pretreatment and Surgery for Cleft Lip/Cleft Palate in Children

José Ferreira da Cunha Filho and Paulo Roberto Leitão de Vasconcelos

Key Points

- Glutamine attenuates surgical trauma-induced inflammatory response and oxidative stress in children submitted to surgical palate repair;
- Glutamine is a conditionally essential nutrient during sepsis or trauma;
- Parenteral nutrition supplemented with the dipeptide alanyl-glutamine in patients in an intensive care unit is associated with a reduction in infection complications and better metabolic tolerance;
- There was no adverse and/or cumulative effect attributed to glutamine;
- Pretreatment with L-alanyl-glutamine attenuates the inflammatory response.

Keywords Oxidative Stress • Metabolism • Palatoplasty • Inflammation • Glutamine

Abbreviations

ASA	Classification American Society of Anesthesiology for the patient's physical status
CG	Control Group
EG	Experimental Group
GLN	Glutamine
GSH	Glutathione (glutamic acid-cysteine-glycine)
GSSG	oxidized glutathione
IL-6	Interleukin-6
L-Ala-Gln	L-alanyl-glutamine
Mg	Milligrams

J.F.D.C. Filho (✉)
Bairro: Dionísio Torres, Fortaleza-CE, Brazil

Department of Surgery, Federal University of Ceará, School of Medicine,
Bairro: Rodolfo Teófilo, Fortaleza, Ceará, Brazil
e-mail: jferreiracf@yahoo.com.br

P.R.L. de Vasconcelos, D.Phil
Department of Surgery, Federal University of Ceará, School of Medicine, Fortaleza, Ceará, Brazil

R. Rajendram et al. (eds.), *Glutamine in Clinical Nutrition*, Nutrition and Health,
DOI 10.1007/978-1-4939-1932-1_22,

T1	First-time blood collection
T2	Second blood collection during induction
T3	Third blood collection soon after the operation
T4	06 h after the operation
T5	12 h after the operation
TBA	Thiobarbituric Acid
TBARS	Thiobarbituric Acid Reactive Substances
UI	International Units

Glutamine

Glutamine (GLN) is a conditionally essential nutrient during sepsis or trauma [1]. GLN is the most abundant amino acid in plasma and skeletal muscle. However, GLN levels fall dramatically after major injury or infection [2]. GLN supplementation in patients submitted to elective surgery attenuates the negative postoperative nitrogen balance, diminishing the dive in intracellular concentration of the amino acid in skeletal muscle and enhancing the synthesis of muscle protein [3, 4].

Glutamine Containing Dipeptides and Cocktails

Glutamine is the most common amino acid found in the organism, corresponding to 25 % of free amino acids. It plays an important role in maintaining muscle metabolism function, representing about 60 % of all amino acids. Its essential function is to allow movements not only in the fast-twitch skeletal muscle but also in the intestinal smooth muscle, thus facilitating the movement of food through the gastrointestinal tract after a meal. In muscle cells, large amounts of glutamine are found freely, meaning that is not related to any other amino acid.

Glutamine is very important to neutralize toxins from the body, establishing itself as the main energy source for the entire immune system, by increasing the ability of the cells of the defense system to do the work to identify and destroy.

Glutamine is an important metabolic fuel for the cells of the gastrointestinal tract, and some evidence shows that all the fast proliferating cells, especially those of the immune system, are strictly dependent on its availability as an energy source. As a non-essential amino acid is neutral in its chemical composition carbon, hydrogen, oxygen and nitrogen, which give important transport characteristics of nitrogen and ammonia carrier to various tissues.

Glutamine plays a vital role in the metabolism of amino acids. Because of its "*biaminação*," it acts as carrier of nitrogen and thus acts on intracellular glutamate transport because the cell membrane is more permeable than glutamine to glutamic acid, being a precursor of several amino acids. It is a great need for the biosynthesis of nucleic acids in all cells, and is a precursor of glutathione, which is an important antioxidant.

The consumer cells have a high concentration of glutamine glutaminase which catalyze the hydrolysis of glutamine to glutamate and ammonia. The glutamine producing make use of glutamine synthetase from glutamate and ammonia.

Glutamine has low aqueous solubility and low stability at elevated temperature. However, when associated with L-alanine, results in a product (L-Ala-Gln), which begins to show high water solubility and stability in the preparation of stable solutions and storage of nutritional solutions. L-ALANYL-GLUTAMINE, when introduced into the body undergoes hydrolysis, releasing free molecules of L-alanine and L-glutamine. L-alanyl-glutamine stimulates increased use of glucose via glycolysis by activation of lactate–malate cycle [5].

The administration of glutamine by the intravenous route is the most reliable method for achieving a prolonged and steady increase in total reserves of free glutamine in the body. There has been no demonstrated adverse effect of glutamine after your employment orally or intravenously.

The transport of glutamine across the muscle cell membrane is very fast, even with greater than all other amino acids speed. The input of glutamine seems to be dependent on Na+ and the conveyor activity can be modulated by membrane potential and intracellular and extracellular amounts of sodium. The parenteral alanyl-glutamine supplementation was associated with improved insulin sensitivity in patients with multiple trauma.

Studies have shown that hypercatabolic and hypermetabolic conditions are associated with profound depletion of glutamine during elective surgery, prolonged fasting and multiple traumas, leading substantially independent intramuscular concentrations of glutamine decrease nutritional status, which makes this amino acid "conditionally essential" mainly during infections and trauma.

The magnitude of the metabolic response to trauma depends on the extent of the damaged tissue. Glutamine seems to be the major energy source for the intestinal epithelium. The use of glutamine has been shown to be of great importance in the treatment of trauma and patients undergoing surgery because it reduces the incidence of infection in these patients. Glutamine is considered a non-essential amino acid. However, recent studies have shown evidence that glutamine may become conditionally essential for inflammatory conditions such as infection and injury.

The mechanism of supplementation with L-alanyl-glutamine in the reversal of some diseases may be due to the support provided by intestinal mucosal immune system, glutathione biosynthesis and, as recently reported, a putative regulatory effect broader due to the modification of the inflammatory response endogenous. These mechanisms may be due to attenuation of pro-inflammatory mediators and/or the regulation of anti-inflammatory factors, as well as its role in the release of insulin by the pancreas.

In experimental studies it was found that interleukin-6 (IL-6) plays an important role in the stimulation of hepatic glutamine transport by burn injuries.

The glutamine supplementation in patients following elective surgery attenuated postoperative negative nitrogen balance, reducing the fall in intracellular glutamine concentration in skeletal muscles and aiding muscle protein synthesis. In addition, glutamine led to beneficial immunological changes for the patient, and has reduced the length of hospital stay by an average of 4 days. Parenteral nutrition supplemented with L-alanyl-glutamine dipeptide in patients at intensive care unit is associated with reduced infectious complications and better metabolic tolerance.

Trauma

Healing of a surgical wound requires local activation of immune cells and secretion of various anti-inflammatory mediators. The process is tightly regulated by anti-inflammatory mediators. Depending on the magnitude of tissue damage and on the vulnerability of the host, the local immune response may fail to control the damage and restore homeostasis. In patients with more severe injury, release of mediators into the circulation occurs with activation of the immune system and systemic release of both pro-inflammatory and, subsequently, anti-inflammatory cytokines [6].

Palatoplasty and Glutamine

Cleft lip and palate are congenital anomalies due to errors in development or in the maturation of embryonic processes [7]. Surgical repair of theses anomalies is a traumatic event due to extensive dissection and bone exposure required for closing the communication between the nasal and oral cavities.

The effect of parenteral glutamine treatment has not been assessed in the setting of palatoplasty in children. The hypothesis that glutamine attenuates the inflammatory response and oxidative stress induced by palatoplasty in children was tested in a clinical study. Thirty patients, aged 2–10 years at the time of surgery, undergoing elective surgical repair of cleft palate (palatoplasty) were included in the study. Children selected for this study showed a homogeneous profile in relation to sex (all males), age, and weight.

All patients were submitted to the same anesthetic procedure with balanced general anesthesia, orotracheal intubation, and controlled ventilation with a semi-open circuit. All surgical procedures were performed at the Albert Sabin Children´s Hospital by a single surgeon using the same technique (Veau-Wardill-Kilner technique) [8] for all the palate repairs.

Allocation of patients to groups A (Control Group—CG) and B (Experimental Group—EG) was made by a software program (*www.lee.dante.br*). Patients who met inclusion criteria were randomly assigned to receive either 100 ml of normal saline solution (Group A or CG) or L-alanyl-glutamine (L-Ala-Gln) 20 % solution (Dipeptiven ®), adding saline solution to complete 100 ml (Group B or EG), delivered intravenously by infusion pump (LF 2001®)—Lifemed Ind. Equip. Artigos Med. Hosp. S/A, São Paulo, Brazil, over 3 h preceding the surgical procedure.

Peripheral venous blood samples were collected at 5 different time-points: T1, at the beginning of the study (3 h prior to the surgical procedure); T2, at the end of the infusion (before the surgical procedure); T3, at the end of the surgical procedure; T4, 6 h postoperative and T5, 12 h postoperative. Parameters analyzed included glutathione (GSH), thiobarbituric acid reactive substances (TBARS), glucose, insulin, C-reactive protein (CRP), and interleukin-6 (IL-6).

L-Ala-Gln (Dipeptiven®) was purchased from Frenesius Kabi Austria GmbH, Graz, Austria. All other chemicals were purchased from standard commercial sources and were of the highest quality available. GSH [9], TBARS [10], and glucose [11], were measured according to biochemical methods published elsewhere. Serum level of insulin was measured by the electrochemiluminescence immunoassay; CRP was measured by an immunonephelometric method and IL6 by ELISA assay.

No statistically significant differences were found in glucose comparing control and L-Ala-Gln-treated patients. Glucose levels were significantly different in T3, T4 and T5 time-points compared with basal (T1) values in control children.

No statistically significant differences were found in insulin levels comparing control and L-Ala-Gln-treated patients, TBARS and glutathione levels were not significantly different comparing control and L-Ala-Gln-treated patients.

CRP levels were significantly different in control patients, comparing T5 with basal values T1. CRP levels in L-Ala-Gln-treated patients were not significantly different (Fig. 22.1 and Table 22.1). IL-6 levels were significantly different in both the groups comparing T4 and T5 with basal values (Fig. 22.2 and Table 22.2).

Safety of glutamine administration has been the aim of several publications [4, 12]. Supplementation with glutamine, using doses of 3–3.5 g/kg/day, for 10 days, did not have significant adverse effects, when administered parenterally in newborns with low birth weight [13]. In a recent publication, Ward et al. [14] evaluated the severity of mucositis in children undergoing chemotherapy, where 0.65 g/kg/day of glutamine was administered orally for 7 days. There was no adverse and/or cumulative effect attributed to glutamine. In this study, children were given L-Ala-Gln 0.5 g/kg using a continuous infusion pump. This dose is equivalent to 0.33 g/kg of GLN, per 3-h period or 0.11 g/kg/h of GLN. No adverse effects were observed.

In this study, glucose levels increased in T3, T4 and T5 time-points compared with basal (T1) values. While the levels of glucose increased gradually in the control group, the absence of significant changes in glucose levels in children treated with L-Ala-Gln suggests a better glycemic control in these patients.

CRP is an acute phase-reactant protein pool produced by the liver as part of the inflammatory response to tissue injury such as infection or trauma [15]. Normal plasma level of CRP is less than

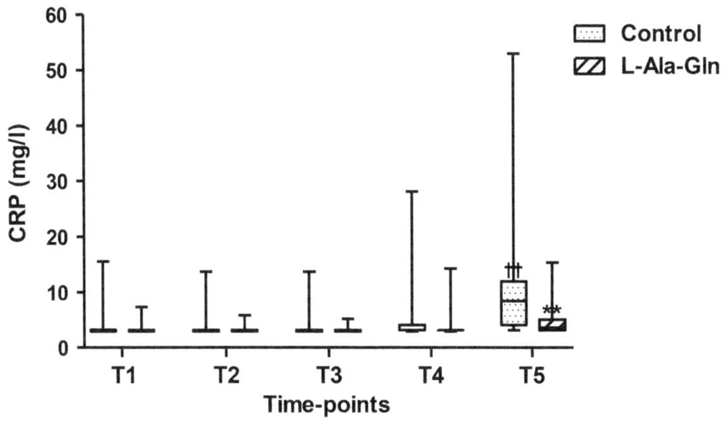

Fig. 22.1 CRP concentrations (mg/l) in the plasma of saline (control) and L-Ala-Gln-treated patients. Bars represent median with interquartile range and minimum and maximum values of 15 subjects of control and L-Ala-Gln groups during different time-points. It was found that L-Ala-Gln treatment significantly reduced CRP concentration at T5 in relation to control ($^{**}P = 0.0037$). However, groups studied are not significantly different, according to Mann–Whitney test, at the other time-points. CRP levels increased significantly in control patients, comparing T5 with basal values (T1). $^{\dagger\dagger}P < 0.05$ compared with T1 (control group)

Table 22.1 CRP concentrations (mg/l) measured in the plasma of saline (control) and L-Ala-Gln-treated patients at T1 (baseline), T2, T3, T4, and T5 time-points. Data correspond to the analysis of 15 patients of both groups at each time-point

	Control ($n = 15$)		L-Ala-Gln ($n = 15$)		Between groups significance
Time-points	Median	Interquartile range	Median	Interquartile range	(Mann–Whitney test)
T1	3.16	2.90–3.16	3.16	2.90–3.16	$P = 0.6805$
T2	3.16	2.90–3.16	3.16	2.90–3.16	$P = 0.9267$
T3	3.16	2.90–3.16	3.16	2.90–3.16	$P = 0.5807$
T4	3.16	3.16–4.10	3.16	3.16–3.16	$P = 0.5185$
T5	8.40††	4.10–11.90	3.60	3.16–5.05	$P = 0.0037$

The symbol †† ($P < 0.01$) denotes statistically significant differences in relation to T1 in the Control group (Friedman test and Dunn's multiple comparison test)

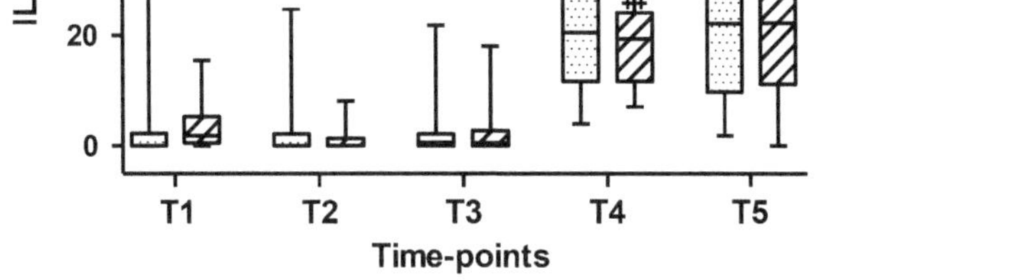

Fig. 22.2 IL-6 concentrations (pg/ml) in the plasma of saline (control) and L-Ala-Gln-treated patients. Bars represent median with interquartile range and minimum and maximum values of 15 subjects of control and L-Ala-Gln groups during different time-points. Groups studied are not significantly different according to Mann–Whitney test. IL-6 levels increased significantly in control and L-Ala-Gln-treated patients, comparing T5 and T4 with basal values (T1). $^{\dagger\dagger}P < 0.01$ compared with T1 (control group); $^{\ddagger\ddagger}P < 0.01$ compared with T1 (L-Ala-Gln group)

Table 22.2 IL-6 concentrations (pg/ml) measured in the plasma of saline (control) and L-Ala-Gln-treated patients at T1 (baseline), T2, T3, T4, and T5 time-points. Data correspond to the analysis of 15 patients of both groups at each time-point

	Control (n = 15)		L-Ala-Gln (n = 15)		Between groups significance
Time-points	Median	Interquartile range	Median	Interquartile range	(Mann–Whitney test)
T1	0.00	0.00–2.27	1.89	0.56–5.30	P = 0.1282
T2	0.00	0.00–2.14	0.00	0.00–1.32	P = 0.6466
T3	0.63	0.00–2.15	0.56	0.00–2.76	P = 0.8796
T4	20.47††	11.64–27.78	19.32‡‡	11.67–24.03	P = 0.4307
T5	22.13††	9.72–33.23	22.18‡‡	11.16–33.41	P = 1.0000

The symbol †† (P < 0.01) denotes statistically significant differences in relation to T1 in the Control group; the symbol ‡‡ (P < 0.01) represents statistically significant differences compared with T1 in the L-Ala-Gln group (Friedman test and Dunn's multiple comparison test)

10 mg/L in healthy adults. The rapid increase in synthesis within hours of tissue injury suggests that it contributes to host defense, and that it is part of the innate immune response [16]. Serum levels of CRP can be used for early detection of surgical complications [17]. In this study the significant increase in CRP levels in control patients, comparing T5 with basal values (T1) and the absence of significant differences in CRP levels in L-Ala-Gln-treated patients point to a possible attenuation of the surgical trauma response in GLN-treated children.

IL-6 is an important cytokine in the early inflammatory response to trauma. This cytokine is produced and detectable within an hour after trauma and it seems to play a dual role in the inflammatory response by acting as both a pro-inflammatory and anti-inflammatory mediator [18, 19]. Parenteral glutamine supplementation had a beneficial effect in reducing the systemic production of IL-6 after abdominal operations. Lower IL-6 levels probably improve nitrogen balance in these patients [20]. In this study, the increase in IL-6 levels in both the groups during the postoperative period signals increased inflammatory response regardless of preoperative use of L-Ala-Gln. Therefore, pretreatment with L-Ala-Gln did not suppress the rise of the pro-inflammatory cytokine IL-6. Based on the observations presented above, there is a rationale for the potential benefit of glutamine.

Conclusions

Pretreatment with L-Ala-Gln attenuates the inflammatory response in early postoperative period and ensures a better glycemic control in children undergoing palatoplasty.

References

1. Lacey JM, Crouch JB, Benfell K, Ringer SA, Wilmore CK, Maguire D, Wilmore DW. The effects of glutamine-supplemented parenteral nutrition in premature infants. JPEN J Parenter Enteral Nutr. 1996;20(1):74–80.
2. Bergström J, Fürst P, Norée LO, Vinnars E. Intracellular free amino acid concentration in human muscle tissue. J Appl Physiol. 1974;36(6):693–707.
3. Wilmore DW. Metabolic response to severe surgical illness: overview. World J Surg. 2000;24(6):705–11.
4. Wilmore DW. The effect of glutamine supplementation in patients following elective surgery and accidental injury. J Nutr. 2001;131(9 Suppl):S2543–9. discussion 2550S-2551S. Review.
5. Déchelotte P, Hasselmann M, Cynober L, Allaouchiche B, Coëffier M, Hecketsweiler B, Merle V, Mazerolles M, Samba D, Guillou YM, Petit J, Mansoor O, Colas G, Cohendy R, Barnoud D, Czernichow P, Bleichner G. L-alanyl-L-glutamine dipeptide-supplemented total parenteral nutrition reduces infectious complications and glucose

intolerance in critically ill patients: the French controlled, randomized, double-blind, multicenter study. Crit Care Med. 2006;34(3):598–604.

6. Lenz A, Franklin GA. Cheadle WG Systemic inflammation after trauma. Injury. 2007;38(12):1336–45.
7. Krost B, Schubert J. Influence of season on prevalence of cleft lip and palate. Int J Oral Maxillofac Surg. 2006;35:215–8.
8. Choudhary S, Cadier MA, Shinn DL, Shekhar K, McDowall RA. Effect of Veau-Wardill-Kilner type of cleft palate repair on long-term midfacial growth. Plast Reconstr Surg. 2003;111(2):576–82. discussion 583-585.
9. Sedlak J, Lindsay RH. Estimation of total, protein-bound, and nonprotein sulfhydryl groups in tissue with Ellman's reagent. Anal Biochem. 1968;25(1):192–205.
10. Buege JA, Aust SD. Microsomal lipid peroxidation. Methods Enzymol. 1978;52:302–10.
11. Trinder P. Determination of blood glucose using 4-amino phenazone as oxygen acceptor. J Clin Pathol. 1969;22(2):246.
12. García-de-Lorenzo A, Zarazaga A, García-Luna PP, Gonzalez-Huix F, López-Martínez J, Mijján A, Quecedo L, Casimiro C, Usán L, del Llano J. Clinical evidence for enteral nutritional support with glutamine: a systematic review. Nutrition. 2003;19(9):805–11.
13. Poindexter BB, Ehrenkranz RA, Stoll BJ, Koch MA, Wright LL, Oh W, Papile LA, Bauer CR, Carlo WA, Donovan EF, Fanaroff AA, Korones SB, Laptook AR, Shankaran S, Stevenson DK, Tyson JE, Lemons JA. Effect of parenteral glutamine supplementation on plasma amino acid concentrations in extremely low-birth-weight infants. Am J Clin Nutr. 2003;77(3):737–43.
14. Ward E, Smith M, Henderson M, Reid U, Lewis I, Kinsey S, Allgar V, Bowers D, Picton SV. The effect of high-dose enteral glutamine on the incidence and severity of mucositis in pediatric oncology patients. Eur J Clin Nutr. 2009;63(1):134–40.
15. Jaye DL, Waites KB. Clinical applications of C-reactive protein in pediatrics. Pediatr Infect Dis J. 1997;16(8):735–46.
16. Black S, Kushner I, Samols D. C-reactive Protein. J Biol Chem. 2004;279(47):487–90.
17. Ackland GL, Scollay JM, Parks RW, de Beaux I, Mythen MG. Pre-operative high sensitivity C-reactive protein and postoperative outcome in patients undergoing elective orthopaedic surgery. Anaesthesia. 2007;62(9):888–94.
18. Xing Z, Gauldie J, Cox G, Baumann H, Jordana M, Lei XF, Achong MK. IL-6 is an antiinflammatory cytokine required for controlling local or systemic acute inflammatory responses. J Clin Invest. 1998;101(2):311–20.
19. Lin E, Calvano SE, Lowry SF. Inflammatory cytokines and cell response in surgery. Surgery. 2000;127(2):117–26.
20. Lin MT, Kung SP, Yeh SL, Liaw KY, Wang MY, Kuo ML, Lee PH, Chen WJ. Glutamine-supplemented total parenteral nutrition attenuates plasma interleukin-6 in surgical patients with lower disease severity. World J Gastroenterol. 2005;11(39):6197–201.

Chapter 23
Use of Perioperative Glutamine Dipeptide in Parenteral Nutrition in Surgical Hospital Patients with Malnutrition

Gabriel Mercadal-Orfila, Josep Manel Llop Talaverón, and Rajkumar Rajendram

Key Points

- Surgical patients at nutritional risk in the 10–14 days before surgery should receive perioperative nutritional support.
- Delaying surgery for those patients at greatest risk of severe undernourishment may be justified in some cases.
- Perioperative administration of glutamine to patients with moderate–severe undernourishment before surgery can effectively reduce the morbidity associated with undernourishment, enhance glycaemic control, reduce the incidence of infections and shorten the length of ICU admission.

Keywords Glutamine dipeptide • Perioperative • Malnutrition • Surgery • Mortality

Introduction

Undernourishment is one of the most important clinical problems in patients admitted to hospital [1]. Undernourishment per se has several consequences and also increases the complications of the disease requiring admission. It also impairs response to treatment and impairs the immune response, increasing the risk of infection. Besides the morbidity and mortality that result from these sequelae of malnutrition, there are significant economic costs associated with any complications and prolonged admission to hospital [2].

In Spain, the prevalence of undernourishment in surgical patients varies from 13 to 48.1 % [3]. In addition, the nutritional status of 25 % of these patients actually gets worse during their hospital admission. This deterioration may be caused by the disease requiring admission to hospital, perioperative fasting, and postoperative complications leading to a protracted catabolic state.

G. Mercadal-Orfila, Pharm D (✉)
Mateu Orfila/Department of Pharmacy, Maó-Menorca, Spain

J.M. Llop Talaverón, Pharm D
Department of Pharmacy, Hospital Universitari Bellvitge/Universitat de Barcelona, Hospitalet de Llobregat, Barcelona, Spain

R. Rajendram, M.R.C.P., F.R.C.A., F.F.I.C.M.
Department of Intensive Care, Barnet and Chase Farm Hospitals, Royal Free London NHS Foundation Trust, London, UK

R. Rajendram et al. (eds.), *Glutamine in Clinical Nutrition*, Nutrition and Health,
DOI 10.1007/978-1-4939-1932-1_23, © Springer Science+Business Media New York 2015

Consumption of energy and protein is often particularly low in the preoperative phase before surgery to the gastrointestinal tract (GIT).

The most significantly malnourished surgical patients benefit most from nutritional supplements (oral and/or parenteral) if supplementation is started 7–10 days before surgery. Nutritional supplementation is associated with a lower incidence of infections and anastamotic leaks in these patients [4].

Elderly patients, patients with chronic diseases and alcohol misusers may have micronutrient deficiencies or ingest vitamins and minerals below recommended doses. These patients may need nutrient supplementation before and after surgery. However, nourishing these individuals requires special consideration because overzealous nutritional support may precipitate the refeeding syndrome.

Thus nutritional supplements are therapies that can provide the patient with sufficient perioperative nutritional support for the stress response to surgery to achieve positive nitrogen and calorie balances. However, careful monitoring of nutritional status and the response to therapy is required to prevent the complications of over and underfeeding.

The focus of clinical nutrition has shifted from simple nutritional support, i.e. just aiming to cover energy and nitrogen requirements, to nutritional therapy, i.e. selecting nutrient supplements for specific pharmacological effects in addition to their nutritional value. Immunonutrition is probably the best example of the application of nutritional therapy in clinical practice [5].

Various diets with different combinations of supplements thought to enhance immune function have been studied in surgical patients. These diets have often contained combinations of arginine, glutamine, omega-3 fatty acids, and nucleotides. The current literature generally suggests that treatment with glutamine has clinically significant benefits. Glutamine reduces the incidence of complications and reduces length of hospital admission in comparison to standard care [5]. Moreover, this treatment is most effective in malnourished patients [4].

Guidelines from both the American (ASPEN; 6) and the European (ESPEN; 7) Societies of Parenteral and Enteral Nutrition recommend the use of nutritional immunomodulators in patients with moderate–severe malnutrition having surgery to the GIT. Of the nutritional immunomodulators currently available, the role of glutamine dipeptides is particularly emphasised [8].

Several meta-analyses and studies [9–32] have demonstrated that large doses of glutamine are associated with a positive nitrogen balance, reduced incidence of infection, shorter hospital admission and lower mortality in critically ill patients and surgical patients. ESPEN guidelines [5] recommend that surgical patients at nutritional risk in the 10–14 days before surgery should receive perioperative nutritional support. Delaying surgery for those patients at greatest risk of severe undernourishment may be justified in some cases.

Investigation of the Effectiveness of Perioperative Intravenous Glutamine Supplementation with Parenteral Nutrition

Few studies have investigated the effect of perioperative intravenous glutamine supplementation on patients having surgery on the gastrointestinal tract (GIT). We therefore conducted a quasi-experimental study [13] of patients over 18 years old having surgery to the GIT who were candidates for perioperative nutritional support.

Methods

We therefore included patients at moderate to severe risk of malnutrition (weight loss over 5–10 % in the last 6 months, or body mass index (BMI) <18.5 kg/m^2, or classified as mildly (B) or severely (C) malnourished patient on subjective global assessment (SGA), or serum albumin <3.5 g/dl, or prealbumin <15 mg/dl (no evidence of kidney or liver disease)). The exclusion criteria were: chronic renal failure requiring dialysis, acute renal failure not treated with haemofiltration (creatinine >2.2 mg/dl), liver failure with encephalopathy, severe metabolic acidosis, pregnant or breast-feeding women, or a psychiatric condition preventing the patient from consenting to the study, and inclusion in another study.

Three cohorts were compared as follows:

Group 1 (control 1; –/–): glutamine was not added to PN before or after surgery (March 2006–March 2007).
Group 2 (control 2; –/G): glutamine (0.4 g/kg/day) was added to PN only in the postoperative period (March 2007–March 2008).
Group 3 follow-up group (G/G): glutamine (0.4 g/kg/day) was added to PN before and after surgery (March 2008–March 2009).

Each patient also received perioperative nutritional support according to their nutritional needs and the expected duration of perioperative fasting. This was given as PN and was started 2–3 days before surgery. Calorific intake was calculated according to the protocol used in the hospital.

The Harris Benedict formula was used to estimate baseline energy expenditure. The values obtained were multiplied by a stress factor (Long) and the activity factor. The groups who received PN without glutamine supplementation received 4 g/kg/day glucose, 1 g/kg/day lipid and 1.5 g/kg/day protein. The groups who received PN with glutamine supplementation received 1.1 g/kg/day protein and 0.4 g/kg/day glutamine when glutamine was given.

The following data were collected:

Demographic data: gender and age.
Anthropometric: weight, height, body mass index (BMI); SGA; weight loss in the preceding 6 months.
Postoperative clinical course: incidence of fistula (suture dehiscence or spontaneous); incidence of intestinal failure (retroperitoneal bleeding, abscess and/or peritonitis); incidence of renal failure (serum creatinine >2.2 mg/dL or serum urea >80 mg/dL), incidence of hyperglycaemia (serum glucose > 160 mg/dL); days on PN, duration of stay in ICU (days); duration of hospital admission (days); respiratory, urinary tract and wound infections (defined as presence of focus of infection, plus two of the following criteria: leucocytes $>12\times10^9$/L; fever >38 °C; heart rate >90 beats per minute; or $PCO_2<31$ mm Hg); death during hospital admission; death at 6 months; biochemistry and haematology on days −1, +3, +7 after surgery and last day of total parenteral nutrition (TPN).

Statistical Analysis

All data are expressed as means, standard deviations and percentages. The statistical software package SPSS 12 for Windows (SPSS Inc., Chicago, IL, USA) was used for all analyses. Univariate analysis of quantitative and qualitative data from the 3 study groups was performed initially. Multivariate analysis was then performed.

The biochemical and haematological data were analysed and compared between groups and within each group using ANOVA and the Wilcoxon signed-rank test for related samples. If the data were normally distributed, parametric tests were used: Student's *t*-test was used for quantitative data and the paired *t*-test was used for paired samples.

If the Kolmogorov–Smirnov test showed that the distribution of the data was not normal, non-parametric tests were used. The chi-squared test was used to analyse categorical data. The Kruskal–Wallis test was used for independent samples, and Wilcoxon signed-rank test for two related samples. $P<0.05$ was considered significant.

We used "Backward Stepwise" logistic regression to analyse the quantitative and categorical data recorded in the study through the predictor variables, to determine the factors which influence the response under investigation.

Results

Sixty-seven patients met the inclusion criteria and were included in the study; 17 patients were excluded from the study by the exclusion criteria. This single-centre sample is relatively small because the Mateu Orfila Hospital where the study was conducted has only 140 beds and the time available for recruitment of patients was short.

Although the sample was small the significant amount of data collected allowed thorough evaluation of the efficacy of perioperative administration of glutamine supplements to patients with moderate to severe undernourishment having surgery to the GIT.

Variance analysis excluded statistically significant differences between the three study groups in age, income, gender, current weight, usual weight, height, weight loss and BMI. The demographics and preoperative anthropometric data of the three groups were therefore similar (Table 23.1). There were no significant differences between the groups' preoperative nutritional assessment, as assessed by the SGA questionnaire. The nutritional status of the groups of patients was therefore similar and comparable.

Table 23.1 Baseline and surgery variables

	Group −/− (n=21)	Group −/G (n=27)	Group G/G (n=19)	P value
Gender (male/female; n, %)	16 (76.2):5 (23.8)	17 (63):10 (37)	14 (73.7):5 (26.3)	0.76
Age (years)	65.19 (12.96)	64.8 (17.03)	65.57 (14.7)	0.986
Height (m; SD)	1.69 (0.07)	1.67 (0.1)	1.66 (0.07)	0.528
BMI (kg/m^2; SD)	24.99 (3.9)	24.42 (3.76)	23.63 (3.72)	0.537
Weight loss (%)	8 (6.63)	8 (6.83)	11.85 (5.01)	0.092
Current weight	71.8 (14.15)	69.03 (14.58)	65.5 (10.18)	0.334
Usual weight	77.73 (12.13)	74.62 (12.34)	78.55 (12.77)	0.519
Subjective Global Assessment				
A	2 (9.5)	0 (0)	0 (0)	0.155
B	13 (61.9)	21 (77.8)	11 (57.9)	
C	6 (28.6)	6 (22.2)	8 (42.1)	
Nutritional Support				
Total Kcal	1920.42 (268.72)	1962 (370.3)	1841.1 (348.33)	0.33
Fat	69.33 (17.34)	74.51 (17.71)	67.36 (16.69)	
Glucose	207.57 (32.22)	211.74 (45.16)	211.74 (45.16)	
Nitrogen	15.47 (2.15)	15.62 (2.81)	15.57 (2.36)	
Operation (n, %)				
Hemicolectomy	6 (28.6)	7 (25.9)	8 (42.1)	0.081
Small bowel resection	7 (33.3)	7 (25.9)	2 (10.5)	
Laparatomy	0 (0)	4 (14.8)	0 (0)	
Hepatectomy	0 (0)	2 (7.4)	0 (0)	
Gastrectomy	7 (33.3)	3 (11.1)	5 (26.3)	
Ileostomy	0 (0)	0 (0)	1 (5.3)	
Cholecystectomy	0 (0)	2 (7.4)	0 (0)	
Others	1 (4.8)	2 (7.4)	3 (15.8)	

Data are expressed as means (SD) or unless otherwise stated. n, number of patients; SD, standard deviation

Table 23.2 Morbidity and mortality data

Complication	Study groups: no. patients (%)			P value	Linear relationship by linear association
	Group –/–	Group –/G	Group G/G		
Hyperglycaemia	11 (52.4)	9 (33.3)	1 (5.3)	0.006	0.002
Urinary infection	3 (14.3)	1 (3.7)	1 (5.3)	0.350	0.269
Wound infection	9 (42.9)	7 (25.9)	3 (15.8)	0.155	0.05
Respiratory infection	4 (19)	6 (22.2)	2 (10.5)	0.587	0.501
Presence of 1 or more infection	13 (619)	12 (44.4)	5 (26.3)	0.078	0.025
Fistula	4 (19)	4 (14.8)	3 (15.8)	0.922	0.776
Renal failure	5 (23.8)	5 (18.5)	1 (5.3)	0.266	0.120
Intestinal failure	6 (28.6)	5 (18.5)	3 (15.8)	0.565	0.319
Mortality	4 (19)	4 (14.8)	3 (15.8)	0.922	0.776
6 month mortality	7 (33.3)	5 (18.5)	3 (15.8)	0.340	0.181
ICU admission	14 (66.7)	18 (66.7)	6 (31.6)	0.033	0.03
Days in ICU (SD)	5.85 (11.41)	6.33 (9)	3.26 (7.4)	0.074	
Days in hospital (SD)	32.57 (27.3)	28.62 (25.96)	24.78 (11.48)	0.886	
Days on TPN (SD)	16 (15.32)	13.7 (13.2)	10.1 (4.64)	0.485	

Data are expressed as number of patients (%) unless expressed otherwise. SD, standard deviation

Table 23.3 COX proportional regression models

Response variable	Variable in equation	B	SE	E^b	1/Eb	95 % CI of 1/ E^b
Duration of admission (days)	Albumin	0.557	0.166	1.745	0.57	0.8–0.41
	Fistula	–1.343	0.434	0.261	3.83	8.9–1.63
	Wound infection	–0.922	0.302	0.398	2.51	4.54–1.39
	Hyperglycaemia	–0.593	0.3	0.553	1.8	3.26–1
ICU admission (days)	Respiratory infection	–1.505	0.498	0.222	4.5	11.9–1.7
Parenteral nutrition (days)	Fistula	–1.378	0.508	0.252	3.9	10.7–1.46
	Renal failure	–1.194	0.39	0.303	3.3	7.08–1.53
	Respiratory infection	–0.954	0.44	0.385	2.6	6.15–1.095
	Wound infection	–0.931	0.345	0.394	2.53	4.9–1.28

B: explanatory variable constant. SE: standard error of constant B
$1/E^b$: inverse exponential function indicative of relative risk

There were no differences in the supply of glucose, nitrogen, lipids or Kcal between the groups. The most common operations were hemicolectomy, small bowel resection and gastrectomy.

Table 23.2 shows that group G/G had shorter admissions to ICU ($P=0.074$) and reduced duration of PN. However, these reductions did not achieve statistical significance. The incidence of hyperglycaemia was lowest in group G/G and the proportion of patients admitted to ICU was also lowest in group G/G.

There was a trend suggesting a lower incidence of infection in patients who received glutamine supplementation but this did not achieve statistical significance ($P=0.078$). Remarkably, the linear tendency test showed a linear relationship between glutamine supplementation and wound infection ($P=0.05$), hyperglycaemia ($P=0.002$), ICU stay ($P=0.03$) and presence of infection ($P=0.025$).

After multivariate analysis (Tables 23.3 and 23.4) group G/G was found to reduce ICU admission, hyperglycaemia and renal failure, but group –/G did not. This suggests that glutamine supplementation before and after surgery is not only more effective than no glutamine supplementation but is also more effective than postoperative glutamine supplementation.

The intergroup analyses of the biochemical and haematological data found that on day +3 there were significant differences in the concentrations of glucose (Fig. 23.1; –/–: 185.7 ± 86 mg/dL vs. –/G: 132.074 ± 31.38 mg/dL vs. G/G: 145.39 ± 62.9 mg/dL; $P=0.001$), and albumin (–/–: 2.38 g/

Table 23.4 Logistic regression models

Complication	Variable in equation	B	SE	E^b^	95 % CI
Fistula	Intestinal failure	2.103	0.866	8.19	3.76–17.533
Intestinal failure	Wound infection	2.4	1.04	11.18	3.77–37.21
	Respiratory infection	2.1	1.02	8.17	2.57–22.94
	Renal failure	3.3	1.09	27.6	9.68–103.9
	Fistula	2.4	1.03	11.25	4.45–44.8
Respiratory infection	Pre-albumin	−0.328	0.119	0.791	0.67–0.9
Renal failure	Group G/G	−1.662	1.12	0.19	0.083–0.74
	Creatinine	0.972	0.414	2.64	1.17–5.9
Wound infection	Intestinal failure	1.87	0.875	6.5	3.4–20.6
	Hyperglycaemia	1.602	0.738	4.96	1.6–7.33
Hyperglycaemia	Group G/G	−2.2	1.1	0.11	0.015 0.286
	Renal failure	1.65	0.816	5.22	2.722–14.31
	Wound infection	1.714	0.745	5.5	1.4–5.8
Death	Intestinal failure	2.34	0.848	10	5.84–30
ICU admission (YES/NO)	Group G/G	−1.24	0.615	0.289	0.135–0.476
	Albumin	−0.98	0.447	0.375	0.23–0.825

B: explanatory variable constant. SE: standard error of constant B

E^b^: exponential function indicative of relative risk (Odds Ratio)

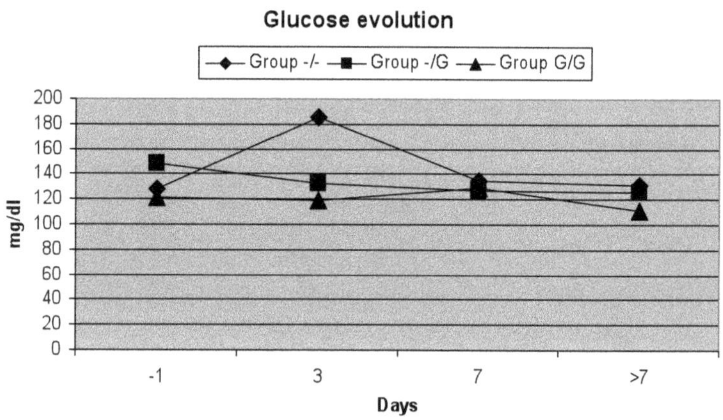

Fig. 23.1 Glucose evolution

dl ± vs. 0.48 g/dl –/G: 2.71 ± 0.55 g/dl vs. G/G: 2.91 ± 0.57 g/dl; $P = 0.013$) between the 3 groups. The groups which received glutamine supplementation (–/G and G/G) had lower serum glucose concentrations and higher albumin concentrations than group –/–. This trend was also observed in the final analysis of the data on glucose and albumin, although these differences were not statistically significant.

In addition, differences in the white cell counts were seen 7 days after surgery. The leucocyte counts of groups –/G and G/G were within the reference range (4–11 × 10^9/L), i.e. normal while the control group –/– had leucocytosis (mean leucocyte count 13.75 × 10^9/L).

Group G/G also had the lowest postoperative fall in plasma albumin (reduction of albumin: –/–: 0.95 g, –/G = 0.86 g; G/G = 0.7 g). In addition, only the –/– group had a significant increase in blood glucose between the preoperative analysis and day + 3 (128.19 ± 40 mg/dL vs. 185.7 ± 86.87 mg/dL; $P = 0.003$). Blood glucose did not increase significantly in groups –/G (148.6 ± 200 mg/dL vs. 132.07 ± 31 mg/dL; $P > 0.05$) or G/G (121.68 vs. ± 39.97 mg/dL vs. 119.12 ± 44.72 mg/dL; $P > 0.05$).

Discussion

Few studies have investigated the effect of perioperative intravenous glutamine supplementation on malnourished human patients having GIT surgery. The end-points of these studies have varied from biomarkers of immune function to more directly clinically relevant endpoints such as risk of infection, length of hospital admission, morbidity and mortality.

Immune Function

Exner et al. [15] were among the first to show that perioperative glutamine administration was associated with more rapid reconstitution of immune function as demonstrated by the recovery of the percentage of TNF-α secretion at 48 h after surgery. Yao et al. [16] found greater restoration of plasma endotoxin inactivation capacity (EIC) and a significant increase in CD4 cell counts on days 1 and 4 after surgery in patients who received perioperative glutamine supplementation. However, there were no differences in infectious complications.

Yeh et al. (2008) reported reduction of postoperative albumin levels, protein C reactive (PCR) and %CD8 cells in patients who received perioperative glutamine supplementation. Fan et al. [18] reported improved maintenance of glutathione (GSH) concentrations, ratio of reduced glutathione to oxidised glutathione (GSH/GSSG ratio), red blood cell counts and albumin concentration, but there were no differences in the laboratory blood markers of liver damage or function.

Asprer et al. [19] provided only preoperative glutamine supplementation and found that leucocyte, granulocyte and lymphocyte counts were increased before surgery, this increase was not sustained after surgery when supplementation was not provided.

These observations suggest that glutamine attenuates inflammation and immunosuppression as well as reducing depletion of nutrients. These effects on immune function are relevant to the effects of glutamine supplementation on risk of infection.

Risk of Infection

Several studies have described the association between glutamine supplementation and reduced risk of infection. For example, the meta-analysis performed by Zheng et al. [12] which included five surgical studies with a total of 215 patients found that the group treated with glutamine had fewer infectious episodes (OR=0.24, 95 % CI=0.06, 0.93; $P=0.04$). Dechelotte et al. [21] also reported less nosocomial pneumonia in the group who received glutamine (17.24 % vs. 33.9 %; $P<0.05$). Bonet et al. [25] also found a lower incidence of nosocomial pneumonia (8.04 % vs. 29.25 % episodes), and fewer urinary tract infections (2.5 % vs. 16.7 % episodes).

In the present study, there were no statistically significant differences between the three groups in the incidence of wound, urinary or respiratory infections. We also analysed incidence of infection as a combined outcome measure; "Presence of one or more infection (respiratory, urinary and/or lower respiratory tract infection)" vs. no infection. Although there was still no statistically significant differences between the three groups studied, there was a trend towards significance ($P=0.078$), and the relationship between glutamine supplementation and reduced incidence of infection was linear ($P=0.025$). Hyperglycaemia is also associated with increased incidence of infections and mortality [21]. The effect of glutamine on glucose metabolism is therefore important and may contribute at least in part to the reduction of infectious complications in patients given glutamine supplements.

Glucose Homeostasis

The prognosis of patients with insulin resistance and persistent hyperglycaemia is poor. It is therefore important to mention note the beneficial role of glutamine in the control of glucose metabolism, which is demonstrated in the results of univariate and multivariate analyses of our present data (Tables 23.2 and 23.4; Fig. 23.1). An earlier study from our group has previously highlighted the protective effect of glutamine (OR: 0.38, CI: 0.19–0.75) against hyperglycaemia in critically ill patients [22]. Reduction of insulin resistance in critically ill patients with glutamine supplementation was also demonstrated by Dechelotte et al. [21]. Dechelotte et al. found that the incidence of hyperglycaemia was lower and less insulin was required in the patients who received glutamine supplements. Bakalar et al. [23] also reported that glycaemic control in patients who had sustained polytrauma was improved when given TPN supplemented with glutamine.

Glutamine has several potential beneficial effects and supplementation also reduces the incidence of some non-infective complications of surgery [22, 26].

Non-infective Complications

When the non-infectious postoperative complications were analysed there were no statistically significant differences between the groups in the incidence of fistulas. However in the present study, supplementation with glutamine before and after GIT surgery was found to protect against intestinal failure (OR = 0.19, 95 % CI = 0.083–0.74). This protective effect of glutamine was previously described in critically ill patients in a study performed by our research group in 2006 [22].

Perioperative complications, infective and non-infective, increase the duration of hospital admission. The beneficial effects of glutamine may therefore reduce duration of hospital admission.

Duration of Hospital Admission

In our study the average length of hospital admission, duration of ICU admission and duration of feeding with TPN of the groups who received glutamine were all less than in the group that did not receive any glutamine. Although these differences did not achieve statistical significance (Table 23.2), logistic regression of data from group G/G suggested that perioperative glutamine supplementation before and after surgery reduced the need for ICU admission (OR = 0.289, CI 95 % = 0.135–0.476) (Table 23.4).

Our observations are consistent with those of previous studies. For example, Yao et al. [16] reported that length of hospital admission was reduced by glutamine (11.7 ± 2 days vs. 10.6 ± 1.2; $P = 0.03$). Yeh et al. [17] also found that length of hospital admission was reduced by glutamine supplementation (16.3 ± 21.3 days vs. 12.2 ± 6.8 days; $P = 0.299$). The meta-analysis by Zheng et al. [12] which included six studies with a total of 291 surgical patients reported that treatment with dipeptides of glutamine in PN reduced duration of hospital admission (−3.55, 95 % CI = −5.26, −1.84; $P < 0.00001$).

This is obviously clinically significant but is also economically important, as reducing duration of admission to hospital and preventing admission to ICU reduces cost. Mertes et al. [27] calculated the potential savings which may be achieved by glutamine supplementation. In the cohort of patients who received glutamine supplementation the mean duration of hospital stay was 4.7 days less and the potential saving was estimated at $42,075. The beneficial effects of glutamine which may contribute to earlier discharge from hospital include acceleration of healing, recovery of intestinal mucosal integrity, improvement of glycaemic control and immune function resulting in prevention of potential infections. Reducing the incidence of postoperative infections improves morbidity and mortality.

Morbidity and Mortality

Although there were no differences in survival at 6 months, our observations suggest that perioperative glutamine supplementation in TPN is associated with less postoperative morbidity in patients at risk of malnutrition and is therefore justified in patients at risk of moderate or severe undernourishment having GIT surgery.

In contrast, Gianotti et al. [20] found that in well-nourished patients having abdominal surgery, perioperative supplementation of glutamine administered in a dextrose carrier solution (rather than TPN), did not reduce morbidity or mortality when compared with the control group. However, it is important to review the methodology of the studies in question. Importantly the patients in our study were at risk of moderate or severe undernourishment before surgery, with rates of weight loss between 8 and 11 %. In contrast, the cohort described by Gianotti et al. were well nourished with weight loss of 1.4 %. Gianotti et al. 2009 also used dextrose 5 % as a carrier solution for dipeptides of glutamine whilst our patients received TPN.

Glutamine supplementation reduces morbidity and mortality in critically ill patients and those who have sustained trauma [7, 23]. These beneficial effects of glutamine supplementation may be explained by increased utilisation of glutamine, increased glutamine metabolism and/or baseline deficits of glutamine in these cohorts of patients.

The meta-analysis performed by Jones et al. [11], which included studies of critically ill patients, found that mortality was significantly reduced by enteral or parenteral glutamine supplementation (RR 0.75, 95 % CI=0.59 –0.96; $P<0.02$). This suggests a beneficial effect of administration of glutamine to critically ill patients, especially if patients receive more than 10 days of TPN with glutamine [25–27]. In our study, there were no significant differences in mortality between the three study groups (19 % vs. 14.8 % vs. 15.8 %). Our findings are consistent with those of Mertes et al. [27] and Jacobi et al. [31] who also investigated the effects of parenteral glutamine in surgical patients.

These data demonstrate a greater reduction of mortality in critically ill patients (who have significant glutamine deficiency) who receive glutamine supplementation than in surgical patients. In addition, several studies have shown increased survival in patients treated with glutamine. Griffiths et al. [29] demonstrated greater survival in critically ill patients when glutamine is added to TPN. Those patients who lived longer had a hospital cost reduced by 50 %. Goeters et al. [32] showed increased survival in critically ill patients at 6 months, when given more than 9 days of TPN.

The risk:benefit ratio of any intervention must be considered. Whilst glutamine has several beneficial effects these must be balanced against any potential side effects.

Side Effects of Glutamine Supplementation

On analysis of laboratory blood tests, Yeh et al. [17] found the lowest fall in serum albumin at day +3 after surgery in group G/G rather than the control groups (0.9 g/dl vs. 0.86 g/dl vs. 0.7 g/dl; $P=0.013$). However in our present data there were no significant changes in the serum markers of hepatic or renal function, suggesting that the use of glutamine dipeptides in TPN is well tolerated. Several other studies have also reported that glutamine supplements are well tolerated and free of side effects [30–33].

Conclusions

Perioperative immunonutrition improves GIT oxygenation and optimises postoperative metabolism. The incidence of postoperative infection and length of admission after elective major GIT surgery are significantly reduced [4]. Perioperative glutamine supplementation should be considered for patients undergoing elective major GIT surgery, even if only provided before surgery, but is more effective if given before and after surgery.

References

1. de Ulibarri JI. Hospital malnutrition. Nutr Hosp. 2003;18:53–6.
2. Stratton RJGC, Elia M. Disease-related malnutrition: an evidence-based approach to treatment: Oxon. UK: CABI Publishing; 2003.
3. Abdel-lah Mohamed AÁHJ. Guia de actuaci6n: Soporte nutricional en el paciente quirúrgico. 2009.
4. Gustafsson UO, Scott MJ, Schwenk W, Demartines N, Roulin D, Francis N, McNaught CE, Macfie J, Liberman AS, Soop M, Hill A, Kennedy RH, Lobo DN, Fearon K, Ljungqvist O. Guidelines for perioperative care in elective colonic surgery: Enhanced Recovery After Surgery (ERAS(®)) Society recommendations. Clin Nutr. 2012;31: 783–800.
5. Braga M. Perioperative immunonutrition and gut function. Curr Opin Clin Nutr Metab Care. 2012;15:485–8.
6. Guidelines for the use of parenteral and enteral nutrition in adult and pediatric patients. J Parenter Enteral Nutr 2002;26(1 Suppl):1SA–138SA
7. Braga M, Ljungqvist O, Soeters P, Fearon K, Weimann A, Bozzetti F. ESPEN Guidelines on Parenteral Nutrition: surgery. Clin Nutr. 2009;28:378–86.
8. Souba W. Nutritional support. N Engl J Med. 1997;336:41–8.
9. Novak F, Heyland DK, Avenell A, Drover JW, Su XY. Glutamine supplementation in serious illness: A systematic review of the evidence. Crit Care Med. 2002;30:2022–9.
10. Jiang Z-M JH, Fürst P. The impact of glutamine dipeptides on outcome of surgical patients: systematic review of randomized controlled trial from Europe and Asia. Clin Nutr. 2004;S1:17–23.
11. Jones NE, Heyland DK. Pharmaconutrition: a new emerging paradigm. Curr Opin Gastroenterol. 2008;24: 215–22.
12. Zheng YM, Li F, Zhang MM, Wu XT. Glutamine dipeptide for parenteral nutrition in abdominal surgery: A meta-analysis of randomized controlled trials. World J Gastroenterol. 2006;12:7537–41.
13. Mercadal Orfila G, Llop Talaver6n JM. Effectiveness of perioperative glutamine in parenteral nutrition in patients at risk of moderate to severe malnutrition. Nutr Hosp. 2011;26:1305–12.
14. Ikeda K, Kimura Y, Iwaya T, Aoki K, Otsuka K, Nitta H, et al. Perioperative nutrition for gastrointestinal surgery. Nippon Geka Gakkai Zasshi. 2004;105:218–22.
15. Exner R, Tamandl D, Goetzinger P, Mittlboeck M, Fuegger R, Sautner T, et al. Perioperative GLY-GLN infusion diminishes the surgery-induced period of immunosuppression - Accelerated restoration of the lipopolysaccharide-stimulated tumor necrosis factor-alpha response. Ann Surg. 2003;237:110–5.
16. Yao GX, Xue XB, Jiang ZM, Yang NF, Wilmore DW. Effects of perioperative parenteral glutamine-dipeptide supplementation on plasma endotoxin level, plasma endotoxin inactivation capacity and clinical outcome. Clin Nutr. 2005;24:510–5.
17. Yeh CN, Lee HL, Liu YY, Chiang KC, Hwang TL, Jan YY, et al. The role of parenteral glutamine supplement for surgical patient perioperatively: result of a single center, prospective and controlled study. Langenbecks Arch Surg. 2008;393:849–55.
18. Fan Y, Yu J, Kang W, Zhang Q. Effects of glutamine supplementation on patients undergoing abdominal surgery. Chin Med Sci J. 2009;24:55–9.
19. Asprer J, Llido L, Sinamban R, Schlotzer E, Kulkarni H. Effect on immune indices of preoperative intravenous glutamine dipeptide supplementation in malnourished abdominal surgery patients in the preoperative and postoperative periods. Nutrition. 2009;25:920–5.
20. Gianotti L, Braga M, Biffi R, Bozzetti F, Mariani L. Perioperative intravenous glutamine supplemetation in major abdominal surgery for cancer: a randomized multicenter trial. Ann Surg. 2009;250:684–90.
21. Dechelotte P, Hasselmann M, Cynober L, Allaouchiche B, Coeffier M, Hecketsweiler B, et al. L-alanyl-L-glutamine dipeptide-supplemented total parenteral nutrition reduces infectious complications and glucose intolerance in

critically ill patients: The French controlled, randomized, double-blind, multicenter study. Crit Care Med. 2006;34:598–604.

22. Mercadal Orfila G, Llop Talaverón J, Gracia García B, Martorell Puigserver C, Badía Tahull M, Tubau Molas M, et al. Glutamine use for parenteral nutrition in the critically ill patient: effects on morbidity and mortality. Nutr Hosp. 2007;22:61–7.
23. Bakalar B, Duska F, Pachl J, Fric M, Otahal M, Pazout J, et al. Parenterally administered dipeptide alanyl-glutamine prevents worsening of insulin sensitivity in multiple-trauma patients. Crit Care Med. 2006;34:381–6.
24. Van den Berghe G, Mesotten D, Vanhorebeek I. Intensive insulin therapy in the intensive care unit. CMAJ. 2009;180:799–800.
25. Bonet AGT, Piñeiro L, Miñambres E, Acosta J, Robles A, Irles JA, Palacios V, Martínez P. La nutrición parenteral total con dipéptido de glutamina disminuye la infección nosocomial de los pacientes de cuidados intensivos:un estudio prospectivo, aleatorio, de doble ciego y multicéntrico. Nutr Hosp. 2008;23:2.
26. Wooley JABI, Good KL. Metabolic and nutritional aspects of acute renal failure in critically ill patients requiring continuous renal replacement therapy. Nutr Clin Pract. 2005;20:176–91.
27. Mertes N, Schulzki C, Goeters C, Winde G, Benzing S, Kuhn KS, et al. Cost containment through L-alanyl-L-glutamine supplemented total parenteral nutrition after major abdominal surgery: a prospective randomized double-blind controlled study. Clin Nutr. 2000;19:395–401.
28. Alpers DH. Glutamine: Do the data support the cause for glutamine supplementation in humans? Gastroenterology. 2006;130:S106–16.
29. Griffiths RD, Jones C, Palmer TEA. Six-month outcome of critically ill patients given glutamine-supplemented parenteral nutrition. Nutrition. 1997;13:295–302.
30. Griffiths RD, Allen KD, Andrews FJ, Jones C. Infection, multiple organ failure, and survival in the intensive care unit: Influence of glutamine-supplemented parenteral nutrition on acquired infection. Nutrition. 2002;18:546–52.
31. Jacobi CAOJ, Zuckermann H. The influence of alanyl-glutamine on immunologic functions and morbidity in post-operative total parenteral nutrition: preliminary results of a prospective randomized trial. Zentralbl Chir. 1999; 124:199–205.
32. Goeters C, Wenn A, Mertes N, Wempe C, Van Aken H, Stehle P, et al. Parenteral L-alanyl-L-glutamine improves 6-month outcome in critically ill patients. Crit Care Med. 2002;30:2032–7.
33. Cynober LA. Metabolic and therapeutic aspects of amino acids in clinical nutrition. 2nd ed. Boca Raton: CRC Press; 2004.

Chapter 24
Therapeutic Use of Glutamine for Diabetic Foot Ulcers and Related Conditions

Annabel E. Barber, Maris S. Jones, and Patrizio Tatti

Key Points

- The economic burden of diabetic foot ulcers is remarkable and the source of these wounds is multifactorial. Glutamine supplementation in diabetics with and without foot wounds has been examined in laboratory and clinical settings.
- Glutamine has been implicated in the improvement of diabetic foot wounds and related conditions. A handful of studies have evaluated a combination of amino acids including glutamine for supplementation in diabetics with foot ulcers with promising results.
- Glutamine has been included in commercially available compounds utilized and studied in surgical and diabetic wounds.
- Glutamine supplementation has been evaluated with respect to surgical wounds. These studies are of particular importance as a basis for evaluating any existing or future literature pertaining to glutamine supplementation in diabetic patients with foot ulcers.
- There exists much literature relating to glutamine supplementation in surgical wounds in non-diabetic patients; however, work still must be done to expand our knowledge regarding glutamine supplementation in diabetic foot wounds.

Keywords Glutamine • Diabetes • Diabetic foot • Wounds and Injuries • Dietary supplements • Amino acids

A.E. Barber, M.D. (✉)
Department of Surgery, University of Nevada School of Medicine,
2040 W Charleston Blvd, Suite 600, Las Vegas, NV 89102, USA
e-mail: aebarber@medicine.nevada.edu

M.S. Jones, M.D.
Department of Surgery, University of Nevada School of Medicine,
2040 W Charleston Blvd, Suite 301, Las Vegas, NV 89102, USA
e-mail: msjones@medicine.nevada.edu

P. Tatti
Department of Endocrinology and Diabetes, ASL RMH, Marino (Roma) 00047, Italy
e-mail: info@patriziotatti.it

R. Rajendram et al. (eds.), *Glutamine in Clinical Nutrition*, Nutrition and Health,
DOI 10.1007/978-1-4939-1932-1_24, © Springer Science+Business Media New York 2015

Abbreviations

CD4	Alpha (α), beta (β), cluster of differentiation 4
CRP	C-Reactive protein
DNA	Deoxyribonucleic acid
g	Grams
HbA1c	Hemoglobin A-1-c
HIF-1	Hypoxia-inducible-factor-1
IgA	Immunoglobulin A (IgA)
IFN	Interferon (IFN)
IL-4	Interleukin-1
IL-4	Interleukin-4
IL-6	Interleukin-6
IV	Intravenous
kg	Kilograms
MHC	Major histocompatibility complex
NV	Nevada
NADPH	Nicotinamide adenine dinucleotide phosphate
PEMF	Pulse electromagnetic field stimulation
RNA	Ribonucleic acid (RNA)
TPN	Total parenteral nutrition
TNF-alpha	Tumor necrosis factor-alpha

Introduction

The incidence of diabetes is increasing throughout the world. Ulcers affecting the lower limbs of diabetics are among the most frequent and costly clinical complications of the disease. Approximately $6–15 billion annually is spent on caring for all chronic wounds in the United States [1]. Among the diabetic population, approximately 1–4 % will develop a foot ulcer per year, with up to 25 % developing an ulcer during their lifetime. Many of these ulcers result in significant morbidity, leading to amputations, disfigurement, sepsis, and sometimes, even death. On average, diabetic foot ulcers exist for 87 ± 83 days [2]. In approximately 15 % of patients, these slow to heal wounds progress to osteomyelitis. Additionally, roughly 16 % of those patients with osteomyelitis progress to amputation [3]. It is clear that diabetic foot ulcers are a highly morbid and costly complication of diabetes mellitus. Despite the fact that many diabetics are obese, decreased lean body mass and an overall catabolic state in diabetics complicate the care of these chronic wounds (see Figs. 24.1 and 24.2). The precise inflammatory milieu at the cellular level in diabetic foot ulcers has yet to be fully elucidated. It is commonly thought that at the macro level, a small skin breakdown or injury from any source along with external factors such as abnormal mechanical load and callus formation due to neuropathy, lead to the initial wound. In this manner, potentially minor injuries are then worsened by diabetes-related factors [4].

Glutamine and Diabetic Wounds

There is in general a paucity of data examining the particular wound healing challenges associated with diabetic foot wounds, and how glutamine may possibly affect these wounds. These wounds are of particular interest to the authors of this chapter and certainly are a morbid problem (see Fig. 24.3).

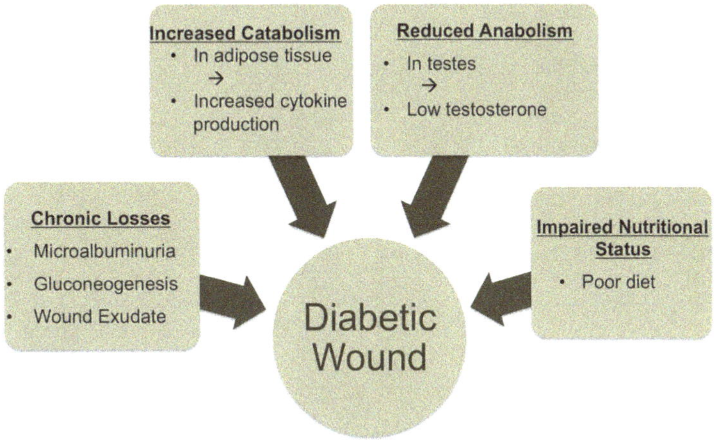

Fig. 24.1 Diabetic wound healing concerns. Constraints on diabetic wound healing include: chronic nutrient losses, increased catabolism, reduced anabolism, and impaired nutritional status

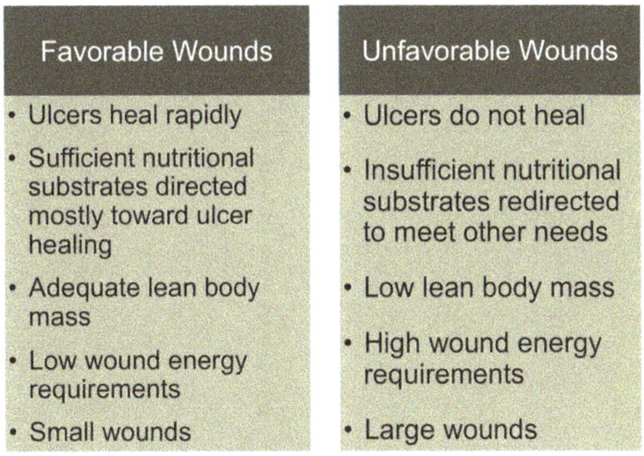

Fig. 24.2 Favorable vs. unfavorable wounds. Physiologic scenarios associated with both favorable and unfavorable wounds

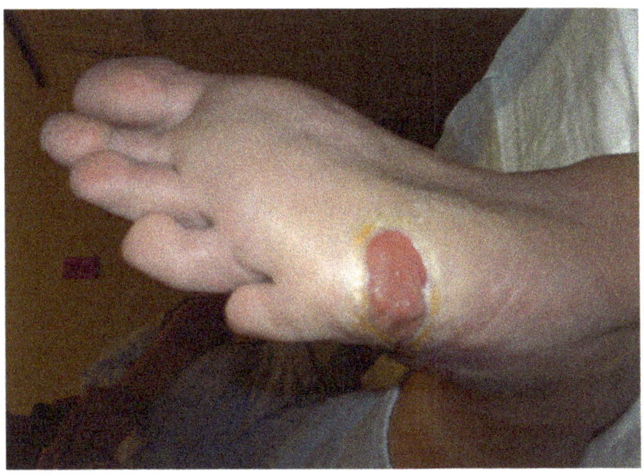

Fig. 24.3 Diabetic foot ulcer

In one paper, published by Tatti et al. in 2012, 22 subjects with type 2 diabetes were evaluated after the administration of an amino acid supplement consisting entirely of glutamine, arginine, and calcium beta-hydroxy beta-methylbutyrate (HMB). In these patients, the cost of antibiotic treatment was reduced by 50 % with use of this particular formula. Additionally, in this study, time to wound healing was shortened, thereby decreasing indirect costs associated with length of stay [5]. Another study

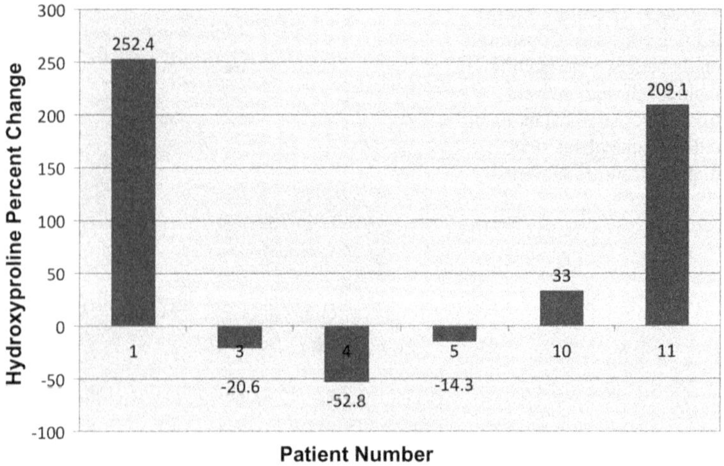

Fig. 24.4 Hydroxyproline percent change with amino acid supplementation. An overall decrease in catabolism noted with arginine, glutamine, and beta-hydroxy-beta-methylbutyrate supplementation in diabetic foot ulcers. Jones MS et al., unpublished data 2013 [8]

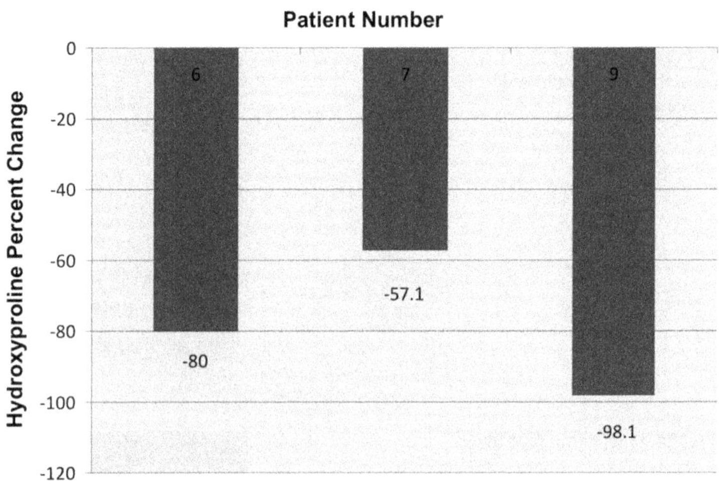

Fig. 24.5 Hydroxyproline percent change with placebo. Effect of placebo on percent change of tissue hydroxyproline concentration in patients with diabetic foot ulcers. Unpublished data, Jones MS, et al. 2013 [8]

conducted by Tatti et al. published in 2011 identified a decrease in microalbuminuria to nearly 50 % of the initial value in patients with diabetic foot ulcers treated with this same dietary supplement containing glutamine (the supplement contained arginine, glutamine, HMB) [6]. A recent study, also identifying nutritional supplementation with the same glutamine-containing compound (glutamine, arginine, HMB) published by this same group, identified a decrease in the progression of diabetes-associated retinal damage during supplementation. Nine diabetic patients with background retinopathy were treated with arginine, glutamine, and HMB. The number of microaneurysms and exudates were counted in these patients. The treatment group exhibited a significant reduction in the number of microaneurysms and exudates [7]. In an ongoing study, conducted by the authors of this chapter (University of Nevada School of Medicine, Department of Surgery, Las Vegas, NV, USA), a significant increase has been noted in tissue hydroxyproline deposition with an amino acid supplement containing arginine, glutamine, and HMB in diabetic human subjects (see pilot data in Figs. 24.4 and 24.5 [8]). Although the activity of this oral supplement is not identical to the activity of glutamine on its own, these data suggest that these amino acids may increase the collagen deposition in human wounds. The research conducted by our group is certainly quite promising, especially given the burden of diabetic foot wounds throughout the developed world.

Glutamine Containing Compounds

In addition to studies of glutamine in isolation and its effect of surgical and diabetic wounds, researchers have investigated commercially available glutamine containing oral supplements given ease of patient access to such compounds. There is generally one commercially available amino acid supplement mixture, and this is the amino acid cocktail examined in the studies discussed previously in this chapter. It is comprised of glutamine, in addition to arginine and HMB. While these cocktails may have differing proprietary names based on country of purchase, they have the same basic formulation, and are from the same manufacturer (Abbott Laboratories, Abbott Park, IL, USA). This cocktail goes by trade names Juven™ and Abound™ (Abbott Laboratories, Abbott Park, IL, USA). They have arisen in response not only to the benefits of glutamine as discussed in this text, but also in response to the benefits of arginine and HMB. Nutritional composition of this commercially available supplement is outlined in Fig. 24.6. HMB is a metabolite of leucine and has been implicated in improved protein metabolism [9]. HMB is presumed to have a beneficial impact on diabetic wounds, however as yet, in isolation that has not been proven. Like glutamine, arginine is a conditionally essential amino acid that is a precursor of nitric oxide. Arginine has been shown to improve vasodilation and as such has been implicated in improved wound outcomes [10, 11]. Given the microcirculatory compromise identified in diabetic wounds, these effects of arginine have been seen as a potential benefit. As with HMB, however, this has not been proven in isolation. Beyond the possible synergistic benefits of arginine and HMB in addition to glutamine, the benefit of studying this commercially available compound is that it is a pleasant tasting, powder-based supplement that is easily utilized and tolerated by patients with surgical or diabetic foot wounds.

Glutamine and Surgical Wounds

Platelets, polymorphonuclear leukocytes, macrophages, and fibroblasts are the main cell types involved in the immune response at the site of tissue injury. Glutamine, as an important source of fuel in these and all rapidly dividing cells, is necessary for DNA and RNA replication before mitosis. Fibroblasts, appearing usually on day 3 in acute wound healing, replace the temporary fibronectin-fibrin framework with collagen. Of note, alpha ketoglutarate (a glutamine metabolite) is taken up via diffusion by these fibroblasts so essential to collagen deposition. There are few in vivo studies and

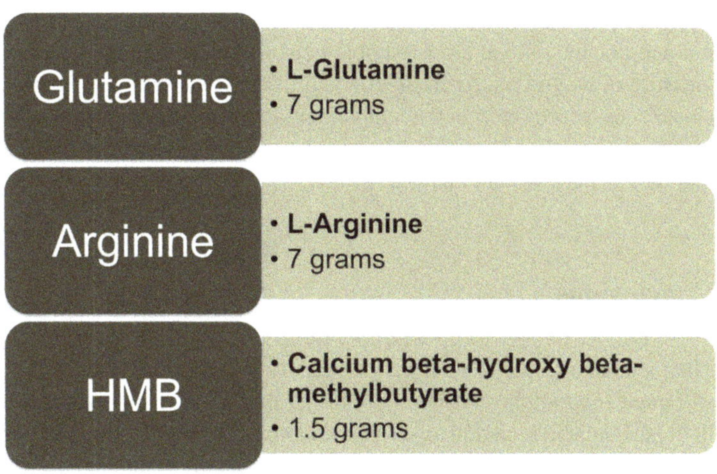

Fig. 24.6 Commercially available glutamine containing amino-acid cocktail. Known by trade names Juven™ and Abound (Abbott Laboratories, Abbott Park, IL, USA), these cocktails contain 7 g each of L-glutamine and L-arginine, and 1.5 g of HMB. They are available in flavored and non-flavored formulations

none have shown a causal link between glutamine and increased collagen deposition [12]. In vitro studies, however, have shown a connectedness between gene expression and glutamine on collagen synthesis in human fibroblast cultures [13, 14]. One particular study examining glutamine's utility in wound healing comes from Polat et al. In 2007, this group used a rat model to investigate bone healing and glutamine supplementation. Glutamine-supplemented rats exhibited more rapid development of primary callus in induced tibial fractures [15]. Kaya et al. in 2007 examined rats with induced colitis to determine if glutamine supplementation (oral and rectal) could improve mucosal healing. This group determined that mucosal DNA contents of both groups were significantly increased, thereby concluding that glutamine supplementation, whether oral or rectal, has a beneficial effect on mucosal regeneration in colitis [16]. Another group, Güven et al. in 2007, studied 40 rats subjected to colorectal anastomoses supplemented with glutamine. Postoperative inflammation and necrosis scores were increased in the rats given delayed feeding (with both normal TPN and glutamine enriched TPN) in comparison to the early feeding groups. Additionally, IGF-I immunoreactivity was increased in the early standard TPN group, and in both early and delayed glutamine supplemented TPN groups. The authors conclude that early feeding plus glutamine supplementation following colorectal anastomosis improves wound healing [17]. Girgan et al. in 2009 studied the effect of pulse electromagnetic field stimulation (PEMF) and glutamine on colorectal anastomoses in rats. Four groups were studied: glutamine alone, PEMF alone, both glutamine and PEMF, and no adjunctive treatments. The groups receiving both glutamine and PEMF exhibited significantly higher mean anastomotic bursting pressures, collagen deposition, and fibroblast infiltration than the glutamine alone and normal resection groups. The glutamine alone group, however, still exhibited higher mean anastomotic bursting pressures than the group with no adjunctive treatment. It appears that even without the addition of PEMF, glutamine aided in the strength of these colorectal anastomoses [18]. Da costa et al. in 2003 also studied the effect of glutamine on colorectal anastomoses. Total anastomotic rupture strength and increased percentage of type I (mature) collagen were significantly increased in the glutamine supplementation group whereas the percent area of type III (immature) collagen was significantly smaller [19]. This is an important finding as submucosa, rich in collagen, is vital to the mechanical strength of the intestinal wall. From these studies in rats we can extrapolate that glutamine-enriched diets have the ability to stimulate anastomotic healing via a number of different mechanisms. These preclinical animal studies are of vital importance for the use of glutamine supplementation in humans. Many of these studies have shown an actual link between glutamine supplementation and increased mature collagen deposition, and thus are extremely topical when thinking about enhancing wound healing in diabetics. A recent human study, conducted by Blass et al., in 2012, supplemented 20 trauma patients with ascorbic acid, α-tocopherol, β-carotene, zinc, selenium and glutamine versus placebo for 2 weeks. These trauma patients preoperatively exhibited a failure of wound healing (i.e. wounds persisting more than 10 days after trauma or surgery), as demonstrated in microcirculation studies done both pre-supplementation and post-supplementation. It was noted that tissue oxygen saturation, which is a measure of wound microcirculation and tissue ischemia, was decreased in the placebo group. Wound closure was more rapid in the supplemental group as compared to the placebo group [20]. This study identifies a potential benefit of glutamine in terms of augmenting factors such as tissue oxygenation that may benefit wound healing.

Conclusions

The metabolic response to injury, especially in diabetic patients, is multifaceted. Additionally, much is still unclear about the continuum of utility of glutamine in health and disease. Looking at the critically ill in particular, a recent prospective randomized study demonstrated a statistically significant increase in in-hospital mortality in addition to 6-month mortality among glutamine-supplemented patients exhibiting multiorgan failure and requiring mechanical ventilation [21]. These are groundbreaking data in that a potential downside to glutamine supplementation has been identified. There is much to be clarified regarding glutamine function not only in non-diabetic patients, but also in the diabetic population. Complicating this topic is the role of insulin sensitivity in obese diabetics versus non-obese diabetics. Is the inflammatory milieu evident in obese diabetics with metabolic syndrome analogous to that present in lean diabetics? How exactly does the tissue microenvironment in diabetics alter wound healing and collagen deposition? These patients appear to exhibit a generally catabolic state, with low lean body mass, and likely depletion of key skeletal and peripheral stores of amino acids including glutamine. The relationship between these nutrient deficits and immunity has yet to be fully elucidated. In numerous animal and human studies, glutamine has been implicated in assisting wound healing and decreasing oxidative stress in the peripheral tissues. More studies looking specifically at glutamine supplementation in diabetics need to be conducted to identify the mechanism of improved wound healing at the cellular level. Hopefully, through this information, we may have a manner of determining an individual's glutamine deficit, so as to precisely replace it. With time and research, the future will allow us to target amino acid therapies on an individual basis as a safe, reliable manner of improving patient outcomes.

References

1. Markova A, Mostow EN. US skin disease assessment: ulcer and wound care. Dermatol Clin. 2012;30(1):107–11, ix.
2. Stockl K, Vanderplas A, Tafesse E, Chang E. Costs of lower-extremity ulcers among patients with diabetes. Diabetes Care. 2004;27(9):2129–34.
3. Driver VR, Fabbi M, Lavery LA, Gibbons G. The costs of diabetic foot: the economic case for the limb salvage team. J Vasc Surg. 2010;52(3 Suppl):17S–22.
4. Eming SA, Hammerschmidt M, Krieg T, Roers A. Interrelation of immunity and tissue repair or regeneration. Semin Cell Dev Biol. 2009;20(5):517–27.
5. Tatti P, Barber AE. The use of a specialized nutritional supplement for diabetic foot ulcers reduces the use of antibiotics. J Endocrinol Metab. 2012;2(1):26–31.
6. Tatti P, Masselli L, Mauro PD, et al. Effect of a nutritional supplement used for diabetic foot ulcers on microalbuminuria. Med J Nutr Metab. 2013;5(1):67–9.
7. Tatti P, Masselli L, di Mauro P. Systemic effects of specific nutrition for wound healing: retinal fundus changes. Clin Nutr Suppl. 2010;5(2):197.
8. Jones MS, Rivera M, Puccinelli CL, et al.: Targeted Amino Acid Supplementation in Diabetic Foot Wounds: Pilot Data and a Review of the Literature. Surg Infect (Larchmt) 2014.
9. Wilson GJ, Wilson JM, Manninen AH. Effects of beta-hydroxy-beta-methylbutyrate (HMB) on exercise performance and body composition across varying levels of age, sex, and training experience: a review. Nutr Metab (Lond). 2008;5:1.
10. Preli RB, Klein KP, Herrington DM. Vascular effects of dietary L-arginine supplementation. Atherosclerosis. 2002;162(1):1–15.
11. Stechmiller JK, Childress B, Cowan L. Arginine supplementation and wound healing. Nutr Clin Pract. 2005;20(1):52–61.
12. Williams JZ, Abumrad N, Barbul A. Effect of a specialized amino acid mixture on human collagen deposition. Ann Surg. 2002;236(3):369–74. discussion 74-5.
13. Bellon G, Monboisse JC, Randoux A, Borel JP. Effects of preformed proline and proline amino acid precursors (including glutamine) on collagen synthesis in human fibroblast cultures. Biochim Biophys Acta. 1987; 930(1):39–47.
14. Bellon G, Chaqour B, Wegrowski Y, Monboisse JC, Borel JP. Glutamine increases collagen gene transcription in cultured human fibroblasts. Biochim Biophys Acta. 1995;1268(3):311–23.
15. Polat O, Kilicoglu SS, Erdemli E. A controlled trial of glutamine effects on bone healing. Adv Ther. 2007;24(1): 154–60.
16. Kaya E, Ceylan A, Kara N, Güven H, Yildiz L. The effect of L-glutamine on mucosal healing in experimental colitis is superior to short-chain fatty acids. Turk J Gastroenterol. 2007;18(2):89–94.

17. Güven A, Pehlivan M, Gökpinar I, Gürleyik E, Cam M. Early glutamine-enriched enteral feeding facilitates colonic anastomosis healing: light microscopic and immunohistochemical evaluation. Acta Histochem. 2007;109(2): 122–9.
18. Girgin S, Gedik E, Ozturk H, Akpolat V, Akbulut V, Kale E, et al. Effects of combined pulse electromagnetic field stimulation plus glutamine on the healing of colonic anastomosis in rats. Dig Dis Sci. 2009;54(4):745–50.
19. da Costa MA, Campos AC, Coelho JC, de Barros AM, Matsumoto HM. Oral glutamine and the healing of colonic anastomoses in rats. J Parenter Enteral Nutr. 2003;27(3):182–5. discussion 5-6.
20. Blass SC, Goost H, Tolba RH, Stoffel-Wagner B, Kabir K, Burger C, et al. Time to wound closure in trauma patients with disorders in wound healing is shortened by supplements containing antioxidant micronutrients and glutamine: a PRCT. Clin Nutr. 2012;31(4):469–75.
21. Heyland D, Muscedere J, Wischmeyer PE, Cook D, Jones G, Albert M, et al. A randomized trial of glutamine and antioxidants in critically ill patients. N Engl J Med. 2013;368(16):1489–97.

Part IV
Clinical Aspects of Glutamine in the Intestine

Chapter 25
Glutamine Protects GI Epithelial Tight Junctions

RadhaKrishna Rao and Kamaljit Chaudhry

Key Points

- Glutamine plays a significant role in the development of gastrointestinal tract.
- Glutamine is required for the preservation of gut mucosal mass under physiologic and pathophysiologic conditions.
- Disruption of gut barrier function has a global impact on the multiple organ systems.
- Glutamine protects intestinal epithelial tight junctions and preserves gut barrier function.
- Specific cellular mechanisms are involved in glutamine-mediated preservation of tight junction integrity.
- Clinical significance of glutamine in diseases associated with gut barrier dysfunction is promising, yet needs further studies to substantiate.

Keywords Glutamine • Intestine • Barrier function • Epithelium • Tight junction • Burn injury • Total parenteral nutrition • Enteral nutrition • Endotoxemia • Bacterial translocation

Abbreviations

AG1478	4-(3-Chloroanillino)-6,7-dimethoxyquinazoline
AIDS	Acquired immune deficiency syndrome
Ala-Gln	Alanine-glutamine dipeptide
Caco-2	Colon adenocarcinoma cell line
DAG	Diacylglycerol
EGF	Epidermal growth factor
EGFR	EGF receptor
ERK	Extracellular signal regulated kinase
FITC	Fluorescein isothiocyanate
Gln	Glutamine

R. Rao, Ph.D., A.G.A.F. (✉) • K. Chaudhry, Ph.D.
Department of Physiology, University of Tennessee Health Science Center,
894 Union Avenue, Nash 426, Memphis, TN 38163, USA
e-mail: rrao2@uthsc.edu; Rkrao-uthsc@gmail.com; kchaudhr@uthsc.edu

R. Rajendram et al. (eds.), *Glutamine in Clinical Nutrition*, Nutrition and Health,
DOI 10.1007/978-1-4939-1932-1_25,

Gln-Gln	Glutamine-glutamine dipeptide
Gly-Gln	Glycine-glutamine dipeptide
IP3	Inositol trisphosphate
IBD	Inflammatory bowel disease
IBS	Irritable bowel syndrome
JAM	Junction adhesion molecule
MAP kinase	Mitogen-activated protein kinase
MMP	Metalloproteinase
PI3K	Phosphatidylinositol 3-kinase
PTEN	Phosphatase and tensin homolog deleted on chromosome 10
PKC	Protein kinase C
TER	Transepithelial electrical resistance
TJ	Tight junction
ZO-1, ZO-2 & ZO-3	Zona occludens-1, -2 and -3

Introduction

L-Glutamine is the most abundant amino acid in blood stream accounting for 30–35 % of the amino acid nitrogen in plasma. It was classified as a non-essential amino acid because it can be readily synthesized in the body from glutamate by glutamine synthetase, which is expressed at high levels in skeletal muscle, liver, brain and stomach tissue. Intracellular concentration of L-glutamine ranges from 2 to 20 mM, and its concentration in the extracellular fluid varies from 0.5 to 0.8 mM. Under conditions of extreme physical exertion, trauma and severe infections, the rate of utilization of glutamine is more than its rate of synthesis, resulting in a significant decline in plasma glutamine concentration. Glutamine is an essential fuel for the gastrointestinal tract. It is required for the synthesis of proteins, nucleic acids and antioxidants, such as glutathione, and involved in the maintenance of acid–base balance with the release of ammonia during its metabolism. Under conditions of reduced plasma glutamine concentration, body depends on the exogenous glutamine to meet its requirements. Therefore, L-glutamine now is reclassified as a conditionally essential amino acid.

If the body requirement of glutamine is not met, the first organ that responds to it is the gastrointestinal tract. Enterocytes prefer glutamine as a source of energy, but it lacks the capacity to synthesize glutamine. Therefore, dietary supply of glutamine is essential to maintain gastrointestinal structure and function. Clinical and experimental studies conducted during the past 25 years have identified glutamine as an important nutrient for the growth and maintenance of intestinal mucosal integrity. Furthermore, glutamine has been recommended for the treatment of burn injury and critically ill patients. Maintenance of gastrointestinal functions, including the barrier function, is not only important to ensure normal gastrointestinal functions, but also essential to prevent injury to other organ systems. A compromised intestinal barrier function may have a global impact on the body due to endotoxemia and bacterial translocation. Therefore, there is a great interest in understanding the role of glutamine in the maintenance and preservation of gut mucosal integrity. This chapter addresses the current understanding of the role of glutamine in intestinal mucosal homeostasis with a focus on its barrier function. Chapter will also make an attempt to distinguish the growth promotional effect of glutamine from its cell signaling effect in regulation of the intestinal epithelial tight junctions and barrier function. Finally, this chapter addresses the clinical implications of glutamine supplementation under health and disease.

Glutamine and the Gastrointestinal Mucosal Homeostasis

Gastrointestinal Mucosa

A functional gastrointestinal tract rapidly develops during the late gestational and neonatal periods. Although a fully functional gut develops at weaning, the epithelial cells continue to proliferate and renew themselves with a high rate of turnover. Intestinal epithelial monolayer lines the luminal surface of mucosa and folded into crypts and villi. Progenitor cells at the bottom of crypts proliferate and differentiate into enterocytes with multiple phenotypes as they migrate upwards to the tips of villi. Due to a continuous renewal of these cells, intestine requires a constant supply of nutrients to maintain cell proliferation and differentiation. Food is an important stimulus for the growth of gut as the enteral nutrients regulate the structure and morphology of the intestinal mucosa. Glutamine is one of the most important components of dietary nutrients that determine the intestinal mucosal integrity. Intestinal mucosa is an adapting tissue. Intestinal failure due to malnutrition is referred to as short bowel syndrome, where functional gut mass is reduced below the level that fails to meet necessary digestive and absorptive functions. But, the intestine bounces back with restoration of enteral nutrition. Three important functions of intestine is digestion, absorption and a defense system against toxins, allergens and pathogens. Therefore, functioning of other organ systems depends on the fully functional gastrointestinal tract.

Glutamine in Development of Gastrointestinal Tract

Glutamine is a major source of energy for the gastrointestinal tract and therefore has a significant influence on the regulation of proliferation and differentiation of intestinal epithelial cells. It appears that glutamine is required for the development as well as maintenance of the gastrointestinal structure and functions. Experimental studies demonstrated that jejunum of developing rats has a greater capacity to oxidize glutamine compared to the jejunum of adults rats [1]. Greater utilization of glutamine in enterocytes of developing intestine was further confirmed in isolated enterocytes from developing pigs [2]. Glutamine depletion in artificially reared rat pups showed that glutamine is essential for the development of gastrointestinal tract [3]. Glutamine supplementation accelerates intestinal growth in hatchling broilers [4] and improves gut development and reduces diarrhea during weaning of piglets [5]. There is an elevated need for glutamine for gastrointestinal growth under challenged conditions. Glutamine improves the intestinal growth in malnourished developing rat pups [6] and prevents retardation of intestinal growth in *E. coli*-challenged piglets [7]. Therefore, glutamine appears to play a crucial role in the development of gastrointestinal tract under normal physiologic and pathophysiologic conditions.

Glutamine in Maintenance of Intestinal Mass

Intestinal epithelial cells continue to proliferate and differentiate even after the development, and therefore, the need for glutamine in the gastrointestinal tract continues. Studies have supported the conclusion that glutamine is essential to maintain the mucosal integrity and gut functions in adults.

Dietary supplementation of glutamine was found to be beneficial in the maintenance of normal intestinal mucosal morphology in weaned piglets [8]. Adult gut mucosa is the major site of glutamine metabolism. It is an important anaplerotic substrate in the mucosal cells and forms important source of energy accounting to about 35 % of the total carbon dioxide produced from various substrates in the intestinal mucosa. In addition to its growth-promoting effects, glutamine seems to have regulatory functions in the intestine. Glutamine promotes electro-neutral sodium chloride absorption in the jejunum of developed pigs, indicating the role of glutamine in functional integrity of the intestine [9]. Glutamine was effective in promoting sodium chloride absorption in animals infected with rotavirus. Therefore, glutamine may help in prevention of fluid loss during diarrhea. In pigs, glutamine supplementation increased the expression of hsp70 in duodenum and jejunum, indicating that it has cytoprotective role in the epithelial cell function and structure [5]. Therefore, in the developed intestine, glutamine is not only important for the proliferation and differentiation of mucosal cells, but also necessary for the regulation of epithelial functions. Therefore, glutamine may have beneficial effects on the intestine under conditions of diarrheal and inflammatory diseases.

The role of glutamine in enterocyte growth was confirmed in cell culture studies. Lack of glutamine attenuates the growth of two types of intestinal epithelial cells, IEC-6 and Caco-2 in culture in vitro. The growth-promoting effects of glutamine was neutralized by the addition of nucleosides, suggesting that glutamine serves as source of amide nitrogen pool for the synthesis of nucleotide and glucosamine in intestine [10]. Glutamine is also necessary during growth factor-mediated enterocyte proliferation. It is required for a maximal stimulation of intestinal epithelial cell proliferation by epidermal growth factor (EGF) [11, 12]. EGF activates glutamine transport activity across the intestinal epithelial membrane through protein kinase C (PKC) and MAP kinase-mediated cell signaling. Therefore, glutamine influences gut in multiple aspects and help maintain the mucosal integrity under normal physiologic conditions.

Gastrointestinal Need for Glutamine Under Pathophysiologic Conditions

The gastrointestinal need for glutamine may be increased during pathophysiologic conditions. Prolonged stress and trauma or therapeutic treatments such as radiation and drugs may lead to drop in body glutamine pool causing mucosal atrophy. Oral glutamine supplementation supports gastrointestinal mucosal growth and prevents mucosal and villous atrophy in patients receiving total parenteral nutrition [13]. Glutamine supplementation in animal models of total parenteral nutrition also showed a dose-dependent increase in mucosal weight. Enteral absorption of nutrients and electrolytes in animals with experimental diarrhea was greatly facilitated by glutamine. It lessens the severity of diarrhea by enhancing water and salt intake, and protects the gut epithelium from ammonia-induced cell death [14]. A mechanism associated with intestinal mucosal atrophy by various factors is increased cell death of epithelial cells. Glutamine-induced prevention of epithelial cell death is likely one of the mechanisms involved in glutamine-mediated mucosal growth.

One of the complications of radiation therapy is intestinal mucosal atrophy. Factors that prevent this side effect of radiation therapy are in search. Evidence indicates that glutamine prevents the radiation-induced gut mucosal injury [15, 16]. Administration of glutamine-rich diet protects gut mucosa from irradiation-induced intestinal injury and ulceration by raising the level of mucosal and plasma glutathione. Oxidative stress is one of the mechanisms involved in radiation-induced gut mucosal injury. Glutamine may promote gut health under such conditions by enhancing the antioxidant defense mechanism.

Glutamine and Gut Barrier Function

Gut Barrier Function

In addition to its important role in digestion, absorption and secretion, the gastrointestinal epithelium serves as a barrier to the diffusion of toxins, allergens and pathogens from the luminal contents into the interstitial tissue. Barrier disruption and diffusion of noxious substances into submucosal region are known to induce inflammation and mucosal injury. In fact, the disruption of gut barrier function plays a crucial role in the pathogenesis of numerous gastrointestinal diseases such as inflammatory bowel disease (IBD), irritable bowel syndrome (IBS), celiac disease, and infectious enterocolitis. Gut barrier dysfunction and increased intestinal permeability appears to be an early factor in the pathogenesis of gastrointestinal diseases. Elevated intestinal permeability was recorded in first-degree relatives of patients with Crohn's disease and ulcerative colitis, although these relatives showed no symptom of IBD. Furthermore, gut barrier dysfunction affects the organs and tissue beyond the gastrointestinal tract. As the consequence of gut barrier dysfunction is endotoxemia and bacterial translocation, all organs are targets of this pathophysiologic condition. Recent studies have demonstrated the presence of increased gut permeability in patients with alcoholic liver disease, diabetes, obesity, and cardiovascular diseases. The specialized junctional complexes called tight junctions provide the intestinal epithelial barrier function. Loss of tight junction integrity and increased intestinal permeability to macromolecules are associated with the pathogenesis of IBD, IBS, and celiac disease. Mucosal protective factors such as growth factors and nutrients preserve the gut barrier integrity and are beneficial in the treatment of various gastrointestinal diseases.

Glutamine in Development and Maintenance of Gut Barrier Function

Lack of enteral nutrition can lead to mucosal barrier dysfunction [17, 18]. Enterocytes prefer glutamine for fuel, and therefore, glutamine is an important dietary component for the maintenance of gut mucosal integrity. The first question is whether glutamine is required for the development and maintenance of gut barrier function. Experimental data from neonatal animal models indicate that glutamine plays an important role in the development of gastrointestinal mucosal barrier function [3]. The effects of endogenous glutamine and the dietary supplementation of glutamine on small intestinal morphology using light and transmission electron microscopy were investigated in artificially reared rat pups. Transmission electron microscopy demonstrated that the intestinal epithelial tight junctions are disrupted in the glutamine-deprived and glutamine synthase inhibitor-treated pups. This study provided the initial evidence that glutamine is required for the formation of tight junction and development of barrier function in the intestinal epithelium. However, the effect of glutamine on the barrier function in this study cannot be distinguished from the glutamine-mediated overall development of gut mucosa. A low level of serum glutamine correlated with the intestinal barrier disruption, inflammation and diarrheal diseases among children [19]. Glutamine supplementation, on the other hand, has been shown to increase intestinal barrier function in malnourished children [20]. These correlative reports do support the role of glutamine in maintenance of normal physiologic barrier function. More direct support to this possibility was provided by studies using Caco-2 cell monolayers. Glutamine depletion by inhibition of glutamine synthetase in cultured Caco-2 cell monolayers increases epithelial permeability and bacterial translocation, indicating that at least the endogenously produced glutamine is essential for the maintenance of barrier function in the intestinal epithelium [21, 22]. Therefore, the current information is convincing that glutamine is necessary for the maintenance of intestinal epithelial barrier function.

Glutamine in Preservation of Gut Barrier Function

Another important question is whether glutamine is required for the maintenance of gut barrier function under physiologic or pathophysiologic conditions. Evidence from clinical studies indicates that glutamine supplementation improves gut barrier function under conditions of total parenteral nutrition [13], burn injury [23–25], gastrointestinal complications in acquired immune deficiency syndrome (AIDS) [26], and malnutrition [27]. These studies are summarized in Table 25.1. The effect of glutamine dipeptide supplementation on intestinal permeability was investigated in critically ill patients who were on support of total parenteral nutrition [13]. Excretion of D-xylose was used as a marker of intestinal permeability. Glutamine dipeptide prevented intestinal atrophy and reduced intestinal permeability. In severe burn injury patients, glutamine supplementation improved plasma glutamine level and reduced intestinal permeability as measured by lactulose-mannitol assay [24]. Intestinal permeability was also measured by lactulose-mannitol assay in malnourished children who were fed enteral formula. Supplementation of formula with glutamine significantly reduced intestinal permeability [27]. Although the clinical studies in support of glutamine response in the gut barrier preservation is handful, these are powerful data in support of the role of glutamine in preservation of gut barrier function at least under challenged conditions.

The role of glutamine in preservation of gut barrier function has been strongly supported by a wide spectrum of experimental studies using mice, guinea pigs, rats, cats and pigs, and applying experimental models of total parenteral nutrition, burn injury, trauma, surgical stress, malnutrition, ischemia–reperfusion injury and biliary obstruction. Glutamine or dipeptides (Gln-Gln, Ala-Gln or Gly-Gln) were used for treatment in different studies. Intestinal permeability and barrier function were evaluated by determining bacterial translocation, endotoxemia, and absorption of fluorescein

Table 25.1 Glutamine-mediated preservation of gut barrier function

Species	Experimental condition	Treatment	Response to L-glutamine supplementation	Reference
Rat	Total parental nutrition	Ala-Gln	Improves intestinal barrier function measured by xylose and FITC-dextran absorption and reduced bacterial translocation	[29, 30, 32]
Pig	Total parenteral nutrition	Gln-Gln	Prevents bacterial translocation	[22]
Human	Total parenteral nutrition (critically ill patients)	Ala-Gln	Reduced gut permeability as measured by D-xylose absorption	[13]
Human	Severe bum injury	Gln	Improvement of gut mucosal barrier function	[23–25]
Guinea pig	TNBS-induced colitis	Gln	Reduced endotoxemia	[33]
Mice	Intestinal obstruction	Gln	Preserves mucosal integrity, barrier disruption, and bacterial translocation	[38]
Rat	Intestinal resection	Gln-Gln Ala-Gln	Prevents bacterial translocation	[36, 37]
Rat	Experimental pancreatitis	Gln	Prevents gut barrier disruption	[34]
Rat	Ischemia–reperfusion	Ala-Gln Gln	Restores small bowel barrier function by increasing the level of intestinal glutathione	[40, 41]
Mice	Ischemia–reperfusion	Gln	No protection; rather worsens condition	[42, 43]
Rat	Experimental biliary obstruction	Gln	Reduced gut permeability and prevents bacterial translocation	[35]
Human	Abdominal radiation-induced toxicity	Gln	Protects systemic immune and gut barrier function by decreasing oxidative stress and increasing mucosal lymphocyte count	[15]
Human	Diarrheal diseases in children	Ala-Gln	Reduces intestinal permeability, endotoxemia, and inflammatory responses	[20, 27]
Human	Surgical stress	Gln	Decreases mucosal atrophy and improves gut barrier function	[36, 37, 39]

(FITC)-conjugated dextran. Total parenteral nutrition in rats increased gut permeability and induced bacterial translocation [28–32]. Administration of glutamine, Ala-Gln or Gly-Gln significantly reduced intestinal permeability and attenuated bacterial translocation. Glutamine supplementation reduced endotoxemia in trinitrobenzoyl sulfonic acid-induced colitis in guinea pigs [33], reduced gut permeability caused by experimental pancreatitis in rats [34], and attenuated bacterial translocation induced by biliary obstruction in rats [35]. Gut barrier function and bacterial translocation caused by surgical stress, such as intestinal resection [36, 37], intestinal obstruction [38], and liver transplantation [39] were also significantly ameliorated by enteral feeding of glutamine or glutamine dipeptide.

Ischemia–reperfusion is a clinically relevant condition that disrupts gut barrier function and increases permeability. However, there are conflicting information present regarding the potential beneficial effect of glutamine in ischemia–reperfusion-induced gut permeability. Two studies showed that administration of glutamine or Ala-Gln dipeptide ameliorates ischemia–reperfusion-induced gut permeability in rats [40, 41]. On the other hand, two other studies showed that intraluminal administration of glutamine worsens the condition and found to be detrimental to gut barrier function during ischemia–reperfusion in mice [42, 43]. It is unclear if this discrepancy was due to the different species used in these studies or some other differences in experimental conditions. Overall, the experimental studies are fairly convincing that glutamine preserves the gut barrier function under conditions of clinically relevant surgical stress, total parenteral nutrition, burn injury, trauma and sepsis.

As glutamine is the preferred fuel for enterocytes it stimulates cell proliferation, differentiation, and mucosal growth. Therefore, the question is whether the glutamine-mediated gut barrier protection seen in all clinical and experimental studies is due to a direct influence on the barrier function, or if it is an indirect effect as a result of improved cell proliferation and mucosal growth. At this time, there are no clear data available to answer this question with confidence. There are no experimental studies reported that directly addressed the regulation of epithelial barrier function by glutamine that is independent of an effect on mucosal growth. However, there are few in vitro studies, using cell lines, indicate that glutamine may have a direct impact on the regulation of epithelial barrier function. Glutamine depletion disrupts epithelial barrier function in Caco-2 cells [21]. Furthermore, glutamine prevents barrier disruption by acetaldehyde in Caco-2 cell monolayers [47]. Figure 25.1 shows the dose-dependent effect of glutamine in preservation of barrier function.

Glutamine and Epithelial Tight Junctions

Epithelial Tight Junctions

The gut barrier function is provided by the epithelial monolayer due to the formation of specialized intercellular junctional complex called tight junctions. Located at the apical end of the lateral membrane, tight junctions seal the intercellular space for a selective barrier to the diffusion of macromolecules across the epithelium. Epithelial tight junctions are size selective and charge selective in allowing diffusion of molecules across the epithelium. Information on the molecular structure of tight junctions in recent studies lead to propose a combination of "leak pathway" and "pore pathway" for the movement of molecules across the tight junctions [44]. Leak pathway represents the impedance to movement of molecules based on the size of the molecule. Diffusion of molecules with a spatial diameter of greater than 4 Å is impeded by the tight junctions. The permeability to larger molecules through the leak pathway is independent of the charge it carries [44]. On the other hand, the pore pathway refers to channel-like pores formed by specific proteins such as claudins that allow diffusion of specific ions. Therefore, tight junctions appear to be a complex structure with specificity of composition varying from epithelium to epithelium.

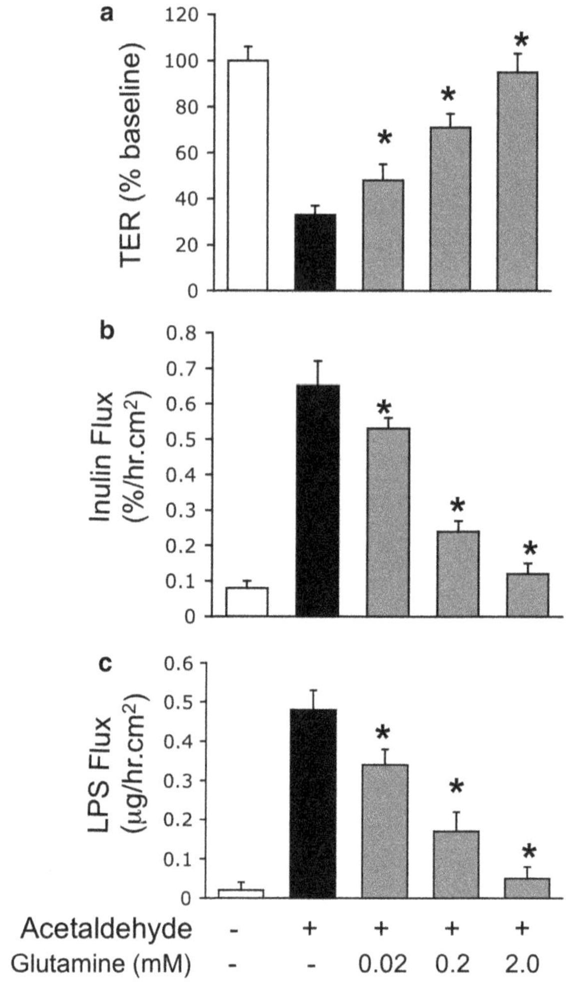

Fig. 25.1 Glutamine prevents acetaldehyde-induced barrier disruption in Caco-2 cell monolayers [47]. In this study, Caco-2 cell monolayers were incubated with varying doses of glutamine prior to exposure to 400 μM acetaldehyde for 4 h. Transepithelial electrical resistance (**a**) and permeability to inulin (**b**) and lipopolysaccharide (LPS) (**c**) were measured. Mean ± SEM are presented and *asterisk* indicates the values are significantly different from the value for acetaldehyde without glutamine

Recent studies have shed light into the molecular structure of tight junctions and the regulation of assembly and disassembly at a greater depth. Tight junction is a multiprotein complex consisting of transmembrane and intracellular plaque proteins. Transmembrane proteins include occludin, claudin, junctional adhesion molecule (JAM), and tricellulin [44]. Several isoforms of occludin, claudin and JAM have been identified that are differentially expressed in different epithelia and contribute to distinct barrier properties of tight junctions in different epithelia. The plaque proteins include the adapter proteins such as ZO-1, ZO-2, and ZO-3. These adapter proteins interact with many other proteins such as 7H6, cingulin, symplekin, ZONAB, etc. The multiprotein complex of tight junction is anchored to the perijunctional actin-myosin belt. The protein–protein and tight junction–actin interactions are essential for the assembly and maintenance of tight junctions. Disruption of interaction between occludin and ZO-1 leads to disruption of tight junctions and barrier dysfunction. Similarly, disruption of actin cytoskeleton results in loss of tight junction integrity and increased paracellular permeability. The protein–protein interactions in the tight junctions are regulated by intracellular signaling elements.

Many signaling molecules either directly interact with the tight junction proteins or localized adjacent to tight junctions [45]. Heterotrimeric G-proteins such as Rab3a and Rab13 interact with ZO-1 and ZO-2 and participate in regulation of tight junction integrity and epithelial barrier function. Tyrosine kinases such as c-Src and c-Yes associate with tight junction protein complex, and induce tyrosine phosphorylation of tight junction proteins. Phosphotidylinositol 3-kinase (PI3-kinase) interacts with occludin and PTEN (phosphatase and tensin homolog deleted on chromosome 10) interacts with ZO-2 and ZO-3. PKCλ interacts with Par3 and Par6, while PKCζ and PKCη interact with the C-terminal domain of occludin. Protein phosphatases, such as PP2A and PP1, also bind to C-terminal domain of occludin and regulate phosphorylation of tight junction proteins on serine and threonine residues. Numerous pharmacologic and molecular studies have demonstrated that these signaling molecules do regulate the tight junction integrity. PKC isoforms such as PKCλ, PKCζ and PKCη are required for the assembly and maintenance of tight junctions. On the other hand, activation of PKCδ leads to disruption of tight junctions. Other PKC isoforms such as PKCβI and PKCε are involved in preservation of tight junction integrity in the intestinal epithelium from toxic effects of acetaldehyde and hydrogen peroxide. Oxidative stress disrupts tight junctions involving multiple signaling molecules such as PI3-kinase, c-Src and PP2A. Prevention of hydrogen peroxide-induced tight junction disruption by EGF involves MAP kinases and PKC. Therefore, multiple signaling pathways are involved in the regulation of tight junctions of different epithelia, including intestinal epithelium.

Influence of Glutamine on Tight Junctions

In vitro studies using Caco-2 cell monolayers demonstrated a direct influence of glutamine on tight junction integrity in the intestinal epithelium. Caco-2 cells were derived from colon adenocarcinoma tissue. In cell culture, these cells differentiate into polarized enterocyte monolayer with well-developed tight junctions. Therefore, this cell line has been extensively used as a model of the intestinal epithelium, especially for the study of gut barrier function. About a decade ago it was first demonstrated that glutamine is essential for the development of barrier function and prevent bacterial translocation in caco-2 cells [46]. Treatment of Caco-2 cells with methionine sulfoximine, an inhibitor of glutamine synthase, caused reduction in transepithelial electrical resistance and increase in permeability to mannitol and FITC-dextran [46]. This effect of methionine sulfoximine was prevented by glutamine supplementation. The extent of the effect of methionine sulfoximine on barrier function was somewhat similar to its effect on overall protein synthesis. Therefore, it is unclear whether the effect was due to its influence on the general protein synthesis or if glutamine had a more specific effect on tight junctions. Another study used Caco-2 cell monolayers to model the luminal starvation to mimic depletion of enteral nutrition. A 24-h apical nutrient deprivation resulted in depletion of intracellular glutamine, glutamate and glutathione, and increased transepithelial permeability to FITC-dextran [21]. Glutamine supplementation restored the barrier function. In this study, the effect of glutamine was attributed to glutamate formation as inhibition of glutaminase by 6-diazo-oxo-L-norLeucine blocked glutamine-mediated restoration of barrier function. Once again, the barrier preservation by glutamine was associated with similar modulation of protein synthesis as well as reduction in glutathione levels. Therefore, it is unclear whether the barrier protective effect of glutamine was related to overall protein synthesis.

Few studies indicated that glutamine has a more specific influence on the integrity of intestinal epithelial tight junctions. Treatment of Caco-2 cell monolayers with methionine sulfoximine resulted in reduced levels of tight junction proteins such as claudin-1, occludin and ZO-1 [22]. This effect of methionine sulfoximine was prevented by glutamine supplementation. The changes in barrier function were associated with corresponding changes in junctional organization of occludin and claudin-1. Disruption of tight junctions and its prevention by glutamine was confirmed by transmission electron microscopy. A direct influence of glutamine on regulation of tight junction integrity was observed in Caco-2 cell monolayers [47]. Glutamine treatment significantly attenuated acetaldehyde-induced disruption of tight junctions and barrier dysfunction. A subsequent study demonstrated that glutamine has a similar protective effect in acetaldehyde-treated human colonic mucosa in vitro [48]. Therefore, glutamine appears to have a specific influence on the intestinal epithelial tight junction integrity that

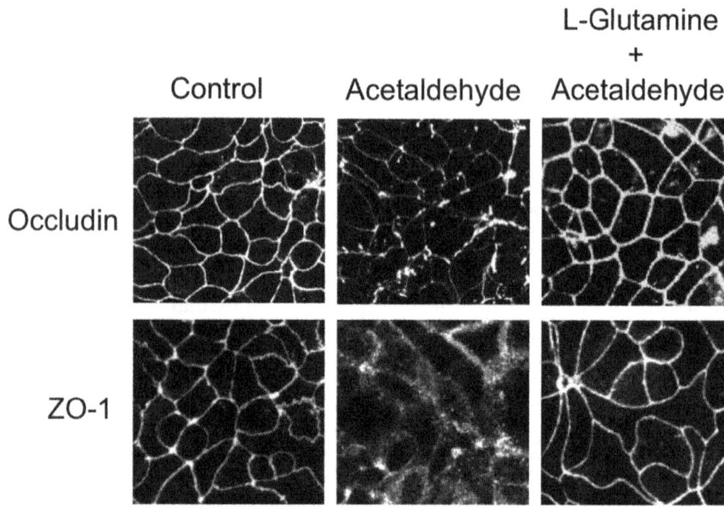

Fig. 25.2 Glutamine prevents acetaldehyde-induced tight junction disruption in Caco-2 cell monolayers [47]. In this study, Caco-2 cell monolayers were incubated with 2 mM glutamine prior to exposure to 400 μM acetaldehyde for 4 h. Fixed cell monolayers were stained for occludin and ZO-1 by immunofluorescence method

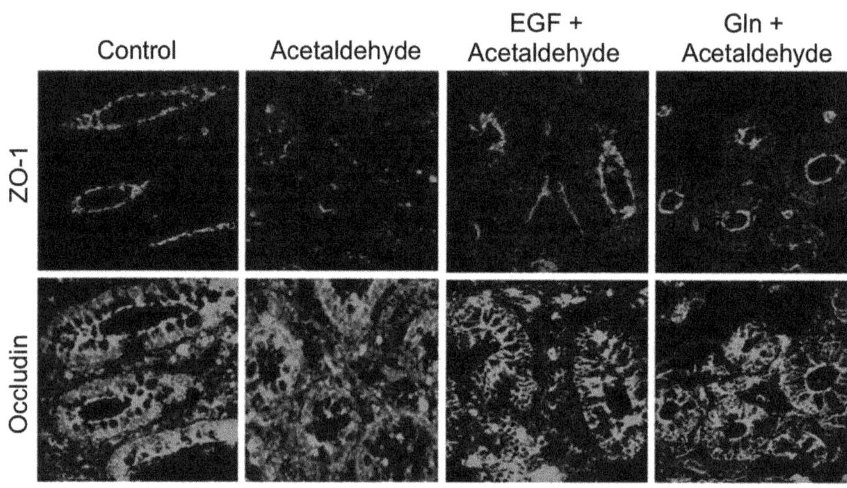

Fig. 25.3 Glutamine prevents acetaldehyde-induced tight junction disruption in human colonic mucosa [50]. In this study, freshly collected human colonic mucosal biopsy tissues were incubated with 2 mM glutamine or 30 μM EGF prior to exposure to 400 μM acetaldehyde for 2 h. Cryosections were stained for occludin and ZO-1 by immunofluorescence method

likely involves specific cellular mechanisms. Figure 25.2 shows glutamine-mediated protection of tight junctions from acetaldehyde in Caco-2 cell monolayers, while Fig. 25.3 shows tight junction protection by glutamine in human colonic mucosal tissue.

Mechanisms of Glutamine-Induced Tight Junction Regulation

Limited information is available regarding the mechanisms involved in glutamine-mediated regulation of intestinal epithelial tight junctions. Treatment of caco-2 cell monolayers with 0.02–2.0 mM glutamine dose-dependently suppressed acetaldehyde-induced decrease in transepithelial electrical

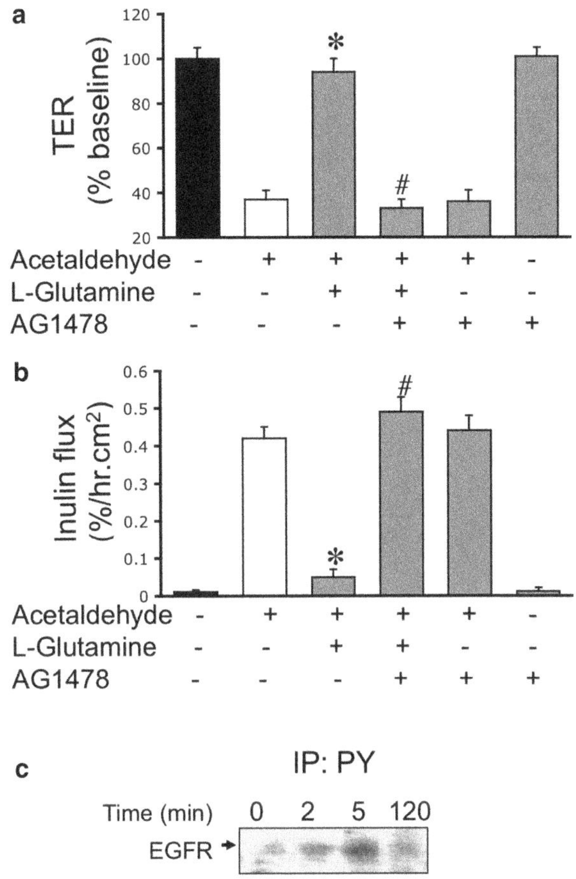

Fig. 25.4 EGF receptor tyrosine kinase is involved in glutamine-mediated prevention of acetaldehyde-induced barrier disruption in Caco-2 cell monolayers [47]. Caco-2 cell monolayers were pretreated with AG1478 prior to glutamine treatment followed by 400 μM acetaldehyde for 4 h. Transepithelial electrical resistance (**a**) and inulin permeability (**b**). Mean ± SEM are presented. *Asterisk* indicates the values are significantly different from the value for acetaldehyde without glutamine and symbol *hash* indicates values that are different from values for acetaldehyde with glutamine

resistance and increase in epithelial permeability to inulin and *E. coli* lipopolysaccharide [47]. D-GLUTAMINE was ineffective, and inhibition of glutaminase by 6-diazo-oxo-L-norLeucine did not alter the protective effect of L-glutamine, indicating that L-glutamine rather than glutamate was responsible for this barrier protective effect. This study showed that glutamine rapidly activates EGF receptor in Caco-2 cells, and that activation of EGF receptor is involved in glutamine-mediated protection of tight junctions [47]. EGF has been previously shown to protect tight junctions in Caco-2 cell monolayers from acetaldehyde [49] and hydrogen peroxide [50]. Inhibition of EGF receptor tyrosine kinase activity by AG1478 significantly blocked glutamine-mediated prevention of acetaldehyde-induced tight junction disruption (Fig. 25.4). This observation suggests that glutamine activates cell to induce a rapid transactivation of EGF receptor, which in turn is involved in the protection of tight junctions in acetaldehyde-treated cell monolayers. EGF-mediated protection of tight junctions involves ERK1/2 and PKC isoforms [49, 50]. Glutamine-mediated protection of tight junctions of human colonic epithelium from acetaldehyde also involves EGF receptor activation. Glutamine reduced acetaldehyde-induced protein tyrosine phosphorylation and attenuated depletion of detergent-insoluble fractions of tight junction and adherens junction proteins [48]. Confocal microscopy indicated that glutamine prevents acetaldehyde-induced disruption of tight junctions and adherens junctions. Pretreatment of colonic mucosal tissues with AG1478 attenuated glutamine-mediated prevention of acetaldehyde-induced depletion of detergent-insoluble fraction of tight junction proteins. These studies indicate that one of the mechanisms by which glutamine may induce barrier protective effect is transactivation of EGF receptor. The mechanism of glutamine-mediated EGF receptor transactivation remains to be uncovered. The potential mechanism is illustrated in Fig. 25.5.

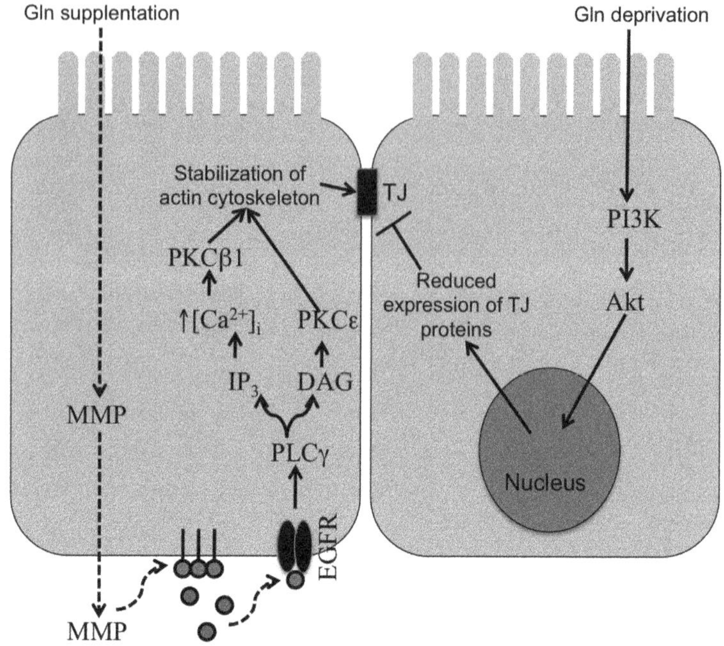

Fig. 25.5 Schematic representation of mechanisms involved in tight junction regulation by glutamine. Part of the scheme with *broken arrows* represents author's speculation. *MMP* metalloproteinase, *EGFR* epidermal growth factor receptor, *PLCγ* phospholipase Cγ, *IP3* inositol trisphosphate, *DAG* diacylglycerol, *PKCβI* protein kinase βI, $[Ca^{2+}]_i$ intracellular calcium, *TJ* tight junction, *PI3K* phosphatidylinositol 3-kinase

A recent study provided some insight into the mechanism involved in tight junction disruption caused by glutamine deprivation (Fig. 25.5). Tight junction disruption and barrier dysfunction induced by glutamine depletion in Caco-2 cell monolayers was blocked by wortmanin and LY294002, selective inhibitors of PI3-kinase [51]. The role of PI3-kinase in glutamine-mediated tight junction disruption was confirmed by knockdown of p85 subunit of PI3-kinase by RNA interference method. This study showed that glutamine induced phosphorylation of Akt, a signaling protein downstream to PI3-kinase. Therefore, tight junction disruption by glutamine depletion involves PI3-kinase-Akt signaling pathway. The current understanding of the mechanisms involved in glutamine-mediated tight junction regulation is illustrated in Fig. 25.5.

Clinical Significance

Most experimental studies have provided positive insight into the potential therapeutic benefit of glutamine in various diseases associated with gut barrier dysfunction. However, clinical studies have not always been encouraging. Improvement of gut barrier function by glutamine or dipeptides in critically ill [13], AIDS [26] and burn injury [23–25] patients, and malnourished children [20] is encouraging. However, lack of an effect of glutamine on barrier function in patients with Crohn's disease, and malnourished Gambian children raised doubt on the potential beneficial effect at the bedside. The information available indicates that glutamine certainly has a beneficial effect in the treatment of critically ill and burn injury patients [13, 23–25]. Additional benefit of glutamine would be in malnourished children and total parenteral nutrition. Therefore, the benefit of glutamine may depend on the type of illness. The high consistency in animal studies and discrepancies in clinical studies begs the question, what is the difference between these two model systems. It is likely that the high consistency in animal studies is due to the fact that experimental animals are maintained under controlled standard conditions, whereas conditions in patients are much more complex with multiple variables.

High turnover of glutamine in the body requires it to be administered at a high dose. The glutamine turnover may further vary in different types and state of illness, and even individualized. Therefore, different doses may be required on an individualized basis. The beneficial effect of glutamine may be improved by optimizing the dosage on an individual basis. The bright side is that so far there is no indication of any harmful effect of glutamine, and therefore is a good candidate to be labeled as a "neutraceutical."

Conclusions

Thus far, it is clear that glutamine is beneficial in maintenance and recovery of gut barrier function. Experimental studies are compelling, and the clinical studies are encouraging. The information that is lacking in this field is the specific effect of glutamine on the development, maintenance, and protection of intestinal epithelial tight junctions. In vivo studies that focus on determining the glutamine effect on tight junctions that separate them from glutamine-induced mucosal growth and in vitro studies that address the cellular and molecular mechanisms involved in tight junction regulation by glutamine are warranted. Such studies are likely to advance our knowledge in the molecular mechanisms of glutamine effect on gut barrier function and help formulate glutamine regimen in therapy of multiple diseases on individualized basis.

Acknowledgements Preparation of this article and some of the studies discussed in it are supported by the National Institutes of Health grants: DK55532 and AA12307.

References

1. Kimura RE. Glutamine oxidation by developing rat small intestine. Pediatr Res. 1987;21(2):214–7.
2. Darcy-Vrillon B, Posho L, Morel MT, Bernard F, Blachier F, Meslin JC, et al. Glucose, galactose, and glutamine metabolism in pig isolated enterocytes during development. Pediatr Res. 1994;36(2):175–81.
3. Potsic B, Holliday N, Lewis P, Samuelson D, DeMarco V, Neu J. Glutamine supplementation and deprivation: effect on artificially reared rat small intestinal morphology. Pediatr Res. 2002;52(3):430–6.
4. Yi GF, Allee GL, Knight CD, Dibner JJ. Impact of glutamine and Oasis hatchling supplement on growth performance, small intestinal morphology, and immune response of broilers vaccinated and challenged with Eimeria maxima. Poult Sci. 2005;84(2):283–93.
5. Zhong X, Zhang XH, Li XM, Zhou YM, Li W, Huang XX, et al. Intestinal growth and morphology is associated with the increase in heat shock protein 70 expression in weaning piglets through supplementation with glutamine. J Anim Sci. 2011;89(11):3634–42.
6. Tannuri U, Carrazza FR, Iriya K. The effects of glutamine-supplemented diet on the intestinal mucosa of the malnourished growing rat. Rev Hosp Clin Fac Med (SP). 2000;55(3):87–92.
7. Yi GF, Carroll JA, Allee GL, Gaines AM, Kendall DC, Usry JL, et al. Effect of glutamine and spray-dried plasma on growth performance, small intestinal morphology, and immune responses of Escherichia coli K88+-challenged weaned pigs. J Anim Sci. 2005;83(3):634–43.
8. Wu G, Meier SA, Knabe DA. Dietary glutamine supplementation prevents jejunal atrophy in weaned pigs. J Nutr. 1996;126(10):2578–84.
9. Rhoads JM, Keku EO, Bennett LE, Quinn J, Lecce JG. Development of L-glutamine-stimulated electroneutral sodium absorption in piglet jejunum. Am J Physiol. 1990;259(1 Pt 1):G99–107.
10. He Y, Sanderson IR, Walker WA. Uptake, transport and metabolism of exogenous nucleosides in intestinal epithelial cell cultures. J Nutr. 1994;124(10):1942–9.
11. Ko TC, Beauchamp RD, Townsend Jr CM, Thompson JC. Glutamine is essential for epidermal growth factor-stimulated intestinal cell proliferation. Surgery. 1993;114(2):147–53. discussion 53–4.
12. Rhoads M. Glutamine signaling in intestinal cells. J Parenter Enteral Nutr. 1999;23(5 Suppl):S38–40.
13. Tremel H, Kienle B, Weilemann LS, Stehle P, Furst P. Glutamine dipeptide-supplemented parenteral nutrition maintains intestinal function in the critically ill. Gastroenterology. 1994;107(6):1595–601.

14. Nakamura E, Hagen S. Role of glutamine and arginase in protection against ammonia-induced cell death in gastric epithelial cells. Am J Physiol Gastrointest Liver Physiol. 2002;283(6):75.
15. Jensen JC, Schaefer R, Nwokedi E, Bevans 3rd DW, Baker ML, Pappas AA, et al. Prevention of chronic radiation enteropathy by dietary glutamine. Ann Surg Oncol. 1994;1(2):157–63.
16. Savarese D, Savy G, Vahdat L, Wischmeyer P, Corey B. Prevention of chemotherapy and radiation toxicity with glutamine. Cancer Treat Rev. 2003;29(6):501–13.
17. Bragg LE, Thompson JS, Rikkers LF. Influence of nutrient delivery on gut structure and function. Nutrition. 1991;7(4):237–43.
18. Inoue Y, Espat NJ, Frohnapple DJ, Epstein H, Copeland EM, Souba WW. Effect of total parenteral nutrition on amino acid and glucose transport by the human small intestine. Ann Surg. 1993;217(6):604–12. discussion 12-4.
19. Guerrant R, OriÃ¡ R, Moore S, OriÃ¡ M, Lima A. Malnutrition as an enteric infectious disease with long-term effects on child development. Nutr Rev. 2008;66(9):487–505.
20. Lima NL, Soares AM, Mota RM, et al. Wasting and intestinal barrier function in children taking alanyl-glutaminyl-supplemented enteral formula. J Pediatr Gastroenterol Nutr. 2007;44(1):365–74.
21. Le Bacquer O, Laboisse C, Darmaun D. Glutamine preserves protein synthesis and paracellular permeability in Caco-2 cells submitted to "luminal fasting". Am J Physiol Gastrointest Liver Physiol. 2003;285(1):G128–36.
22. Li N, Lewis P, Samuelson D, Liboni K, Neu J. Glutamine regulates Caco-2 cell tight junction proteins. Am J Physiol Gastrointest Liver Physiol. 2004;287(3):G726–33.
23. Peng X, Yan H, You Z, Wang P, Wang S. Effects of enteral supplementation with glutamine granules on intestinal mucosal barrier function in severe burned patients. Burns. 2004;30(2):135–9.
24. Zhou Y, Jiang Z, Sun Y. Glutamine dipeptide enriched enteral nutrition improving gut permeability in sever burns. Zhonghua Yi Xue Za Zhi. 1999;79(11):825–7.
25. Zhou YP, Jiang ZM, Sun YH, Wang XR, Ma EL, Wilmore D. The effect of supplemental enteral glutamine on plasma levels, gut function, and outcome in severe burns: a randomized, double-blind, controlled clinical trial. J Parenter Enteral Nutr. 2003;27(4):241–5.
26. Noyer CM, Simon D, Borczuk A, Brandt LJ, Lee MJ, Nehra V. A double-blind placebo-controlled pilot study of glutamine therapy for abnormal intestinal permeability in patients with AIDS. Am J Gastroenterol. 1998; 93(6):972–5.
27. Lima AA, Brito LF, Ribeiro HB, Martins MC, Lustosa AP, Rocha EM, et al. Intestinal barrier function and weight gain in malnourished children taking glutamine supplemented enteral formula. J Pediatr Gastroenterol Nutr. 2005;40(1):28–35.
28. Ding LA, Li JS. Effects of glutamine on intestinal permeability and bacterial translocation in TPN-rats with endotoxemia. World J Gastroenterol. 2003;9(6):1327–32.
29. Haque SM, Chen K, Usui N, Iiboshi Y, Okuyama H, Masunari A, et al. Alanyl-glutamine dipeptide-supplemented parenteral nutrition improves intestinal metabolism and prevents increased permeability in rats. Ann Surg. 1996;223(3):334–41.
30. Khan J, Iiboshi Y, Cui L, Wasa M, Sando K, Takagi Y, et al. Alanyl-glutamine-supplemented parenteral nutrition increases luminal mucus gel and decreases permeability in the rat small intestine. J Parenter Enteral Nutr. 1999; 23(1):24–31.
31. Li YS, Li JS, Jiang JW, Liu FN, Li N, Qin WS, et al. Glycyl-glutamine-enriched long-term total parenteral nutrition attenuates bacterial translocation following small bowel transplantation in the pig. J Surg Res. 1999;82(1):106–11.
32. Ma Y, Jiang Z, Bai M. The change of gut barrier function and gene expression after surgical stress and parenteral nutrition. Zhonghua Wai Ke Za Zhi. 1995;33(6):371–3.
33. Fujita T, Sakurai K. Efficacy of glutamine-enriched enteral nutrition in an experimental model of mucosal ulcerative colitis. Br J Surg. 1995;82(6):749–51.
34. Foitzik T, Stufler M, Hotz HG, Klinnert J, Wagner J, Warshaw AL, et al. Glutamine stabilizes intestinal permeability and reduces pancreatic infection in acute experimental pancreatitis. J Gastrointest Surg. 1997;1(1):40–6. discussion 6-7.
35. White JS, Hoper M, Parks RW, Clements WD, Diamond T. Glutamine improves intestinal barrier function in experimental biliary obstruction. Eur Surg Res. 2005;37(6):342–7.
36. Bai M, Jiang Z, Ma Y. Glutamine dipeptide enriched nutritional solutions attenuate bacterial translocation in rats after 60 % intestinal resections. Zhonghua Yi Xue Za Zhi. 1996;76(2):116–9.
37. Liu YW, Bai MX, Ma YX, Jiang ZM. Effects of alanyl-glutamine on intestinal adaptation and bacterial translocation in rats after 60 % intestinal resection. Clin Nutr. 1997;16(2):75–8.
38. dos Santos R, Viana ML, Generoso SV, Arantes RE, Davisson Correia MI, Cardoso VN. Glutamine supplementation decreases intestinal permeability and preserves gut mucosa integrity in an experimental mouse model. J Parenter Enteral Nutr. 2010;34(4):408–13.
39. Jiang JW, Ren ZG, Chen LY, Jiang L, Xie HY, Zhou L, et al. Enteral supplementation with glycyl-glutamine improves intestinal barrier function after liver transplantation in rats. Hepatobiliary Pancreat Dis Int. 2011; 10(4):380–5.

40. Kozar RA, Schultz SG, Bick RJ, Poindexter BJ, DeSoignie R, Moore FA. Enteral glutamine but not alanine maintains small bowel barrier function after ischemia/reperfusion injury in rats. Shock. 2004;21(5):433–7.
41. Tazuke Y, Wasa M, Shimizu Y, Wang HS, Okada A. Alanyl-glutamine-supplemented parenteral nutrition prevents intestinal ischemia-reperfusion injury in rats. J Parenter Enteral Nutr. 2003;27(2):110–5.
42. Fukatsu K, Ueno C, Hashiguchi Y, Hara E, Kinoshita M, Mochizuki H, et al. Glutamine infusion during ischemia is detrimental in a murine gut ischemia/reperfusion model. J Parenter Enteral Nutr. 2003;27(3):187–92. discussion 92.
43. Omata J, Fukatsu K, Ueno C, Maeshima Y, Saitoh D, Mochizuki H. Intraluminal glutamine administration during ischemia worsens survival after gut ischemia-reperfusion. J Surg Res. 2007;143(2):260–4.
44. Anderson JM, Van Itallie CM. Physiology and function of the tight junction. Cold Spring Harb Perspect Biol. 2009;1(2):a002584.
45. Rao R. Oxidative stress-induced disruption of epithelial and endothelial tight junctions. Front Biosci. 2008;13:7210–26.
46. DeMarco VG, Li N, Thomas J, West CM, Neu J. Glutamine and barrier function in cultured Caco-2 epithelial cell monolayers. J Nutr. 2003;133(7):2176–9.
47. Seth A, Basuroy S, Sheth P, Rao RK. L-Glutamine ameliorates acetaldehyde-induced increase in paracellular permeability in Caco-2 cell monolayer. Am J Physiol Gastrointest Liver Physiol. 2004;287(3):G510–7.
48. Basuroy S, Sheth P, Mansbach CM, Rao RK. Acetaldehyde disrupts tight junctions and adherens junctions in human colonic mucosa: protection by EGF and L-glutamine. Am J Physiol Gastrointest Liver Physiol. 2005; 289(2):G367–75.
49. Suzuki T, Seth A, Rao R. Role of phospholipase Cgamma-induced activation of protein kinase Cepsilon (PKCepsilon) and PKCbetaI in epidermal growth factor-mediated protection of tight junctions from acetaldehyde in Caco-2 cell monolayers. J Biol Chem. 2008;283(6):3574–83.
50. Basuroy S, Seth A, Elias B, Naren AP, Rao R. MAPK interacts with occludin and mediates EGF-induced prevention of tight junction disruption by hydrogen peroxide. Biochem J. 2006;393(Pt 1):69–77.
51. Li N, Neu J. Glutamine deprivation alters intestinal tight junctions via a PI3-K/Akt mediated pathway in Caco-2 cells. J Nutr. 2009;139(4):710–4.

Chapter 26
Glutamine Therapy in Colitis Models

Hongyu Xue

Key Points

- A complex interplay between genetic, enteric microbiota, environmental, and immunological factors has been believed to contribute to disease initiation and progression.
- Glutamine deficiency has been found in active IBD lesions of human biopsies, providing theoretical niche for glutamine supplementation in IBD.
- Preclinical data are generally supportive of a positive role of glutamine to prevent or attenuate intestinal inflammatory in the experimental IBD models.
- Glutamine is shown to modulate multiple interrelated mechanistic factors, e.g., intestinal barrier integrity, tissue oxidative burden/stress, cytokine network, and innate cytoprotective mechanisms.
- A limited body of clinical trials examining therapeutic potential of glutamine in IBD patients, however, produced considerably mixed results.
- A gap still remains between experimental findings and a practical clinical strategy for glutamine use, and basic questions on how to administer this nutrient in a clinically relevant and effective paradigm still remain poorly answered in IBD settings.

Keywords Inflammatory bowel disease • Glutamine • Gut barrier • Oxidative stress • Immunity • Cytokine • Heat shock protein

Abbreviations

B_{reg}	Regulatory B cells
CD	Crohn's disease
DSS	Dextran sulfate sodium
GI	Gastrointestinal
HCl	Hydrochloric acid

H. Xue, M.D., Ph.D. (✉)
Department of Anesthesiology, University of Colorado Denver,
Anschutz Medical Campus, RC2, P15, Box 8602, 12700 E 19th Ave, Aurora, CO 80045, USA
e-mail: Hongyu.Xue@ucdenver.edu

R. Rajendram et al. (eds.), *Glutamine in Clinical Nutrition*, Nutrition and Health,
DOI 10.1007/978-1-4939-1932-1_26, © Springer Science+Business Media New York 2015

HSR	Heat shock response
HSP	Heat shock protein
HO	Heme oxygenase
IBD	Inflammatory bowel disease
IFN	Interferon
IKK	IκB kinase
IL	Interleukin
iNOS	Inducible nitric oxide synthase
IP	Intestinal permeability
MCP	Monocyte chemoattractant protein
MIP	Macrophage inflammatory protein
MPO	Myeloperoxidase
MyD88	Myeloid differentiation primary response gene 88
NFκB	Nuclear factor (NF)-κB
LPS	Lipopolysaccharides
NSAID	Nonsteroid anti-inflammatory drugs
T_H	T-Helper lymphocyte
TJ	Tight junction
TLR	Toll-like receptor
TNBS	trinitrobenzene sulfonic acid
TNF	Tumor necrosis factors
TPN	Total parental nutrition
TRAIL	Tumor necrosis factor-alpha-related apoptosis-inducing ligand
T_{reg}	Regulatory T cells
UC	Ulcerative colitis
YAMC	Young adult mouse colonic epithelial cells
ZO	Zonula occludens

Introduction

Inflammatory bowel disease (IBD) is an idiopathic chronic condition of the gastrointestinal (GI) tract characterized by intermittent periods of inflammation and remission. It comprises two major forms, i.e., Crohn's disease (CD) and ulcerative colitis (UC), with distinct clinical and histopathological features. Although the etiology and pathogenesis of IBD is not fully understood, a complex interplay between genetic, enteric microbiota, environmental, and immunological factors has been believed to contribute to disease initiation and progression (Fig. 26.1) [43]. In genetically susceptible individuals, an exaggerated host immune response toward commensal bacteria is crucially essential to the pathogenesis of IBD [43]. This belief lays the framework for the current paradigm for IBD treatment, which is aimed to correct the disrupted intestinal immune-microbial axis or the imbalance between inflammatory insults/environmental injurious factors and the cytoprotective response. Growing evidence suggests that a variety of dietary elements may extensively influence immune-microbial axis and/or favor the host cytoprotection against inflammatory injury. This creates a unique niche for potential use of these nutrients as therapeutics for IBD.

Glutamine figures very prominently in the literature on nutritional modulation of the GI tract and appears to be among the most functionally versatile immunonutrients for regulating intestinal immunity and promoting GI protective mechanisms in a variety of settings of inflammatory stress and injury [8]. The aim of this review is to investigate the therapeutic potential of glutamine in in vitro cell cultures and in vivo animal IBD models.

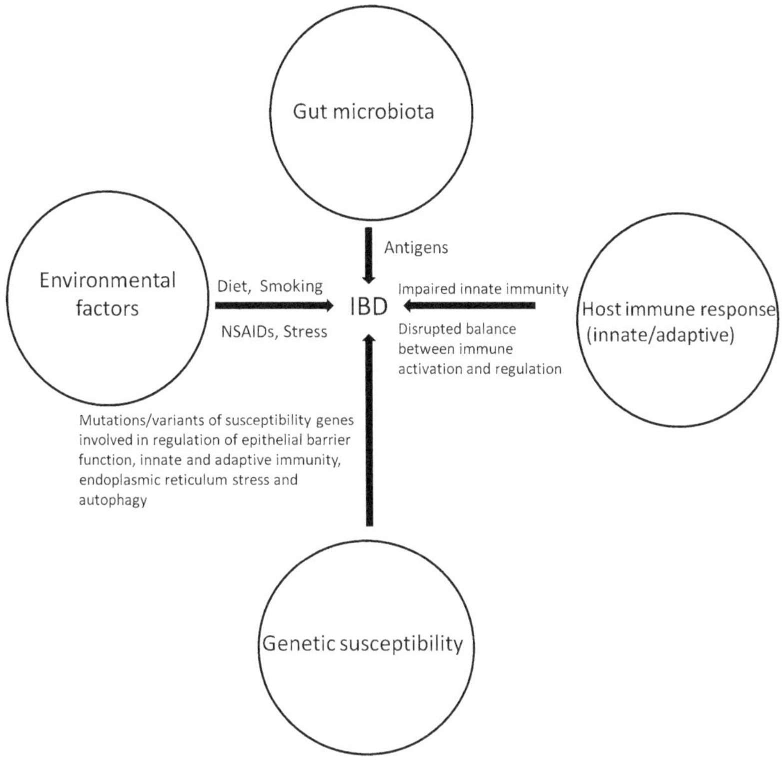

Fig. 26.1 Schematized interaction of contributing etiological factors involved in the inflammatory bowel disease pathogenesis

Pathogenesis of IBD

It is widely hypothesized that the intestinal inflammation and mucosal damage characterized of IBD is triggered and perpetuated by excessive host immune responses to a subset of commensal enteric bacteria in genetically susceptible hosts.

Growing evidence indicates that IBD are, at least in part, the result of a genetic predisposition [54]. A number of susceptibility genes important to regulation of immune response, mucosal barrier function and microbial clearance are suggested to be implicated in the pathogenesis of IBD [54]. Mutations or variants of these genes (e.g., *NOD2/CARD15*, *DLG5*, *MDR1*, *IBD5*, *IL23R*, and *ATG16L1*) are found to be associated with CD and/or UC and may cause deficient downregulation of the innate intestinal immune response and altered microbial homeostasis [43, 54].

A variety of studies using murine models show that the development of spontaneous chronic colitis are directly dependent on the presence of a luminal flora, which supports a pivotal role of enteric flora in the pathogenesis of IBD [45]. The intestinal immune-microbial axis, characterized by a dynamic balance between enteric microbes, particularly commensal flora, and host mucosal defense is key to the initiation and development of chronic IBD.

One hand, a disrupted compositional balance between beneficial and aggressive species of the enteric flora could render a pro-inflammatory milieu in the intestinal lumen of a susceptible host [44]. Accumulating evidence shows dysbiosis, an unfavorable alteration in the microbial composition of microbial commensal flora, is present in patients with IBD (11). Certain probiotics such as *Lactobacillus* and *Bifidobacterium* species are protective against a variety of experimental colitis [44], whereas organisms such as *E. coli*, *Enterococcus* and *Klebsiella* species have been implicated in the pathogenesis of human IBD and experimental colitis [44].

Nonetheless, colitis can be induced in a genetically susceptible host with normal commensal bacteria species [44]. These findings indicate that the nature of the host defensive response, rather than the biological properties of an enteric bacterial species per se, may more crucially determine the role of microbe × host interaction in the initiation of IBD. The sophisticated interplay of genetic, microbial, and other environmental factors culminates in an excessive host immune response against antigens of the enteric commensal flora (Fig. 26.1). The sustained and exaggerated mucosal immune response serves as primary trigger of chronic intestinal inflammation and tissue damage that are manifest in IBD patients [43].

An excessive innate and adaptive immune response is a more common feature in human IBD [43]. Sustained immune activation is arguably the driver of tissue damage and has been a primary target that a large body of therapeutic endeavors has been focusing on [43, 54]. Compromised intestinal barrier function may lead to increased uptake of antigens, thus constantly prime the immune activation and tune the mucosal immune homeostasis toward a pro-immune milieu. Increased gut permeability has been found in families with CD, indicating a role of gut barrier function in IBD predisposition. Genetic mutation or polymorphism in key genes (e.g., *NOD2/CARD15*) involved in epithelial function may result in altered intestinal barrier integrity.

The innate immune system constitutes the first line of immune defense and provides immediate defense against infection. Recruitment of activated innate immune cells (i.e., neutrophils, macrophages, and dendritic cells) into the target site generally favors a pro-immune milieu, as these cells produce key effectors such as reactive oxygen species that result in inflammation and increased IP. Macrophages and dendritic cells in the lamina propria are activated and increased in quantities in human and experimental IBD. Functionally, monocyte and polymorphonuclear cell-derived production of pro-inflammatory cytokines is also augmented in IBD. Although most pro-inflammatory cytokines and chemokines are upregulated in both CD and ulcerative colitis, cytokines induce type 1 T-helper lymphocyte (T_H1) and T_H17 responses (e.g., interleukin (IL)-12, IL-23, and IL-27) are only selectively upregulated in CD but not in UC [39] (Table 26.1).

Table 26.1 Cytokine profile in Crohn's disease and ulcerative colitis

Innate immune response		
Cytokine/chemokine	CD	UC
IL-1β	I	I
IL-6	I	I
IL-8 (CXCL8)	I	I
IL-12	I	N
IL-18	I	I
IL-23 (p40/p19)	I	N
IL-27	I	N
TNF-α	I	I
Monocyte chemoattractant protein (MCP)-1	I	I
MCP-2	I	I
Macrophage inflammatory protein (MIP)-1α	I	I
(MIP)-1β	I	I
Adaptive immune response		
Cytokine	CD	UC
IL-5	N	I
IL-13	N	I
IL-17	I	N
IL-21	I	N
IFN-γ	I	N

I increase, *N* normal, *CD* Crohn's disease, *UC* ulcerative colitis

NFκB pathway is the converging point for the signals initiated by these receptors when binding to their specific bacterial adjuvants [44]. Enhanced expression and activation of NFκB is strongly induced in the inflamed mucosal tissue of IBD patients [42]. NFκB is the master transcriptional regulator of a variety of pro-inflammatory mediators including cytokines (e.g., IL-1β, tumor necrosis factors (TNF), IL-6, and IL-8), adhesion molecules (e.g., Intercellular Adhesion Molecule 1) and co-stimulatory molecules (e.g., CD40, CD80, CD86). Biological and pharmacological targeting therapeutics to block NFκB activation has been shown to ameliorate the spontaneous colitis in IL-10-deficient mice [12]. Of note, NFκB signaling in the intestinal epithelium also has a key role in sustaining normal mucosal homeostasis via its anti-apoptotic action. Given the divergent functions of NFκB pathway in different cell types, downregulation of NFκB-controlled inflammatory cytokines via blocking NFκB in immune cells may not be sufficient to counteract the compromised epithelial barrier integrity due to the loss of pro-survival NFκB action in the epithelial cells [40].

The mucosal tissue damage characterized in IBD is more attributable to the excessive activation of adaptive immunity, which is primed by the innate immune responses [39]. The effectors of adaptive immune responses include a variety of lymphocyte populations, i.e., T cells polarized with a T_H1, T_H17 or T_H2 phenotype, immunoglobulin-secreting B cells, regulatory T (T_{reg}) and B (B_{reg}) cells. CD and UC have distinct T-cell cytokine profiles with former exhibiting a $T_H1$polarization and the latter dominated by a T_H2 phenotype [39].

As the key mediator for T_H1 response, interferon (IFN)-γ increases the production of IL-12 produced by antigen-presenting cells (i.e., dendritic cells and macrophages), and via positive feedback, IL-12 stimulates the production of IFN-γ in helper T cells, thereby promoting the T_H1 profile. The T_H2 response promotes its own profile primarily via cytokine IL-4, which acts on T_H cells to promote the production of T_H2 cytokines (i.e., IL-4, IL-5, IL-10, and IL-13). The T-cell profile of UC has been generally believed to have a T_H2 polarization, although levels of key T_H2 mediators (e.g., IL-4 and IL-5) are not necessarily elevated in UC as reported in some studies [21]. In addition to T_H1/ T_H2 polarization paradigm, the T_H17 response has recently been identified to play a role in IBD [1]. The T_H17 cells are maintained by the IL-12 family member IL-23. Both IL-23 and IL-17 levels are upregulated in mucosal tissue of CD patients [47].

In addition to activated innate and acquired immune responses, loss of tolerance to commensals is a common feature to both CD and UC. It is a vital task for the intestinal immune system to mount protective immune responses against harmful intestinal pathogens while preventing excessive responses to innocuous commensal microbiome. Tolerance is an active physiological mechanism to sustain immune "unresponsiveness" to commensal bacterial antigens and is crucial for preventing harmful hypersensitivity responses in the intestine. Regulatory T cells (T_{reg}) are the primary executors for maintaining tolerance to commensal microbes. Recent research has shown that these T_{reg} cells are crucial in preventing intestinal inflammation and even have a key role in reverse established colitis [37]. In addition to T_{reg} cells, regulatory B cells (B_{reg}) have also been reported. By contrast to T_{reg} cells, B_{reg} cells are only observed in conditions of inflammation and suppress progression rather than initiation of experimental colitis [36].

Given the genetic heterogeneity of human IBD and the multi-factorial nature of IBD pathogenesis, much of our current understanding of IBD pathogenesis has come from the studies of various animal and cell models which resemble several key immunological and histopathological aspects of human IBD. Examples of animal IBD models are listed in Table 26.2 representing a multifold of targeting mechanistic points of pathobiology.

Evidence for Nutritional Modulation of IBD by Glutamine

Glutamine is proposed to become conditionally essential during stress states where demand for glutamine outstrips its synthesis from endogenous precursors. In patients with CD at the remission stage, the splanchnic glutamine utilization does not seem to be altered, and there is no glutamine deficiency

Table 26.2 Examples of experimental animal inflammatory bowel disease models

Chemically-induced colitis
Trinitrobenzene sulfonic acid-induced colitis
Dextran sulfate sodium-induced colitis
Iodoacetamide-induced colitis
Acetic-acid-induced colitis
Spontaneously occurring
C3H/HeJBir mice
SAMP1/Yit mice
Compromised intestinal barrier function
Mutated multidrug-resistant gene mice
Intestinal trefoil factor knockout mice
Altered cytokine balance
IL-10 knockout mice
Interleukin-2 knockout/IL-2 receptor (R)α knockout mice
TNF-3' untranslated region knockout mice
STAT-4 transgenic mice
Altered T-cell function
T0cell receptor mutant mice
HLA-B27 transgenic rat

at the whole-body level as reflected by the plasma level of glutamine [7]. However, local intestinal glutamine deficiency has been consistently reported in active CD and UC lesions of human biopsies [4]. The latter findings also furnish a theoretical niche for glutamine supplementation in IBD, which may potentially improve the outcomes by correcting the local intestinal glutamine deficiency.

Clinical Evidence

Clinical research has emerged exploring the therapeutic use of glutamine in IBD patients. Results from this limited body of clinical trials are, however, considerably mixed (Table 26.3). Topical administration of glutamine and butyrate was compared on pouchitis secondary to ileal pouch-anal anastomosis in a pilot study. During the 21-day treatment, 6 of the 10 patients receiving glutamine suppository had no recurrence of pouchitis, whereas only 3 of the 9 patients receiving butyrate suppository had no recurrence [52]. Compromised gut barrier function is a common feature of IBD. In a randomized controlled trial, patients with CD in the remission phase with an abnormal intestinal permeability (IP) received oral glutamine treatment at 0.5 g/kg/day. At the end of the 2-month study, glutamine treatment significantly improved IP and intestinal morphometry assessed by villous crypt ratio [5]. Another uncontrolled pilot study investigated effects of oral glutamine treatment at 6 g/day on patients with inactive or moderate CD. Glutamine treatment significantly improved IP and overall nutritional status compared to pretreatment values [58]. In terms of glutamine's effect on IP, an earlier clinical trial also reported that total parental nutrition (TPN) enriched with glycyl-glutamine maintained the normal LMR which was otherwise abnormally increased with standard TPN treatment not containing glutamine [49].

Nonetheless, a number of clinical trials also show an absence of clear benefits by glutamine supplementation in outcomes of IBD. A glutamine-enriched polymeric diet (42 % of amino acid composition, ~8.5 g/day glutamine delivered) given to pediatric patients with active CD for 4 weeks offered no benefits in disease activity index, weight and acute-phase reactants, compared to a standard polymeric diet with a low glutamine content (4 % of amino acid composition) [2]. In another

Table 26.3 Clinical trials of glutamine supplementation in inflammatory bowel disease

Total number of subjects	Subject features	Design	Form of glutamine	Dose of glutamine	Route of glutamine administration	Duration of glutamine treatment	Control	Glutamine's effects on examined endpoints	Reference
28 ($n=14$ for each group)	Patients with CD in the remission phase with an abnormal IP	Randomized, controlled	Free glutamine	0.5 g/kg/day	Oral	2 months	Whey protein at 0.5 g/kg/day via oral administration	Glutamine increased IP and villous crypt ratio compared to pretreatment values; whey protein equally improved these endpoints	[5]
19 ($n=10$ for glutamine; $n=9$ for butyrate)	Patients with pouchitis secondary to ileal pouch	Pilot, controlled	Free glutamine		Topical via suppository	21 days	Butyrate administered via suppository	Six of the 10 patients receiving glutamine treatment showing no recurrence of pouchitis vs. 3 of the 9 patients receiving butyrate suppository having no recurrence	[52]
11 (all receiving glutamine treatment)	Patients with inactive or moderate CD	Uncontrolled	Free glutamine	6 g/day (3 g twice a day)	Oral	Not known	No control	Glutamine improved IP and nutritional status compared to pretreatment values	[58]
16 ($n=7$ for glutamine treatment, $n=9$ for control)	Pediatric patients with active CD	Randomized, double-blind, controlled	Not specified (free glutamine or protein-bound)	Approximately 8.5 g/day	Glutamine-enriched polymeric diet (42 % of amino acid composition)	4 weeks	Isocaloric, isonitrogenous, standard polymeric diet with a low glutamine content (4 % of its amino acid content as glutamine, the amount naturally occurring in foods)	Glutamine-enriched diet was less effective than the standard low-glutamine polymeric diet in improving disease activity index	[2]
14 ($n=7$ for glutamine, $n=7$ for placebo)	Patients with CD with increased IP	Randomized, double-blind, placebo-controlled	Free glutamine	Oral: 21 g/day (7 g three times a day)	Oral or given in TPN when TPN became necessary	4 weeks	Glycine as placebo at 21 g/d (7 g three times a day)	Neither glutamine nor placebo treatment improved IP, CD activity index, C-reactive protein, or nutritional status; plasma levels of glutamine, glutamate and ammonia were not changed after glutamine treatment	[14]
24 ($n=12$ for glutamine$^+$, and $n=12$ for glutamine$^-$)	Patients with active IBD (19 CD; five ulcerative colitis) who needed to be on TPN for at least a week	Randomized, double-blind, controlled	Alanyl-glutamine	0.3 g/kg/day, equivalent to 0.2 g/kg/day glutamine	0.3 g/kg/day alanyl-glutamine added to 1.2 g/kg/day of glutamine-free standard amino-acid solution	≥7 days	Isonitrogenous, isocaloric TPN with 1.5 g/kg/day of a glutamine-free standard amino acid mixture	Glutamine treatment did not change glutamine plasma levels, IP, disease activity, length of TPN, hospital stay	[38]

CD Crohn's disease, *IBD* inflammatory bowel disease, *IP* intestinal permeability, *TPN* total parental nutrition

study, oral glutamine in single form at 21 g/day (7 g, three times a day) was not able to improve the IP or other endpoints such as CD activity index and C-reactive protein in patients with CD. Of note, plasma levels of glutamine and glutamate were not changed after glutamine treatment, which may suggest that glutamine administration as factored by dose, administration schedule and duration, could be insufficient [14]. Compared to glutamine-free standard TPN, glutamine-enriched (0.2 g/kg/day) TPN was also found unable to improve the IP or other outcomes examined in patients with active IBD. Parental glutamine in this administration paradigm was also found unable to change glutamine plasma levels [38].

Preclinical Evidence from Experimental IBD Models

A relatively small number of preclinical studies have explored the therapeutic potential of glutamine in a variety of experimental IBD models. Although limited, these preclinical data are generally supportive of a positive role of glutamine in the experimental settings of IBD (Table 26.4). Multiple inter-related key players in IBD pathogenesis could be potentially modulated by glutamine treatments. In these preclinical models, glutamine treatments exert direct or indirect effects on these mechanistic factors, such as improving intestinal barrier integrity, reducing tissue oxidative burden/stress, correcting cytokine imbalance, modulating immune-microbial axis and promoting inherent cytoprotective mechanisms (i.e., heat shock response (HSR)), and overall favors an ameliorated functional, structural and immune homeostasis in the intestinal mucosa (Fig. 26.2).

Improving Intestinal Barrier Integrity

Compromised gut barrier function has a vital role in the initiation and progression of intestinal inflammation characteristic of IBD [44]. In a guinea-pig model of carrageenan-induced UC-like colitis, glutamine-enriched elemental diet at 2 % (w/v) was shown to reduce gut-derived endotoxin translocation compared to a standard elemental diet with low glutamine content (0.64 % (w/v)) [20]. In an ex vivo study using isolated rat colonic mucosa, glutamine supplied from only serosal side diminished mannitol permeability of the colonic mucosa injured by hydrochloric acid (HCl). Even though glutamine added to both luminal and serosal sides seems to be superior to supplementation from the serosal side alone, a beneficial effect with glutamine-supplemented parental nutrition is still indicated [46]. Dugan et al. [15] studied effects of luminal glutamine on IP using isolated ileum loops perfused with or without glutamine. Ileal perfusion with a glutamine solution effectively prevents endotoxin-induced increases in mucosal permeability [15].

Mechanistically, glutamine's modulation on gut barrier function may stem from a multiplicity of action on factors vital in upholding intestinal epithelial homeostasis. Splanchnic perfusion and intestinal microcirculation is essential to preservation of mucosal structural integrity. Compromised intestinal microcirculation has been observed in intestinal segments in colitis models. Glutamine, either administered enterally or parentally, can affect intestinal microcirculation [18, 19, 29]. Glutamine luminal perfusions helped to reestablish microvascular circulation after hemorrhagic shock in a rat model [18]. In a trinitrobenzene sulfonic acid (TNBS) colitis model, glutamine-supplemented TPN increased colonic capillary blood flow [29, 19], indicating a protection in the intestinal microcirculation, though the glutamine treatment in a 48-h duration was not able to translate these benefits in intestinal microcirculation into improved gut barrier function at large [19].

Tight junctions (TJ), which are multi-protein complexes composed of integral membrane proteins including occludin, claudins, and zonula occludens (ZO)-1, ZO-2, and ZO-3 that are in turn bound to

Table 26.4 Preclinical studies of glutamine supplementation in inflammatory bowel disease models

Reference	Animal/cell line/tissue	Glutamine dose	Administration route	Form of glutamine	Duration of treatment	Control treatment	Results
[20]	Guinea-pig model of carrageenan-induced UC-like colitis	The same elemental control diet supplemented with 2 % (w/v) glutamine	Oral	Free glutamine	5 days	Chemically defined elemental diet containing 0.644 % (w/v) glutamine	Glutamine-enriched elemental diet reduced endotoxin level of portal vein
[15]	Isolated distal ileum loops in piglets in vivo	Ringer's lactate solution supplemented with 2 % glutamine	Luminal perfusion	Free glutamine	280 min	Ringer's lactate solution without glutamine	Glutamine perfusion prevented endotoxin-induced increases in mucosal permeability, but did not alter intestinal myeloperoxidase (MPO) activity
[19]	TNBS-induced colitis in Sprague-Dawley rats	Glutamine at 0.5 g/kg/day	Via TPN	Alanyl-glutamine	48 h	Alanyl-glycine-enriched iso-caloric and iso-nitrogenous standard TPN solution	Glutamine treatment increased colonic capillary blood flow, but had no effect on IP or bacterial translocation
[46]	Ex vivo isolated rat colonic injured by luminal hydrochloric acid and resealing was studied with or without added glutamine or butyrate	Glutamine 2 mM added to incubation medium (Krebs-Ringer solution)	Ex vivo, both luminal and serosal exposure as compared to single serosal exposure	Free glutamine	4 h	Equimolar NaCl added to Krebs-Ringer solution	Glutamine supplied from both luminal and serosal sides decreased IP and permeation of *Escherichia coli* Glutamine supplied from serosal side alone diminished IP. Both glutamine treatments promoted colonocyte proliferation
[55]	Sprague-Dawley rat model of DSS-induced colitis (via oral 5 % DSS) for 7 days)	Concurrent glutamine (0.75 g/kg/day) treatment throughout the 7-day DSS treatment	Oral gavage	Free glutamine	7 days	Sham (water)	Glutamine attenuated DSS-induced colitis by decreasing area under curve for bleeding and diarrhea, associated with enhanced HSP25 and HSP70 in colonic mucosa

(continued)

Table 26.4 (continued)

Reference	Animal/cell line/tissue	Glutamine dose	Administration route	Form of glutamine	Duration of treatment	Control treatment	Results
[26]	TNBS-induced colitis in Sabra rats	Glutamine enemas (50 mg in 1 ml saline, once a day)	Topical	Free glutamine	Schedule 1[a]: day −2 to day +7 ; Schedule 2: day −2 to day +3; Schedule 3: day 0 to day +7	Saline enemas	Only prophylactic topical glutamine treatment (Schedule 1 and 2, but not Schedule 3) reduced macroscopic inflammation, histological index, and MPO activity, reduced tissue oxidative injury, increased ascorbic acid and energy-rich phosphates in colonic mucosa
[22]	TNBS-induced colitis in Wistar-Albino rats	1 g/kg/day	Intragastric gavage	Free glutamine	Day −3 to day 15	Saline	Glutamine Treatment preserved mucosal structural integrity, increased GSH store and HO-1 expression and decreased oxidative injury, apoptosis and NFκB p50 expression
[28]	TNBS-induced colitis in Wistar rats	25 mg/kg/day	Rectal administration	Free glutamine	4 h after the induction of colitis till day 7	Receiving TNBS treatment alone	Glutamine preserved structural and functional integrity, reduced colonic myeloperoxidase activity, tissue TNF-α and IFN-γ levels, and NFκB activation
[17]	Acetic acid-induced colitis in Wistar rats	25 mg/kg/day	Rectal administration	Free glutamine	48 and 24 before acetic acid instillation	Receiving acetic acid alone	Glutamine preserved structural and functional integrity, decreased tissue oxidative injury, and NFκB activation
[3]	TNBS-induced colitis in Sprague-Dawley rats	2 and 4 % glutamine-enriched (w/w) casein-based (20 %, w/w) semipurified diet	Glutamine-enriched diet	Free glutamine	Day[a] −14 till the end of study (day +14)	Iso-nitrogenous and iso-caloric diet with glutamine substituted by glycine	Both glutamine-enriched diets attenuated weight loss, improved intestinal histological integrity, prevented bacterial translocation and reduced IL-8 and TNF-α levels in inflamed tissue. Four percent glutamine-diet was associated with better benefits compared to 2 % glutamine-diet

[27]	Endotoxemia in Sprague-Dawley rats induced by LPS injections on two consecutive days	Glutamine in drinking water (2 %)	Glutamine-contained drinking water	Free glutamine	Starting 2 days before LPS injection till 1 day after the 2nd dose of LPS	Rats receiving LPS alone	Glutamine treatment protected endotoxemia-induced intestinal mucosal injury, reduced expression of TLR4 and MyD88
[24]	DSS-induced colitis in C57BL/6 mice	Alanyl-glutamine at 0.75 g/kg/day, which provided 0.5 g glutamine/kg/day	Intraperitoneal injection	Alanyl-glutamine	Preventive schedule: glutamine (Day −3 to Day 0[b]) then saline (Day 0 to day +2); interventional schedule: saline (Day −3 to Day 0[b]) then glutamine (Day 0[b] to Day +2)	Isovolumic saline	Either pre- or post-DSS Glutamine treatment diminished structural destruction, reduced expression of TLR4 and IL-17A expression, increased IκB/NFκB ratio. Compared to the post-DSS schedule, pre-DSS glutamine better preserved structural integrity associated with increased expression of mucin 2, trefoil factor 3, and Hsp70

DSS dextran sulfate sodium, *HSP* heat shock protein, *IP* intestinal permeability, *LPS* lipopolysaccharides, *TNBS* trinitrobenzene sulfonic acid, *TPN* total parental nutrition, *UC* ulcerative colitis

[a]Day −*n* and +*n* designated as *n* days before or after TNBS instillation respectively

[b]Day 0 designated as the day when DSS treatment was initiated

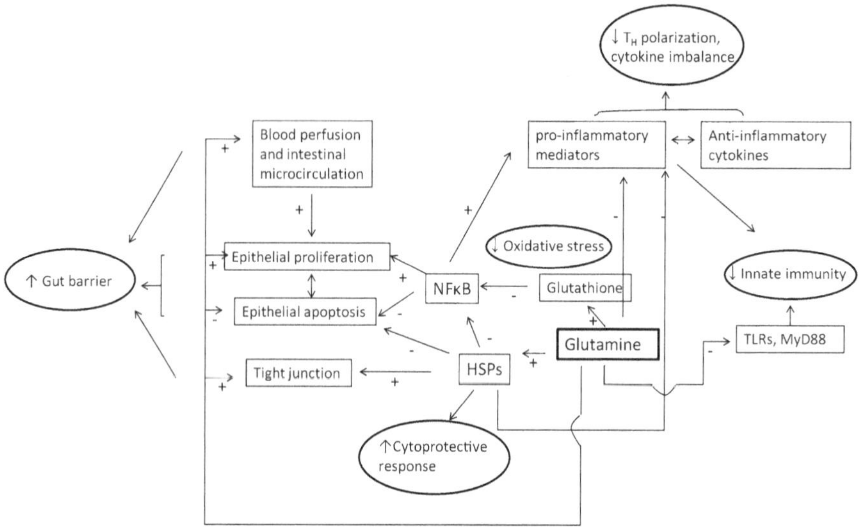

Fig. 26.2 Glutamine modulates multiple interrelated key players in inflammatory bowel disease pathogenesis, which may overall favor an ameliorated functional, structural and immune homeostasis in the intestinal mucosa. HSP: heat shock protein; MyD88: myeloid differentiation primary response gene 88; T_H: T-helper lymphocyte; TLR: toll-like receptor

the perijunctional ring of cytoskeletal actin, form the paracellular apical junctions of intestinal epithelia. They serve as a vital cellular component of mucosal barrier and are the principal determinant of mucosal permeability. TJ alterations are found to contribute to the barrier defects in IBD. TJs appear to be abnormal with a substantial loss of occluding and other TJ proteins such as ZO-1, JAM-A, and claudin-1 [30]. Disrupted integrity of TJ may result in paracellular transport of bacterial lipopolysaccharides (LPS) and luminal antigens, which may culminate in a constantly stimulated pro-inflammatory milieu in the intestinal mucosal tissue [45]. Li et al. show that glutamine is essential to TJ protein expression and cellular localization in cultured Caco-2 cell monolayers [32, 33]. Deprivation of glutamine from cell culture medium and inhibition of glutamine synthetase (GS) using methionine sulfoximine led to increased permeability of Caco-2 cell monolayers [13]. This was associated with reduced expression of claudin-1, occludin, and ZO-1 and abnormal subcellular re-localization of claudin-1 and irregular junctional complexes formation [32]. We lack an understanding of how glutamine potentially affects TJ functional and structural integrity during intestinal inflammation. Given the glutamine deficiency commonly found in the local intestinal mucosal tissue of IBD patients, which may jeopardize the mucosal tissue into a condition that renders an altered TJ protein expression and/or localization, exogenous glutamine supplementation may conceivably help to preserve TJ integrity and thus maintain mucosal homeostasis.

On the other hand, gut barrier is also dependent on epithelial homeostasis determined by the balance between epithelial proliferation and death. Epithelial apoptosis is a prominent feature of the epithelial barrier disturbance in intestinal inflammation. Glutamine has long been proposed as a gut-trophic factor which stimulates enterocyte proliferation, prevents excessive apoptosis and thus promotes epithelial homeostasis recovery during a variety of acute and chronic stresses/injuries [41]. In Scheppach et al.'s ex vivo study using isolated rat colonic mucosa injured by HCl, glutamine exposure at the serosal side with and without luminal glutamine exposure, improved IP, which was also associated with an increase in crypt cell proliferation [46]. In a rat model with dextran sulfate sodium (DSS)-induced colitis, we report that pharmacologic-dose, oral bolus glutamine (0.75 g/kg/day) attenuated colitis disease activity [55]. This was associated with decreased apoptosis in colonic mucosa (unpublished data). In cultured non-transformed young adult mouse colonic epithelial cells (YAMC) exposed to concurrent cytokine (IFN-γ + TNF-α) and glutamine treatment, glutamine deprivation or insufficient glutamine supply (glutamine supplanted at 0 or 0.25 mM) renders the cells more vulnerable to cytokine injury with increased apoptosis and diminished cell proliferation, whereas this effect can be blunted with adequate glutamine supply at 0.5 mM or higher [55]. Likewise, in cultured human colon carcinoma HT-29 cells injured with a combination of IFN-γ + TNF-α or a single cytokine, tumor necrosis factor-alpha-related apoptosis-inducing ligand (TRAIL), cytokine-induced apoptosis was attenuated by glutamine treatment in a dose-dependent manner and was completely blocked when glutamine was supplied at 0.5 mM [16].

Reducing Tissue Oxidative Burden/Stress

Of note, amongst the immunoregulatory factors, reactive oxygen molecules are produced in abnormally high levels in IBD. A role of these reactive oxygen species and enhanced oxidative stress in the initiation and/or propagation of the disease has been identified [56]. The notion that oxidative stress has a key role in triggering and propagating and/or propagation of IBD leads to theoretical basis for using antioxidants or compounds that can evoke or boost antioxidant defense during IBD conditions. Glutamine (via glutamate) is a precursor for glutathione synthesis and has been suggested to be rate limiting for glutathione synthesis during stress [51]. Enteral or topical glutamine supplementation has been consistently shown to preserve the glutathione store in models of TNBS and acetic acid-induced colitis [17, 22, 28]. In addition to GSH, glutamine treatment has been shown to increase other players of host antioxidant defense. Topical use of glutamine enemas which was initiated 2 days before induction of colitis by TNBS instillation reduced tissue oxidative damage and increased tissue ascorbic acid levels in colonic mucosa [26].

NFκB pathway, primarily via activating pro-inflammatory mediator expression, is intimately involved in the pathogenesis of IBD. It is noteworthy that activation of NFκB pathway is sensitive to the intracellular redox state. The activation of NFκB by most of the extracellular inducers is dependent on the phosphorylation and subsequent degradation of IκB, inhibitor of NFκB, which results in release of p65/p50 complex and its rapid nuclear translocation where it activates the target gene transcription. The increase in intracellular GSH by glutamine can reduce the activity of the redox-sensitive IκB kinases (IKK) which subsequently stabilizes IκB and downregulates activation of NFκB [48]. This pinpoints a mechanistic target point by which glutamine may potentially affect inflammatory mediator network. In TNBS or acetic acid-induced colitis, glutamine administered via a rectal route was shown to reduce oxidative stress associated with inhibited NFκB signaling [17, 28]. Giriş et al. also demonstrated that glutamine treatment at 1 g/kg/day via intragastric gavage could reduce tissue oxidative stress, increase GSH store and reduce colonic p50 expression in rats with TNBS-induced colitis [22]. We also show that in cultured YAMC cells, exogenous glutamine could reduce cytokine-induced nuclear translocation of NFκB p65 subunit and inducible nitric oxide synthase (iNOS) expression [55].

Regulating Intestinal Innate Immunity

A defective suppression of innate immunity is implicated in IBD initiation and progression [54]. Toll-like receptors (TLRs) have emerged as a central point in innate immunity [35]. Activation of these receptors via binding to their microbial ligands, such as LPS or double-stranded RNA, initiates an inflammatory cascade that attempts to clear the offending pathogen and further helps shaping specific adaptive immune response [35]. Expression of TLRs, especially TLR4 and TLR2, is upregulated on intestinal epithelial cells and the intestinal macrophages of patients with IBD [23]. Kessel et al. demonstrated that oral glutamine treatment protected endotoxemia-induced intestinal mucosal injury, associated with downregulation of expression of TLR4 and myeloid differentiation primary response gene 88 (MyD88), a key adaptor protein recruiting downstream kinase which leads to NFκB activation [27]. In a DSS-induced colitis model, intraperitoneal administration of alanyl-glutamine was also shown to attenuate colitis associated with reduced colonic TLR4 expression [24].

Modulating Cytokine Balance and T-Cell Polarization

The immune homeostasis of intestinal mucosa is regulated by a delicate balance of pro-inflammatory and anti-inflammatory cytokines. It has been well recognized that modulation of the gut cytokine milieu profoundly affects the nature of the response by effector immune cells to luminal microbes and their products [9]. In both entities of IBD (CD and ulcerative colitis) this intricate balance between pro-inflammatory and anti-inflammatory mediators is severely impaired and shifted toward the pro-inflammatory side [39]. This belief constitutes a foundation for targeting pro-inflammatory cytokines, such as using the neutralizing TNF antibodies in the clinic [6].

Coeffier et al. investigated how glutamine affected the cytokine network in cultured biopsies from human duodenum or colon ex vivo [11, 31]. Glutamine treatment at a physiological dose of 0.5 mM could effectively decrease the basal production of IL-6 and IL-8 of cultured biopsies as compared to isonitrogenous amino acid mixture [11]. These authors showed that supra-physiological doses up to 10 mM compared to physiological dose at 0.5 mM further suppressed IL-1β induced production of IL-6 and IL-8 and at the same time increased production of the anti-inflammatory cytokine IL-10 [10]. Further, glutamine at the pharmacological dose decreased IL-6 and IL-8 spontaneous production and NFκB p65 subunit expression, as compared to the physiological dose at 0.6 mM, in cultured inflamed colonic biopsies from patients with active CD [31]. These ex vivo models enable an in-depth mechanistic pursue of glutamine's regulations on related signaling pathways in human gut tissue [31]. In a TNBS-induced colitis model, pretreatment with semi-purified diet enriched with 2 and 4 % glutamine (w/w) for 2 weeks before TNBS instillation attenuated the disease activity associated with suppressed levels of pro-inflammatory cytokines IL-8 and TNF-α in inflamed tissue [3]. The same authors also show that IL-17A expression in the colonic tissue could be reduced by glutamine treatment in the same model [24].

Enhancing Intestinal Cytoprotective Heat Shock Response

During the course of evolution, cells have developed inherent stress-responsive mechanisms to dampen the many physiological and environmental insults they encounter. These are largely accomplished by a class of stress proteins, also termed as heat shock proteins (HSP). Induction of HSPs is a key innate mechanism to protect cells against stress/injury, and adequate expression of HSPs (e.g., HSP25, HSP70, heme oxygenase (HO)-1). Multiple lines of evidence reveal a key protective role of HSPs against inflammatory injury in IBD. Chang et al. [25] have shown that the HSP expression is markedly suppressed in human IBD lesions, which may contribute to the dysregulated pro-inflammatory response seen in IBD patients. HSPs could potentially modulate a gamut of interrelated processes or factors contributing to IBD pathogenesis, suggesting a multiplicity of HSPs' action. During a variety of stress conditions, HSPs preserve intestinal epithelial cytoskeletal integrity, maintain integrity of intestinal TJ [34] and preventing permeability changes [34], which ultimately leads to better preserved intestinal barrier function. Further, activation of intestinal HSP expression has been shown to be a potent anti-inflammatory signal through downregulation of NFκB pathway [50].

Mucosal injury associated with IBD is in nature a result from the unbalanced interplays between cytotoxic factors/conditions and cell inherent defense capacity. Promoting HSP expression appears to be a promising therapeutic target for preventing intestinal inflammatory injury. However, laboratory approaches using chemical or hyperthermia are not practical for clinical application due to their inherent toxicities. We demonstrated for the first time that oral bolus glutamine administration in pharmacological dose (0.75 g/kg/day) enhanced colonic epithelial expression of inducible HSPs in DSS-induced colitis model associated with mitigated disease activity and decreased colonic epithelial apoptosis [55]. Further, in cultured YAMC cells, glutamine increased cellular HSP 25 and HSP 70 in a dose-dependent manner and attenuated cytokine-induced injury [55]. Echoed with our study, Hou et al. also showed that parental administration (intraperitoneal) of glutamine at 0.5 g/kg/day also enhanced colonic epithelial HSP70 expression and attenuated DSS-induced colitis [24]. Thus, given the safe profile of its clinical use, glutamine has the potential to be developed as the first clinically relevant enhancer of heat shock response and may further elicit benefits in improving outcomes in IBD.

Conclusions

In experimental IBD models, glutamine seems to be a promising pharmaco-nutrient therapeutic to modulate a multifold of interrelated mechanistic factors, e.g., intestinal barrier integrity, tissue oxidative burden/stress, cytokine network, and innate cytoprotective mechanisms (i.e., HSP), and thus overall to prevent or attenuate intestinal inflammatory injury related to IBD. Despite significant clinical data supporting its use in conditions such as trauma, sepsis, burns and cancer chemotherapies, its therapeutic use in the setting of IBD has been inadequately explored because the importance of basic pharmacological principles (i.e., route, dose, and schedule) have not been considered. Basic questions on how to administer this nutrient in a clinically relevant and effective paradigm, which have been defined in conditions such as critical illness, still remain poorly answered in IBD settings.

Topical administration of glutamine, which conceivably ensures a great bioavailability of glutamine to local inflamed tissue, is associated with relatively consistent positive results in both clinical and experimental settings [17, 26, 28, 52]. Considerable debate has taken place regarding whether enteral or parental administration of glutamine provides a greater benefits. Direct communication between gut mucosa and enteral glutamine has irreplaceable benefits to the GI tract as a whole via preferential use as fuel source or precursors of important biomolecules via direct luminal absorption of upper small intestine, modifying mucosal immunity, and stimulating splanchnic blood perfusion and intestinal blood microcirculation. Compared to the enteral route, parenteral administration of glutamine would presumably result in a greater bioavailability to lower small intestine and large intestine, which are most frequently involved in IBD, as enteral glutamine supply is subject to a great deal of first-pass metabolism in the upper small bowel. Available evidence is not adequate to support one route as opposed to the other.

In in vitro cytokine-induced injury models, we and others demonstrated that insufficient glutamine supply at concentrations less than 0.5 mM in the media, which mimics tissue glutamine deficiency in vivo, renders the cells more sensitive to cytokine-induced cell death [16, 55]. In light of this, large pharmacological doses of glutamine (at or approaching 0.5 g/kg/day), when supplied enterally in vivo, may thus pharmacokinetically lead to an adequate and sustained elevation of tissue glutamine level in lower small intestine and large intestine, which is likely essential for correcting glutamine deficiency and overcoming the threshold to elicit benefits (e.g., HSR). Markedly insufficient (or non-pharmacologic) doses of glutamine used in some of these clinical trials, which is evidenced by the failure to increase plasma glutamine concentrations, may thus not able to result in an adequate increase in tissue-free glutamine pool size. Of note, in conditions such as critical illness or bone marrow transplant, "pharmacological" glutamine doses which exceed the usual physiological requirements consistently produce positive results in terms of clinical and mechanistic outcomes [53, 57]. The newly emerged conception of administering glutamine in "pharmaco-nutrition" paradigm thus warrants more experimental and clinical trials in the settings of IBD.

References

1. Abraham C, Cho J. Interleukin-23/Th17 pathways and inflammatory bowel disease. Inflamm Bowel Dis. 2009;15:1090–100.
2. Akobeng AK, Miller V, Stanton J, et al. Double-blind randomized controlled trial of glutamine-enriched polymeric diet in the treatment of active Crohn's disease. J Pediatr Gastroenterol Nutr. 2000;30:78–84.
3. Ameho CK, Adjei AA, Harrison EK, et al. Prophylactic effect of dietary glutamine supplementation on interleukin 8 and tumour necrosis factor alpha production in trinitrobenzene sulphonic acid induced colitis. Gut. 1997;41:487–93.
4. Balasubramanian K, Kumar S, Singh RR. Metabolism of the colonic mucosa in patients with inflammatory bowel diseases: an in vitro proton magnetic resonance spectroscopy study. Magn Reson Imaging. 2009;27:79–86.
5. Benjamin J, Makharia G, Ahuja V, et al. Glutamine and whey protein improve intestinal permeability and morphology in patients with Crohn's disease: a randomized controlled trial. Dig Dis Sci. 2012;57:1000–12.
6. Bosani M, Ardizzone S, Porro GB. Biologic targeting in the treatment of inflammatory bowel diseases. Biologics. 2009;3:77–97.
7. Bourreille A, Humbert B, Maugere P. Glutamine metabolism in Crohn's disease: a stable isotope study. Clin Nutr. 2004;23:1167–75.
8. Calder PC. Immunonutrition in surgical and critically ill patients. Br J Nutr. 2007;98 Suppl 1:S133–9.
9. Chahine BG, Bahna SL. The role of the gut mucosal immunity in the development of tolerance against allergy to food. Curr Opin Allergy Clin Immunol. 2010;10:220–5.
10. Coeffier M, Marion R, Ducrotte P, et al. Modulating effect of glutamine on IL-1beta-induced cytokine production by human gut. Clin Nutr. 2003;22:407–13.
11. Coeffier M, Marion R, Leplingard A, et al. Glutamine decreases interleukin-8 and interleukin-6 but not nitric oxide and prostaglandins e(2) production by human gut in-vitro. Cytokine. 2002;18:92–7.
12. Dave SH, Tilstra JS, Matsuoka K. Amelioration of chronic murine colitis by peptide-mediated transduction of the IkappaB kinase inhibitor NEMO binding domain peptide. J Immunol. 2007;179:7852–9.
13. DeMarco VG, Li N, Thomas J, et al. Glutamine and barrier function in cultured Caco-2 epithelial cell monolayers. J Nutr. 2003;133:2176–9.
14. Den Hond E, Hiele M, Peeters M. Effect of long-term oral glutamine supplements on small intestinal permeability in patients with Crohn's disease. J Parenter Enteral Nutr. 1999;23:7–11.
15. Dugan ME, McBurney MI. Luminal glutamine perfusion alters endotoxin-related changes in ileal permeability of the piglet. J Parenter Enteral Nutr. 1995;19:83–7.
16. Evans ME, Jones DP, Ziegler TR. Glutamine prevents cytokine-induced apoptosis in human colonic epithelial cells. J Nutr. 2003;133:3065–71.
17. Fillmann H, Kretzmann NA, San-Miguel B, et al. Glutamine inhibits over-expression of pro-inflammatory genes and down-regulates the nuclear factor kappaB pathway in an experimental model of colitis in the rat. Toxicology. 2007;236:217–26.
18. Flynn Jr WJ, Gosche JR, Garrison RN. Intestinal blood flow is restored with glutamine or glucose suffusion after hemorrhage. J Surg Res. 1992;52:499–504.
19. Foitzik T, Kruschewski M, Kroesen AJ, et al. Does glutamine reduce bacterial translocation? A study in two animal models with impaired gut barrier. Int J Colorectal Dis. 1999;14:143–9.
20. Fujita T, Sakurai K. Efficacy of glutamine-enriched enteral nutrition in an experimental model of mucosal ulcerative colitis. Br J Surg. 1995;82:749–51.
21. Fuss IJ, Neurath M, Boirivant M. Disparate CD4+ lamina propria (LP) lymphokine secretion profiles in inflammatory bowel disease. Crohn's disease LP cells manifest increased secretion of IFN-gamma, whereas ulcerative colitis LP cells manifest increased secretion of IL-5. J Immunol. 1996;157:1261–70.
22. Giris M, Erbil Y, Dogru-Abbasoglu S, et al. The effect of heme oxygenase-1 induction by glutamine on TNBS-induced colitis. The effect of glutamine on TNBS colitis. Int J Colorectal Dis. 2007;22:591–9.
23. Hausmann M, Kiessling S, Mestermann S, et al. Toll-like receptors 2 and 4 are up-regulated during intestinal inflammation. Gastroenterology. 2002;122:1987–2000.
24. Hou YC, Chu CC, Ko TL, et al. Effects of alanyl-glutamine dipeptide on the expression of colon-inflammatory mediators during the recovery phase of colitis induced by dextran sulfate sodium. Eur J Nutr. 2013;52:1089–98.

25. Hu S, Ciancio MJ, Lahav M, et al. Translational inhibition of colonic epithelial heat shock proteins by IFN-gamma and TNF-alpha in intestinal inflammation. Gastroenterology. 2007;133:1893–904.
26. Israeli E, Berenshtein E, Wengrower D, et al. Prophylactic administration of topical glutamine enhances the capability of the rat colon to resist inflammatory damage. Dig Dis Sci. 2004;49:1705–12.
27. Kessel A, Toubi E, Pavlotzky E, et al. Treatment with glutamine is associated with down-regulation of Toll-like receptor-4 and myeloid differentiation factor 88 expression and decrease in intestinal mucosal injury caused by lipopolysaccharide endotoxaemia in a rat. Clin Exp Immunol. 2008;151:341–7.
28. Kretzmann NA, Fillmann H, Mauriz JL, et al. Effects of glutamine on proinflammatory gene expression and activation of nuclear factor kappa B and signal transducers and activators of transcription in TNBS-induced colitis. Inflamm Bowel Dis. 2008;14:1504–13.
29. Kruschewski M, Perez-Canto S, Hubotter A. et al [Protective effect of glutamine on microcirculation of the intestine in experimental colitis]. Langenbecks Arch Chir Suppl Kongressbd. 1998;115:229–31.
30. Kucharzik T, Walsh SV, Chen J, et al. Neutrophil transmigration in inflammatory bowel disease is associated with differential expression of epithelial intercellular junction proteins. Am J Pathol. 2001;159:2001–9.
31. Lecleire S, Hassan A, Marion-Letellier R. Combined glutamine and arginine decrease proinflammatory cytokine production by biopsies from Crohn's patients in association with changes in nuclear factor-kappaB and p38 mitogen-activated protein kinase pathways. J Nutr. 2008;138:2481–6.
32. Li N, Lewis P, Samuelson D, et al. Glutamine regulates Caco-2 cell tight junction proteins. Am J Physiol Gastrointest Liver Physiol. 2004;287:G726–33.
33. Li N, Neu J. Glutamine deprivation alters intestinal tight junctions via a PI3-K/Akt mediated pathway in Caco-2 cells. J Nutr. 2009;139:710–4.
34. Liu TS, Musch MW, Sugi K, et al. Protective role of HSP72 against Clostridium difficile toxin A-induced intestinal epithelial cell dysfunction. Am J Physiol Cell Physiol. 2003;284:C1073–82.
35. Medzhitov R. Toll-like receptors and innate immunity. Nat Rev Immunol. 2001;1:135–45.
36. Mizoguchi A, Bhan AK. A case for regulatory B cells. J Immunol. 2006;176:705–10.
37. Mottet C, Uhlig HH, Powrie F. Cutting edge: cure of colitis by CD4+CD25+ regulatory T cells. J Immunol. 2003;170:3939–43.
38. Ockenga J, Borchert K, Stuber E. Glutamine-enriched total parenteral nutrition in patients with inflammatory bowel disease. Eur J Clin Nutr. 2005;59:1302–9.
39. Sartor RB, Hoentjen F. Proinflammatory cytokines and signaling pathways in intestinal innate immune cells. In: Mestecky J, Lamm ME, Mayer L, McGhee JR, et al., editors. Mucosal immunology. Philadelphia, PA: Elsevier; 2005. p. 681–701.
40. Rakoff-Nahoum S, Paglino J, Eslami-Varzaneh F. Recognition of commensal microflora by toll-like receptors is required for intestinal homeostasis. Cell. 2004;118:229–41.
41. Reeds PJ, Burrin DG. Glutamine and the bowel. J Nutr. 2001;131:2505S–8. discussion 2523S–2504S.
42. Rogler G, Brand K, Vogl D, et al. Nuclear factor kappaB is activated in macrophages and epithelial cells of inflamed intestinal mucosa. Gastroenterology. 1998;115:357–69.
43. Sartor RB. Mechanisms of disease: pathogenesis of Crohn's disease and ulcerative colitis. Nat Clin Pract Gastroenterol Hepatol. 2006;3:390–407.
44. Sartor RB. Microbial-host interactions in inflammatory bowel diseases and experimental colitis. Nestle Nutr Workshop Ser Pediatr Program. 2009;64:121–32. discussion 132–127, 251–127.
45. Sartor RB, Muehlbauer M. Microbial host interactions in IBD: implications for pathogenesis and therapy. Curr Gastroenterol Rep. 2007;9:497–507.
46. Scheppach W, Dusel G, Kuhn T, et al. Effect of L-glutamine and n-butyrate on the restitution of rat colonic mucosa after acid induced injury. Gut. 1996;38:878–85.
47. Schmidt C, Giese T, Ludwig B, et al. Expression of interleukin-12-related cytokine transcripts in inflammatory bowel disease: elevated interleukin-23p19 and interleukin-27p28 in Crohn's disease but not in ulcerative colitis. Inflamm Bowel Dis. 2005;11:16–23.
48. Sen CK, Packer L. Antioxidant and redox regulation of gene transcription. F J. 1996;10:709–20.
49. van der Hulst RR, van Kreel BK, von Meyenfeldt MF, et al. Glutamine and the preservation of gut integrity. Lancet. 1993;341:1363–5.
50. Voegeli TS, Wintink AJ, Chen Y, et al. Heat shock proteins 27 and 70 regulating angiotensin II-induced NF-kappaB: a possible connection to blood pressure control? Appl Physiol Nutr Metab. 2008;33:1042–9.
51. Welbourne TC. Ammonia production and glutamine incorporation into glutathione in the functioning rat kidney. Can J Biochem. 1979;57:233–7.
52. Wischmeyer P, Pemberton JH, Phillips SF. Chronic pouchitis after ileal pouch-anal anastomosis: responses to butyrate and glutamine suppositories in a pilot study. Mayo Clin Proc. 1993;68:978–81.
53. Wischmeyer PE. Glutamine: role in critical illness and ongoing clinical trials. Curr Opin Gastroenterol. 2008;24:190–7.
54. Xavier RJ, Podolsky DK. Unravelling the pathogenesis of inflammatory bowel disease. Nature. 2007;448:427–34.

55. Xue H, Sufit AJ, Wischmeyer PE. Glutamine therapy improves outcome of in vitro and in vivo experimental colitis models. J Parenter Enteral Nutr. 2011;35:188–97.
56. Zhu H, Li YR. Oxidative stress and redox signaling mechanisms of inflammatory bowel disease: updated experimental and clinical evidence. Exp Biol Med (Maywood). 2012;237:474–80.
57. Ziegler TR, Ogden LG, Singleton KD, et al. Parenteral glutamine increases serum heat shock protein 70 in critically ill patients. Intensive Care Med. 2005;31:1079–86.
58. Zoli G, Care M, Falco F, et al. Effect of oral glutamine on intestinal permeability and nutritional status in Crohn's disease. Gastroenterology. 1995;108:A766.

Chapter 27
Glutamine Supplementation and *Helicobacter pylori* Infection

Susan J. Hagen

Key Points

- Supplemental glutamine is a potent gastroprotective agent. It protects nearly fully against stress ulceration and mucosal lesions caused by a number of injurious substances.
- Supplemental glutamine protects against ulceration by buffering gastric acid and by transcriptionally regulating protective proteins in gastric epithelial cells.
- Supplemental glutamine has been evaluated in animal models as a potential alternative therapy in *H. pylori* infection. This work had mixed results.
- Supplemental glutamine in *H. pylori* infection blocks some of the important mucosal changes and reduces inflammation.
- Supplemental glutamine is also utilized by *H. pylori* for growth, colonization, and survival and as such, supports the persistence of infection.
- Ammonia/ammonium is one important product of glutamine metabolism by *H. pylori.* This product is cytotoxic to gastric epithelial cells.
- Long-term, mucosal pathogenesis during *H. pylori* infection (atrophy, metaplasia, dysplasia) occurs at about the same rate with or without supplemental glutamine.

Keywords Mucosal protection • Stomach • Gastric • Ammonia • Mucosal injury

Abbreviations

AA	Ammonia/ammonium
ER	Endoplasmic reticulum
GLDH	Glutamate dehydrogenase
Glu	L-Glutamate
Gln	L-Glutamine

S.J. Hagen, Ph.D. (✉)
Roberta and Stephen R. Weiner Department of Surgery, Beth Israel Deaconess Medical Center, Harvard Medical School, E/RW-871, 330 Brookline Avenue, Boston, MA 02215, USA
e-mail: shagen@bidmc.harvard.edu

R. Rajendram et al. (eds.), *Glutamine in Clinical Nutrition*, Nutrition and Health,
DOI 10.1007/978-1-4939-1932-1_27, © Springer Science+Business Media New York 2015

H. pylori	*Helicobacter pylori*
HP-Glts	*H. pylori*-specific glutamate transporter
HP-GTT	*H. pylori*-specific g-glutamyltranspeptidase
NH_4Cl	Ammonium chloride
NMDA	*N*-Methyl D-aspartate
RGM1	Rat gastric mucosal 1 cells
wkPI	Weeks post infection

Introduction

Helicobacter pylori (*H. pylori*) infection of the stomach is associated with mucosal injury and ulceration, inflammation that increases over time with concomitant pro-inflammatory cytokine production, defects in tight junction barrier function, abnormal repair mechanisms, and an increase in epithelial cell death and proliferation. Due to the potent gastroprotective properties of L-glutamine (Gln), this amino acid has been proposed as a potential therapeutic agent during *H. pylori* infection. Gln may also be an attractive alternative therapy because of increasingly antibiotic-resistant bacteria and the adverse effects of eradication regimes on esophageal homeostasis. Animal studies done to test this idea, however, suggest that supplemental Gln affects, both positively and negatively, mucosal pathogenesis and disease outcome. Further confounding the use of supplemental Gln in *H. pylori* infection is Gln metabolism by *H. pylori* itself, which is robust and is utilized to support cell survival mechanisms, colonization, and growth of the organism. Constitutive Gln metabolism by *H. pylori* contributes to the production of ammonia/ammonium (AA), which is one of the cellular cytotoxins liberated during infection. Long-term exposure to AA in the absence of infection induces cell injury and mucosal atrophy, and increases inflammation in vivo. In this review, we focus on the balance of processes that utilize supplemental Gln in a beneficial and detrimental way (see Fig. 27.1) to influence the course of *H. pylori* infection.

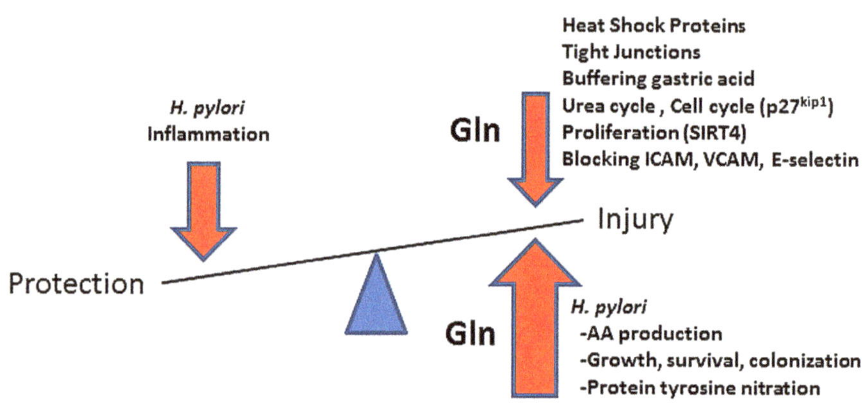

Fig. 27.1 Effects of supplemental L-glutamine on gastric mucosal protection versus injury during *H. pylori* infection. The positive and negative features of L-glutamine shift the balance of protection and injury such that the later predominates during infection, resulting in mucosal pathogenesis and cancer progression

Glutamine and Mucosal Protection in the Stomach: *A Historical Perspective*

It has been known for some time that Gln is a potent mucosal protective compound in the stomach. The pioneering work of Takagi and Okabe [1], who developed the stress-induced ulcer model in rats, showed that Gln was the most effective amino acid at curing existing stress-induced ulcers (61.8 % curative), while Gln had no effect on the severity of ulcers if given prior to the experimental stress. This same group reported the curative effects of Gln on ulcers formed by other mechanisms as well, for instance on ulcers induced by indomethacin [2, 3]. Further work with aspirin-, acetic acid-, or taurocholate-induced gastric lesions demonstrated that (1) high doses of Gln (750–1,500 mg/kg) resulted in nearly full protection from injury and ulceration [4–8]; (2) ulceration occurred in these different models by a common mechanism that involves the back-diffusion of gastric acid due to barrier defects. Gln protected against ulceration by buffering gastric acid so that acid back-diffusion and thus mucosal injury was attenuated [5]; (3) protection occurred when Gln remained in the stomach for the duration of injury and repair rather than being provided as an oral gavage once or twice daily [3, 4]; and (4) the protective effects of Gln on ulceration and mucosal lesions did not seem to be a specific effect on cell function because both L- and D-Gln provided similar protection [9]. These studies suggested that oral dietary supplementation with Gln would protect against ulceration and mucosal injury that were the result of acid hypersecretion in patients with ulcer disease or other similar gastric disorders. In fact, Kotobuki Pharmaceutical Co. Ltd. launched the therapeutic drug Marzulene-S in 1969, which is an oral agent containing 99 % L-glutamine and 1 % sodium azulene sulfonate (azulene) and is prescribed to combat gastric and duodenal ulcers, and acute and chronic gastritis. Marzulene-S and new generation drugs in this class are also thought to attenuate chronic gastritis, ulceration, and mucosal injury that occur during *H. pylori* infection due to the potent protective properties of Gln and anti-inflammatory properties of sodium azulene sulfonate. One study supports this premise experimentally in gerbils infected with *H. pylori* [10], although the Gln concentration given as a dietary supplement (20 % dietary Gln or Marzulene-S supplementation, approximately 45 % dietary protein) was not controlled so it is unclear whether the protective effects of Gln with or without azulene are specific for Gln and azulene or are due to high protein levels, changes in energy balance, or changes in food consumption.

H. pylori Infection of the Stomach

Numerous review articles have outlined aspects of the pathogenesis of *H. pylori* infection [11, 12] and will not be covered in this review. It should be noted, however, that infection with *H. pylori* occurs in 50 % of the world's population and is a major risk factor for gastric cancer development, which is the fourth most common cancer and the second most common cause of cancer deaths worldwide [13–15]. *H. pylori* infection is associated with increasing levels of inflammation and pro-inflammatory cytokine production, along with the liberation of a number of cytotoxins including members of the *cag* pathogenicity island, *vacA* producing vacuolating cytotoxin, lipopolysaccharide, and AA, which individually or together are thought to facilitate cancer development. The *ure* genes from *H. pylori* are required for the expression of urease, which facilitates the production of AA from the metabolism of urea in the gastric juice [16]. *H. pylori* also express enzymes that hydrolyze asparagine and Gln, further increasing AA production [17, 18]. AA production is essential for *H. pylori* colonization and the persistence of infection [19], but is cytotoxic to gastric epithelial cells. Although other *H. pylori* virulence factors are essential components of mucosal pathogenesis and cancer development, Gln specifically affects the production of AA by *H. pylori*. Luminal AA in the absence of infection causes gastritis, superficial erosions, enterochromaffin-like cell hyperplasia, mucosal thickening, increased levels of gastrin, mucosal atrophy, and accelerated cell migration in vivo [20, 21]. Increased production of AA by *H. pylori* is thus likely to be an important factor in shifting the balance of protection versus injury and cancer development (see Fig. 27.1) with supplemental Gln administration.

Glutamine Protects Against AA Cytotoxicity in Gastric Epithelial Cells

The concentration of AA is normally about 0.5–0.7 mM in the gastric juice but can increase to more than 20 mM in patients infected with *H. pylori* [22, 23]. When cultured human gastric cells were incubated with *ure*⁺ *H. pylori* in the presence of urea, about 20 mM AA was generated in 2 h and 40 mM in 24 h and the viability of cells was reduced as the AA concentration increased [24]. In vivo [21, 20] and in vitro [25–27] studies confirmed that AA also reduced the viability of gastric epithelial cells.

Using ammonium chloride (NH_4Cl) as the source of AA and rat gastric mucosal (RGM)1 cells in vitro, it was recently shown that NH_4Cl caused a dose-dependent increase in cell death and vacuolation, which were both inhibited by Gln [26]. RGM1 cells metabolize ammonia to urea via arginase (see Fig. 27.2), a process that is stimulated by Gln and results in reduced AA cytotoxicity [26]. Gln also protects mitochondria directly (see Fig. 27.2), by preventing the loss of membrane potential and maintaining cellular ATP levels [28]. Further mechanistic work using RGM1 cells to study AA cytotoxicity (see Fig. 27.3), with AA that was generated from NH_4Cl or from *ure* + *H. pylori*, showed that AA kills gastric epithelial cells by activating Ca^{2+} uptake via *N*-methyl-D-aspartate (NMDA) channels, resulting in Ca^{2+}-mediated mitochondrial injury and ATP depletion, calpain and cathepsin D activation, and endoplasmic reticulum (ER) stress/injury [29]. Although not tested experimentally, Gln administration must protect against injury from one or more of these Ca^{2+}-mediated pathways or it blocks NMDA channel activation by AA altogether.

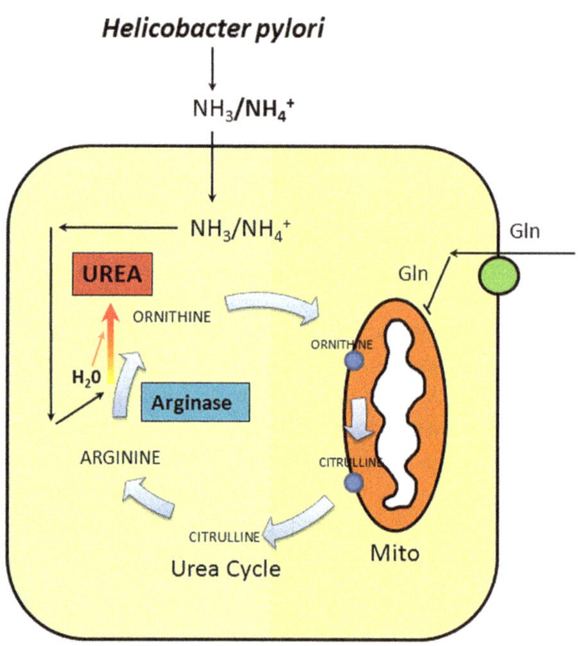

Fig. 27.2 Glutamine protects against ammonia (NH_3)/ammonium (NH_4^+)-induced injury in gastric epithelial cells. Ammonia/ammonium, generated by *H. pylori* (or chemically by exposure to NH_4Cl) is detoxified in the urea cycle by the enzyme arginase, which converts L-arginine plus ammonia to L-ornithine and urea. L-Glutamine also protects against the loss of mitochondrial membrane potential in mitochondria (Mito) and the concomitant reduction in cellular ATP levels that occur in the presence of ammonia/ammonium

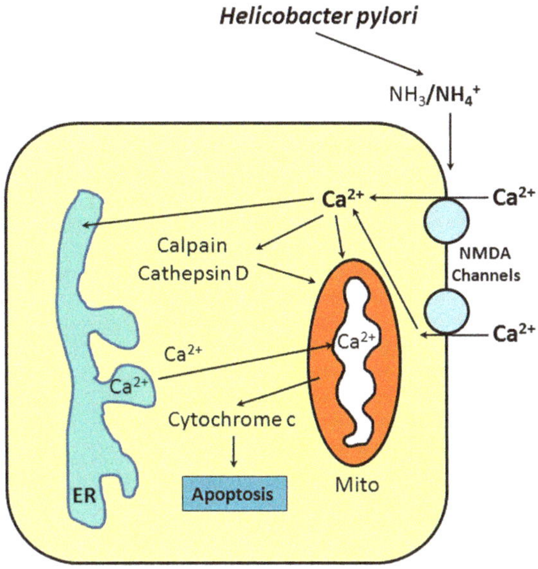

Fig. 27.3 Ammonia (NH_3)/ammonium (NH_4^+) generated by *H. pylori* damages cells by *N*-methyl-D-aspartate (NMDA)-mediated calcium (Ca^{2+}) cytotoxicity. Ammonia/ammonium generated by *H. pylori* activates NMDA-channel-mediated Ca^{2+} permeation in gastric epithelial cells. This intracellular Ca^{2+} damages mitochondria (Mito), activates calpain and cathepsin D, reduces mitochondrial membrane potential resulting in the leakage of cytochrome c and apoptosis induction, and causes stress of the endoplasmic reticulum (ER) followed by the transfer of Ca^{2+} from ER to mitochondria. Overall, L-glutamine inhibits one or more of these pathways in vitro to confer protection against ammonia/ammonium-induced injury

Glutamine Supplementation as an Alternative Therapy for H. pylori Infection

The protective effects of Gln against stomach ulceration in vivo and against AA-induced injury to gastric epithelial cells in vitro, suggested that Gln supplementation may be effective as an alternative therapy for reducing mucosal pathogenesis during *H. pylori* infection. To show feasibility for this idea, it would be important to limit the supplemental Gln concentration to 5 % or less and the study must use a Gln-containing diet with purified components that maintains an energy balance. To this end, a mouse model of *H. pylori* infection was used to demonstrate that 5 % supplemental Gln (6.9 % total Gln) had both a positive and negative impact on gastric histopathology over time [30].

One unexpected result in *H. pylori*-infected mice was that supplemental dietary Gln significantly increased inflammation early in infection (see Fig. 27.4) that was correlated with high levels of IL-1β expression [30]. Because dietary Gln alone was insufficient to produce gastric inflammation, the combination of Gln and *H. pylori* was responsible for this negative effect of Gln [30]. Gln increases MAPK signaling as does *H. pylori*, suggesting that Gln, in combination with *H. pylori*, increases IL-8/CXC chemokine expression early in infection resulting in greater inflammation than occurs with *H. pylori* alone. Although it is unclear what long-term effects the high initial IL-1β expression causes early in infection, IL-1β affects gastric epithelial cells by disrupting tight junction integrity [31, 32], and it induces IL-6 and TNF-α mRNA expression, facilitates the development of atrophy, metaplasia, and dysplasia, and enhances neutrophil chemotaxis [33, 34]. Additionally, IL-1β inhibits gastric acid secretion by parietal cells [35]. Correlated with the increase in inflammation was a significant increase in anti-inflammatory cytokine expression, particularly IL-4, IL-10, and TGF-β [30]. Anti-inflammatory cytokine expression in *H. pylori* infection may modulate the immune response to *H. pylori* and additionally have protective effects on currently unidentified downstream targets.

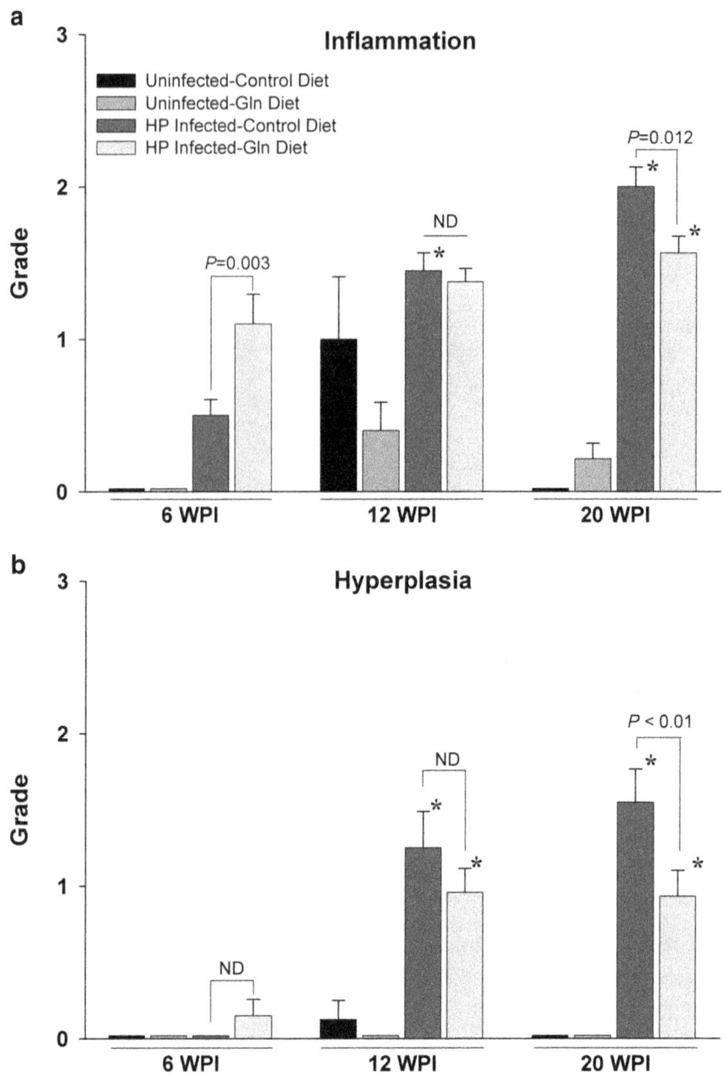

Fig. 27.4 Inflammation and hyperplasia histopathology scores in *H. pylori*-infected mice with or without supplemental L-glutamine. (**a**) Inflammation was significantly greater at 6 weeks post-infection (wkPI) and was significantly lower at 20 wkPI in *H. pylori*-infected mice fed supplemental L-glutamine compared to *H. pylori*-infected mice fed a control diet. Furthermore, the high level of inflammation at 6 wkPI did not increase significantly at 12 wkPI or from 12–20 wkPI in *H. pylori*-infected mice fed supplemental L-glutamine. This result was in contrast to *H. pylori*-infected mice fed a control diet, who showed a significant increase in inflammation from 6–12 wkPI and from 12–20 wkPI. There was multifocal-to-coalescing leukocyte infiltration by 20 wkPI in contrast to the diffuse pattern of inflammation found in *H. pylori*-infected mice fed supplemental L-glutamine at all time points. (**b**) Hyperplasia in *H. pylori*-infected mice fed supplemental L-glutamine was reduced at 12 wkPI and was reduced significantly at 20 wkPI compared to *H. pylori-infected* mice fed a control diet. The hyperplastic glands were significantly longer in *H. pylori*-infected mice fed a control diet compared to *H. pylori*-infected mice fed supplemental L-glutamine. $*P<0.05$ compared to control, comparisons as indicated by brackets after 2-way analysis of variance; ND, not significantly different. Reproduced from Table 3 [30]

In contrast to the early effects of Gln supplementation in *H. pylori*-infected mice, the course of inflammation and foveolar hyperplasia later in infection remained constant rather than increasing over time (see Fig. 27.4), suggesting that mucosal injury and immune cell recruitment are positively impacted by Gln supplementation long-term [30]. Although not tested experimentally, important protective mechanisms in epithelial cells may be induced by Gln supplementation during *H. pylori* infection including arginase and ammonia detoxification pathways [26] and heat shock protein expression [36]. Pathways that utilize Gln to regulate proliferation (SIRT4) and cell cycle progression (p27^{kip1} protein) may also be affected by supplemental Gln [37, 38]. Gln also modulates inflammation by inhibiting the expression of ICAM-1, VCAM-1, and E-selectin on vascular endothelial cells, and may reduce IL-8 expression as it does in intestine [39].

Other unexpected results with the supplemental Gln diet were (1) a significant increase in *H. pylori* colonization later in infection, and (2) continued mucosal injury, atrophy, and metaplasia development despite having adequate supplemental Gln to elicit a protective response in the mucosa [30]. Although inflammation, per se, can transcriptionally silence protective pathways initially supported by Gln [40], the changes may also be explained on the basis of Gln metabolism by *H. pylori. H. pylori* utilize Gln dose-dependently to generate AA, which induces protein nitration and inactivation of key enzymes that may be protective for gastric epithelial cells [41]. One example is that glutamine synthetase undergoes protein nitration and enzyme inactivation in the presence of AA [41]. Thus, Gln metabolism by *H. pylori* is likely to be an additional factor in shifting the balance of protection versus injury and cancer development (see Fig. 27.1) with supplemental Gln administration.

Glutamine Utilization by H. pylori

H. pylori have the unique capability, compared to other *Campylobacter*-like bacteria, to metabolize glucose by the pentose phosphate and Entner-Doudoroff pathways [42–44]. However, *H. pylori* preferentially metabolize a subset of amino acids as an energy source, particularly Glu/Gln [17, 18]. In fact, *H. pylori* consume Glu/Gln at a rate of 0.483 mM/h in liquid culture [18]. When glutamine is provided as the sole amino acid source in culture, glutamate and its products of metabolism (succinate, acetate, and formate) are derived from this amino acid [18]. Additionally, in the presence of Gln and low levels of urea, *H. pylori* produce approximately 2 mM of AA per day [17]. This level of AA production cannot be explained on the basis of urease activity alone, and is thus amplified by amino acid metabolism including that of Gln [17]. Gln serves, at the least, two important metabolic functions in *H. pylori.* First, Gln catabolism and synthesis are linked to energy production and nitrogen assimilation and second, Gln is essential for nucleotide synthesis, particularly pyrimidine synthesis.

Glutamine Transport by H. pylori

Although genomic analysis of the *H. pylori* genome contains annotation of a putative Gln transporter, they are unable to transport this amino acid directly [45]. Rather, Gln in the extracellular environment (see Fig. 27.5) is transported for use by indirect means after deamidation to Glu by an *H. pylori-specific* γ-glutamyltranspeptidase (HP-GTT) [45]. HP-GTT is an enzyme with conserved function throughout the *Helicobacter* genus [46] and an enzyme that is active in the bacterial periplasm [47]. Once Gln is deaminated to Glu, the *H. pylori*-specific glutamate transporter (HP-Glts) that is localized to the bacterial inner membrane (see Fig. 27.5) transports Glu into the cytoplasm [19]. HP-GGT and HP-GltS activity are responsible for the high level of Gln consumption from the environment (for instance from the culture media, as described above) and may be responsible for maintaining a constant level of ammonia when the *H. pylori* urease is inactivated. Gln acts as a positive transcriptional regulator of HP-GGT expression [48], suggesting that Gln supplementation would support the expression of high levels of this protein. Furthermore, at acidic pH (pH 4–5) when HP-GTT is inactive, the addition of ammonium and other cations like K^+ and Na^+ dramatically increases HP-GTT activity [48].

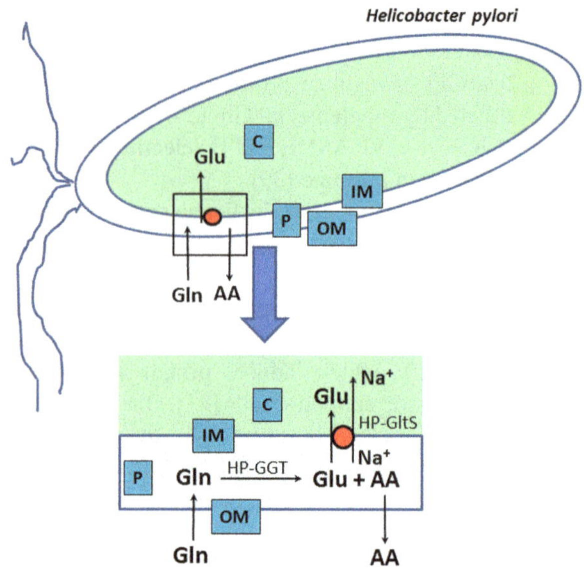

Fig. 27.5 Glutamine transport by *H. pylori. H. pylori* are gram-negative bacteria with flagella. They have an outer membrane (OM) and an inner membrane (IM), between which is the periplasm (P). The cytoplasm/cytosol (C) constitutes the interior of the bacterium. Glutamine (Gln) diffuses across the OM and in the periplasm is deamidated to glutamate (Glu) and ammonia/ammonium (AA) by the *H. pylori*-specific γ-glutamyltranspeptidase (HP-GGT). Glutamate is transported into the cytoplasm across the IM by an *H. pylori*-specific glutamate transporter, HP-GltS. This transporter is a Na^+/Glu symporter and as such, co-transports Na^+ into the cytosol. AA produced from the deamidation of glutamine diffuses across the OM into the environment and contributes further to the AA produced by *H. pylori* urease activity

Gln deamidation followed by Glu transport, and the expression of HP-GTT and HP-GltS are essential for colonization of *H. pylori* in the gastric mucosa [19, 49]. Gln supplementation would thus support *H. pylori* colonization of the gastric mucosa by providing an essential substrate for these important metabolic functions to occur. Recent data in mice support this conclusion because the mean colonization of *H. pylori* was significantly greater in infected mice that received supplemental Gln compared to mice receiving a control diet [30].

The Importance of Gln as a Nitrogen Source for H. pylori

Nitrogen is essential for the growth of *H. pylori* and it derives this essential component from only a few sources (see Fig. 27.6); from ammonium (produced from urea/urease) and Gln/Glu [45]. Because *H. pylori* have no ability to transport Gln (previous section), they must utilize the deaminated Gln that is transported into the cytoplasm as Glu and then synthesize Gln by assimilating ammonia in the presence of glutamine synthetase (see Fig. 27.6). Annotation of the *H. pylori* genome identified HP0512 as the gene similar to *glnA* in *E. coli* with a putative role similar to GS in mammals [45]. This reaction requires ATP and as such, must occur in an energy-rich environment [45]. Glu that was produced from Gln and then transported into the cytoplasm can also be converted to a-ketoglutarate by glutamate dehydrogenase (GLDH). Annotation of the *H. pylori* genome identified HP0380 as a gene similar to *gdhA* in *E. coli*, with a putative role similar to GLDH in mammals [45]. The conversion of Glu to a-ketoglutarate also assimilates ammonia (see Fig. 27.6) and can occur in an energy-depleted environment [45]. Together, these two pathways derived from extracellular Gln are important for the assimilation of

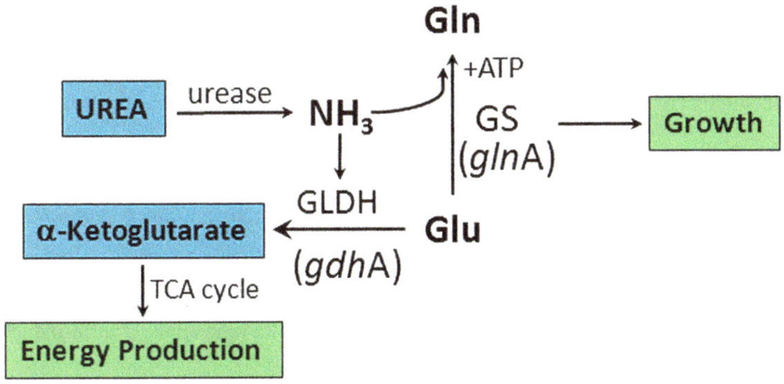

Fig. 27.6 Assimilation of ammonia as a nitrogen source for *H. pylori*. Glutamate (Glu) that is transported into the cytoplasm (Fig. 27.5) is converted to glutamine (Gln) by glutamine synthetase (GS), which is encoded by the gene *glnA*. Glutamate can also be converted to a-ketoglutarate, in the presence of ammonia (NH_3) that is generated from urease activity in the presence of urea, and enter the TCA cycle where it is used for energy production

ammonia as a nitrogen source for *H. pylori*. It is likely that supplemental Gln increases use of these nitrogen assimilation pathways, resulting in improved growth characteristics of this pathogen.

Essential Role of Gln in Nucleotide Synthesis

H. pylori have no orthologous pyrimidine salvage genes and thus are thought to exclusively use de novo synthetic pathways that require Gln to produce pyrimidines, resulting in UTP and CTP synthesis [45]. Annotation of the *H. pylori* genome identified HP1237 and HP0919 as the genes similar to *pyrAa* in *Salmonella cholerasius* and *pyrAb* in *Bacillus caldolyticus* that encode carbamoyl-phosphate synthetases, which with Gln and bicarbonate, produce the first intermediate in the pyrimidine synthetic pathway [45]. Using a set of nine *pyr* genes, *H. pylori* then synthesizes CTP and UTP [45]. Deletion mutants of *pyrB*, another gene in the pyrimidine synthetic pathway, were lethal for *H. pylori*, demonstrating that this pathway is essential for survival of the organism [50]. It is likely that supplemental Gln supports nucleotide synthesis in the de novo synthetic pathway, additionally contributing to improved survival and the persistence of infection.

Conclusion

Supplemental Gln significantly decreases the risk of ulcer formation by protecting against acid-induced mucosal injury. Supplemental Gln, particularly when combined with sodium azulene sulfonate (azulene), also reduces acute and chronic gastritis that is associated with ulcer disease. Although supplemental Gln has been proposed to limit mucosal injury and gastritis during *H. pylori* infection, the use of supplemental Gln during infection is complicated by the positive effects of Gln on mucosal protection and the negative effects of Gln on growth, colonization, and survival by *H. pylori*. Additionally, Gln is an important amino acid that regulates the rate of ammonia production by *H. pylori*, which suggests that increasing dietary Gln increases ammonia production and cytotoxicity during infection. Overall, the available data suggest that the course of mucosal pathogenesis is unaffected by the use of supplemental Gln during *H. pylori* infection because the balance of these positive and negative factors favor mucosal injury and continued cancer development.

References

1. Takagi K, Okabe S. The effects of drugs on the production and recovery process of the stress ulcer. Jpn J Pharmacol. 1968;18:9–18.
2. Urushidani T, Okabe S, Takeuchi K. Effects of various amino acids on indomethacin-induced gastric ulcers in rats. Jpn J Pharmacol. 1977;27:316–9.
3. Okabe S, Ohtsu K, Takeuchi K, et al. Effect of L-glutamine on indomethacin-induced gastric lesions in the rat. Jpn J Pharmacol. 1974;24:169–71.
4. Okabe S, Takeuchi K, Takata Y, et al. Effects of L-glutamine on various gastric lesions in rats and guinea pigs. Digestion. 1976;14:325–31.
5. Okabe S, Takeuchi K, Nakamura K, et al. Inhibitory effects of L-glutamine on the aspirin-induced gastric lesions in the rat. J Pharm Pharmacol. 1974;26:605–11.
6. Okabe S, Takeuchi K, Honda K, et al. Effects of acetylsalicylic acid (ASA), ASA plus L-glutamine, and L-glutamine on healing of chronic gastric ulcer in the rat. Digestion. 1976;14:85–8.
7. Okabe S, Hung C-R, Takeuchi K, et al. Effects of L-glutamine on acetylsalicyclic acid or taurocholic acid-induced gastric lesions and secretory changes in pylorus-ligated rats under normal or stress conditions. Jpn J Pharmacol. 1976;26:455–60.
8. Okabe S, Honda K, Takeuchi K, et al. Inhibitory effect of L-glutamine on gastric irritation and back diffusion of gastric acid to aspirin in the rat. Am J Dig Dis. 1975;20:626–31.
9. Okabe S, Takeuchi K, Honda K, et al. Effects of various amino acids on gastric lesions induced by acetylsalicyclic acid (ASA) and gastric secretion in pylorus-ligated rats. Drug Res. 1976;26:534–7.
10. Nakamura E, Hayashi S, Amagase K, et al. Prophylactic effect of glutamine and marzulene against *Helicobacter pylori*-related gastric diseases in Mongolian gerbils. Jpn Pharmacol Ther. 2007;35:479–88.
11. Wroblewski LE, Peek RM, Wilson KT. *Helicobacter pylori* and gastric cancer: factors that modulate disease risk. Clin Microbiol Rev. 2010;23:713–39.
12. Correa P, Houghton J. Carcinogenesis of *Helicobacter pylori*. Gastroenterology. 2007;133:659–72.
13. Anderson WF, Camargo MC, Fraumeni JF, et al. Age-specific trends in incidence of noncardia gastric cancer in US adults. JAMA. 2010;303:1723–8.
14. Parkin DM, Bray F, Ferlay J, et al. Global cancer statistics, 2002. CA Cancer J Clin. 2005;55:74–108.
15. Parkin DM. The global health burden of infection-associated cancers in the year 2002. Int J Cancer. 2006;118:3030–44.
16. Sachs G, Weeks DL, Melchers K, et al. The gastric biology of *Helicobacter pylori*. Annu Rev Physiol. 2003;65:349–69.
17. Stark RM, Suleiman MS, Hassan IJ, et al. Amino acid utilisation and deamination of glutamine and asparagine by *Helicobacter pylori*. J Med Microbiol. 1997;46:793–800.
18. Mendz GL, Hazell SL. Amino acid utilization by *Helicobacter pylori*. Int J Biochem Cell Biol. 1995;27:1085–93.
19. Leduc D, Gallaud J, Stingl K, et al. Coupled amino acid deamidase-transport systems essential for *Helicobacter pylori* colonization. Infect Immun. 2010;78:2782–92.
20. Tsujii M, Kawano S, Tsuji S, et al. Cell kinetics of mucosal atrophy in rat stomach induced by long-term administration of ammonia. Gastroenterology. 1993;104:796–801.
21. Lichtenberger LM, Dial EJ, Romero JJ, et al. Role of luminal ammonia in the development of gastropathy and hypergastrinemia in the rat. Gastroenterology. 1995;108:320–9.
22. Triebling AT, Korsten MA, Dlugosz JW, et al. Severity of *Helicobacter*-induced gastric injury correlates with gastric juice ammonia. Dig Dis Sci. 1991;36:1089–96.
23. Verdu EF, Armstrong D, Sabovcikova L, et al. High concentrations of ammonia, but not volatile amines, in gastric juice of subjects with *Helicobacter pylori* infection. Helicobacter. 1998;3:97–102.
24. Smoot DT, Mobley HLT, Chippendale GR, et al. *Helicobacter pylori* urease activity is toxic to human gastric epithelial cells. Infect Immun. 1990;58:1992–4.
25. Suzuki H, Yanaka A, Shibahara T, et al. Ammonia-induced apoptosis is accelerated at higher pH in gastric surface cells. Am J Physiol Gastrointest Liver Physiol. 2002;283:G986–95.
26. Nakamura E, Hagen SJ. Role of glutamine and arginase in protection against ammonia-induced cell death in gastric epithelial cells. Am J Physiol Gastrointest Liver Physiol. 2002;283:1264–75.
27. Hagen SJ, Takahashi S, Jansons R. The role of vacuolation in the death of gastric epithelial cells. Am J Physiol Cell Physiol. 1997;272:C48–58.
28. Ahmad S, White CW, Chang L-Y, et al. Glutamine protects mitochondrial structure and function in oxygen toxicitity. Am J Physiol. 2001;280:L779–91.
29. Seo JH, Fox JG, Peek RM, et al. *N*-methyl D-aspartate channels link ammonia and epithelial cell death mechanisms in *Helicobacter pylori* infection. Gastroenterology. 2011;141:2064–75.

30. Hagen SJ, Ohtani M, Zhou J-R, et al. Inflammation and foveolar hyperplasia are reduced by supplemental dietary glutamine during *Helicobacter pylori* infection in mice. J Nutr. 2009;139:912–8.
31. Al-Sadi RM, Ma TY. IL-1β causes an increase in intestinal epithelial tight junction permeability. J Immunol. 2007;178:4641–9.
32. Al-Sadi RM, Ye D, Dokladny K, et al. Mechanism of IL-1β-induced increase in intestinal epithelial tight junction permeability. J Immunol. 2008;180:5653–61.
33. Yamada H, Takeshi Y, Okabe S. Mechanism for *Helicobacter pylori* stimulation of interleukin-8 production in a gastric epithelial cell line (MKN 28): roles of mitogen-activated protein kinase and interleukin-1β. Biochem Pharmacol. 2001;61:1595–604.
34. Tu S, Bhagat G, Cui G, et al. Overexpression of interleukin-β induces gastric inflammation and cancer and mobilizes myeloid-derived supressor cells in mice. Cancer Cell. 2008;14:408–19.
35. Padol IT, Hunt RH. Effect of Th1 cytokines on acid secretion in pharmacology characterised gastric glands. Gut. 2004;53:1075–81.
36. Wischmeyer PE, Musch MM, Madonna MB, et al. Glutamine protects intestinal epithelial cells: role of inducible HSP70. Am J Physiol Gastrointest Liver Physiol. 1997;272:G879–84.
37. Kuzushita N, Rogers AB, Monti NA, et al. $p27^{kip1}$ deficiency confers susceptibility to gastric carcinogenesis in *Helicobacter pylori*-infected mice. Gastroenterology. 2005;129:1544–56.
38. Csibi A, Fendt S-M, Li C, et al. The mTORC1 pathway stimulates glutamine metabolism and cell proliferation by repressing SIRT4. Cell. 2013;153:840–54.
39. Xhou Z, Connell MC, MacEwan DJ. TNFR1-induced NF-kB, but not ERK, p38MAPK or JNK activation, mediates TNF-induced ICAM-1 and VCAM-1 expression on endothelial cells. Cell Signal. 2007;19:1238–48.
40. Hu S, Zhu X, Triggs JR, et al. Inflammation-induced, 3'-UTR-dependent translation inhibition of Hsp70 mRNA impairs intestinal homeostasis. Am J Physiol Gastrointest Liver Physiol. 2009;296(5):G1003–11.
41. Schliess F, Görg B, Fischer R, et al. Ammonia induces MK-801-sensitive nitration and phosphorylation of protein tyrosine residues in rat astrocytes. FASEB J. 2002;16:739–41.
42. Mendz GL, Hazell SL, Burns BP. The Entner-Doudoroff pathway in *Helicobacter pylori*. Arch Biochem Biophys. 1994;312:349–56.
43. Mendz GL, Hazell SL, Burns BP. Glucose ulilization by *Helicobacter pylori*. J Gen Microbiol. 1993;139:3023–8.
44. Mendz GL, Hazell SL. Glucose phosphorylation in *Helicobacter pylori*. Arch Biochem Biophys. 1993; 300:522–5.
45. Marais A, Mendz GL, Hazell SL, et al. Metabolism and genetics of *Helicobacter pylori*: the genome era. Microbiol Mol Biol Rev. 1999;63:642–74.
46. Rossi M, Bolz C, Revez J, et al. Evidence for conserved function of γ-glutamyltranspeptidase in *Helicobacter* genus. PLoS One. 2012;7:e30543.
47. Shibayama K, Wachino J, Arakawa Y, et al. Metabolism of glutamine and gluathione via gamma-glutamyltranspeptidase and glutamate transport in *Helicobacter pylori*: possible significance in the pathophysiology of the organism. Mol Microbiol. 2007;64:396–406.
48. Ki MR, Yun NR, Hwang SY. Glutamine-induced production and secretion of *Helicobacter pylori* gamma-glutamyltranspeptidase at low pH and its putative role in glutathione transport. J Microbiol Biotechnol. 2013;23: 467–72.
49. Kavermann H, Burns BP, Angermüller K, et al. Identification and characterization of *Helicobacter pylori* genes essential for gastric colonization. J Exp Med. 2003;197:813–22.
50. Burns BP, Hazell SL, Mendz GL, et al. The *Helicobacter pylori pyrB* gene encoding aspartate carbamoyltransferase is essential for bacterial survival. Arch Biochem Biophys. 2000;380:78–84.

Chapter 28
Small Intestinal Hypoxic Injury and Use of Arginyl-Glutamine Dipeptide: Applications to Pediatrics

Liya Ma, Nan Li, and Josef Neu

Key Points

- Hypoxia-associated small intestinal injury may occur in a variety of severe pathophysiologic conditions in pediatric patients such as perinatal asphyxia, shock, or other hypoxic–ischemic states.
- Hypoxic/ischemic injury of the bowel has been thought to be one of the main risk factors in term infants with necrotizing enterocolitis, which is one of the most common and devastating diseases in newborn infants.
- Pathogenesis of small intestinal hypoxic injury may include toxic oxygen-derived free radicals, inflammatory mediators, intestinal barrier damage, and vascular dysfunction.
- Glutamine and arginine deficiency may occur in very preterm and critically ill infants.
- Supplementation of glutamine and arginine has been shown to be helpful in reducing hypoxic small intestinal injury in animal and clinical studies.
- Arginyl-glutamine dipeptide combines theoretical benefits of both amino acids and has been shown safe and effective in a rodent model of hyperoxia-induced retinopathy, lung, and intestinal damage. It may have similar effects on hypoxic small intestinal injury. With the positive animal studies, it would be tempting to carry out control clinical studies in the future.

Keywords Small intestine • Hypoxic injury • Necrotizing enterocolitis • Arginine • Glutamine • Arginyl-glutamine • Dipeptide • Neonate

Abbreviations

Arg-Gln	Arginyl-glutamine
ELBW	Extremely low birth weights
ET-1	Endothelin-1
H/R	Hypoxia/reoxygenation

L. Ma, M.D.
Shenzhen Baoan Maternity and Child Health Hospital, Shenzhen, China
e-mail: maliya226@qq.com

N. Li, M.D. • J. Neu, M.D. (✉)
Department of Pediatrics, University of Florida, 1600 SW Archer Road, Gainesville, FL 32610, USA
e-mail: linan@peds.ufl.edu; neuj@peds.ufl.edu

R. Rajendram et al. (eds.), *Glutamine in Clinical Nutrition*, Nutrition and Health,
DOI 10.1007/978-1-4939-1932-1_28, © Springer Science+Business Media New York 2015

IL	Interleukin
LDH	Lactate dehydrogenase
NEC	Necrotizing enterocolitis
NICU	Neonatal intensive care units
NO	Nitric oxide
PAF	Platelet-activating factor
SIRS	Systemic inflammatory response syndrome
TNF	Tumor necrosis factor
TPN	Total parenteral nutrition
VLBW	Very low birth weight

Introduction

Premature infants are exposed to various perinatal stresses, including hypotension, hypoxia, hyperoxia, hypothermia, feeding, anemia, and umbilical vessel catheterization. Hypoxia-associated small intestinal injury may occur in a variety of severe pathophysiologic conditions in pediatric patients such as perinatal asphyxia, shock, or other hypoxic–ischemic states. It has been speculated that when such events occur, intestinal blood flow will diminish [1] via the diving seal reflex (reflex with circulatory shunting to selectively perfuse the brain, heart, and kidneys at the expense of other "nonvital" organs such as intestine and extremities), which can result in intestinal injury, systemic inflammatory response syndrome (SIRS), bacterial translocation, distal organ injury, and even multiple organ failure. Hypoxic intestinal injury-related diseases can have a profound impact on children's health. For example, necrotizing enterocolitis (NEC) is one of the most common and devastating diseases found in premature infants in neonatal intensive care units (NICU) with high mortality, long hospitalization, and high financial cost [2]. It can also affect distant organs such as the brain and place affected infants at substantially increased risk for neurodevelopmental delays. Although evidence shows that the most common form of NEC seen in preterm infants is not triggered by a primary hypoxic–ischemic event [3], hypoxic/ischemic injury of the bowel has been thought to be one of the main risk factors in term infants, especially those with congenital heart disease who have low blood flows to the gastrointestinal tract.

The possible mechanisms involved in hypoxia-mediated gut injury include inadequate tissue and cellular oxygen delivery, oxygen-derived toxic free radicals generating after reoxygenation/reperfusion, and the production of inflammatory mediators. Interventions to prevent hypoxic intestinal injury in animal and clinical researches include cytoprotective agent such as sucralfate [4], antiapoptotic factor such as insulin-like growth factor [5], antioxidants such as Ginkgo biloba extract [6], and so on. In this review, we will focus on the potential use of arginine, glutamine, and arginyl-glutamine (Arg-Gln) dipeptide to prevent and treat small intestinal hypoxic injury in pediatric patients especially in neonates.

Pathogenesis of Small Intestinal Hypoxic Injury (Fig. 28.1)

Hypoxia/Reoxygenation (H/R): The Role of Oxidative Stress

Oxidative stress plays an important role in the pathogenesis of small intestinal hypoxic injury [7]. Upon reoxygenation/reperfusion of ischemic intestine, reactive oxygen metabolites are generated and are responsible for both intestinal cell apoptosis (programmed cell death) and necrosis.

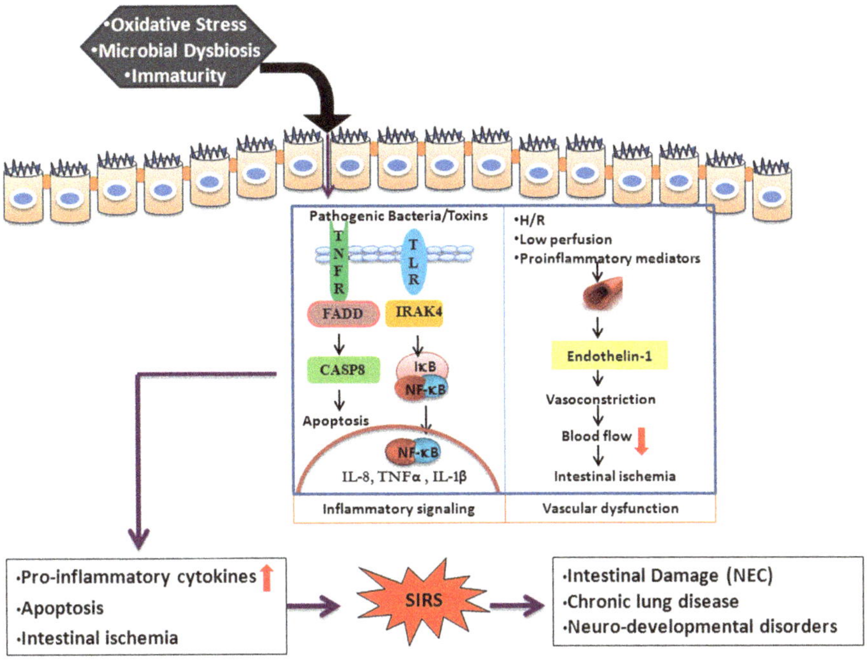

Fig. 28.1 Small intestinal injury induced by oxidative stress. Under oxidative or other stress conditions, disruption of epithelial integrity causes the pathogenic bacteria or toxin translocate through the epithelial barrier and activates TLRs. Activation of TLRs interact with adaptors to induce a cascade of signaling transduction, including activations of IRAKs, IκB/NFκB, and caspases-associated apoptosis. A translocation of NFκB from cytoplasm into nuclear may result in cytokine and chemokine production. In addition, hypoxia/reperfusion, low-flow perfusion, or pro-inflammatory mediators alter the ET-1–NO balance in favor of vasoconstriction, generating a cascade wherein ischemia rapidly extends into larger portions of the intestine. These changes may cause systematic inflammatory response syndrome, including necrotizing enterocolitis, chronic lung disease, and neurodevelopmental disorders

The involvement of oxidative stress or free radicals in gastrointestinal injury observed after H/R has been widely reported [7]. Previous study has demonstrated that the oxidant formation significantly increased right after 2–5 min of reperfusion of the ischemic intestine by using electron spin resonance spectrometry and low-level chemiluminescence [8]. Intestinal tissue malondialdehyde level, a product of lipid peroxidation, was increased after H/R-induced intestinal injury in a mice model [9].

Evidence that apoptosis is involved in this process includes an increase in intestinal apoptotic cells and products after H/R exposure and antiapoptosis interventions attenuating intestinal injury [5].

Intestinal Barrier Damage

Multiple defense layers against bacterial invasion comprise the whole intestinal barrier, including the mucus layer, the epithelium, and the underlying mucosal immune system. Intestinal epithelial cells produce pro-inflammatory cytokines and other mediators when stimulated, acting as both antigen processing and immune effector cells. Several factors related to H/R that may affect gut barrier integrity include enterocyte apoptosis, necrosis, and disruption of tight junctions. H/R itself can also directly impair intestinal cellular function by increasing monolayer permeability and decreasing trans epithelial electrical resistance values [10].

Inflammation

Animals exposed to hypoxia followed by hyperoxia resuscitation develop small intestinal edema, localized hemorrhagic necrosis, and extensive inflammation in intestinal tissue manifested by invasion of polymorphonuclear neutrophils and production of inflammatory mediators such as tumor necrosis factor (TNF), platelet-activating factor (PAF), leukotriene, and nitric oxide (NO) [11]. Anti-inflammatory agents can reduce intestinal injury induced by H/R in animal models [12]. Clinical studies have also shown that inflammatory mediators, such as TNF-α, interleukin(IL)-1, IL-6, IL-8, IL-12 and 18, PAF produced by enterocytes and inflammatory cells, contribute to the pathogenesis of NEC [13].

Intestinal Vascular Dysfunction

Regulation of vascular resistance is determined by a balance between the vasoconstrictor peptide endothelin-1 (ET-1) and the vasodilatory free radical NO produced by endothelial cells. In the newborn, this balance heavily favors vasodilation and thus blood and oxygen can be delivered to the rapidly growing intestine. However, factors disrupting endothelial cell function, such as hypoxia–ischemia/reperfusion, sustained low-flow perfusion, or pro-inflammatory mediators, alter the ET-1–NO balance in favor of vasoconstriction. The ET-1–NO interaction thereafter might facilitate rapid extension of this constriction, generating a cascade wherein ischemia rapidly extends into larger portions of the intestine. Evidence obtained from animal models and infant tissue with NEC implicates NO and ET-1 dysregulation in the pathogenesis of H/R injury, and a diminished NO production may be involved in the pathophysiology of NEC [14, 15]. It may be helpful to use approaches focused on maintaining the delicate balance favoring vasodilation in the newborn intestinal circulation in the prevention and treatment of H/R injury diseases like NEC.

Protective Effects of Glutamine or Arginine on Small Intestinal Hypoxic Injury

Glutamine in Early Life and Effects on Small Intestinal Injury

Glutamine is the predominant amino acid providing to the fetus through the placenta. For the healthy term newborn infant breastfed ad libitum, plasma glutamine concentrations normally increase during the first days of life and glutamine deficiency rarely occurs. For the very preterm and critically ill infants especially for those with intestinal injury, glutamine deficiency may become a significant issue. While normally present in the enteral diet, free glutamine is not a component of parenteral amino acid solutions because of low solubility and instability. Premature infants in the first weeks of life and infants with gut problems will receive most of their nutrients from glutamine-free parenteral nutrition solution [16], making them vulnerable to glutamine deficiency and related diseases. During catabolic stress, glutamine consumption rate would exceed the supply, and both plasma and skeletal muscle pools of free glutamine are severely reduced. Under catabolic conditions, premature and ill infants are not able to synthesize sufficient glutamine to meet demand, and glutamine becomes a conditionally essential amino acid. Low plasma concentrations of glutamine have been associated with a higher incidence of NEC [17].

As demonstrated by previous studies, mechanisms of glutamine action related to preventing H/R intestinal injury may include tissue protection [18], preservation of glutathione and antioxidant capacity [18], preservation of mucosal integrity [19] and intestinal barrier functions [20], anti-inflammation [12], decreased intestinal apoptosis [21], and enhancement of heat shock proteins [22]. Glutamine protects intestinal epithelial cells against H/R-induced apoptosis through increasing Bcl-2 expression [23]. In an infant rat pup-in-the-cup model, glutamine significantly decreased lipopolysaccharide-induced inflammatory mediators in the intestine, liver, and lung [24]. Therefore, there appears to be a strong relationship between gut-derived systemic inflammation and glutamine. The ability of glutamine to decrease gut-derived systemic inflammation has especially significant implications for premature infants.

Arginine in Early Life and Effects on Small Intestine Injury

Arginine is the substrate for NO synthesis, a potent vasodilator and anti-inflammatory. Arginine also serves as a precursor for the synthesis of other amino acids, including glutamine, and vice versa (Fig. 28.2). The hospitalized premature newborn experiences various stresses which increase the utilization of critical amino acids while simultaneously exceeding endogenous biosynthetic pathways [25].

Free arginine is provided in parenteral amino acid solutions. However, the amount administered may be inadequate to meet the needs of the critically ill premature or very low birth weight (VLBW) infants. In preterm infant formula, the recommended minimum and maximum concentrations of arginine are 72 mg/100 kcal and 104 mg/100 kcal, respectively [26]. These requirements are higher in stressed infants with higher utilization conditions such as NEC or pulmonary hypertension. The concentration of arginine found in the current formulas is 47–51 mg/100 kcal according to the manufacturer's specifications. Thus, preterm infants have low arginine intakes and levels. Low plasma arginine concentrations are associated with NEC [15, 17].

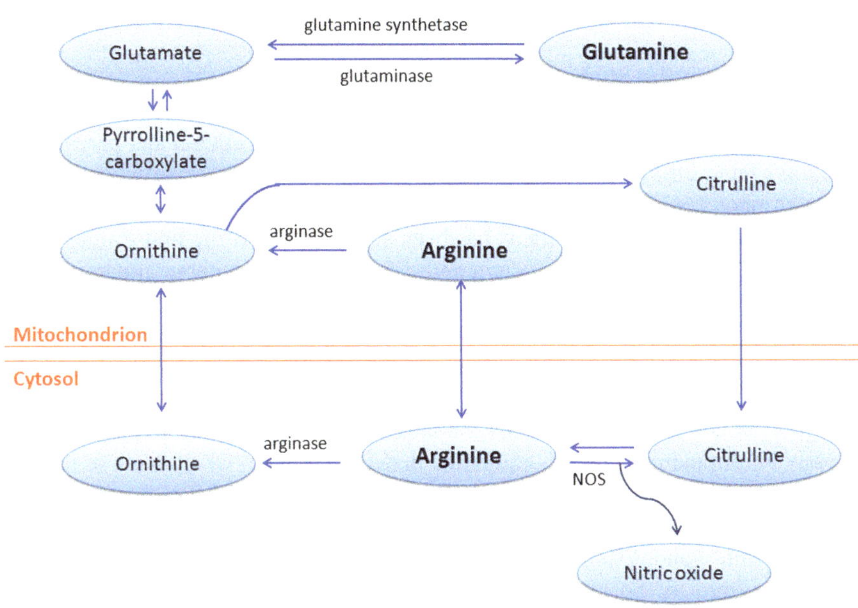

Fig. 28.2 Glutamine and arginine synthesis

Although there are conflicting data about increase of NO production in the presence of intestinal injury [27], NO has been known to be able to influence mucosal integrity, gut healing and blood pressure regulation, and intestinal blood flow regulation. Endogenous NO also plays a role in protection of the intestine from hypoxia-induced inflammation and injury [11]. Different from other organs, inhibition of NO synthesis increased intestinal lipid peroxidation in hypoxia-induced changes in newborn rats [28]. Arginine can protect intestinal epithelial integrity via a mechanism dependent on NO donation [28].

Animal Studies of Glutamine and Arginine on Hypoxic Intestinal Injury

NEC-like intestinal injury induced by H/R has been widely studied in animal models. In a H/R-induced experimental NEC model, glutamine oral supplementation reduced the histologic evidence of intestinal injury in young mice by inhibiting intestinal cytokine release [11]. Glutamine also has protective effects on ischemia/reperfusion-induced intestinal injury in animal models through attenuating neutrophil infiltration, P-selectin and ICAM-1 upregulation in the ileum, tyrosine residues nitration, PARP activation, NF-κB expression, apoptosis, and Bax and Bcl-2 expression [30].

As previously mentioned, arginine can protect intestinal hypoxic injury through NO donation. In a newborn mice model, supply of L-arginine increased tissue NO levels and reduced morphologic intestinal injury in mice with H/R [31]. Other animal studies also supported the protective effects of arginine on hypoxic intestinal injury [9].

Enteral glutamine supplementation alone or with arginine has favorable effects on oxidative stress in both experimental models of H/R and healthy newborn rats [32], suggesting that in premature neonates with inadequate oxidative resistance, glutamine and arginine supplementation may help prevent hypoxia-related diseases including NEC.

Clinical Studies of Glutamine and Arginine

Glutamine Supplementation Studies

Clinical studies in premature infants have proved the safety of both enteral and parenteral glutamine supplementation (Table 28.1). Because the majority VLBW infants receive most of their nutrition parenterally with poor feeding tolerance during the first several weeks of life, supplementation of glutamine parenterally in premature infants has been studied. One of the first studies was in 44 randomized low birth weight infants (birth weight 530–1,250 g) with or without glutamine supplementation via total parenteral nutrition (TPN) [33]. The results show that glutamine supplementation reduced days of TPN, shortened length of time to full enteral feedings, and decreased periods of ventilator support in the infants less than 800 g. The length of stay in the NICU also tends to be shorter. This study suggests that glutamine was safe and probably conditionally essential in extremely low birth weights (ELBW) premature infants. Another study was conducted to evaluate the safety and efficacy of early PN supplemented with glutamine in decreasing the risk of death or late-onset sepsis in a large multicenter, randomized, double-masked clinical trial in ELBW infants. Within 72 h of birth, infants between 401 and 1,000 g were randomized into either Troph Amine (control) group or 20 % glutamine isonitrogenous study amino acid solution group to receive PN up to 120 days of age, death, or discharge from the hospital. No significant adverse events were observed with glutamine supplementation. Glutamine had no effect on tolerance of enteral feeds, NEC, or growth [34].

Table 28.1 Randomized and controlled prospective glutamine clinical studies in infants and other pediatric patients

Participants	n	Amino acid	Dose and duration	Route	Outcome
VLBW preterm infants, Birth weight between 530 and 1,250 g [33]	44	Glutamine	20 % gln solution for more than 7 days	Parenteral	Shortened days of TPN, time to full enteral feedings, and periods of ventilator support in babies less than 800 g
ELBW infants, Birth weight between 401 and 1,000 g [34]	721	Glutamine	20 % gln solution for 120 days, or until death, discharge from the hospital	Parenteral	No effect on feeding tolerance, NEC, and growth
VLBW infants, Birth weight 500–1,250 g and gestational age 24–32 weeks [35]	68	Glutamine	From 0.08 to 0.31 g/kg/day for 11 days, then 0.3 g/kg/day for 16 days	Enterally by glutamine supplemented formula	Reduced hospital cost
VLBW infants, Birth weight 500–1,250 g and gestational age 24–32 weeks [36]	68	Glutamine	From 0.08 to 0.31 g/kg/day for 11 days, then 0.3 g/kg/day for 16 days	Enterally by glutamine supplemented formula	Decreased morbidity
Critically ill babies aged 1 month to 2 years in ICU [37]	9	Glutamine	0.3 g/kg/day for more than 5 days	Enteral	Well tolerated by critically ill infants and tended to be associated with less infectious morbidity and mortality
Preterm infants, Birth weight no more than 1,500 g [38]	69	Glutamine	0.3 g/kg/day for 4 months	Enteral	Improved growth with higher mean weight, length, head circumference, left upper mid-arm, and left mid-thigh circumference
VLBW infants, Gestational age <32 weeks and/or birth weight <1,500 g [39]	88	Glutamine	0.3 g/kg/day for 27 days	Enteral	Decreased the risk of atopic dermatitis and gastrointestinal tract infections at 6 years of age
VLBW infants, Gestational age <32 weeks [40]	52	Glutamine	0.3 g/kg/day for 27 days	Enteral	Improved brain development with increased white matter, hippocampus, and brain stem volumes at 6 years of age
VLBW infants less than 7 days old [41]	649	Glutamine	0.3 g/kg/day for 28 days	Enteral	Less often had gastrointestinal dysfunction
Preterm infants less than 34 weeks and 2,000 g [42]	101	Glutamine	0.3 g/kg/day for no more than 30 days	Enteral	Decreased intestinal permeability and NEC/septicemia
VLBW infants gestational age <32 weeks or birth weight <1,500 g [43]	102	Glutamine	0.3 g/kg/day Between day 3 and day 30 of life	Enteral	Did not alter plasma levels of glutamine, glutamate, or other amino acids. Safe for VLBW infants
VLBW neonates, Birth weight 580–1,250 g, gestational age 26–32 week [57]	55	Glutamine dipeptide	20 % of total amino acid From day 4 to day 14	Enteral	Decreased the incidence of NEC, but did not affect the incidence of hospital-acquired sepsis, the length of NICU stay, and total time of hospitalization

The methods used in this study have been questioned [16], but because of the largely negative results, it will be unlikely that a similar study with more appropriate controls will be repeated.

Since the fetus comes from an environment where approximately 450 mL of amniotic fluid is swallowed daily, postnatally even the premature infant is capable of tolerating at least small volumes of enteral intake. Based on this rationale, studies have been done to investigate the efficacy of glutamine using the enteral route to deliver glutamine to preterm. In premature or VLBW infants, glutamine supplementation enterally administered has been reported to reduce hospital costs [35], decrease morbidity [36], be well tolerated in critically ill infants, and tended to be associated with less infectious morbidity and mortality in this high-risk population [37]. Other studies have suggested long-term benefits of enteral glutamine supplementation in neonatal period including improvements in growth [38], decrease in the risk of atopic dermatitis and gastrointestinal tract infections at childhood [39], and improvements in brain development at school age mediated by a decrease in serious neonatal infections [40]. In a multicenter clinical trial, with 649 VLBW infants less than 7 days old involved, neonates supplied with glutamine at a dose of 0.3 g/kg/day enterally for the first 28 days less often had gastrointestinal dysfunction, indicating gut protective effect of glutamine [41]. Recently Sevastiadou and coworkers reported a placebo-controlled randomized trial about the impact of oral glutamine supplementation on the intestinal permeability and incidence of NEC/septicemia in premature neonates. One hundred and one preterm neonates with gestational age <34 weeks and birth weight <2,000 g were recruited. Oral glutamine supplementation with 0.3 g/kg/day for no more than 30 days results in decreased intestinal permeability and less NEC/septicemia [42].

The benefit of using the enteral route is that more glutamine can be delivered directly to the intestine when exposed to hypoxia, where it may reach a concentration of >20 mM and can be rapidly used by the intestinal epithelium. Intravenous infusions rarely result in plasma (basolateral) concentration of more than 1 mM, which is also proved by study in which no differences were shown between groups for plasma concentrations of glutamine during the enteral supplementation of glutamine [43]. Panigrahi et al. reported that glutamine decreased bacterial translocation when supplied by the apical versus the basolateral route (mucosal and arterial supplies, respectively) using Caco-2 monolayers [44]. It is not clear if the enteral route offers a greater capability to modulate inflammation. However, enteral supplementation could reduce the amount taken up from the arterial supply by the intestine, therefore leaving more substrates, including essential amino acids for nonsplanchnic organs.

A recent Cochrane review identified 11 randomized and a total of 2,771 preterm infants participated controlled trials [45]. Five of them evaluated enteral glutamine supplementation and six of them evaluated parenteral glutamine supplementation. Glutamine supplementation did not show a significant effect on mortality [typical relative risk 0.98 (95 % confidence interval 0.80–1.18); risk difference 0.00 (95 % confidence interval −0.03–0.02)] or major neonatal morbidities including the incidence of invasive infection or NEC by meta-analysis. It is concluded that the available trial data do not provide evidence that glutamine supplementation provides significant benefits for preterm infants. In another review related to glutamine randomized studies in early life, the author also concluded that "although apparently safe in animal models (pups), premature infants, and critically ill children, glutamine supplementation does not reduce mortality or late-onset sepsis, and its routine use cannot be recommended in these sensitive populations. Large prospectively stratified trials are needed" [46]. Based on the controversial results, some investigators suggest that further study in this area is no longer necessary. However, in van Zwol's review, more recent research in the area of glutamine supplementation is described and the authors suggest additional studies are still warranted [47], especially with a suggestion for neurodevelopmental benefits.

In summary, studies done so far have suggested that in infants glutamine supplementation is safe both enterally and parenterally. However, the results for efficacy on a limited number of outcomes have been controversial. The use of glutamine alone has not become routine. In infants and critically ill children, the effects are unknown since less data is available during childhood.

Table 28.2 Randomized and controlled prospective arginine clinical studies in infants and other pediatric patients

Participants	*n*	Amino acid	Dose and duration	Route	Outcome
Preterm infants Birth weight ≤1,250 g and gestational age ≤32 week [48]	152	L-arginine	1.5 mmol/kg/day First 28 days of life	Enteral or parenteral	Reduced the incidence of all stages of NEC
Preterm infants Birth weight ≤1,250 g at 36 months adjusted age [51]	132	L-arginine	1.5 mmol/kg/day First 28 days of life	Enteral or parenteral	A long-term evaluation for about study at 36 months adjusted age. L-arginine did not increase neurodevelopmental disability
VLBW infants Birth weight ≤1,500 g and gestational age ≤34 week [52]	83	L-arginine	1.5 mmol/kg/day bid Between 3rd and 28th day of life	Enteral	Safe for VLBW neonates Reduced the incidence of stage III NEC

Arginine Supplementation Studies

Arginine supplementation has been reported to decrease the incidence of NEC in several studies (Table 28.2). In an earlier randomized, double-blind, placebo-controlled study reported in 2002 with 152 premature neonates <32 weeks and <1,250 g involved, supplementation of L-arginine (1.5 mmol/kg per day) with oral feeds/parenteral nutrition during the first 28 days of life increased blood level of arginine at 14 and 28 days of age and reduced the incidence of all stages of NEC [48]. This study is also regarded as the only eligible one by Shah et al. in the Cochrane reviews in both 2004 and 2007 [49, 50]. The reviewers concluded that multicenter randomized controlled studies of arginine supplementation in preterm neonates are needed, focusing on the incidence of NEC, stage 2 or 3. A long-term study was done in this same group of patients at 36 months adjusted age by the same group of investigators. They demonstrated that L-arginine supplementation for prevention of NEC in premature infants did not increase neurodevelopmental disability in later life [51]. Recently Polycarpou et al. [52] conducted a parallel blind randomized pilot study, comprising VLBW infants with birth weight ≤1,500 g and gestational age ≤34 weeks. In this study, 40 neonates received enteral L-arginine supplementation (1.5 mmol/kg per day, bid) and 43 neonates received placebo between the 3rd and 28th day of life. No adverse effects were reported in infants receiving L-arginine supplementation. Arginine supplementation significantly reduced the incidence of NEC stage III (2.5 % vs. 18.6 %).

In conclusion, available data indicates that arginine supplementation in premature neonates is safe and appears to decrease the incidence of NEC in VLBW infants. However, larger multicenter studies are needed to further access the effect of arginine supplementation in preventing NEC in VLBW infants.

Use of Arg-Gln Dipeptide to Protect Small Intestine from Hypoxic or Hyperoxic Injury

Glutamine or arginine as an individual amino acid each has its own advantages in the prevention of intestinal injury; however, they both also have limitations. Low solubility (35 g/L at 20 °C) and instability during heat sterilization and prolonged storage limit the use of free glutamine in the routine clinical setting. Thus it would be desirable to search for alternative substrates to overcome the drawbacks of free glutamine and integrate the advantages of both amino acids. Arg-Gln dipeptide is such an agent. Glutamine-containing dipeptide is an aqueous stable source of glutamine with greater solubility compared with individual amino acid [53]. It is stable under heat sterilization. There is a theoretical advantage of improved absorption of the dipeptide compared with single amino acids by virtue of oligopeptide transporters located in the intestinal brush border membrane in both the small and large intestine [54].

As the glutamine carrier, several glutamine dipeptides such as alanyl-glutamine [55] and glycyl-glutamine [56] have been used to study various diseases in animal models and in human trials that supported its safety and efficacy. In a pilot study, standard amino acid solution with an addition of glutamine dipeptide (20 % of total amount of amino acids) from day 4 to day 14 among VLBW neonates increased blood levels of glutamine and decreased the incidence of NEC compared with control group [57]. In other clinical studies, nitrogen balance was shown to be more positive in catabolic patients receiving a glutamine-containing dipeptide, L-alanyl-L-glutamine solution than in control patients receiving isonitrogenous, isoenergetic TPN [58].

Arg-Gln dipeptide, containing both glutamine and arginine (Structure 28.1), should be able to exert the effects of both amino acids. Several animal studies have shown that intraperitoneal or oral administration of Arg-Gln dipeptide reduced abnormal retinal neovascularization and vascular leakage, pulmonary or intestinal injury induced by hyperoxia in neonatal mice model [59–61].

Premature newborns often need high concentrations of oxygen. However, hyperoxia could be considered as an oxidative stress condition that affects the development of the intestine [62]. By using a hyperoxia-induced retinopathy mouse model, a study was conducted to evaluate the effect of the dipeptide Arg-Gln on levels of vascular endothelial cell growth factor (VEGF) in primary human retinal pigment epithelial cell cultures and on retinal neovascularization in mice [59]. Arg-Gln significantly reduced retinal neovascularization in the oxygen-induced retinopathy mouse model. This effect was associated with a decreased retinal VEGF mRNA levels. Similarly, Arg-Gln decreased VEGF expression in human retinal pigment epithelial cells, a retinal cell type likely to respond to retinal hypoxia by expressing VEGF. Dipeptide Arg-Gln appears to be safe and may prove beneficial in the prevention of retinopathy of prematurity with future human infants studies [59]. In the same mouse hyperoxia model, which produces hyperoxia-induced lung injury, Arg-Gln prevented the development of important indicator of lung injury, including histologic changes, myeloperoxidase, lactate dehydrogenase (LDH), and inflammatory cytokines IL-6 and C-X-C motif ligand 1/keratinocyte-derived chemokine. This beneficial effect of Arg-Gln on the reversal of oxygen-induced lung injury was associated with restoration of levels of nuclear factor-kappaB inhibitor. These results suggested that Arg-Gln is a promising nutritional adjunct that may prevent lung damage due to oxygen toxicity in infants [61]. In a similar hyperoxic intestinal injury study, mice exposed to hyperoxia then room air

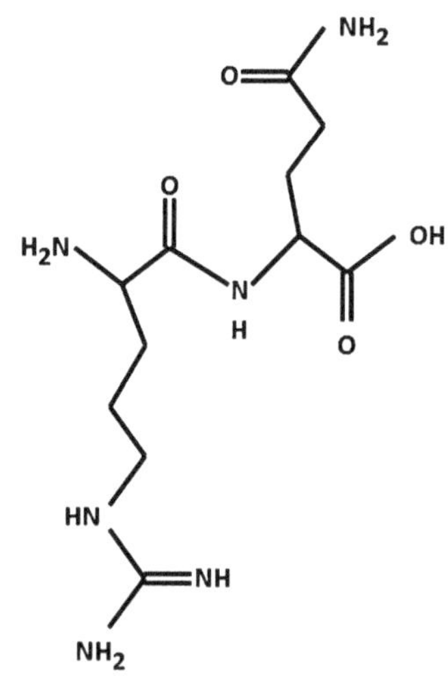

Structure 28.1 Arginyl-glutamine dipeptide

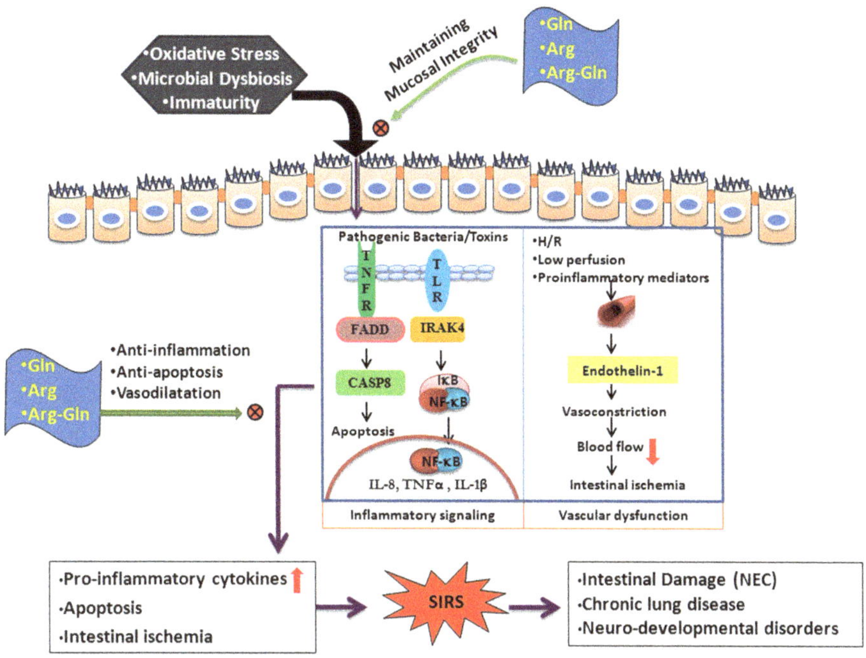

Fig. 28.3 Effects of glutamine, arginine, and Arg-Gln dipeptide on small intestinal injury. Glutamine, arginine, or Arg-Gln dipeptide supplementations show beneficial effects in small intestinal injury by maintaining mucosal integrity, anti-inflammation, antiapoptosis, and vasodilatation

showed a greater distortion of overall villus structure with higher injury scores. Arg-Gln supplementation groups were more similar to the room air control group. Arg-Gln inhibited hyperoxia-induced myeloperoxidase activity and returned LDH activity to levels of control. In addition, Arg-Gln reversed hyperoxia-induced apoptotic cell death in distal small intestine, suggesting that supplementation of Arg-Gln may limit certain inflammatory and apoptotic processes involved in hyperoxic-induced intestinal injury in neonatal mice [60]. It may have similar effects on hypoxic small intestinal injury. With the positive animal studies, it would be tempting to carry out control clinical studies in the future. Figure 28.3 illustrates effects of glutamine, arginine, and dipeptide Arg-Gln on small intestinal injury.

Conclusions

Supplementation of glutamine or arginine may protect small intestinal hypoxic injury through preservation of glutathione and antioxidant capacity, preservation of mucosal integrity and intestinal barrier functions, anti-inflammation, decreased intestinal apoptosis, and decreasing vascular dysfunction (Fig. 28.3).

Glutamine and arginine have been shown to provide benefit in several models of intestinal injury and both are safe in infants. However, the use of each amino acid alone has not become routine since the results for efficacy on a limited number of outcomes have been controversial. The long-term effects of glutamine on neurodevelopment in preterm infants should prompt additional scrutiny.

Combining these two amino acids as a dipeptide has several theoretical benefits, and preliminary studies support that it is safe and effective in a rodent model of hyperoxia-induced retinopathy, lung, and intestinal damage. It may have similar effects on hypoxic small intestinal injury. With the positive animal studies, it would be tempting to carry out control clinical studies in the future.

References

1. Koc E, Arsan S, Ozcan H, et al. The effect of asphyxia on gut blood flow in term neonates. Indian J Pediatr. 1998;65(2):297–302.
2. Neu J, Walker WA. Necrotizing enterocolitis. N Engl J Med. 2011;364(3):255–64.
3. Young CM, Kingma SD, Neu J. Ischemia-reperfusion and neonatal intestinal injury. J Pediatr. 2011;158(2 Suppl):e25–8.
4. Sencan AB, Sencan A, Aktas S, et al. Treatment and prophylaxis with sucralfate ameliorates hypoxia/reoxygenation-induced intestinal injury in pup rats. Med Sci Monit. 2005;11(4):BR126–30.
5. Ozen S, Akisu M, Baka M, et al. Insulin-like growth factor attenuates apoptosis and mucosal damage in hypoxia/reoxygenation-induced intestinal injury. Biol Neonate. 2005;87(2):91–6.
6. Ozdemir OM, Ergin H, Yenisey C, et al. Protective effects of Ginkgo biloba extract in rats with hypoxia/reoxygenation-induced intestinal injury. J Pediatr Surg. 2011;46(4):685–90.
7. Sasaki M, Joh T. Oxidative stress and ischemia-reperfusion injury in gastrointestinal tract and antioxidant, protective agents. J Clin Biochem Nutr. 2007;40(1):1–12.
8. Turrens JF, Giulivi C, Pinus C, et al. Low level chemiluminescence from isolated rat hepatocytes, intact lung and intestine in situ. Basic Life Sci. 1988;49:239–42.
9. Kabaroglu C, Akisu M, Habif S, et al. Effects of L-arginine and L-carnitine in hypoxia/reoxygenation-induced intestinal injury. Pediatr Int. 2005;47(1):10–4.
10. Xu DZ, Lu Q, Kubicka R, et al. The effect of hypoxia/reoxygenation on the cellular function of intestinal epithelial cells. J Trauma. 1999;46(2):280–5.
11. Caplan MS, Hedlund E, Hill N, et al. The role of endogenous nitric oxide and platelet-activating factor in hypoxia-induced intestinal injury in rats. Gastroenterology. 1994;106(2):346–52.
12. Akisu M, Baka M, Huseyinov A, et al. The role of dietary supplementation with L-glutamine in inflammatory mediator release and intestinal injury in hypoxia/reoxygenation-induced experimental necrotizing enterocolitis. Ann Nutr Metab. 2003;47(6):262–6.
13. Markel TA, Crisostomo PR, Wairiuko GM, et al. Cytokines in necrotizing enterocolitis. Shock. 2006;25(4):329–37.
14. Gellen B, Kovacs J, Nemeth L, et al. Vascular changes play a role in the pathogenesis of necrotizing enterocolitis in asphyxiated newborn pigs. Pediatr Surg Int. 2003;19(5):380–4.
15. Richir MC, Siroen MP, van Elburg RM, et al. Low plasma concentrations of arginine and asymmetric dimethylarginine in premature infants with necrotizing enterocolitis. Br J Nutr. 2007;97(5):906–11.
16. Neu J. Glutamine supplements in premature infants: why and how. J Pediatr Gastroenterol Nutr. 2003;37(5):533–5.
17. Becker RM, Wu G, Galanko JA, et al. Reduced serum amino acid concentrations in infants with necrotizing enterocolitis. J Pediatr. 2000;137(6):785–93.
18. Neu J, Li N. Pathophysiology of glutamine and glutamate metabolism in premature infants. Curr Opin Clin Nutr Metab Care. 2007;10(1):75–9.
19. Li J, Langkamp-Henken B, Suzuki K, et al. Glutamine prevents parenteral nutrition-induced increases in intestinal permeability. JPEN J Parenter Enteral Nutr. 1994;18(4):303–7.
20. Li N, Neu J. Glutamine deprivation alters intestinal tight junctions via a PI3-K/Akt mediated pathway in Caco-2 cells. J Nutr. 2009;139(4):710–4.
21. Ban K, Kozar RA. Glutamine protects against apoptosis via downregulation of Sp3 in intestinal epithelial cells. Am J Physiol Gastrointest Liver Physiol. 2010;299(6):G1344–53.
22. Wischmeyer PE, Musch MW, Madonna MB, et al. Glutamine protects intestinal epithelial cells: role of inducible HSP70. Am J Physiol. 1997;272(4 Pt 1):G879–84.
23. Yuan ZQ, Zhang Y, Li XL, et al. HSP70 protects intestinal epithelial cells from hypoxia/reoxygenation injury via a mechanism that involves the mitochondrial pathways. Eur J Pharmacol. 2010;643(2–3):282–8.
24. Li N, Liboni K, Fang MZ, et al. Glutamine decreases lipopolysaccharide-induced intestinal inflammation in infant rats. Am J Physiol Gastrointest Liver Physiol. 2004;286(6):G914–21.
25. Wu G, Jaeger LA, Bazer FW, et al. Arginine deficiency in preterm infants: biochemical mechanisms and nutritional implications. J Nutr Biochem. 2004;15(8):442–51.
26. Klein CJ. Nutrient requirements for preterm infant formulas. J Nutr. 2002;132(6 Suppl 1):1395S–577S.
27. Chokshi NK, Guner YS, Hunter CJ, et al. The role of nitric oxide in intestinal epithelial injury and restitution in neonatal necrotizing enterocolitis. Semin Perinatol. 2008;32(2):92–9.
28. Kilic I, Kilic BA, Guven C, et al. Role of nitric oxide in hypoxia-induced changes in newborn rats. Biol Neonate. 2000;78(3):191–7.
29. Chapman JC, Liu Y, Zhu L, et al. Arginine and citrulline protect intestinal cell monolayer tight junctions from hypoxia-induced injury in piglets. Pediatr Res. 2012;72(6):576–82.

30. Mondello S, Galuppo M, Mazzon E, et al. Glutamine treatment attenuates the development of ischaemia/reperfusion injury of the gut. Eur J Pharmacol. 2010;643(2–3):304–15.
31. Cintra AE, Martins JL, Patricio FR, et al. Nitric oxide levels in the intestines of mice submitted to ischemia and reperfusion: L-arginine effects. Transplant Proc. 2008;40(3):830–5.
32. Kul M, Vurucu S, Demirkaya E, et al. Enteral glutamine and/or arginine supplementation have favorable effects on oxidative stress parameters in neonatal rat intestine. J Pediatr Gastroenterol Nutr. 2009;49(1):85–9.
33. Lacey JM, Crouch JB, Benfell K, et al. The effects of glutamine-supplemented parenteral nutrition in premature infants. JPEN J Parenter Enteral Nutr. 1996;20(1):74–80.
34. Poindexter BB, Ehrenkranz RA, Stoll BJ, et al. Parenteral glutamine supplementation does not reduce the risk of mortality or late-onset sepsis in extremely low birth weight infants. Pediatrics. 2004;113(5):1209–15.
35. Dallas MJ, Bowling D, Roig JC, et al. Enteral glutamine supplementation for very-low-birth-weight infants decreases hospital costs. JPEN J Parenter Enteral Nutr. 1998;22(6):352–6.
36. Neu J, Roig JC, Meetze WH, et al. Enteral glutamine supplementation for very low birth weight infants decreases morbidity. J Pediatr. 1997;131(5):691–9.
37. Barbosa E, Moreira EA, Goes JE, et al. Pilot study with a glutamine-supplemented enteral formula in critically ill infants. Revista do Hospital das Clinicas. 1999;54(1):21–4.
38. Korkmaz A, Yurdakok M, Yigit S, et al. Long-term enteral glutamine supplementation in very low birth weight infants: effects on growth parameters. Turk J Pediatr. 2007;49(1):37–44.
39. van Zwol A, Moll HA, Fetter WP, et al. Glutamine-enriched enteral nutrition in very low birthweight infants and allergic and infectious diseases at 6 years of age. Paediatr Perinat Epidemiol. 2011;25(1):60–6.
40. de Kieviet JF, Oosterlaan J, Vermeulen RJ, et al. Effects of glutamine on brain development in very preterm children at school age. Pediatrics. 2012;130(23071202):1121–7.
41. Vaughn P, Thomas P, Clark R, et al. Enteral glutamine supplementation and morbidity in low birth weight infants. J Pediatr. 2003;142(6):662–8.
42. Sevastiadou S, Malamitsi-Puchner A, Costalos C, et al. The impact of oral glutamine supplementation on the intestinal permeability and incidence of necrotizing enterocolitis/septicemia in premature neonates. J Matern Fetal Neonatal Med. 2011;24(21463215):1294–300.
43. van den Berg A, van Elburg RM, Teerlink T, et al. A randomized controlled trial of enteral glutamine supplementation in very low birth weight infants: plasma amino acid concentrations. J Pediatr Gastroenterol Nutr. 2005;41(1):66–71.
44. Panigrahi P, Gewolb IH, Bamford P, et al. Role of glutamine in bacterial transcytosis and epithelial cell injury. JPEN J Parenter Enteral Nutr. 1997;21(2):75–80.
45. Moe-Byrne T, Wagner JV, McGuire W. Glutamine supplementation to prevent morbidity and mortality in preterm infants. Cochrane Database Syst Rev. 2012;3:CD001457.
46. Briassouli E, Briassoulis G. Glutamine randomized studies in early life: the unsolved riddle of experimental and clinical studies. Clin Dev Immunol. 2012;2012:749189.
47. van Zwol A, Neu J, van Elburg RM. Long-term effects of neonatal glutamine-enriched nutrition in very-low-birth-weight infants. Nutr Rev. 2011;69(1):2–8.
48. Amin HJ, Zamora SA, McMillan DD, et al. Arginine supplementation prevents necrotizing enterocolitis in the premature infant. J Pediatr. 2002;140(4):425–31.
49. Shah P, Shah V. Arginine supplementation for prevention of necrotising enterocolitis in preterm infants. Cochrane Database Syst Rev. 2004;4:CD004339.
50. Shah P, Shah V. Arginine supplementation for prevention of necrotising enterocolitis in preterm infants. Cochrane Database Syst Rev. 2007;3:CD004339.
51. Amin HJ, Soraisham AS, Sauve RS. Neurodevelopmental outcomes of premature infants treated with l-arginine for prevention of necrotising enterocolitis. J Paediatr Child Health. 2009;45(4):219–23.
52. Polycarpou E, Zachaki S, Tsolia M, et al. Enteral L-arginine supplementation for prevention of necrotizing enterocolitis in very low birth weight neonates: a double-blind randomized pilot study of efficacy and safety. JPEN J Parenter Enteral Nutr. 2013;37:617.
53. Furst P. New developments in glutamine delivery. J Nutr. 2001;131(9 Suppl):2562S–8S.
54. Adibi SA. The oligopeptide transporter (Pept-1) in human intestine: biology and function. Gastroenterology. 1997;113(1):332–40.
55. Tazuke Y, Wasa M, Shimizu Y, Wang HS, et al. Alanyl-glutamine-supplemented parenteral nutrition prevents intestinal ischemia-reperfusion injury in rats. JPEN J Parenter Enteral Nutr. 2003;27(2):110–5.
56. Jiang JW, Zheng SS, Xue F, et al. Enteral feeding of glycyl-glutamine dipeptide improves the structure and absorptive function of the small intestine after allogenetic liver transplantation in rats. Hepatobiliary Pancreat Dis Int. 2006;5(2):199–204.
57. Bober-Olesinska K, Kornacka MK. Effects of glutamine supplemented parenteral nutrition on the incidence of necrotizing enterocolitis, nosocomial sepsis and length of hospital stay in very low birth weight infants. Med Wieku Rozwoj. 2005;9(3 Pt 1):325–33.

58. Furst P, Albers S, Stehle P. Glutamine-containing dipeptides in parenteral nutrition. JPEN J Parenter Enteral Nutr. 1990;14(4 Suppl):118S–24S.
59. Neu J, Afzal A, Pan H, et al. The dipeptide Arg-Gln inhibits retinal neovascularization in the mouse model of oxygen-induced retinopathy. Invest Ophthalmol Vis Sci. 2006;47(7):3151–5.
60. Li N, Ma L, Liu X, et al. Arginyl-glutamine dipeptide or docosahexaenoic acid attenuates hyperoxia-induced small intestinal injury in neonatal mice. J Pediatr Gastroenterol Nutr. 2012;54(4):499–504.
61. Ma L, Li N, Liu X, et al. Arginyl-glutamine dipeptide or docosahexaenoic acid attenuate hyperoxia-induced lung injury in neonatal mice. Nutrition. 2012;28(11–12):1186–91.
62. Giannone PJ, Bauer JA, Schanbacher BL, et al. Effects of hyperoxia on postnatal intestinal development. Biotech Histochem. 2007;82(1):17–22.

Chapter 29
Dipeptide-Bound Glutamine and the Intestinal Microcirculation in Sepsis

Nadia A. Al-Banna and Christian Lehmann

Key Points

- Glutamine is a conditionally essential amino acid for critically ill patients.
- Intestinal microcirculatory dysfunction is a key factor in the development of sepsis.
- Proposed mechanisms by which glutamine affects intestinal microcirculation include effects on functional capillary density, microvascular integrity, leukocyte rolling, and adherence to intestinal microcirculation.
- Glutamine also influences the expression of adhesion molecules, and production of cytokines, oxidation stress and nitric oxide-related mechanisms, heat shock proteins and other effectors.
- Glutamine should be examined in the future as a therapeutic strategy for patients with sepsis.

Keywords Glutamine • Sepsis • Intestinal microcirculation • Leukocytes • Endothelium

Abbreviations

AlaGln	L-alanyl-L-glutamine dipeptide
CAM	Cell adhesion molecules
CASP	Colon ascendens stent peritonitis
CCL	Chemokine CC ligand
CLP	Cecal ligation peritonitis

N.A. Al-Banna, Ph.D.
Department of Pharmacology, Dalhousie University,
5850 College Street, Tupper Medical Building, Lab 6H, Halifax, NS, Canada B3H 1X5
e-mail: Nadia.al-banna@dal.ca; Nadiaali_99@yahoo.com

C. Lehmann, M.D., Ph.D., F.R.C.P.C. (✉)
Department of Anesthesia, Pain Management and Perioperative Medicine, QE II Health Sciences Centre,
Dalhousie University, 10 West Victoria, 1276 South Park St., Halifax, NS, Canada B3H 2Y9

Department of Pharmacology & Microbiology and Immunology, Dalhousie University,
10 West Victoria, 1276 South Park St., Halifax, NS, Canada B3H 2Y9

Department of Anesthesiology and Operative Intensive Care Medicine, Charité - Universitätsmedizin,
Berlin, Germany
e-mail: chlehmann@dal.ca; chlehmann@mac.com

R. Rajendram et al. (eds.), *Glutamine in Clinical Nutrition*, Nutrition and Health,
DOI 10.1007/978-1-4939-1932-1_29,

DIP	L-alanyl-L-glutamine dipeptide
DSS	Dextran sodium sulfate
FCD	Functional capillary density
GLN or Gln	Glutamine
HSP	Heat shock proteins
HUVECs	Human umbilical vein endothelial cells
ICAM-1	Intracellular adhesion molecule-1
ICU	Intensive care unit
IL	Interleukin
iNOS	Inducible nitric oxide synthase
LPS	Lipopolysaccharide
MAdCam-1	Mucosal addressin cell adhesion molecule-1
MOF	Multiorgan failure
NO	Nitric oxide
PMNs	Polymorphonuclear neutrophils
TNBS	Trinitrobenezene sulfonic acid
TNF	Tumor necrosis factor

Introduction: Glutamine in Sepsis

Glutamine is made from glutamine and ammonia through a biochemical reaction, catalyzed by enzyme glutamine synthetase [1]. In fact, GLN is crucial in the regulation of amino acid homeostasis. GLN provides the amide-group required for the synthesis of metabolites, such as the amino-sugars, purines, pyrimidines and nucleotides. In addition, Gln is an important nutrient for rapidly proliferating cells, including enterocytes and lymphocytes [2]. The relevance of GLN is also related to enhancing the availability of these metabolites, e.g. the synthesis of the antioxidant glutathione, and the synthesis of citrulline and arginine [3], and the resultant production of the vasodilator nitric oxide.

Depletion of endogenous GLN stores has been reported. During clinical sepsis, intracellular levels of GLN are reduced by ~50 % and plasma levels by ~20 % [4]. During endotoxemia, glutamine utilization is reduced in mucosal cells [5]. Similarly in rats treated with interleukin-1, the uptake of GLN is reduced and the metabolism of GLN is lowered by 25 % [6]. Consequently, the metabolism of GLN metabolites, namely glutathione, and cysteine, is affected in patients with sepsis [7, 8]. This leads to a number of events including a decreased radical defense, suppressed immune response, a delayed wound healing, intestinal hyperpermeability and enhanced bacterial translocation. Because of the insufficient metabolism of GLN, the depletion of its endogenous stores and the increased demand during tissue injury, GLN becomes “conditionally essential” for critically ill patients [2, 9].

Therefore, the use of GLN supplementation by the parenteral route has been suggested in order to counteract the demand for GLN and its metabolites in patients [10], and in rats [11]. GLN administration is recommended (grade A) whenever ICU patients require parenteral nutrition [12]. The administration of GLN has been reported to improve intestinal barrier, reduce the frequency of infections, control the inflammatory response, and result in better prognosis for patients with critical illnesses [13, 14]. Studies have considered the administration of L-alanyl-L-glutamine (AlaGln) for improved stability of GLN in ready-to-use solutions to replace GLN in tissues, as shown in rats [11]. The administration of AlaGln with total parenteral nutrition was shown to provide Gln in a stable form and replenish the decline in Gln that was induced in skeletal muscles after surgical trauma [15]. The use of this form of GLN, L-alanyl-L-glutamine dipeptide, in total parenteral nutrition was shown to reduce infectious morbidities and glucose intolerance in critically ill patients [16, 17].

Importance of Intestinal Microcirculation in Sepsis

Sepsis, and the systemic inflammation associated with septic shock represent the most frequent cause of mortality among patients of the surgical intensive care units [18]. During sepsis, the functional and structural microvascular changes present in the intestine are reported in the early stages and are more prominent in most severely ill patients [19–23]. These disturbances in the microcirculation are known to contribute to the pathogenesis of intestinal inflammation. The intestinal microcirculation participates in several processes such as hypoperfusion/ischemia, increased leukocyte recruitment, platelet adhesion, edema, remodeling of the vascular bed, and ulceration/tissue necrosis [24, 25]. Earlier studies illustrated the reduced microvascular volume as an indication of ischemia in patients with segmental Crohn's disease, by assessing the microvasculature using microradiography after barium perfusion [26].

An association between leukocyte recruitment and endothelial changes has been made by Goddard and colleagues, who showed a prolonged capillary transit time and a retention of leukocytes in the coronary capillaries in endotoxemia models of sepsis [27]. Thus, the structural changes of the coronary endothelial cells might contribute to the inflammatory process [28]. In fact, one of the significant sequelaes in intestinal inflammation is tissue hypoxia, which leads to a breakdown of the mucosal barrier function and increased bacterial translocation (via transcellular and/or paracellular route) [29]. Because the loss of mucosal integrity induces a multitude of events, including bacterial translocation and leukocyte activation, it is considered the driving force in the pathogenesis of sepsis [30]. The immune response triggered by the presence of the bacteria from the gut involves the recruitment of leukocytes, through a process of tethering, rolling, adhesion and transmigration [31].

In addition, the increased adhesion and transmigration of leukocytes induced by intestinal inflammation is associated with changes in the blood flow in the microcirculation, such as slowing of the velocity of flow and an increase in volumetric flow, as assessed by intravital microscopy investigations in mice with TNBS-induced colitis [32]. In fact, changes in the microcirculation, such as the impaired colonic capillary blood flow, were shown to precede histological changes in TNBS-induced colitis in mice. This explains why the improvement in the capillary blood flow in these mice was followed by an enhancement in the gut barrier function [33].

During sepsis, the increased interaction of leukocytes and the endothelium and the leukocyte transmigration across the intestinal microvessels coincides with the release of inflammatory mediators, e.g. cytokines and chemokines. Using intravital microscopy, the role of microcirculation in promoting the inflammatory response was illustrated; the inhibition of leukocyte–endothelial cell interactions by blocking either adhesion molecules like ICAM-1 [34] and MAdCam-1, or chemokines like CCL20 [35], was found to inhibit leukocyte adhesion and recruitment in DSS-induced colitis.

In addition, the increased rolling and adherence of leukocytes with endothelium in intestinal microvessels during the inflammatory response leads to a reduction in capillary perfusion, assessed as functional capillary density (i.e. the length of capillaries with observable perfusion) in animals with colon ascendens stent peritonitis (CASP) [36]. The induction of TNF in the intestine after ischemia/reperfusion injury was suggested to contribute to remote organ dysfunction [37].

Therefore, the changes in the intestinal microcirculation have been suggested to affect the systemic immune response and contribute to the development of multiorgan failure (MOF) in sepsis [37–43].

Proposed Mechanisms by Which Glutamine Affects Intestinal Microcirculation

Glutamine Improves Functional Capillary Density (FCD) in Gut Microcirculation

The administration of Gln and AlaGln in rats with endotoxemia improved the capillary perfusion in the intestine as shown by our studies in the rats [44]. Endotoxemia induced after LPS administration in rats lead to an impaired microperfusion of the intestine, with a reduced FCD and an increased number of non-functional capillaries in the muscular sublayers and the mucosal layers of the intestine (Fig. 29.1) [44]. When Gln and AlaGln were administered prior to the induction of endotoxemia, the FCD was increased and the number of non-functional capillaries was reduced. The endotoxin-induced FCD decreases was completely reversed in the longitudinal muscle layer, and was significantly improved in the circular muscle layer and the mucosa (Fig. 29.1) [44]. This improvement of intestinal microperfusion was similarly observed when Gln or AlaGln were administered after the induction of endotoxemia (administered as a post-treatment after LPS challenge) (Fig. 29.1) [44]. It is interesting to note that the beneficial effect of AlaGln on the intestinal microperfusion was similar to that of Gln for both regimens (pre-treatment or post-treatment).

Glutamine Protects Microvascular Integrity

Significant changes to the microvascular integrity occur during sepsis [42, 45]. The administration of glutamine has been shown to improve the intestinal hyperpermeability and protect structural changes in the small intestine, as shown in rats with turpentine-induced tissue injury [46]. The ability of Gln to improve the histopathological changes, like villus heights, was associated with a restored concentration of glutathione in the jejunum [47]. The intestinal structural changes and enterocyte apoptosis that is induced by endotoxemia were shown to be reversed, when animals were provided with Gln in the drinking water [48]. The histopathological changes in the intestinal structure was improved even when Gln was administered intravenously in a rat model of endotoxemia [49].

The ability of Gln supplementation to protect the microvascular integrity was also reflected in studies where the gut barrier function, and bacterial translocation was examined. Gut permeability was improved by Gln administration in rats with pancreatitis, as assessed by electrophysiological measurements. This was demonstrated as an increase in the colonic transmucosal resistance and a significant reduction in mannitol flux through the epithelium [50]. In our own studies, we have observed that the treatment of Gln or AlaGln had completely reversed the LPS-induced increase in plasma extravasation in endotoxemic animals compared to control animals. AlaGln (DIP) was shown to have similar effect in that it significantly reduced the plasma extavasation across intestinal microvessels in endotoxemic animals. It should be noted that this effect can be observed as early as 2 h after administration of Gln or AlaGln (Fig. 29.2) [51].

The enhanced gut barrier function after Gln administration resulted in a reduction in bacterial infections and mortality rates. Prevalence of pancreatic infections was lower in animals that received Gln-enriched diet by ~33 % and this corresponded to a reduction in mortality by ~32 % [50]. However, it should be noted that in other models, namely turpentine-induced tissue injury, the beneficial effects of Gln supplementation of microvascular integrity did not translate into any effect on bacterial translocation [47].

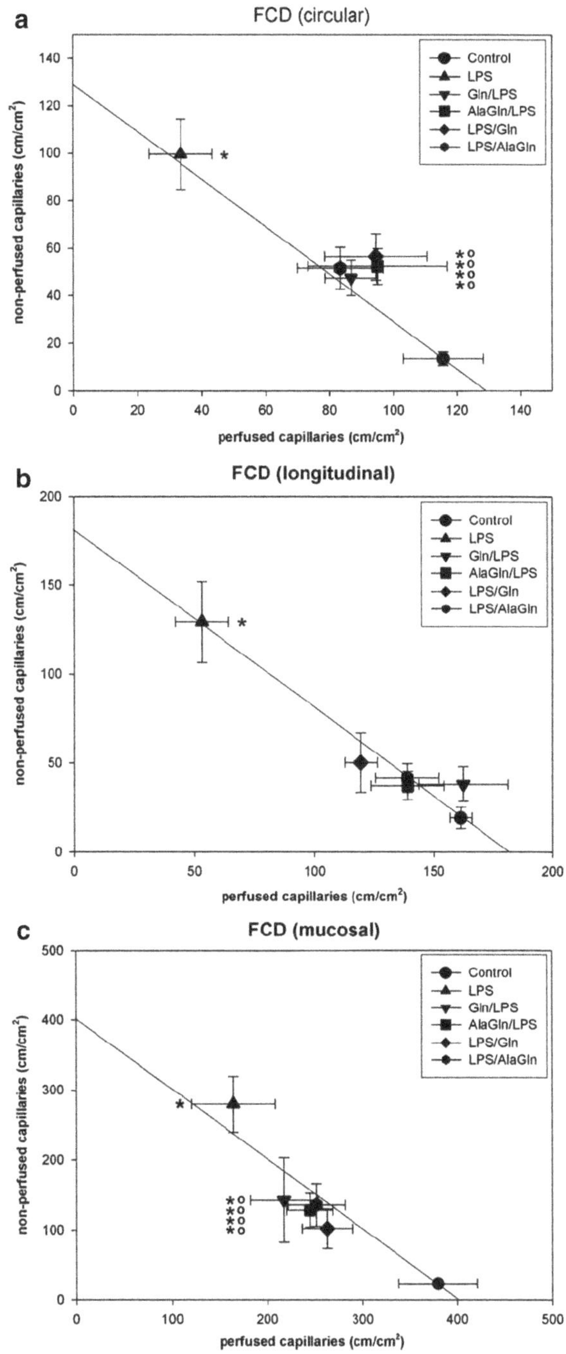

Fig. 29.1 Functional capillary density. (**a**) Circular muscular layer (cm/cm^2). (**b**) Longitudinal muscular layer (cm/cm^2). (**c**) Mucosal layer (cm/cm^2). °$P<0.05$ versus LPS group; *$p<0.05$ versus control group. *AlaGln* L-ALANYL-L-glutamine, *FCD* functional capillary density, *Gln* glutamine, *LPS* lipopolysaccharide (Reprinted from ref. [44] with permission from Elsevier)

Glutamine Reduces Leukocyte Rolling and Adherence to Intestinal Microcirculation

Leukocyte recruitment is one of the factors that influence intestinal microvasculature [42, 45]. The rolling and adherence of leukocyte are known to increase during intestinal inflammation. The administration of Gln by oral gavage over a period of 14 days prior to and/or after the administration

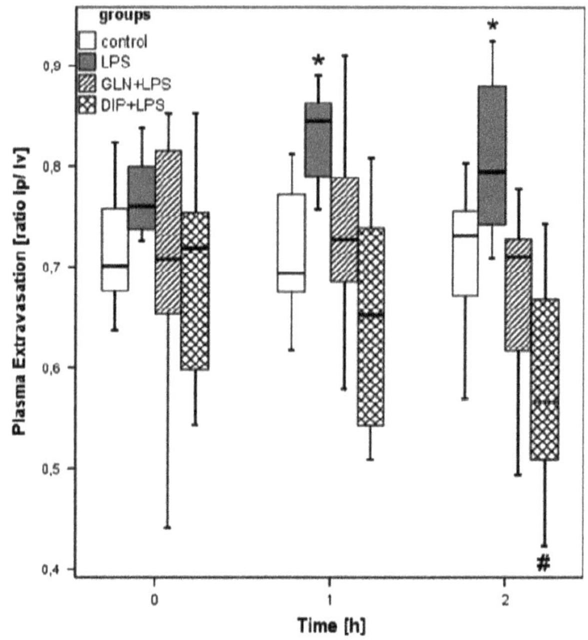

Fig. 29.2 Plasma extravasation. Fluorescence activity in the venule under the study (Iv) and in contiguous areas of the perivenular interstitium (Ip), expressed as the ratio Ip/Iv; Significances: * $p<0.05$ for LPS group vs. other groups; # $p<0.05$ for DIP+ LPS group vs. LPS group or control group. Median, 10th, 25th, 75th, 90th percentiles (Reprinted from ref. [51] with permission)

of indomethacin was performed to determine the effects of leukocyte–endothelial interactions. In this study, Gln-treated rats had 35–55 % reduction in the number of rolling and adhesion of leukocytes on mesenteric venules during indomethacin-induced ileitis compared to nontreated animals [52].

In our studies, endotoxemia induced increases in leukocyte rolling and adhesion in 6–8-fold in mesenteric venules after 1 h (Fig. 29.3). The administration of Gln before LPS challenge inhibited the increase in leukocyte rolling and adherence to mesenteric venules (Fig. 29.3). Similar to Gln, the administration of AlaGln (DIP) prior to LPS challenge prevented the LPS-induced increase in leukocyte rolling and adhesion (Fig. 29.3) [51]. Thus, the prior administration of either Gln or AlaGln (DIP) had inhibitory effects on leukocyte recruitment in intestinal inflammation, an effect observed as early as 1 h post-administration.

In addition, the effect of Gln or AlaGln administration on leukocyte adhesion to intestinal venules was observed in endotoxemic rats. The number of leukocytes adhering submucosal collecting venules (V1 venules) and the smaller, postcapillary venules (V3 venules) is increased by threefold after 2 h of LPS administration (Fig. 29.4). As we had observed in mesenteric venules (Fig. 29.3), the administration of Gln or AlaGln prior to LPS challenge reduced the number of adherent leukocytes (Fig. 29.4). In addition, the administration of these compounds after LPS challenge halved the LPS-induced increases in leukocyte adherence to V1 and V3 intestinal venules (Fig. 29.4). Thus, our studies have clearly demonstrated the beneficial effects of Gln and AlaGln (DIP) whether they are administered before or after endotoxemia, in both cases the increase in leukocyte adherence to mesenteric and intestinal microvasculature is significantly inhibited.

Impaired capillary blood flow in intestinal inflammation was shown to be reversed after Gln administration in several animal studies. In a study where intestinal disturbances were assessed Gln-administered animals with pancreatitis using intravital microscopy, it was found that Gln improved colonic capillary blood flow (by ~25 % in the colonic mucosa) [50]. Similarly, in animals with indomethacin-induced long-lasting ileitis in rats, the blood flow, shear rate and the velocity of rolling leukocytes was normalized after oral administration of Gln [52]. The beneficial effects of Gln administration on the intestinal microcirculatory disturbances lead to an improved macroscopic damage in intestine [52].

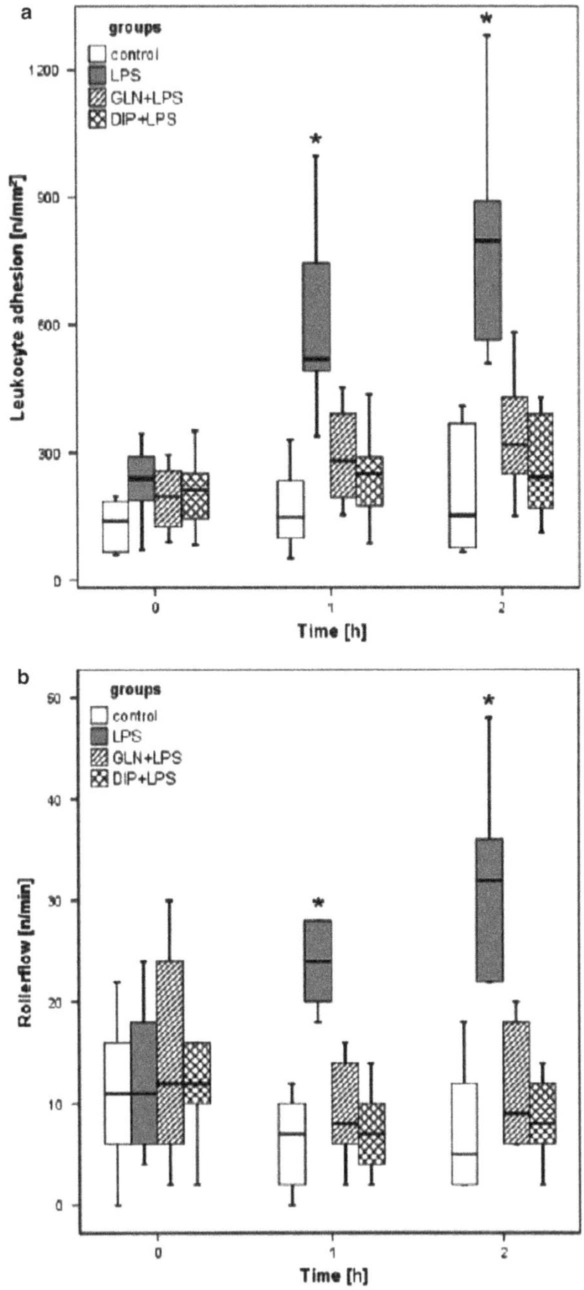

Fig. 29.3 Leukocyte–endothelial interactions. (**a**) Leukocyte adhesion (n/mm^2); (**b**) Rollerflow (n/min); Significances: * $p<0.05$ for LPS group vs. other groups. Median, 10th, 25th, 75th, 90th percentiles (Reprinted from ref. [51] with permission)

Glutamine Modulates the Expression of Adhesion Molecules

One of the mechanisms by which leukocytes adhere involves the cell adhesion molecules (CAM) [35, 53]. While a reduced Gln concentration enhances the transendothelial migration of neutrophils, it also increases the expression of cell adhesion molecules. This has been demonstrated in vitro using arsenic-activated human umbilical vein endothelial cells (HUVECs) and polymorphonuclear neutrophils (PMNs). When cells were treated at higher concentration of Gln (1,000 μM), PMNs were shown

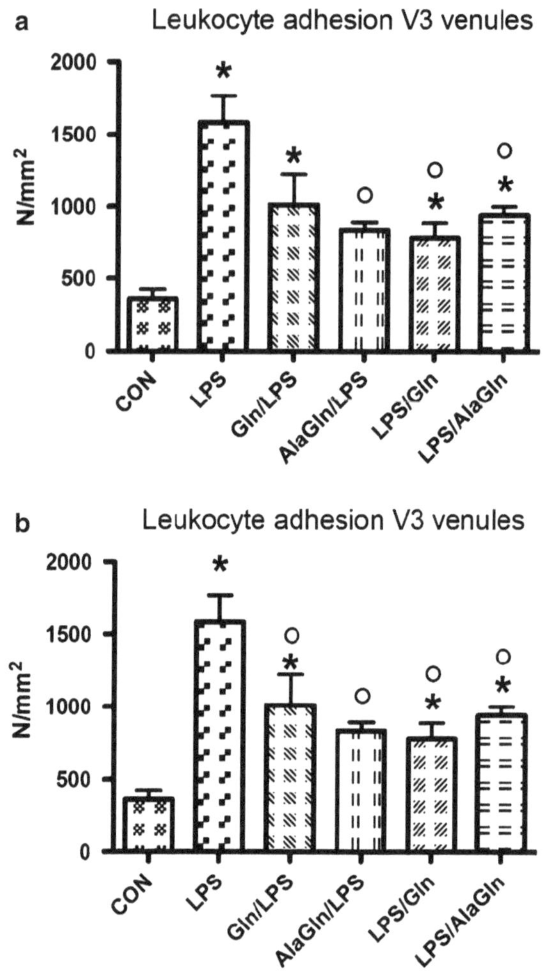

Fig. 29.4 Leukocyte adhesion. (**a**) Submucosal collecting (V1) venules (n/mm^3). (**b**) Submucosal postcapillary (V3) venules (n/mm^3). °$P<0.05$ versus LPS group; *$p<0.05$ versus control group. *AlaGln* L-alanyl-L-GLUTAMINE, *CON* control, *Gln* glutamine, *LPS* lipopolysaccharide (Reprinted from ref [44] with permission from Elsevier)

to express lower levels of certain cell adhesion molecules (e.g. CD11b) and the endothelial cells expressed lower levels of Vascular CAM-1, and this may explain the ability of those Gln-treated cells to have reduced transmigration across the endothelium [54]. The inhibitory effect of higher Gln concentrations on the endothelial expression of CAMs and on the transendothelial migration of PMNs was also confirmed when a different inflammatory stimuli was used to activate the endothelial cells in vitro (namely plasma or peritoneal drain fluid from a surgical patient) [55]. These results was also confirmed in mouse model of sepsis, whereby Gln supplementation reduced expression of CAMs and reduced the infiltration of neutrophils (reflected by a decrease in the myeloperoxidase activity) after tissue injury [56].

Glutamine Influences Cytokine Production

Additional inflammatory signals, such as cytokine production, are induced during sepsis in concurrence with the increased leukocyte–endothelial interaction in the intestinal microcirculation.

In vitro studies examined the effect of Gln on cytokine production by adding high concentrations of Gln (1,000 μM) to cells. The production of the pro-inflammatory cytokine, IL-8, was found to be reduced by GLn-treated HUVECs and this corresponded to a reduced expression of IL-8 receptor on PMNs [54, 55].

	Control	LPS	GLN+LPS	DIP+LPS
TNF- α	79 (64-152)	* 958 (834-1270)	*# 678 (490-1004)	*# 697 (617-1034)
IL - 1β	145 (128-173)	* 1809 (1369-2305)	* 1856 (1760-2142)	* 2063 (1416-2526)
IL - 6	740 (405-1220)	* 13034 (12923-13148)	* 13023 (12917-13144)	* 12890 (12814-13036)
IL - 10	226 (157-434)	* 496 (401-733)	* 476 (425-797)	* 505 (399-604)

Fig. 29.5 Cytokine levels in serum of animals after Gln treatment (Reprinted from ref. [51] with permission)

As an in vivo model of sepsis, endotoxemia enhances the circulating levels of inflammatory cytokines, inducing a 8-fold increase in TNF-alpha, 12-fold increase in IL-1β and 15-fold increase in IL-6 (Fig. 29.5) [51]. When animals received Gln or AlaGln (DIP), prior to the induction of endotoxemia, there was a significant reduction in the level of systemic TNF-alpha (Fig. 29.5). This effect did not extend to the other cytokines (e.g. IL-1β, IL-6, or IL-10) within the observation time of the study [51].

The observed reduction in pro-inflammatory cytokine level after Gln supplementation is crucial, as it has been shown to correlate with improved survival of animals with endotoxemia. Intravenous supplementation of Gln reduced the release of TNF and IL-6 within 2–4 h and reduced mortality of the animals with endotoxemia within 72 h [49]. It should be noted that these beneficial effects were reported when Gln was provided at onset of endotoxemia, rather than after the induction of endotoxemia (i.e. as a treatment) [49]. This effect is likely related to the inhibitory effect of Gln on NF-kappaB pathway, an important transcription factor for inflammatory mediators, as was shown in Gln-treated rats with experimental colitis [57]. Interestingly, the inhibitory effect of Gln on the mechanisms related to the cytokine release (e.g. TNF, IL-6, and IL-18) was linked to its role in preventing the development of lung injury following cecal ligation peritonitis in rats [58]. Therefore, these Gln-treated septic animals had attenuated mortality rates [58]. It should be noted that Gln supplementation did not appear to influence the cytokine profile of lymphocytes isolated from peyer's patches in animals with CLP [59], suggesting that other cell types may be responsible for the anti-inflammatory effect of Gln administration.

Glutamine Activates T-Cell and B-Cell Immune Response

Gln can act on multiple mechanisms related to leukocyte–endothelial cell interaction, and therefore it is reasonable to consider that it can influence immune response induced by T and B cells. Although the topic of immunomodulatory effects of Gln is beyond the scope of this chapter, it is important to consider a study by Lai et al., where the effect of Gln supplementation (both in diets before the induction of CLP model of sepsis, and in total parenteral nutrition after the induction of CLP model of sepsis) was examined. In this study, Gln-supplemented rats with sepsis were shown to have a higher number of lymphocytes in the peyer's patches and this effect appeared to be primarily restricted to CD4 T cells [59], which may indicate their proliferation in the gut-associated lymphoid tissue. In addition, Gln-supplemented septic rats were shown to have higher levels of plasma immunoglobulin A than the control group [59], reflecting yet another way by which Gln can improve the immunologic response and reduce mortality in rodents with sepsis.

Glutamine Regulate Oxidation Stress and Nitric Oxide-Related Mechanisms

Glutamine is known to upregulate the amino acid transport, and the synthesis of intracellular glutathione in human intestinal epithelial cells during ischemia–reperfusion in human intestinal epithelial cells [60]. In addition to being a precursor for the cellular antioxidant glutathione, glutamine is known to participate in the regulation of the cellular redox potential, and the production of reactive oxygen species [61–63]. The increased availability of glutamine and therefore increased ratio of intracellular content of reduced glutamine to oxidized glutathione is important to reducing oxidative stress in the cell. It is shown that the oxidative stress is associated with the induction of some inflammatory pathways: the activation of transcription factor Nuclear factor-kappa B (NF-kappaB), and the production of several pro-inflammatory cytokines, including TNF in animals with endotoxemia [64]. As a result, the participation of glutathione in a multitude of cellular effects is reported during many clinical conditions [65]. Several studies have demonstrated that the administration of glutamine was shown to downregulate NF-kappaB and inhibit the pro-inflammatory response in animals with colitis [57]. Treatment of Gln was shown to reduce the degree of oxidative stress in the mucosa of small intestine, corresponding increases in free radical scavenging enzymes in rats with indomethacin-induced ileitis [66].

The nitric oxide (NO) system is another central component in the autoregulatory control of microcirculatory patency. This is severely disturbed in sepsis by the increased expression of inducible nitric oxide synthase (iNOS), thus resulting in pathological shunting of flow [42] and the development of the inflammatory reaction [67]. Several studies demonstrated the ability of glutamine treatment to reduce the oxidative stress via a partial reduction in protein levels of iNOS, as demonstrated in rats with experimental colitis [57], and in rats with CLP [58]. In both studies, the anti-inflammatory effect of Gln treatment also occurred in conjunction with Gln-inhibition of the NF-kappaB pathway [57, 58].

In addition to its ability to activate glutathione and inhibit NF-kappaB pathway and the NOS systems, the gut-protective effects of enteral glutamine have been explained by other mechanisms, e.g. the activation of anti-inflammatory transcription factor named peroxisome proliferator-activated receptor-γ [68].

Glutamine Induces Heat Shock Proteins (HSPs)

Heat shock response is one of the defense mechanisms against stress conditions, as occurs in intestinal inflammation, and is involved in restoring intestinal homeostasis. The increase of HSP response can attenuate the oxidative stress pathway and the release of pro-inflammatory cytokines, like TNF and IL-1β [69]. One of the mechanisms that have been suggested for the gut-protective role of Gln involves its ability to induce heat shock proteins.

In rats with endotoxin shock, Gln supplementation was shown to induce the increased expression of HSP25 and HSP72 in different organs, and thus control the tissue damage and limit the mortality rates. It should be noted that these protective effects were induced when Gln was used at the initiation of sepsis, rather than later after sepsis [70]. Gln treatment of mice with sepsis was shown to specifically increase the level of HSP72 and reduce the level of TNF-alpha in peritoneal macrophages in vivo [71]. In addition to HSP72, the induction of HSP 70 after Gln treatment may explain why it can protect from sepsis and lung injury. In fact, Gln-treated $HSP70^{-/-}$ mice were not protected from lung injury, or inflammatory cytokine response induced after CLP-induced sepsis [72]. This is not limited to intestinal microenvironment, as it has been also demonstrated in rats after cardiopulmonary bypass [73].

In vitro studies have examined the increase in the expression of HSPs induced by Gln in different cell types. An increased expression of HSP70 was demonstrated after the addition of Gln to intestinal endothelial cell lines in vitro and protected them from cell lethal heat and oxidant-induced injury [74]. Gln-induced expression of HSP70 was also reported in fibroblasts [75]. The induction of HSPs was also shown in Gln-treated circulating cells. For instance, polymorphonuclear cells had an increased

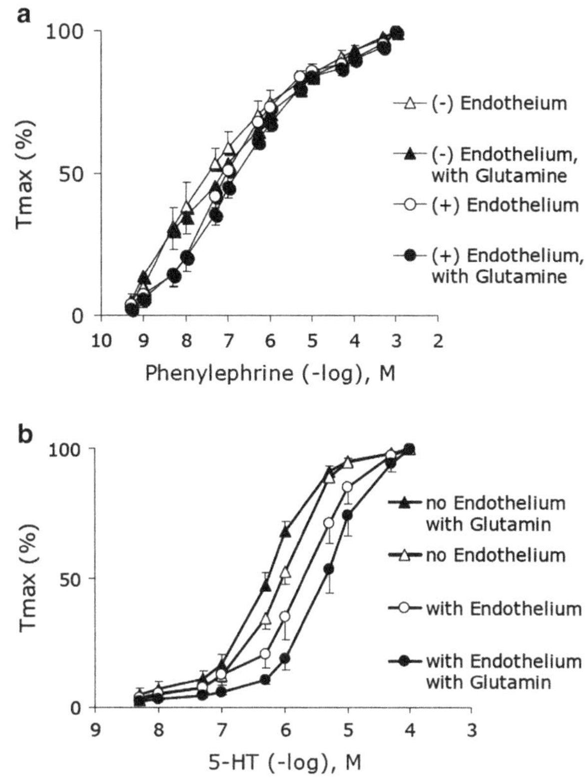

Fig. 29.6 Dose–response curves. The responses to phenylephrine (**a**) and 5-HT (**b**) were obtained following 30 min preincubation of rat aorta in vitro with glutamine preparations. Significances: phenylephrine, controls vs. glutamine with endothelium, $p<0.05$; for 5-HT differences were not significant; mean ± SEM (Reprinted from ref. [51] with permission)

expression of HSP 72 and a reduced production of TNF [76]. This observation was also made when LPS-activated macrophage cell lines were treated with Gln in vitro [71].

In addition, it was reported that Gln treatment can enhance the expression of heat shock factor-1, which is required for the attenuation of iNOS expression [77], and is involved in the inhibition of LPS-induced transcription of IL-1β and IL-6 [78].

Glutamine Induces Other Effectors

When Gln was added to intestinal epithelial cells that underwent hypoxia-reoxygenation, these cells had a reduced permeability and enhanced cell growth, which was associated with increased expression of Syndecan, a predominant heparan sulfate proteoglycan. In vivo studies confirmed that the ability of Gln treatment to reverse the gut ischemia–reperfusion-induced intestinal inflammation and hyperpermeability is dependent on Syndecan-1, as observed using Syndecan$^{-/-}$ mice [79]. In addition, Gln treatment induces other effectors in epithelial cells. For instance, in our studies, we observed that Gln-treated rat aortic endothelial cells did not influence dose response of phenylephrine and of 5-HAT (Fig. 29.6) [51].

Future Direction for the Effect of Glutamine on Intestinal Microcirculation

Studies have examined the kinetics of Gln administration in patients and rats. For instance, when Gln excretion was studied in patients of ICU after peripheral administration of Gln, rapid hydrolysis of the dipeptide was reported, with the half-life of the dipeptide being 0.26 h [80], and the rate of appearance

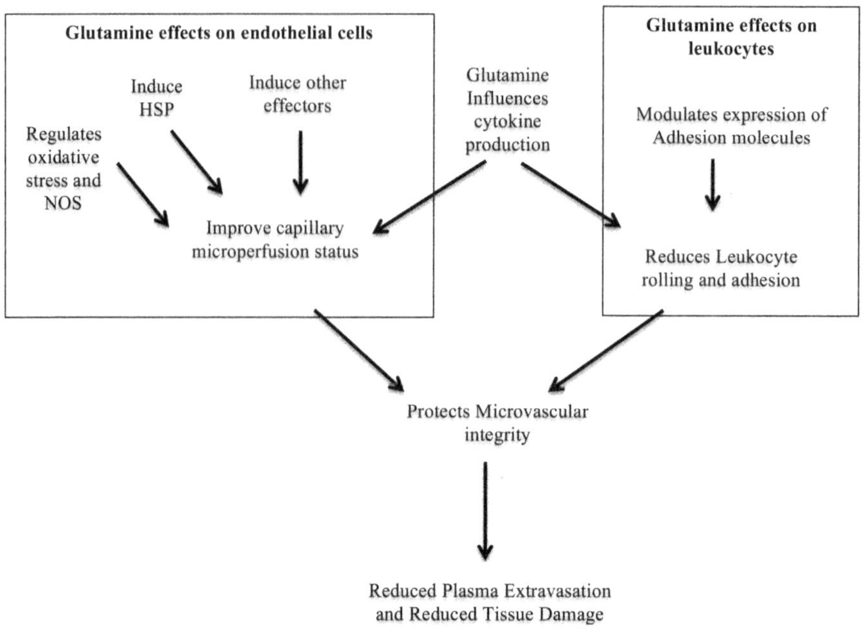

Fig. 29.7 Schematic summary of major effects of glutamine, including dipeptide-bound glutamine, on the endothelial cell and leukocytes. Proposed therapeutic benefits are based on changes in intestinal microcirculation and leukocyte–endothelial cell interaction. Not depicted here are the effects on T- and B-cell responses

of Gln was 54 g/h [81]. Kinetics of Gln uptake was also measured in rats with LPS-induced sepsis. It was found that dipeptide constituents of alanine and Gln increased at 20 min and approached baseline at 120 min [44]. Other studies also examined the kinetics in rats with CLP within the first 5 h of administration [82].

Several studies indicated the beneficial effects of Gln administration for patients with intestinal diseases, including Crohn's disease, as reviewed elsewhere [83]. ICU patients were shown to have improved long-term survival after Gln treatment, making this strategy of great interest [83, 84]. The use of dipeptide as therapeutic strategy is likely useful for patients with AIDS and celiac disease, due to the ability of Gln to restore AIDs-associated increased intestinal permeability [85]. Therapeutic applications of Gln with other patients, e.g. those receiving cancer chemotherapy, are discussed elsewhere [83, 86]. In the future, it is necessary to examine the impact of Gln supplementation in patients with sepsis in clinical trials. Although we have discussed that the effect of Gln or dipeptide supplementation on intestinal microcirculation can occur via a number of mechanisms, it is important to note that other factors can affect the intestinal microcirculation in sepsis, but are not well described.

Conclusions

Glutamine (Gln) is an important nutrient for rapidly proliferating cells, and is critically required during sepsis. Since dysfunctional intestinal microcirculation is considered a driving force in the pathogenesis of sepsis, we and others have examined the impact of Gln and/or dipeptide administration on intestinal microcirculation [44, 51]. As reviewed in this chapter, several mechanisms are shown to explain the beneficial effects of Gln on intestinal microcirculation (summarized in Fig. 29.7): Glutamine (1) Improves the functional capillary density (FCD) in gut microcirculation, (2) Protects microvascular integrity, (3) Reduces leukocyte rolling and adherence to intestinal microcirculation, (4) Affects the expression of adhesion molecules, (5) Modulates cytokine production, (6) Activates T-cell and B-cell immune response, (7) Regulates oxidation stress and nitric oxide-related mechanisms, (8) Induces heat shock proteins (HSPs), and (9) Induces other effectors.

Since Gln improved the status of gut microcirculation, there was significant interest in identifying Gln kinetics in patients and in animal models of sepsis. Several studies suggested that beneficial impact of Gln on intestinal microcirculation could extend to several populations of patients. It is therefore necessary to assess the microcirculatory changes in the intestine in clinical trials for glutamine use in patients with sepsis. Future studies should determine how to utilize the benefits of Gln supplementation on maintaining intestinal integrity in these critically ill patients.

References

1. Kovacevic Z, McGivan JD. Mitochondrial metabolism of glutamine and glutamate and its physiological significance. Physiol Rev. 1983;63(2):547–605.
2. Lacey JM, Wilmore DW. Is glutamine a conditionally essential amino acid? Nutr Rev. 1990;48(8):297–309.
3. Ligthart-Melis GC, Van de Poll MCG, Boelens PG, Dejong CHC, Deutz NEP, Van Leeuwen PA. Glutamine is an important precursor for de novo synthesis of arginine in humans. Am J Clin Nutr. 2008;87(5):1282–9.
4. Askanazi J, Carpentier YA, Michelsen CB, et al. Muscle and plasma amino acids following injury. Influence of intercurrent infection. Ann Surg. 1980;192(1):78–85.
5. Souba WW, Herskowitz K, Klimberg VS, et al. The effects of sepsis and endotoxemia on gut glutamine metabolism. Ann Surg. 1990;211(5):543–9.
6. Austgen TR, Chen MK, Dudrick PS, Copeland EM, Souba WW. Cytokine regulation of intestinal glutamine utilization. Am J Surg. 1992;163(1):174–9. discussion 179–80.
7. Lyons J, Rauh-Pfeiffer A, Ming-Yu Y, et al. Cysteine metabolism and whole blood glutathione synthesis in septic pediatric patients. Crit Care Med. 2001;29(4):870–7.
8. Biolo G, Antonione R, De Cicco M. Glutathione metabolism in sepsis. Crit Care Med. 2007;35(9 Suppl):S591–5.
9. Furst P, Stehle P. What are the essential elements needed for the determination of amino acid requirements in humans? Am Soc Nutr Sci. 2004;134:1558S–65.
10. Wernerman J. Clinical use of glutamine supplementation. J Nutr. 2008;138(10):2040S–4.
11. Cruzat VF, Tirapegui J. Effects of oral supplementation with glutamine and alanyl-glutamine on glutamine, glutamate, and glutathione status in trained rats and subjected to long-duration exercise. Nutrition. 2009;25(4):428–35.
12. Singer P, Berger MM, Van den Berghe G, et al. ESPEN Guidelines on Parenteral Nutrition: intensive care. Clin Nutr. 2009;28(4):387–400.
13. De-Souza DA, Greene LJ. Intestinal permeability and systemic infections in critically ill patients: effect of glutamine. Crit Care Med. 2005;33(5):1125–35.
14. Wischmeyer PE. Glutamine: role in gut protection in critical illness. Curr Opin Clin Nutr Meta Care. 2006;9(5):607–12.
15. Hammarqvist F, Wernerman J, Von der Decken A, Vinnars E. Alanyl-glutamine counteracts the depletion of free glutamine and the postoperative decline in protein synthesis in skeletal muscle. Ann Surg. 1990;212(5):637–44.
16. Grau T, Bonet A, Miñambres E, et al. The effect of L-alanyl-L-glutamine dipeptide supplemented total parenteral nutrition on infectious morbidity and insulin sensitivity in critically ill patients. Crit Care Med. 2011;39(6):1263–8.
17. Déchelotte P, Hasselmann M, Cynober L, et al. L-alanyl-L-glutamine dipeptide-supplemented total parenteral nutrition reduces infectious complications and glucose intolerance in critically ill patients: the French controlled, randomized, double-blind, multicenter study. Crit Care Med. 2006;34(3):598–604.
18. Vincent J-L, Rello J, Marshall J, et al. International study of the prevalence and outcomes of infection in intensive care units. JAMA. 2009;302(21):2323–9.
19. Xu D, Qi L, Guillory D, Cruz N, Berg R, Deitch EA. Mechanisms of endotoxin-induced intestinal injury in a hyperdynamic model of sepsis. J Trauma. 1993;34(5):676–83.
20. Klemm K, Moody FG. Regional intestinal blood flow and nitric oxide synthase inhibition during sepsis in the rat. Ann Surg. 1998;227(1):126–33.
21. Lush CW, Kvietys PR. Microvascular dysfunction in sepsis. Microcirculation. 2000;7(2):83–101.
22. Dyson A, Cone S, Singer M, Ackland GL. Microvascular and macrovascular flow are uncoupled in early polymicrobial sepsis. Br J Anaesth. 2012;108(6):973–8.

23. Spanos A, Jhanji S, Vivian-Smith A, Harris T, Pearse RM. Early microvascular changes in sepsis and severe sepsis. Shock. 2010;33(4):387–91.
24. Deban L, Correale C, Vetrano S, Malesci A, Danese S. Multiple pathogenic roles of microvasculature in inflammatory bowel disease: a Jack of all trades. Am J Pathol. 2008;172(6):1457–66.
25. Hatoum OA, Miura H, Binion DG. The vascular contribution in the pathogenesis of inflammatory bowel disease. Am J Physiol Heart Circ Physiol. 2003;285(5):H1791–6.
26. Carr ND, Pullan BR, Schofield PF. Microvascular studies in non-specific inflammatory bowel disease. Gut. 1986; 27(5):542–9.
27. Goddard CM, Allard MF, Hogg JC, Herbertson MJ, Walley KR. Prolonged leukocyte transit time in coronary microcirculation of endotoxemic pigs. Am J Physiol. 1995;269(4 Pt 2):H1389–97.
28. Goddard CM, Poon BY, Klut ME, et al. Leukocyte activation does not mediate myocardial leukocyte retention during endotoxemia in rabbits. Am J Physiol Heart Circ Physiol. 1998;275:H1548–57.
29. MacFie J. Current status of bacterial translocation as a cause of surgical sepsis. Br Med Bull. 2004;71:1–11.
30. Gatt M, Reddy BS, MacFie J. Review article: bacterial translocation in the critically ill–evidence and methods of prevention. Aliment Pharmacol Ther. 2007;25(7):741–57.
31. Liu Y, Shaw SK, Ma S, Yang L, Francis W, Parkos CA. Regulation of leukocyte transmigration: cell surface. J Immunol. 2004;172:7–13.
32. Ravnic DJ, Konerding MA, Tsuda A, et al. Structural adaptations in the murine colon microcirculation associated with hapten-induced inflammation. Gut. 2007;56(4):518–23.
33. Foitzik T, Kruschewski M, Kroesen A, Buhr HJ. Does microcirculation play a role in the pathogenesis of inflammatory bowel diseases? Answers from intravital microscopic studies in animal models. Int J Colorectal Dis. 1999; 14(1):29–34.
34. Farkas S, Herfarth H, Rössle M, et al. Quantification of mucosal leucocyte endothelial cell interaction by in vivo fluorescence microscopy in experimental colitis in mice. Clin Exp Immunol. 2001;126(2):250–8.
35. Teramoto K, Miura S, Tsuzuki Y, et al. Increased lymphocyte trafficking to colonic microvessels is dependent on MAdCAM-1 and C-C chemokine mLARC/CCL20 in DSS-induced mice colitis. Clin Exp Immunol. 2005; 139:421–8.
36. Lustig MK, Bac VH, Pavlovic D, et al. Colon ascendens stent peritonitis – a model of sepsis adopted to the rat: physiological, microcirculatory and laboratory changes. Shock. 2007;28(1):59–64.
37. Yao Y, Yu Y, Wu Y, Shi Z, Sheng Z. The role of gut as a cytokine-generating organ in remote organ dysfunction after intestinal ischemia and reperfusion. Chin Med J. 1998;111(6):514–8.
38. Meakins JL, Marshall JC. The gastrointestinal tract: the "motor" of MOF. Arch Surg. 1986;121(2):197–201.
39. Adams JM, Hauser CJ, Adams CA, Xu DZ, Livingston DH, Deitch EA. Entry of gut lymph into the circulation primes rat neutrophil respiratory burst in hemorrhagic shock. Crit Care Med. 2001;29(11):2194–8.
40. Gong J-P, Wu C-X, Liu C-A, et al. Intestinal damage mediated by Kupffer cells in rats with endotoxemia. World J Gastroenterol. 2002;8(5):923–7.
41. Schmidt H, Martindale R. The gastrointestinal tract in critical illness. Curr Opin Clin Nutr Meta Care. 2001; 4(6):547–51.
42. Ince C. The microcirculation is the motor of sepsis. Crit Care. 2005;9 Suppl 4:S13–9.
43. Stechmiller J, Treloar D, Allen N. Gut dysfunction in critically ill patients: a review of the literature. Am J Crit Care. 1997;6(3):204–9.
44. Lehmann C, Pavlovic D, Zhou J, et al. Intravenous free and dipeptide-bound glutamine maintains intestinal microcirculation in experimental endotoxemia. Nutrition. 2012;28(5):588–93.
45. Spronk PE, Zandstra DF, Ince C. Bench-to-bedside review: sepsis is a disease of the microcirculation. Crit Care. 2004;8(6):462–8.
46. Wusteman M, Tate H, Weaver L, Austin S, Neale G, Elia M. The effect of enteral glutamine deprivation and supplementation on the structure of rat small-intestine mucosa during a systemic injury response. JPEN. 1995;19(1):22–7.
47. Belmonte L, Coëffier M, Le Pessot F, et al. Effects of glutamine supplementation on gut barrier, glutathione content and acute phase response in malnourished rats during inflammatory shock. World J Gastroenterol. 2007;13(20): 2833–40.
48. Sukhotnik I, Agam M, Shamir R, et al. Oral glutamine prevents gut mucosal injury and improves mucosal recovery following lipopolysaccharide endotoxemia in a rat. J Surg Res. 2007;143(2):379–84.
49. Wischmeye PE, Kahana M, Wolfson R, Ren H, Musch M, Chang EB. Glutamine reduces cytokine release, organ damage, and mortality in a rat model of endotoxemia. Shock. 2001;16(5):398–402.
50. Foitzik T, Kruschewski M, Kroesen AJ, Hotz HG, Eibl G, Buhr HJ. Does glutamine reduce bacterial translocation? A study in two animal models with impaired gut barrier. Int J Colorectal Dis. 1999;14(3):143–9.
51. Scheibe R, Schade M, Gründling M, et al. Glutamine and alanyl-glutamine dipeptide reduce mesenteric plasma extravasation, leukocyte adhesion and tumor necrosis factor-alpha (TNF-α) release during experimental endotoxemia. J Physiol Pharmacol. 2009;60 Suppl 8:19–24.

52. Arndt H, Kullmann F, Reuss F, Scholmerich J, Palitzsch KDD, ReuB F. Glutamine attenuates leukocyte-endothelial cell adhesion in indomethacin-induced intestinal inflammation in the rat. J Parenter Enteral Nutr. 1999;23(1):12–8.
53. Moser B, Loetscher P. Lymphocyte traffic control by chemokines. Nat Immunol. 2001;2(2):123–8.
54. Hou Y-C, Hsu C-S, Yeh C-L, Chiu W-C, Pai M-H, Yeh S-L. Effects of glutamine on adhesion molecule expression and leukocyte transmigration in endothelial cells exposed to arsenic. J Nutr Biochem. 2005;16(11):700–4.
55. Yeh CL, Hsu CS, Chen SC, Pai MH, Yeh SL. Effect of glutamine on cellular adhesion molecule expression and leukocyte transmigration in endothelial cells stimulated by plasma or peritoneal drain fluid from a surgical patient. Shock. 2006;25(3):236–40.
56. Yeh C-L, Hsu C-S, Yeh S-L, Lin M-T, Chen W-J. Dietary glutamine supplementation reduces cellular adhesion molecule expression and tissue myeloperoxidase activity in mice with gut-derived sepsis. Nutrition. 2006;22(4): 408–13.
57. Fillmann H, Kretzmann NA, San-Miguel B, et al. Glutamine inhibits over-expression of pro-inflammatory genes and down-regulates the nuclear factor kappaB pathway in an experimental model of colitis in the rat. Toxicology. 2007;236(3):217–26.
58. Singleton KD, Beckey VE, Wischmeyer PE. Glutamine prevents activation of NF-kappaB and stress kinase pathways, attenuates inflammatory cytokine release, and prevents acute respiratory distress syndrome following sepsis. Shock. 2005;24(6):583–9.
59. Lai YN, Yeh SL, Lin MT, Shang HF, Yeh CL, Chen WJ. Glutamine supplementation enhances mucosal immunity in rats with Gut-Derived sepsis. Nutrition. 2004;20(3):286–91.
60. Wasa M, Soh H, Shimizu Y, Fukuzawa M. Glutamine stimulates amino acid transport during ischemia-reperfusion in human intestinal epithelial cells. J Surg Res. 2005;123(1):75–81.
61. Matés JM, Pérez-Gómez C, Núñez de Castro I, Asenjo M, Márquez J. Glutamine and its relationship with intracellular redox status, oxidative stress and cell proliferation/death. Int J Biochem Cell Biol. 2002;34(5):439–58.
62. Barth A, Bauer R, Gedrange T, Walter B, Klinger W, Zwiener U. Influence of hypoxia and hypoxia/hypercapnia upon brain and blood peroxidative and glutathione status in normal weight and growth-restricted newborn piglets. Exp Toxicol Pathol. 1998;50(4–6):402–10.
63. Barth A, Bauer R, Gedrange T, Walter B, Linss C, Klinger W. Influence of hypoxia and hyperthermia upon peroxidative and glutathione status in growth-restricted newborn piglets. Exp Toxicol Pathol. 1998;50(1):31–3.
64. Blackwell TS, Blackwell TR, Holden EP, Christman BW, Christman JW. In vivo antioxidant treatment suppresses nuclear factor-kappa B activation and neutrophilic lung inflammation. J Immunol. 1996;157(4):1630–7.
65. Roth E, Oehler R, Manhart N, et al. Regulative potential of glutamine–relation to glutathione metabolism. Nutrition. 2002;18(3):217–21.
66. Basivireddy J, Jacob M, Balasubramanian KA. Oral glutamine attenuates indomethacin-induced small intestinal damage. Clin Sci. 2004;107(3):281–9.
67. Guzik TJ, Korbut R, Adamek-Guzik T. Nitric oxide and superoxide in inflammation and immune regulation. J Physiol Pharmacol. 2003;54(4):469–87.
68. Ban K, Kozar RA. Enteral glutamine: a novel mediator of PPARγ in the postischemic gut. J Leuk Biol. 2008; 84(3):595–9.
69. Sikora A, Girzesiuk E. Heat shock response in gastrointestinal tract. J Physiol Pharmacol. 2007;58 Suppl 3: 43–62.
70. Wischmeyer PE, Kahana M, Wolfson R, Ren H, Musch MM, Chang EB. Glutamine induces heat shock protein and protects against endotoxin shock in the rat. J Appl Physiol. 2001;90(6):2403–10.
71. Liang M, Wang X, Yuan Y, Zhou Q, Tong C, Jiang W. Different effect of glutamine on macrophage tumor necrosis factor-alpha release and heat shock protein 72 expression in vitro and in vivo. Acta Biochim Biophys Sin. 2009; 41(2):171–7.
72. Singleton KD, Wischmeyer PE. Glutamine's protection against sepsis and lung injury is dependent on heat shock protein 70 expression. Am J Physiol Reg Integ Compar Physiol. 2007;292(5):R1839–45.
73. Hayashi Y. Preoperative glutamine administration induces heat-shock protein 70 expression and attenuates cardiopulmonary bypass-induced inflammatory response by regulating nitric oxide synthase activity. Circulation. 2002; 106(20):2601–7.
74. Wischmeyer PE, Musch MW, Madonna MB, Thisted R, Chang EB. Glutamine protects intestinal epithelial cells: role of inducible HSP70. Am J Physiol. 1997;272(4 Pt 1):G879–84.
75. Hamiel CR, Pinto S, Hau A, Wischmeyer PE. Glutamine enhances heat shock protein 70 expression via increased hexosamine biosynthetic pathway activity. Am J Physiol Cell Physiol. 2009;297(6):C1509–19.
76. Wischmeyer PE, Riehm J, Singleton KD, et al. Glutamine attenuates tumor necrosis factor-alpha release and enhances heat shock protein 72 in human peripheral blood mononuclear cells. Nutrition. 2003;19(1):1–6.
77. Peng Z-Y, Hamiel CR, Banerjee A, Wischmeyer PE, Friese RS, Wischmeyer P. Glutamine attenuation of cell death and inducible nitric oxide synthase expression following inflammatory cytokine-induced injury is dependent on heat shock factor-1 expression. JPEN. 2006;30(5):400–7.

78. Xie Y, Chen C, Stevenson MA, Auron PE, Calderwood SK. Heat shock factor 1 represses transcription of the IL-1beta gene through physical interaction with the nuclear factor of interleukin 6. J Biol Chem. 2002;277(14): 11802–10.
79. Peng Z, Ban K, Sen A, et al. Syndecan 1 plays a novel role in enteral glutamine's gut-protective effects of the post-ischemic gut. Shock. 2012;38(1):57–62.
80. Berg A, Rooyackers O, Norberg A, Wernerman J. Elimination kinetics of L-alanyl-L-glutamine in ICU patients. Amino Acids. 2005;29(3):221–8.
81. Berg A, Norberg A, Martling CR, Gamrin L, Rooyackers O, Wernerman J. Glutamine kinetics during intravenous glutamine supplementation in ICU patients on continuous renal replacement therapy. Intensive Care Med. 2007; 33(4):660–6.
82. Nose K, Wasa M, Okada A. Gut glutamine metabolism at different stages of sepsis in rats. Surg Today. 2002;32(8): 695–700.
83. Ziegler TR, Bazargan N, Leader LM, Martindale RG. Glutamine and the gastrointestinal tract. Curr Opin Clin Nutr Metab Care. 2000;3(5):355–62.
84. Wernerman J, Hammarqvist F. Glutamine: a necessary nutrient for the intensive care patient. Int J Colorectal Dis. 1999;14(3):137–42.
85. Thomson AB, Keelan M, Thiesen A, Clandinin MT, Ropeleski M, Wild GE. Small bowel review: diseases of the small intestine. Dig Dis Sci. 2001;46(12):2555–66.
86. Miller AL. Therapeutic considerations of L-glutamine: a review of the literature. Altern Med Rev. 1999;4(4): 239–48.

Part V
Clinical Aspects of Glutamine in Certain Patient Populations

Chapter 30
Manganese Toxicity and the Glutamine–Glutamate Cycle

Marta Sidoryk-Wegrzynowicz and Michael Aschner

Key Points

- Manganese is required for the proper maintenance and function of many biochemical and cellular reactions.
- Overdose and excessive Mn accumulation may be toxic to the CNS and cause a neurological disorder, referred to as manganism.
- Mn toxicity is associated with dyshomeostasis in glutamine (Gln) metabolism and with the disruption of the Gln/glutamate (Glu) GABA cycle (GGC) between astrocytes and neurons, leading to changes in Glu-ergic or GABA-ergic neurotransmission.
- The effects of Mn on astrocytes may culminate in pathology, affect their protective properties and resulting in impaired astrocyte–neuronal integrity.
- In this chapter, we discuss the mechanistic commonalities inherent to Mn-neurotoxicity related to the astrocyte pathology and GGC impairment.

Keywords Manganese • Neurotoxicity • Glutamine • Glutamate • Transporter • PKC signaling • Ubiquitination

Abbreviations

ASP	Aspartate
BBB	Blood–brain barrier
BIS II	Bisindolylmaleimide II
CNS	Central nervous system
CSF	Cerebrospinal fluid

M. Sidoryk-Wegrzynowicz, Ph.D. (✉)
Department of Pediatrics, Vanderbilt University School of Medicine,
11415 MRB IV, 2215-B Garland Avenue, Nashville, TN 37232, USA
e-mail: martasidoryk@gmail.com

M. Aschner, Ph.D.
Department of Molecular Pharmacology, Albert Einstein College of Medicine,
Forchheimer 209, 1300 Morris Park Avenue, Bronx, NY 10461, USA
e-mail: michael.aschner@einstein.yu.edu

R. Rajendram et al. (eds.), *Glutamine in Clinical Nutrition*, Nutrition and Health,
DOI 10.1007/978-1-4939-1932-1_30, © Springer Science+Business Media New York 2015

DAT	Dopamine transporter
ECF	Extracellular fluid
GABA	γ-Amino butyric acid
GAD	Glutamic acid decarboxylase
GFAP	Glial fibrillary acidic protein
GGC	The glutamate–glutamine γ-amino butyric acid cycling
GLAST	Glutamate–aspartate transporter
Glc	Glucose
GLN	Glutamine
GLT1	Glutamate transporter
GLU	Glutamate
GS	Gln synthetase
GSH	Glutathione
HECT	Homology to the E6-associated protein C terminus
iNOS	Nitric oxide synthase
MeAIB	Methyl-amino-iso-butyric acid
MMT	Methylcyclopentadienyl manganese tricarbonyl
Mn	Manganese
Nedd4-2	Neuronal precursor cell expressed developmentally downregulated 4-2 activity
NO	Nitric oxide
PAG	Phosphate-activated glutaminase
PC	Pyruvate carboxylase
PKC	Protein kinase C
PKCδ CF	PKCδ catalytic fragment
PMA	Activator α-phorbol 12-myristate 13-acetate
ROS	Reactive oxygen species
SGK1	Serum- and glucocorticoid-regulated kinase 1
TCA	Tricarboxylic acid cycle

Introduction

Glutamine (Gln) is abundantly expressed in the central nervous system (CNS), where it participates in a variety of metabolic pathways. Gln metabolism proceeds via the glutamine/glutamate (Glu)-γ-aminobutyric acid (GABA) cycle (GGC), and the reactions within this cycle are carried out both in astrocytic and neuronal compartments. The GGC appears to have an important, albeit not exclusive role, in the recycling of Glu and GABA. Disruption of GGC between astrocytes and neurons contributes to changes in Glu-ergic and/or GABA-ergic transmission, and is associated with several neuropathological conditions, including manganese (Mn) toxicity.

Mn exposure and accumulation causes dysfunction of carriers transporting Gln and Glu, which may impact on neurotransmitter generation and have profound effects on synaptic plasticity. In general, Mn mediates astrocytic pathology and impairs astrocyte–neuronal integrity. This chapter addresses interaction between neurons and astrocytes and emphasizes the role of GGC in both normal physiological functions and pathology associated with Mn toxicity.

Table 30.1 Manganese and glutamine transport

Gln transporter (System)	Neutral amino acid substrates	Direction of transport	Principal cellular localization	Targets of Mn action
SNAT3 (System N)	Gln, Asn, His	Bidirectional (outward preferred)	Astrocytes	mRNA and protein expression; function (uptake and efflux)
SNAT2 (System A)	Short-chain	Inward	Neurons	mRNA and protein expression
LAT2 (System L)	Bulky	Bidirectional	Astrocytes; neurons; endothelial cells	mRNA and protein expression; function (uptake and efflux)
ASCT2 (System ASC)	Short-chain	Bidirectional	Astrocytes	Protein expression; function (uptake and efflux)

General characteristic of glutamine carriers. Distribution and properties, and the manganese (Mn)-induced effects on the glutamine/glutamate-γ-aminobutyric acid (GGC) cycle associated with the glutamine (Gln)-transporting systems A, N, ASC and L

Glutamine (Gln) Content and Regional Distribution and Its Role in Central Nervous System (CNS)

Gln concentrations in mammalian brain are 5–9 nmol/mg wet weight or 6–11 mM, with slight regional differences [1]. Gln content in the extracellular fluid (microdialysates) (ECF) or in the cerebrospinal fluid (CSF) (~0.5–1 mM) exceeds, by at least one order of magnitude, the extracellular contents of other amino acids in these compartments. Gln is the most abundant amino acid in the plasma (at 600–800 μmol) and exhibits extremely rapid cellular turnover rates [2]. This ubiquitous amino acid serves in multiple roles in the mammalian brain; as cycler in multiple metabolic pathways, essential precursor in nucleotide, glucose and amino sugar biosynthesis, glutathione homeostasis and protein synthesis. Moreover, the growth of proliferating cells, such as fibroblasts, lymphocytes, enterocytes and neoplastic tissue depends on Gln, which provides oxidative energy fuel [3]. In the CNS Gln supports tissue homeostasis by participation in intercellular substrate cycles. Gln metabolism generates compounds that serve as direct precursors of the tricarboxylic acid cycle (TCA), thus contributing to the supply of the high-energy demand in the brain. Gln serves as a precursor of the amino acid neurotransmitters glutamate (Glu), γ-amino butyric acid (GABA) and aspartate (Asp) [4]. Furthermore, the nitrogen-rich character and unique metabolism of this amino acid allow it to serve as the major inter-organ ammonia shuttle. Notably, Gln synthesis from Glu and ammonia in a reaction catalyzed by Gln synthetase (GS), a glia-specific enzyme, is an important pathway for detoxification of ammonia upon hepatic failure associated with hyperammonemia.

Glutamine Transport

In mammalian cells, Gln is transported by several transport systems, characterized by their overlapping substrate specificities, substrate affinities and cellular distributions. At least four systems have been identified: A (alanine-preferring), L (leucine-preferring), ASC (alanine-, serine-, cysteine) and N (glutamine-, asparagine-, histidine). Systems A, ASC and N are sodium-dependent, while system L is sodium-independent. Systems A and N tolerate lithium as a substitute for sodium. All of the Systems, N, L, A and ASC, have been identified in brain [5], indicating that the CNS possesses multiple pathways for Gln uptake and/or efflux across the plasma membrane (Table 30.1). System A transporters: SNAT2 and SNAT1 recognize the prototypic substrate methyl-amino-iso-butyric acid,

MeAIB and a broad range of neutral amino acids [6]. Both transporters are pH-sensitive. SNAT2 is expressed in neurons and other cells, but has relatively low affinity for Glu compared to other amino acids. SNAT1 expression is restricted to brain and heart, suggesting its specialized properties are congruent with the function of these organs [7]. Moreover, this transporter has higher affinity for Gln than for other amino acids. The mRNA for SNAT1 and SNAT2 is expressed in cultured astrocytes, but the transporters remain inactive unless stimulated by amino acid depletion [8]. Both SNAT1 and SNAT2 share about 60 % homology with SNAT3, a variant of System N [9].

Among all thus far identified transporters, SNAT3 possess the highest affinity for Gln. Functional analysis shows that SNAT3 transports neutral amino acid and Na^+ in exchange for H^+, and mediates Gln uptake as well as efflux. Gln transport via SNAT3 is electroneutral and reversible, and involves the co-transport of 1 Na^+ and the antiport of one H^+. Efflux of Gln is particularly favored at high intracellular Na^+ and low extracellular pH [10]. Structurally and mechanistically, another variant of system N, SNAT5, is closely related to the SNAT3 transporter. The SNAT5 transporter differs in substrate profile; SNAT3 can recognize classic System N substrates such as Gln, asparagine and histidine, while SNAT5 favors serine [11].

System ASC mediates a wide-spectrum of neutral amino acids, showing a preference for shorter-chain substrates, such as alanine, serine, cysteine and threonine [12]. System ASC is represented by ASCT1 and ASCT2; however, only ASCT2 accepts Gln. ASCT2 efficiently transports Gln in cell lines and neoplastic tissues. ASCT2 take up Gln with high affinity and transport a wide panel of other zwitterionic amino acids as well as bulky/branch-chain. In addition, this transporter is able to mediate the efflux of intracellular neutral amino acids in exchange with extracellular neutral amino acids [13].

Low-affinity, high-capacity uptake of Gln mediated by system L is observed both in astrocytes and neurons, although Gln is not recognized as a preferred substrate. System L is an amino acid antiporter comprised of two isoforms, LAT1 and LAT2, of which LAT2 shows a much higher affinity for Gln. This system can mediate Gln release in the presence of extracellular amino acid substrates, such as alanine and leucine. Both LAT1 and LAT2 mediate Gln transport at the blood–brain barrier (BBB) [14].

The Glutamine (Gln)/Glutamate (Glu)-γ-Aminobutyric Acid (GABA) Cycle (GGC): Involvement of Carriers Transporting Glu and Gln in GGC

Gln functions via the glutamine/glutamate-γ-aminobutyric acid cycle (GGC) and the reactions within the cycle are carried out in both astrocytic and neuronal compartments. After exocytotic release at synaptic terminals, Glu is taken up by surrounding astrocytes via the glia-specific Glu transporter 1 (GLT-1)/EAAT2 and Glu–aspartate transporter (GLAST)/EAAT1. Gln synthetase, which is exclusively expressed in glia converts the Glu into Gln. Glu accumulation at high concentrations is oxidatively degraded after conversion to α-ketoglutarate [15]. Gln carriers, transport a portion of Gln formed within astrocytes into the extracellular space with a predominant role for the SNAT3 and ASCT2 transporters, belonging to the bidirectional transporter System N and ASC, respectively [13]. A portion of astroglial-derived Gln transport across the BBB to the periphery is mediated by system N transporters with some additional contribution from System L transporters [16]. Extracellular Gln is transported into GABA-ergic and Glu-ergic neurons by the unidirectional System A transporters, SNAT1 and SNAT2 [17]. In neurons, Gln is converted to Glu by the mitochondrial enzyme phosphate-activated glutaminase (PAG) [18]. It should be noted that the activity of PAG is much higher in neurons than in astrocytes [19] and that differential cellular compartmentation of PAG and GS forms the basis for the GGC pathway. Inhibition of GS reduces levels of GABA in the nerve terminal, which is consistent with the generation of GABA from Glu in a reaction mediated by glutamic acid decarboxylase (GAD). Additionally, Glu is packaged into synaptic vesicles by the vesicular VGLUT

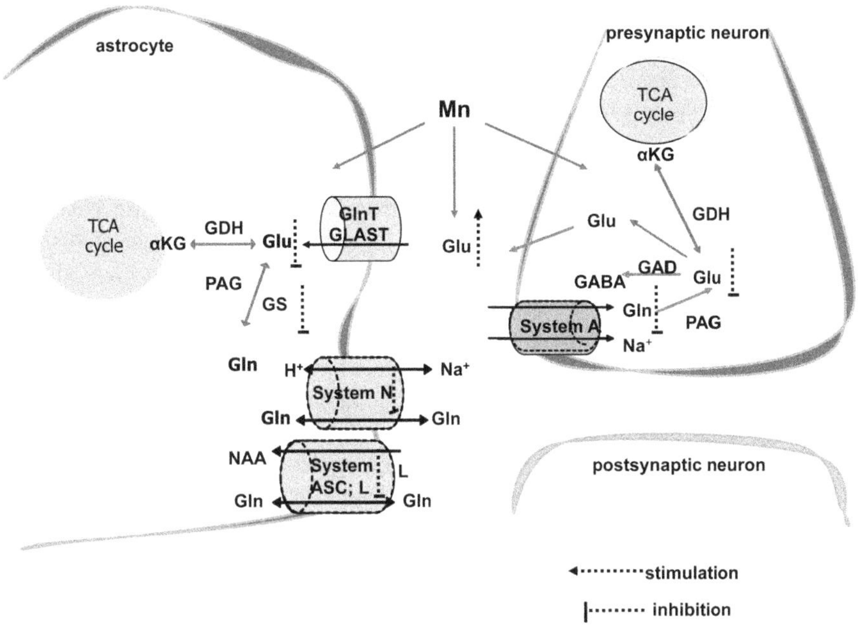

Fig. 30.1 Glutamine and glutamate transport systems related to the Gln/Glu–GABA cycle and potential sites for interference by Mn. Schematic representation showing the Gln and Glu transport and metabolism cycling between astrocytes and neurons. Glu released from presynaptic terminals is translocated to the astrocytes via GLAST and GlnT-1 transporters. In astrocyte Gln is converted to Gln by the Gln synthetase (GS). Astrocytic Gln transporters mediate its release into the extracellular space. In turn Gln is transferred into the neurons mainly by transporters belonging to the System A. In neurons Gln is regenerated via phosphate-dependent glutaminase (PAG). Glu is subsequently converted into GABA via decarboxylation by glutamic acid decarboxylase (GAD). In both astrocytes and neurons Glu is used for the synthesis of alpha-ketoglutaric acid (α KG), a substrate for the tricarboxylic acid cycle (TCA), by oxidative deamination mediated by Glu dehydrogenase (GDH)

transporter [20], released into the extracellular space and taken up by astrocytes where it is re-synthesized into Gln. The Gln and Glu cycling between astrocytes and neurons is critical for optimal CNS function, thus maintaining proper levels of the amino acid neurotransmitters Glu and GABA (Fig. 30.1).

Manganese and the Glutamine/Glutamate-γ-Aminobutyric Acid Cycle

Essentiality and Toxicity of Manganese

Manganese (Mn) is a trace metal commonly found in the environment. It is an essential dietary nutrient, and as such is required for normal physiological function. Mn-regulated enzyme families include oxidoreductases, transferases, hydrolases, isomerases, and ligases. Mn metalloenzymes include glutamine synthetase, arginase, phosphoenolpyruvate decarboxylase and Mn superoxide dismutase [21]. Nonetheless, chronic exposure to Mn may be toxic and lead to a neurological disorder, referred to as manganism. Exposure to Mn in the general population occurs from consumption of well-water containing high levels of the metal and from soy-based infant formulas. Mn is found in methylcyclopentadienyl manganese tricarbonyl (MMT), a fuel additive used in some unleaded gasoline [22]. Humans may also be exposed to organic Mn-containing pesticides, such as manganese ethylene-bis-dithiocarbamate [23]. Manganism commonly occurs in workers chronically exposed to aerosols or dusts that contain extremely high levels (>1–5 mg Mn/m^3) of Mn [24]. Occupational exposure to Mn has been identified as a health hazard for miners, battery manufacturers ferroalloy workers and automotive repair technicians [25]. Recent studies demonstrate a distinctive extrapyramidal syndrome, changes in magnetic resonance imaging (MRI) signal in the basal ganglia and elevated blood Mn levels in methcathinone abusers [26]. Manganism is characterized by neuropsychiatric symptoms resembling those observed in idiopathic Parkinson's disease [27]. Typically, individuals affected by manganism exhibit extrapyramidal changes with hypokinesia, rigidity and tremor, postural instability, dystonia and bradyskinesia, micrographia, mask-like facial expression, and speech disturbance [24]. Mn-mediated neuropathological changes are also manifested by neuronal loss and gliosis predominately in the globus pallidus and the substantia nigra pars reticulata or the striatum [28].

Mn transport within the CNS is mediated by several transporter proteins as a free ion or a nonspecific protein-bound species. Mn^{3+} binds to the transferrin receptor (TfR) and its transport competes with iron (Fe) [29]. Transport of Mn^{2+} is mediated by the family of natural resistance-associated macrophage proteins (Nramp), the divalent metal transporter-1 (DMT-1) [30]. Moreover additional channels/transporters have been identified, as potential Mn-recognizing transporters, including the divalent metal/bicarbonate ion symporters ZIP8 and ZIP14, various calcium channels, the solute carrier-39 (SLC39) family of zinc transporters, park9/ATP13A2, the magnesium transporter hip14, and the transient receptor potential melastatin 7 (TRPM7) [31].

At the cellular level, Mn specifically concentrates in mitochondria [32]. Overexposure or accumulation of Mn leads to mitochondrial disruption. Mn clearance from mitochondria is slow, thus leading to the accumulation of intra-mitochondrial Ca^{2+} [33]. Mn also promotes mitochondrial respiratory dysfunction, inducing reactive oxygen species (ROS) and inhibiting the antioxidant defense mechanisms by depleting glutathione (GSH) and glutathione peroxidase [34]. Mitochondrial function is tightly coupled to cellular energy production, thus compromised brain energy metabolism leading to decreased oxidative phosphorylation likely represents a crucial feature of Mn-induced neurotoxicity [35].

Manganese Effects on Astrocytes Function

Astrocytes express high-capacity transporters for Mn [36], and are considered a primary target for Mn-induced neurotoxicity [37]. Chronic exposure to Mn leads to selective neuronal loss in basal ganglia structures concomitant with gliosis and Alzheimer type II astrocytes with enlarged, pale nuclei and margination of chromatin. Furthermore, Mn decreases the expression of the astrocytic markers S100 and glial fibrillary acidic protein (GFAP) in several rat brain structures [37]. Approximately 60–70 % of Mn is sequestered in mitochondria while the rest is localized to the cytosol [38]. Mn causes oxidative stress in primary cultures of astrocytes, leading to mitochondrial dysfunction and energy depletion [39]. Mn leads to failure of astrocytes to maintain antioxidant defense mechanisms via disruption of GSH synthesis [40]. Treatment of astrocytes with Mn also results in increased uptake of L-arginine, a substrate for the inducible form of nitric oxide synthase (iNOS), which may lead to increased ROS generation as a consequence of nitric oxide (NO) production [41]. Astrocytic exposure to Mn is also associated with cell swelling secondary to NOS activation. Moreover, increased expression of the water channel protein aquaporin-4, a predominantly astrocytic isoform, has been implicated in Mn-mediated cell swelling [40].

Adult mammalian brain energy metabolism depends on the oxidation of glucose (Glc). Sodium–coupled transfer of Glu into astrocytes and activation of Na^+/K^+-ATPase stimulate Glc uptake and glycolytic processing [42]. The stoichiometry between oxidative Glc metabolism and Glu cycling in the cerebral cortex is close to 1:1, suggesting that the majority of cortical energy production supports functional Glu-ergic neuronal activity [43]. It is well accepted that Glc metabolism via TCA activity leads to the biosynthesis of the neurotransmitters Glu and GABA [39]. Homeostasis of these neurotransmitters

Table 30.2 Manganese and glutamate transport in astrocytes

Glu transporter	Catalytic mechanism	Principal cellular localization	Targets of Mn action
GLAST	Inward transport of one Glu is coupled to co-transport of three Na^+ and one H^+ with one K^+ being counter-transported	Astrocytes; endothelial cells	protein expression; function (uptake)
GLT-1	Inward transport of one Glu is coupled to co-transport of three Na^+ and one H^+ with one K^+ being counter-transported	Astrocytes; endothelial cells	mRNA and protein expression; function (uptake)

General characteristic of glutamate transporters and Manganese (Mn)-induced effects on glutamate carriers and signaling associated with the glutamine/glutamate-γ-aminobutyric acid cycle (GGC)

is essentially dependent upon neuronal–astrocytic interactions via the GGC. Mn mediates changes in astrocytic Glc metabolism by inhibiting the astrocyte-specific enzyme, GS [34]. Furthermore, Mn plays an important role in brain energy metabolism by affecting the key anaplerotic glial-specific enzyme, pyruvate carboxylase (PC) [44]. These effects of Mn may cause changes in astrocytic and neuronal integrity and affect astrocyte-mediated neuronal support. For example, Mn-induced neuronal injury in the striatum and the globus pallidus is associated with primary dysfunction of astrocytes via mechanisms involving NO. In addition, Mn inhibits the ability of astrocytes to promote neuronal differentiation by a mechanism that involves oxidative stress and a reduction in levels of the extracellular matrix protein, such as fibronectin.

Manganese and Glutamate Transport

Glu is the principal excitatory neurotransmitter of mammalian brain. Glu uptake by astrocytes is essential for maintaining optimal extracellular Glu concentrations that do not activate Glu transporters [45]. Extracellular accumulation of Glu causes toxicity in the CNS [46], playing an essential role in neurodegenerative diseases, such as Huntington's disease or Alzheimer's disease [47]. Furthermore, acute insults such as stroke or traumatic injury are associated with elevation of the extracellular Glu content [48].

Glu transfer is largely dependent upon neuronal–astrocytic interactions and is essential for proper functioning of the GGC cycle [4]. Moreover, pharmacological studies suggest that a significant proportion of Glu is recycled by GGC. For example in the retina, Glu levels and electrophysiological responses to light are rapidly ablated by inhibition of GS with methionine sulfoximine [49]. Glu removal from the synaptic cleft is mediated by two major astrocytic transporters: GLAST and GLT-1 [50]. The inward transport of one Glu is coupled to co-transport of three Na^+ and one H^+, with one K^+ being counter-transported. Downregulation of GLAST and GLT-1, both at the mRNA and protein levels, has been described in non-human primate brain after long-term airborne Mn exposure [51]. In agreement, impairment in Glu transport has been observed in Chinese hamster ovary cells transfected with GLAST or GLT-1 upon Mn exposure (Table 30.2). Although the underlying mechanisms responsible for the loss of Glu transporter are not completely understood, activation of the lysosomal, rather than the proteasomal pathway, is likely responsible for downregulation of Glu transporter activity in response to Mn exposure [52].

Furthermore, PKC signaling involvement has been identified in Mn-induced downregulation of Glu turnover. A recent study revealed that PKC stimulation by α-phorbol 12-myristate (PMA) significantly decreases astrocytic Glu uptake, while treatment with the general PKC inhibitor, bisindolylmaleimide II (BIS II), protects astrocytes from the Mn-induced downregulation of Glu transport. The same study also established that the PKCδ and PKCα isoforms, as well as caspase 3, are involved in Mn-dependent downregulation of astrocytic Glu uptake or GLT1 expression [52].

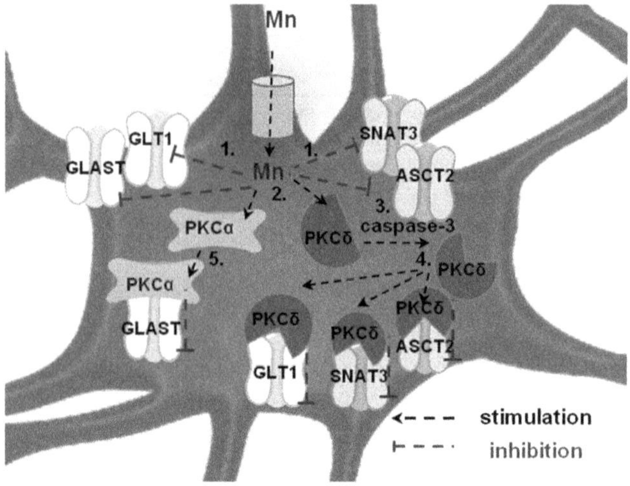

Fig. 30.2 Proposed model for Mn-induced disruption of glutamine/glutamate-γ-aminobutyric acid cycle involving PKCs signaling. Mn treatment impairs Glu and Gln transporters expression and functions (*1*) and activates PKCs isoforms: PKCδ and PKCα (*2*); Mn mediates activation of PKCδ by promoting caspase-3-dependent proteolytic cleavage (*3*); caspase-3 activation of PKCδ increases its binding with ASCT2, SNAT3 and GLT-1 transporters leading to their inactivation/dysfunction (*4*); Mn-dependent activation of PKCα triggers downregulation of GLAST transporter (*5*)

Co-immunoprecipitation studies demonstrated association between GLT-1 and the PKCδ and PKCα isoforms, and Mn-induced increases in PKCδ–GLT-1 interaction [52]. Reversal of the Mn-induced downregulation of GLAST protein expression was observed in the presence of PKCα and casapase-3 inhibitors. Moreover, no interaction between GLAST and the PKC isoforms was observed in control conditions or upon Mn exposure in primary cultures of astrocytes [52]. Several groups have demonstrated contradictory effects of PKCs on GLAST-mediated transport, showing that activation of PKC increases, decreases or has no effect on GLAST expression and activity [53]. More consistent observation has been observed in the case of the GLT-1 transporter. These studies show that activation of PKC rapidly decreases GLT-1 cell surface expression in C6 glioma stably transfected with GLT-1 and in primary cultures that endogenously express GLT-1 [54]. It appears that both GLAST and GLT-1 are regulated via the PKC-dependent pathway; however, with different contribution of the α and δ PKC isoforms for each of these transporters [55] (Fig. 30.2).

Manganese and PKCδ

Protein kinase C (PKC) isozymes comprise a family of at least ten related serine-threonine kinases that play crucial roles in the regulation of various cellular processes, including differentiation, proliferation, tumorigenesis and apoptosis [56]. Members of this family have been shown to be either pro- or antiapoptotic. PKCδ has been implicated in many cellular processes, including regulation of apoptotic cell death [57]. Mn has been shown to promote the specific phosphorylation of PKCδ isozyme, and increase PKC activity [52]. Astrocytes transfected with shRNA against PKCδ are less sensitive to Mn compared to those transfected with control shRNA. Mn also promotes the nuclear translocation of PKCδ [52]. These findings suggest that Mn affects PKCδ signaling (Fig. 30.3).

Proteolytic cleavage, mediated by caspase-3 gives rise to the PKCδ catalytic fragment (PKCδ CF), which has been invoked as a putative mechanism for kinase activation [58]. Overexpression of the PKCδ CF induces chromatin condensation and DNA fragmentation, which supports a role for

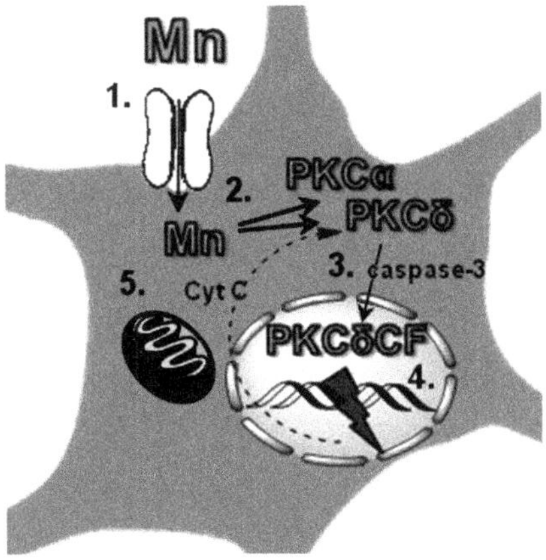

Fig. 30.3 Putative mechanism of PKC signaling in Mn-induced apoptosis and the associated mitochondrial dysfunction. (*1*) Mn exposure activates PKC isoforms: PKCδ and PKCα; (*2*) activation of PKCδ by Mn requires its proteolytic cleavage mediated by active caspase-3; (*3*) Proteolytic cleavage, mediated by caspase-3 gives rise to the PKCδ catalytic fragment (PKCδ CF), which in turn translocates to the nucleus and mediates DNA fragmentation; (*4*) PKCδ regulates key apoptotic events, including cytochrome *c* (Cyt C) release into the cytosol from mitochondria; (*5*) Cyt *c* activates caspase cascade via positive feedback loop, which leads to the amplification of the apoptotic signals

PKCδ cleavage in the induction of apoptosis. Furthermore, nuclear translocation of PKCδ is strictly dependent upon its caspase-3-mediated cleavage [57]. Notably, Mn toxicity is associated with caspase-3 activation in several in vitro and in vivo models, and as mentioned before, with increased PKCδ's nuclear translocation [52]. Moreover, a mechanism implicating caspase-3 and PKCδ inhibition has been invoked for the Mn-mediated disruption of Glu transport [52]. PKCδ plays a crucial role in the cellular response to ROS and oxidative stress-mediated PKCδ activation by caspase-3 [59]. Notably, oxidative stress particularly in mitochondria is a common feature of Mn toxicity [60]. Moreover, it has been established that caspase-3-dependent PKCδ activation not only contributes to neuronal apoptosis, but also has a significant feedback regulatory role in amplification of the apoptotic cascade during neurotoxic stress upon Mn treatment [58]. Combined, these findings suggest that caspase-3-dependent PKC activation is required for PKCδ/Mn-mediated deregulation of glutamate turnover.

Manganese and Glutamine Transport

Mn inhibits the initial net uptake of Gln in a concentration-dependent manner in primary culture of astrocyte [61]. Mn induces deregulation in the expression of SNAT3, SNAT2, ASCT2, and LAT2 transporters. These observations are consistent with Mn-mediated decrease in Gln uptake by carriers belonging to Systems N and ASC, and a decrease in Gln efflux mediated by Systems N, ASC and L in astrocytes [62].

The contribution of PKC signaling to Mn-induced dyshomeostasis in Gln transport has been investigated in cultured astrocytes [63]. A recent study revealed that PKC inhibition by BIS II blocked the Mn-induced downregulation in Glu uptake. Treatment of primary astrocyte cultures with a PKC stimulator decreases Gln uptake mediated by Systems ASC and N, and decreases expression of ASCT2 and SNAT3 protein levels in cell lysates and in plasma membranes [63]. It is noteworthy that both Mn-affected transporters contain putative PKC phosphorylation sites, which are conserved in the human, rat and mouse [64] A recent in situ study has revealed that PKC activation induces phosphorylation and internalization of SNAT3 [65]. Furthermore, increased binding of PKCδ to ASCT2 and SNAT3 upon exposure to Mn has been identified by co-immunoprecipitation. Taken together, these findings suggest a prominent role for PKCδ in Mn-mediated disruption of Gln turnover. The above-described studies combined with findings on Mn's influence on Glu transport are consistent with aberrant GGC function by Mn at two key steps, including Gln and Glu transport, via similar PKC signaling events (Fig. 30.2).

Manganese Involvement in SNAT3 Expression and Function

Ubiquitination is as an important mechanism for controlling surface expression of membrane proteins. This post-translational modification involves the sequential action of several enzymes, including an ubiquitin-activating enzyme E1, an ubiquitin-conjugating enzyme E2 and an ubiquitin-protein ligase E3. Nedd4-2 (neuronal precursor cell expressed, developmentally downregulated 4-2), a member of the HECT (homology to the E6-associated protein C terminus) family of E3 ubiquitin ligases is a physiologically important regulator of numerous membrane channels and transporters by promoting their ubiquitination [66]. Polyubiquitination triggers transporter sorting and targeting for lysosomal degradation, which also involves the proteasome. In general, phosphorylation of Nedd4-2 and E3 ligases represents a powerful regulatory mechanism for altering the fate of ion channels and other targets for ubiquitination [67]. It has been confirmed that SGK1 (serum- and glucocorticoid-regulated kinase 1) decreases the interaction between Nedd4-2 and target proteins by phosphorylation of ubiquitin ligase at three residues [68]. Furthermore, in a *Xenopus laevis* oocyte expression system, SNAT3 is downregulated by Nedd4-2 and that this effect is blocked by SGK1 [69]. It is interesting to note that Mn decreases SGK1 expression and phosphorylation, suggesting Nedd4-2/SGK1 involvement in Mn-mediated degradation of SNAT3. These findings, concomitant with those that chronic Mn exposure alters the expression of genes associated with the ubiquitin/proteasome system [70, 71], suggest that Mn-mediated disruption of SNAT3 expression or function precedes its ubiquitination [63].

It has also been shown that PKC activation regulates dopamine transporter (DAT) function by its internalization and degradation in an ubiquitin-dependent manner. Furthermore, RNA interference (RNAi) analysis shows the essential and specific role of Nedd4-2 in PKC-mediated endocytosis of DAT. Downregulation of Nedd4-2 results in a significant reduction in PKC-dependent ubiquitination of DAT. A recent study has demonstrated that PKC activation induces hyper-ubiquitination, and increases the association of SNAT3 with Nedd4-2. PKC stimulation decreases Gln uptake mediated by System N in astrocytes and significantly downregulates SNAT3 at protein levels, while Mn exposure activates PKCs [63]. In addition, prolonged stimulation of PKC with phorbol ester leads to the degradation of SNAT3 [65]. Combined, these findings demonstrate that Mn-induced deregulation of SNAT3 function is likely mediated via PKC signaling and ubiquitin-mediated proteolysis.

Conclusions

The GGC represents a complex process, because Gln efflux from astrocytes must be met by its uptake in neurons. Disturbances in Gln delivery to neurons and/or its metabolism to Glu or GABA likely contribute to neurotransmission imbalances in different neuropathological conditions. In light of the above, the key role of Mn in the GGC appears beyond doubt (Figs. 30.1 and 30.2). Mn toxicity is associated with the disruption of Gln and Glu transport in astrocytes, and consequentially with the development of secondary Glu-mediated neurotoxicity, which may modulate the activity of neuronal circuits. Mn also affects astrocytic Glc metabolism by inhibiting the astrocyte-specific enzymes GS and PC.

These effects may lead to alterations in neuronal excitatory and inhibitory inputs. In general, astrocytes are involved at multiple levels in brain (patho) physiology via their interaction with neurons, and Mn disrupts astrocyte–neuronal integrity. Thus, future studies should focus on uncovering therapeutic strategies that reverse astrocyte pathology mediated by Mn and restore optimal GGC in the astrocyte–neuron unit.

Acknowledgements The authors wish to acknowledge partial support by grants from the National Institute of Environmental Health Sciences (NIEHS) ES R01 10563 and ES P30 000267.

References

1. Erecinska M, Silver IA. Metabolism and role of glutamate in mammalian brain. Prog Neurobiol. 1990;35:245–96.
2. Darmaun D, Matthews DE, Bier DM. Glutamine and glutamate kinetics in humans. Am J Physiol. 1986;251: E117–26.
3. Eagle H. Nutrition needs of mammalian cells in tissue culture. Science. 1955;122:501–14.
4. Bak LK, Schousboe A, Waagepetersen HS. The glutamate/GABA-glutamine cycle: aspects of transport, neurotransmitter homeostasis and ammonia transfer. J Neurochem. 2006;98:641–53.
5. Sershen H, Lajtha A. Inhibition pattern by analogs indicates the presence of ten or more transport systems for amino acids in brain cells. J Neurochem. 1979;32:719–26.
6. Christensen HN, Oxender DL, Liang M, et al. The use of N-methylation to direct route of mediated transport of amino acids. J Biol Chem. 1965;240:3609–16.
7. Melone M, Quagliano F, Barbaresi P, et al. Localization of the glutamine transporter SNAT1 in rat cerebral cortex and neighboring structures, with a note on its localization in human cortex. Cereb Cortex. 2004;14:562–74.
8. Heckel T, Broer A, Wiesinger H, et al. Asymmetry of glutamine transporters in cultured neural cells. Neurochem Int. 2003;43:289–98.
9. Reimer RJ, Chaudhry FA, Gray AT, et al. Amino acid transport system A resembles system N in sequence but differs in mechanism. Proc Natl Acad Sci U S A. 2000;97:7715–20.
10. Broer A, Albers A, Setiawan I, et al. Regulation of the glutamine transporter SN1 by extracellular pH and intracellular sodium ions. J Physiol. 2002;539:3–14.
11. Nakanishi T, Sugawara M, Huang W, et al. Structure, function, and tissue expression pattern of human SN2, a subtype of the amino acid transport system N. Biochem Biophys Res Commun. 2001;281:1343–8.
12. Bode BP. Recent molecular advances in mammalian glutamine transport. J Nutr. 2001;131:2475S–85. discussion 2486S–2477S.
13. Broer A, Brookes N, Ganapathy V, et al. The astroglial ASCT2 amino acid transporter as a mediator of glutamine efflux. J Neurochem. 1999;73:2184–94.
14. Arriza JL, Kavanaugh MP, Fairman WA, et al. Cloning and expression of a human neutral amino acid transporter with structural similarity to the glutamate transporter gene family. J Biol Chem. 1993;268:15329–32.
15. Yu AC, Schousboe A, Hertz L. Metabolic fate of 14C-labeled glutamate in astrocytes in primary cultures. J Neurochem. 1982;39:954–60.
16. Xiang J, Ennis SR, Abdelkarim GE, et al. Glutamine transport at the blood-brain and blood-cerebrospinal fluid barriers. Neurochem Int. 2003;43:279–88.
17. Broer S, Brookes N. Transfer of glutamine between astrocytes and neurons. J Neurochem. 2001;77:705–19.
18. Kvamme E, Torgner IA, Roberg B. Kinetics and localization of brain phosphate activated glutaminase. J Neurosci Res. 2001;66:951–8.
19. Schousboe A, Hertz L, Svenneby G, et al. Phosphate activated glutaminase activity and glutamine uptake in primary cultures of astrocytes. J Neurochem. 1979;32:943–50.
20. Bellocchio EE, Hu H, Pohorille A, et al. The localization of the brain-specific inorganic phosphate transporter suggests a specific presynaptic role in glutamatergic transmission. J Neurosci. 1998;18:8648–59.
21. Wedler FC, Denman RB. Glutamine synthetase: the major Mn(II) enzyme in mammalian brain. Curr Top Cell Regul. 1984;24:153–69.
22. Finkelstein MM, Jerrett M. A study of the relationships between Parkinson's disease and markers of traffic-derived and environmental manganese air pollution in two Canadian cities. Environ Res. 2007;104:420–32.
23. Ferraz HB, Bertolucci PH, Pereira JS, et al. Chronic exposure to the fungicide maneb may produce symptoms and signs of CNS manganese intoxication. Neurology. 1988;38:550–3.
24. Pal PK, Samii A, Calne DB. Manganese neurotoxicity: a review of clinical features, imaging and pathology. Neurotoxicology. 1999;20:227–38.

25. Roth JA, Garrick MD. Iron interactions and other biological reactions mediating the physiological and toxic actions of manganese. Biochem Pharmacol. 2003;66:1–13.
26. Stepens A, Logina I, Liguts V, et al. A Parkinsonian syndrome in methcathinone users and the role of manganese. N Engl J Med. 2008;358:1009–17.
27. Kim Y, Kim JW, Ito K, et al. Idiopathic Parkinsonism with superimposed manganese exposure: utility of positron emission tomography. Neurotoxicology. 1999;20:249–52.
28. Yamada M, Ohno S, Okayasu I, et al. Chronic manganese poisoning: a neuropathological study with determination of manganese distribution in the brain. Acta Neuropathol. 1986;70:273–8.
29. Aschner M, Aschner JL. Manganese neurotoxicity: cellular effects and blood-brain barrier transport. Neurosci Biobehav Rev. 1991;15:333–40.
30. Fitsanakis VA, Au C, Erikson KM, et al. The effects of manganese on glutamate, dopamine and gamma-aminobutyric acid regulation. Neurochem Int. 2006;48:426–33.
31. Aschner M, Gannon M. Manganese (Mn) transport across the rat blood-brain barrier: saturable and transferrin-dependent transport mechanisms. Brain Res Bull. 1994;33:345–9.
32. Maynard LS, Cotzias GC. The partition of manganese among organs and intracellular organelles of the rat. J Biol Chem. 1955;214:489–95.
33. Kowaltowski AJ, Castilho RF, Vercesi AE. Ca(2+)-induced mitochondrial membrane permeabilization: role of coenzyme Q redox state. Am J Physiol. 1995;269:C141–7.
34. Erikson KM, Dorman DC, Fitsanakis V, et al. Alterations of oxidative stress biomarkers due to in utero and neonatal exposures of airborne manganese. Biol Trace Elem Res. 2006;111:199–215.
35. Gavin CE, Gunter KK, Gunter TE. Mn2+ sequestration by mitochondria and inhibition of oxidative phosphorylation. Toxicol Appl Pharmacol. 1992;115:1–5.
36. Aschner M, Gannon M, Kimelberg HK. Manganese uptake and efflux in cultured rat astrocytes. J Neurochem. 1992;58:730–5.
37. Henriksson J, Tjalve H. Manganese taken up into the CNS via the olfactory pathway in rats affects astrocytes. Toxicol Sci. 2000;55:392–8.
38. Wedler FC, Ley BW, Grippo AA. Manganese(II) dynamics and distribution in glial cells cultured from chick cerebral cortex. Neurochem Res. 1989;14:1129–35.
39. Chen CJ, Liao SL. Oxidative stress involves in astrocytic alterations induced by manganese. Exp Neurol. 2002;175:216–25.
40. Rama Rao KV, Reddy PV, Hazell AS, et al. Manganese induces cell swelling in cultured astrocytes. Neurotoxicology. 2007;28:807–12.
41. Hazell AS, Norenberg MD. Ammonia and manganese increase arginine uptake in cultured astrocytes. Neurochem Res. 1998;23:869–73.
42. Magistretti PJ. Regulation of glycogenolysis by neurotransmitters in the central nervous system. Diabete Metab. 1988;14:237–46.
43. Sibson NR, Dhankhar A, Mason GF, et al. Stoichiometric coupling of brain glucose metabolism and glutamatergic neuronal activity. Proc Natl Acad Sci U S A. 1998;95:316–21.
44. Zwingmann C, Leibfritz D, Hazell AS. Energy metabolism in astrocytes and neurons treated with manganese: relation among cell-specific energy failure, glucose metabolism, and intercellular trafficking using multinuclear NMR-spectroscopic analysis. J Cereb Blood Flow Metab. 2003;23:756–71.
45. Mayer ML, Westbrook GL. The physiology of excitatory amino acids in the vertebrate central nervous system. Prog Neurobiol. 1987;28:197–276.
46. Sheldon AL, Robinson MB. The role of glutamate transporters in neurodegenerative diseases and potential opportunities for intervention. Neurochem Int. 2007;51:333–55.
47. Zoia C, Cogliati T, Tagliabue E, et al. Glutamate transporters in platelets: EAAT1 decrease in aging and in Alzheimer's disease. Neurobiol Aging. 2004;25:149–57.
48. Faden AI, Demediuk P, Panter SS, et al. The role of excitatory amino acids and NMDA receptors in traumatic brain injury. Science. 1989;244:798–800.
49. Pow DV, Robinson SR. Glutamate in some retinal neurons is derived solely from glia. Neuroscience. 1994; 60:355–66.
50. Sims KD, Robinson MB. Expression patterns and regulation of glutamate transporters in the developing and adult nervous system. Crit Rev Neurobiol. 1999;13:169–97.
51. Erikson KM, Dorman DC, Lash LH, et al. Duration of airborne-manganese exposure in rhesus monkeys is associated with brain regional changes in biomarkers of neurotoxicity. Neurotoxicology. 2008;29:377–85.
52. Sidoryk-Wegrzynowicz M, Lee E, Aschner M. Mechanism of Mn(II)-mediated dysregulation of glutamine-glutamate cycle: focus on glutamate turnover. J Neurochem. 2012;122:856–67.
53. Conradt M, Stoffel W. Inhibition of the high-affinity brain glutamate transporter GLAST-1 via direct phosphorylation. J Neurochem. 1997;68:1244–51.

54. Gonzalez-Gonzalez IM, Garcia-Tardon N, Gimenez C, et al. PKC-dependent endocytosis of the GLT1 glutamate transporter depends on ubiquitylation of lysines located in a C-terminal cluster. Glia. 2008;56:963–74.
55. Sidoryk-Wegrzynowicz M, Lee E, Mingwei N, et al. Disruption of astrocytic glutamine turnover by manganese is mediated by the protein kinase C pathway. Glia. 2011;59:1732–43.
56. Nishizuka Y. The role of protein kinase C in cell surface signal transduction and tumour promotion. Nature. 1984;308:693–8.
57. Reyland ME. Protein kinase C isoforms: Multi-functional regulators of cell life and death. Front Biosci. 2009; 14:2386–99.
58. Latchoumycandane C, Anantharam V, Kitazawa M, et al. Protein kinase Cdelta is a key downstream mediator of manganese-induced apoptosis in dopaminergic neuronal cells. J Pharmacol Exp Ther. 2005;313:46–55.
59. Sun X, Wu F, Datta R, et al. Interaction between protein kinase C delta and the c-Abl tyrosine kinase in the cellular response to oxidative stress. J Biol Chem. 2000;275:7470–3.
60. Rivera-Mancia S, Rios C, Montes S. Manganese accumulation in the CNS and associated pathologies. Biometals. 2011;24:811–25.
61. Milatovic D, Yin Z, Gupta RC, et al. Manganese induces oxidative impairment in cultured rat astrocytes. Toxicol Sci. 2007;98:198–205.
62. Sidoryk-Wegrzynowicz M, Lee E, Albrecht J, et al. Manganese disrupts astrocyte glutamine transporter expression and function. J Neurochem. 2009;110:822–30.
63. Sidoryk-Wegrzynowicz M, Lee ES, Ni M, et al. Manganese-induced downregulation of astroglial glutamine transporter SNAT3 involves ubiquitin-mediated proteolytic system. Glia. 2010;58:1905–12.
64. Pawlik TM, Souba WW, Sweeney TJ, et al. Phorbol esters rapidly attenuate glutamine uptake and growth in human colon carcinoma cells. J Surg Res. 2000;90:149–55.
65. Nissen-Meyer LS, Popescu MC, el Hamdani H, et al. Protein kinase C-mediated phosphorylation of a single serine residue on the rat glial glutamine transporter SN1 governs its membrane trafficking. J Neurosci. 2011;31: 6565–75.
66. van Bemmelen MX, Rougier JS, Gavillet B, et al. Cardiac voltage-gated sodium channel Nav1.5 is regulated by Nedd4-2 mediated ubiquitination. Circ Res. 2004;95:284–91.
67. Debonneville C, Flores SY, Kamynina E, et al. Phosphorylation of Nedd4-2 by Sgk1 regulates epithelial Na(+) channel cell surface expression. EMBO J. 2001;20:7052–9.
68. Rotin D, Staub O. Nedd4-2 and the regulation of epithelial sodium transport. Front Physiol. 2012;3:212.
69. Boehmer C, Okur F, Setiawan I, et al. Properties and regulation of glutamine transporter SN1 by protein kinases SGK and PKB. Biochem Biophys Res Commun. 2003;306:156–62.
70. Guilarte TR, Burton NC, Verina T, et al. Increased APLP1 expression and neurodegeneration in the frontal cortex of manganese-exposed non-human primates. J Neurochem. 2008;105:1948–59.
71. Sidoryk-Wegrzynowicz M, Aschner M. Manganese toxicity in the CNS: the glutamine/glutamate-gamma-aminobutyric acid cycle. J Intern Med. 2013;273:466.

Chapter 31
Glutamine and Epilepsy

Weiwei Hu and Zhong Chen

Key Points

- Although the tissue content of glutamine is similar to other major amino acids, the concentration of glutamine in the cerebrospinal fluid and extracellular space of brain is at least one order of magnitude higher than other amino acids.
- The transport of glutamine from blood to the brain is insufficient to reach the requirement of the brain, and the synthesis from glutamate by glutamine synthetase in astrocytes supplements the demand.
- The glutamine synthesis is crucial to the glutamate clearance in interstitial space and neuronal glutamate and GABA synthesis by participating in the glutamine–glutamate–GABA cycle between astrocytes and neurons.
- The deficiency of glutamine synthesis due to the loss of glutamine synthetase may result in a seizure or the development of epilepsy.
- The accumulation of glutamate in interstitial space and the deficit of GABA synthesis could be the main reasons for the hyperexcitability, following the inhibition of glutamine synthetase.

Keywords Glutamine • Glutamine–glutamate–GABA cycle • Glutamine synthetase • Epilepsy • Seizure

Abbreviations

AAV	Adeno-associated virus
CNS	Central nervous system
eGFP	Enhanced green fluorescent protein
eIPSC	Evoked inhibitory post-synaptic currents
GAD	Glutamate decarboxylase
GDH	Glutamate dehydrogenase

W. Hu, Ph.D. • Z. Chen, Ph.D. (✉)
Department of Pharmacology, Key Laboratory of Medical Neurobiology of the Ministry of Health of China, Zhejiang Province Key Laboratory of Neurobiology, School of Basic Medical Sciences, Zhejiang University, Yuhangtang Road 866#, Hangzhou, Zhejiang 310058, P. R. China
e-mail: huww@zju.edu.cn; chenzhong@zju.edu.cn

R. Rajendram et al. (eds.), *Glutamine in Clinical Nutrition*, Nutrition and Health,
DOI 10.1007/978-1-4939-1932-1_31, © Springer Science+Business Media New York 2015

GS	Glutamine synthetase
MSO	L-methionine sulfoximine
MTLE	Mesial temporal lobe epilepsy
PAG	Phosphate-activated glutaminase
SAT	System A type transporter
TCA	Tricarboxylic acid cycle
TLE	Temporal lobe epilepsy
VGAT	Vesicular GABA transporter protein
VGLUT	Vesicular glutamate transporters

Introduction

The amount of glutamine is abundant in the central nervous system (CNS) and it is evenly distributed in the different brain regions [1, 2]. The transport of glutamine from blood to the brain is insufficient to reach the requirement of the brain, and the synthesis from glutamate by glutamine synthetase (GS) in astrocytes supplements the demand [2]. Glutamine is required for several physiological processes, including synthesis of proteins, osmoregulation and synthesis of glutamate and GABA [3]. So, glutamine is crucial to the glutamine–glutamate–GABA cycle in the brain, which may largely affect the balance between the excitatory and inhibitory transmission. However, the excessive accumulation of glutamine in the brain may result in CNS dysfunction, due to cerebral edema and mitochondrial damage. For instance, hyperammonemia can cause such disturbance by facilitating the formation of glutamine. Yet, this chapter focuses on the participation of glutamine in the glutamine–glutamate–GABA cycle, and the association between the disruption of the cycle and seizure or epilepsy.

Glutamine and Glutamine–Glutamate–GABA Cycle

Although the tissue content of glutamine is similar to other major amino acids, the concentration of glutamine in the cerebrospinal fluid and extracellular space of brain is at least one order of magnitude higher than other amino acids (Table 31.1) [2, 4]. The extracellular concentrations of most amino acids in the brain are at the range of low micromole, which are much lower than their plasma level. In contrast, the extracellular concentration of glutamine varies from 0.06 to 0.5 mM, and the upper of the range is close to its level in CSF, plasma and serum [4]. The distinction of the concentration among different amino

Table 31.1 Concentrations (μM) of amino acids in cerebrospinal fluid, plasma and serum

	CSF	Plasma	Serum
Glutamate	3.3 ± 0.3	43 ± 26	67 ± 36
Aspartate	2.1 ± 0.7	3.3 ± 1.6	10 ± 7
Glutamine	378 ± 67	416 ± 200	416 ± 200
Asparagine	4.7 ± 33	43 ± 27	47 ± 27
Glycine	8.4 ± 0.9	153 ± 74	155 ± 73
Alanine	26 ± 9	218 ± 130	230 ± 124
Serine	44 ± 4	107 ± 61	117 ± 56
Threonine	5.1 ± 0.9	139 ± 82	149 ± 81
Taurine	19 ± 0.4	178 ± 105	284 ± 38
Citrulline	5.5 ± 1.9	72 ± 39	83 ± 35

Adapted from [4] and reproduced with permission from Neuroscience\Elsevier B.V.

acids in interstitial space may be partially due to the difference in the ability of crossing the blood–brain barrier, for example the rate of glutamate penetration is 5–10 folds less than that of glutamine [5].

In the CNS, the glutamine participates in the glutamine–glutamate–GABA cycle (Fig. 31.1), which is crucial to glutamate clearance in interstitial space and maintenance of excitatory and inhibitory transmissions. In this cycle, glutamine comes from a reaction catalyzed by GS, which metabolize glutamate and ammonia to glutamine with consumption of a molecule ATP:

$$\text{Glutamate} + \text{NH}^4 + \text{ATP} \rightarrow \text{Glutamine} + \text{ADP} + \text{Pi}.$$

As glutamine transported from the periphery does not reach the demand of the brain tissues, a majority of CNS glutamine is synthesized by GS endogenously. GS is preferentially located in the cytoplasm of astrocytes, but varies in different regions with the greatest degree noted in the hippocampus and cerebellar cortex, while the least is found in brain stem, deep cerebellar nuclei and spinal cord [6]. In the hippocampus, GS-immunoreactivity is strongest in astrocyte processes that engulf glutamatergic nerve terminals [7] and displays a layer specific distribution corresponding to the glutamate binding sites [8], highlighting its critical role in glutamate metabolism. The formed glutamine then leaves the cytoplasm of astrocytes to extracellular space mostly via glutamine transporter system N transporters 1 [9]. Subsequently, glutamine is imported into GABAergic and glutamatergic neurons via the system A type transporter, SAT1 and SAT2, respectively [10, 11].

In the glutamatergic neurons, glutamine is converted to glutamate via mitochondrial enzyme phosphate-activated glutaminase (PAG) [12], and then packaged into synaptic vesicles by vesicular

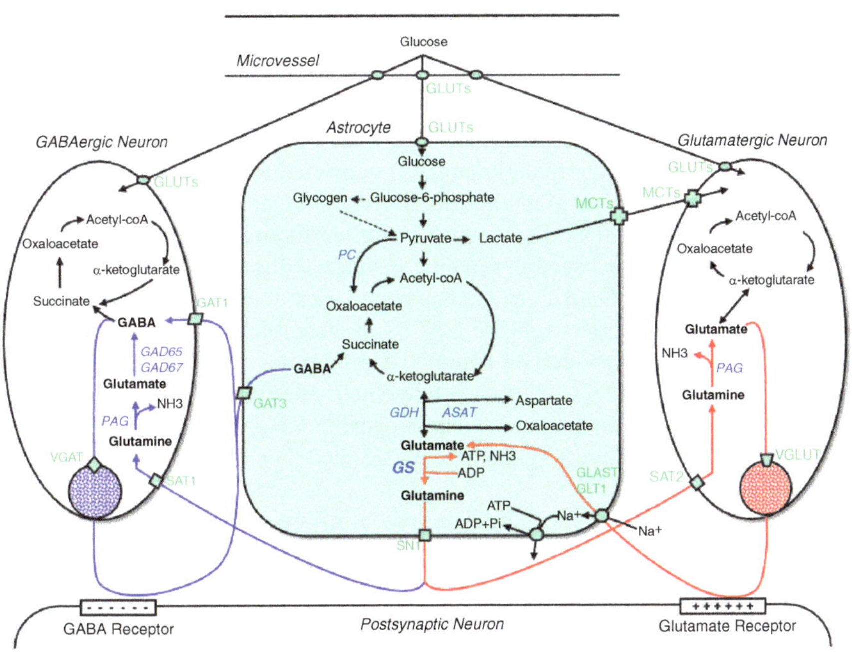

Fig. 31.1 Diagram of GS and its role in the glutamine–glutamate–GABA cycle and ammonia metabolism. Key enzymes, transporter molecules, and metabolic intermediates are shown. Note the metabolic relationship among astrocytes, GABAergic neurons, and glutamatergic neurons as indicated by the glutamine–glutamate–GABA cycle (*purple arrows* to the *left*) and the glutamine–glutamate cycle (*red arrows* to the *right*). *ADP* adenosine diphosphate, *ASAT* aspartate aminotransferase, *ATP* adenosine triphosphate, *GABA* c-aminobutyric acid, *coA* coenzyme A, *GAT3* GABA transporter subtype 3, *GAD65/67* glutamate decarboxylase isoforms 65/67, *GDH* glutamate dehydrogenase, *MCTs* monocarboxylate transporters, *PAG* phosphate-activated glutaminase, *SAT1/2* system A transporter subtypes 1/2, *SN1* system N transporter subtype 1, *VGAT* vesicular GABA transporter, *VGLUT* vesicular glutamate transporter (Adapted from [36] and reproduced with permission from Neurochem Res\Springer)

glutamate transporters (VGLUT) [13, 14]. After release from synaptic vesicles, glutamate binds to glutamate receptors in neurons and glial cells. The extracellular glutamate is mainly taken up by glutamate transporters in astrocytes. There are Na^+-independent and Na^+-dependent glutamate uptake systems, among which astrocyte Na^+-dependent systems show high affinity for glutamate and are the predominant glutamate uptake mechanism in the brain [15]. Overall, five Na^+-dependent glutamate transporters have been identified, that are EAAT1 (GLAST), EAAT2 (GLT-1), EAAT3, EAAT4 and EAAT5. Among them, GLAST and GLT-1 are almost exclusive glial glutamate transporters but with different location. In adult brain, GLT-1 expression is most abundant in forebrain regions [16], whereas GLAST is prevalent in cerebellum [17]. EAAT3 is mainly expressed in glutamatergic and GABAergic neurons, showing lower density compared with astrocytic glutamate transporters [16]. The less efficiency of neuronal glutamate uptake results in the uptake of most neuronally released glutamate by astrocytes to reduce extracellular glutamate at 3–4 μM under resting status, compared with cytosolic glutamate at the range from 1 to 10 mM in different cell types [15]. EAAT4 and EAAT5 are found in Purkinje cells and retina, respectively, which are less related to the cerebral glutamine–glutamate–GABA cycle addressed here.

The imported glutamate is converted back to glutamine by the reaction mentioned before, so as to complete the glutamine–glutamate metabolic cycle. On the other hand, glutamate is an important metabolic fuel, which is oxidatively degraded to carbon dioxide and water, besides being the most important excitatory transmitter [18]. It has been estimated that two-thirds of glutamate is converted to glutamine, while one-third enters the tricarboxylic acid cycle (TCA) to participate in oxidative metabolism which also exists in neurons [19]. In astrocytes, glutamate is also metabolized to glutathione, which is exported to the extracellular space to provide neurons with the glutathione precursor L-cysteinylglycine [20]. Because of the low penetration of the blood–brain barrier, glutamate degradation must be compensated for by net synthesis of glutamate from glucose. However, neurons lack the enzyme pyruvate carboxylase which mediates the effective synthesis of precursors for glutamate synthesis in TCA, so neurons need net formation of glutamate from glucose in astrocytes to maintain their glutamate activity [21].

In GABAergic neurons, the imported glutamine is converted to glutamate via PAG catalysis and then further converted to GABA via glutamate decarboxylase isoenzymes GAD65, which is concentrated in the nerve terminals, and GAD67, which is present throughout the cytoplasm [22]. GABA used for neurotransmission is packaged in synaptic vesicles by the vesicular GABA transporter protein (VGAT) [23]. The released GABA can be transported back to neurons or to astrocytes by GABA transporters. The GABA transporters subtype GAT3 is preferentially present on astrocytes, whereas GAT1 and GAT2 are mainly expressed on neurons. A proportion of GABA is not metabolized and may be released back into extracellular space, while others enter the TCA cycle as succinate, which may be converted to glutamate by glutamate dehydrogenase (GDH) [24]. In astrocytes, the synthesized glutamate can be metabolized to glutamine by GS, and then the glutamine–glutamate–GABA cycle is completed.

It has been suggested that astrocytic glutamine synthesis is essential for maintaining neuronal glutamate release. In hippocampal slice cultures, inhibition of GS with L-methionine sulfoximine (MSO), reduced glutamate-like immunoreactivity by 52 % in terminals and increased nearly fourfold in glias, meanwhile glutamine-like immunoreactivity was reduced by 66 % in glias [25]. However, recent studies suggested that the astrocyte mediated cycle may primarily support the inhibitory GABA neurotransmission. In a hippocampal slice study, it is found that blocking steps during glutamate–glutamine cycle can reduce synaptic GABA release in hippocampus [26]. High-titer transduction of astrocytes with enhanced green fluorescent protein (eGFP) via adeno-associated virus (AAV 2/5) induced reactive astrocytosis and downregulated expression of GS in hippocampus, which reduced inhibitory, but not excitatory, synaptic currents [27]. Blocking the glutamate–glutamine cycle by MSO could mimic this phenomenon, while exogenous glutamine administration enhanced inhibitory synaptic currents [27] (Fig. 31.2). Moreover, oral L-glutamine increased GABA levels in striatal tissue

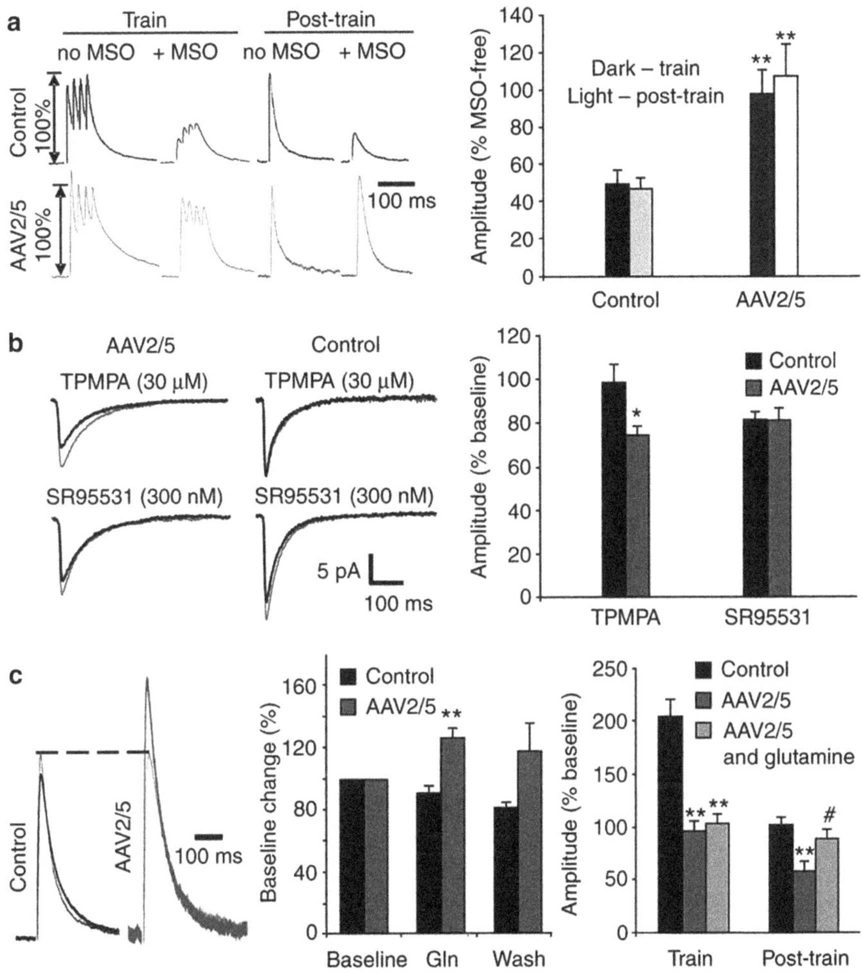

Fig. 31.2 Glutamate–glutamine cycle deficits reduce the concentration of vesicular GABA. (**a**) *Left*, eIPSCs of MSO-treated cells compared with cells that were not exposed to MSO during and following train stimulation. *Right*, effect of train stimulation on eIPSC amplitudes following incubation in MSO (1.5 mM) is expressed as the percentage change from eIPSCs recorded in the absence of MSO. MSO triggered an activity-dependent decrease of eIPSC amplitude in control cells, but not AAV2/5 cells (**$P<0.001$ relative to control). (**b**) *Left*, miniature inhibitory postsynaptic currents (mIPSC) averages in the absence (*thin traces*) and presence (*thick traces*) of TPMPA (low-affinity $GABA_A$ antagonist) and SR95531 (high-affinity $GABA_A$ antagonist). *Right*, TPMPA significantly reduced mIPSC amplitude in neurons from AAV2/5 eGFP-positive cells (AAV2/5 (+/–TPMPA), 9.5±1.2 pA/7.1±0.9 pA, $n=6$, $P=0.005$, paired t test; control (+/–TPMPA), 12.5±1.6 pA/12.2±2 pA, $n=6$, $P=0.87$, paired t test). SR95531 reduced mIPSC amplitude to a similar extent in both groups of cells (AAV2/5 (+/–SR95531), 12.3±1.4 pA/9.9±1.4 pA, $n=5$, $P=0.033$, paired t test; control (+/–SR95531), 13.6±2.1 pA/11.1±1.8 pA, $P=0.004$, paired t test). *$P=0.027$ compared with controls. (**c**) *Left*, current traces before (*thin trace*) and during (*thick trace*) application of 10 mM glutamine. *Middle*, supplementation with glutamine partially reversed eIPSC failure in a subset of AAV2/5 cells (**$P<0.001$ relative to control; AAV2/5, $n=7$; control, $n=7$). *Right*, bath-applied glutamine restored eIPSC amplitudes to control levels following train stimulation, but failed to prevent eIPSC failure during the train (**$P\leq0.003$ relative to control, #$P=0.04$ relative to AAV2/5). Cell numbers (train/post-train) are as follows: control, $n=12/10$; AAV2/5, $n=10/6$; AAV2/5 and glutamine, $n=6/5$. Error bars represent s.e.m (Adapted from [27] and reproduced with permission from Nat Neurosci\Nature Publishing Group)

and extracellular fluid, but not glutamate [28]. Since GS converts glutamate to glutamine in astrocytes, it has been proposed that the deficiency in GS may lead to an increase of glutamate in astrocytes, which could result in the accumulation of glutamate in the extracellular space. This hypothesis is based on that rapid metabolism of intracellular glutamate is a prerequisite for efficient glutamate clearance form extracellular space [29]. Thus, the inhibition of glutamine synthesis in astrocytes could induce either glutamate or GABA synaptic perturbations, leading to broader functional disorders associated with neurologic disease.

Glutamine/Glutamine–Glutamate–GABA Cycle and Epilepsy

Epilepsy is a common and diverse set of chronic neurological disorders characterized by recurring seizures. Epileptic seizures result from abnormal, excessive or hypersynchronous neuronal activity in the brain that may be due to the imbalance between excitability and inhibition in neurotransmission. Therefore, it is reasonable to propose that the glutamine–glutamate–GABA cycle is involved in the induction of seizure or the development of epilepsy. Indeed, abundant evidence showed that the dysfunction of this cycle associates with epilepsy, especially the temporal lobe epilepsy (TLE). TLE is one of the most common forms of drug-resistant focal epilepsies in humans. The recurrent epileptic seizures of TLE may arise from mesial temporal lobe structures, involving the hippocampus, entorhinal cortex and amygdala [30]. One of its characteristics is the hippocampal sclerosis, showing a pattern of neuronal loss, gliosis, mossy fiber sprouting and granule cell dispersion [31]. At present, there is still no effective treatment to control TLE, which may be due to an incomplete understanding of the pathophysiology of TLE.

In microdialysis studies to measure the extracellular levels of glutamate and glutamine in the hippocampus of epileptic patients during the interictal period, it is found that the epileptogenic hippocampus had surprisingly high basal glutamate levels and low glutamine/glutamate ratio [32], and the increased glutamate level associates with epileptogenic hippocampal atrophy [33]. Moreover, during seizures extracellular glutamate increased 6-fold above interictal level and 30-fold higher than normal, which remained at high level for several hours after the cessation of seizure [34]. In the febrile seizure which may be related to the development of TLE, glutamate release increased before onset of seizures in rats and this increase correlated with a decrease in seizure threshold temperature, indicating that increased cortical extracellular glutamate induced by hyperthermia contributes to the onset of seizures [35]. The mechanism may be same as that in clinical seizures induced by fever in patients with febrile convulsions or epilepsy. The reason for the pronounced increase could result from the slow rates of glutamate–glutamine cycling, although the release of glutamate from astrocytes into extracellular space may also be involved [36]. By magnetic resonance spectroscopy, the epileptogenic, gliotic human hippocampus appears to be characterized metabolically by an increase in glutamate content, decreased glutamine content, and slow rates of glutamate–glutamine cycling [37].

The deficiency of GS is proposed to account for the low rate of glutamate–glutamine cycling that leads to a failure of glial glutamate detoxification and continuing excitotoxicity. A study of surgically resected tissue from mesial temporal lobe epilepsy (MTLE) patients indicated that the expression of GS in the hippocampus was 40 % lower than that in non-MTLE samples, and the enzyme activity was lower by 38 % vs. non-MTLE [38]. The loss of GS was particularly pronounced in CA1 of the MTLE hippocampus (Fig. 31.3), where showed obvious astroglial proliferation [38]. In the TLE patients with hippocampal sclerosis, GS was markedly downregulated in the hippocampus in areas with severe neuron loss [39].

The roles of GS in epilepsy are also revealed by animal studies. In seizure prone gerbils (*Meriones unguiculatus*), it was found that seizures were related to a deficiency in cerebral GS [40]. Also, the expression of GS was strongly correlated to electroconvulsive threshold in a gene expression and

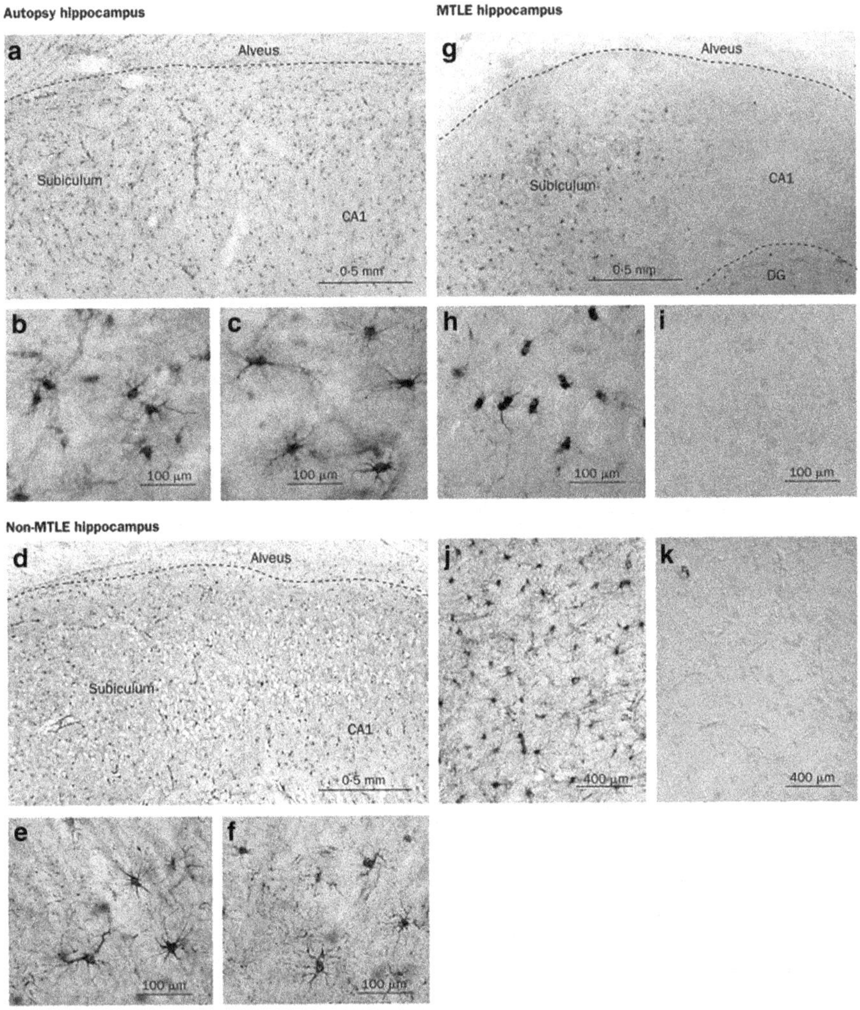

Fig. 31.3 GS immunoreactivity of representative autopsy (**a**–**c**), non-MTLE (**d**–**f**), and MTLE (**g**–**i**) hippocampi. There is dense and even distribution of GS-positive cells in subiculum and area CA1 of autopsy (**a**) and non-MTLE hippocampi (**d**). High-power fields of subiculum in autopsy (**b**) and non-MTLE (**e**) hippocampi show that staining is confined to astroglial cells. High-power fields of area CA1 in autopsy (**c**) and non-MTLE (**f**) hippocampi also show many positive astroglial cells. In MTLE hippocampus (**g**), there are many GS-positive cells in the subiculum but area CA1 is severely deficient in staining for GS. High-power field of subiculum in G (**h**) confirms presence of staining in astroglial cells, which have somewhat fewer processes than positive astrocytes in the corresponding area of autopsy (**b**) and non-MTLE hippocampi (**e**). High-power field of area CA1 in G (**i**) confirms lack of staining in this region. Specificity controls with GS antiserum (**j**) and preimmune serum (**k**) on adjacent sections of the non-MTLE hippocampus shown in (**d**–**f**) reveal no staining in (**k**). DG = dentate gyrus (Adapted from [38] and reproduced with permission from Lancet\Elsevier B.V.)

phenotype correlation study [41]. The causative action of GS in epilepsy was suggested from genetically modified animals and pharmacological inhibition. In GS haploinsufficiency mice, partial knockdown of GS increased the susceptibility to febrile seizures by measuring the latencies to four behavioral febrile seizure characteristics [42]. MSO is an irreversible inhibition of GS, which causes depletion of glutamine and accumulation of glutamate in astrocytes [25]. Systemic single injection of MSO promoted acute convulsive seizures in rodents [43]. Sustained brain microinfusion of MSO into the hippocampus in rats induced the recurrent seizures continuously for several weeks, along with a deficiency

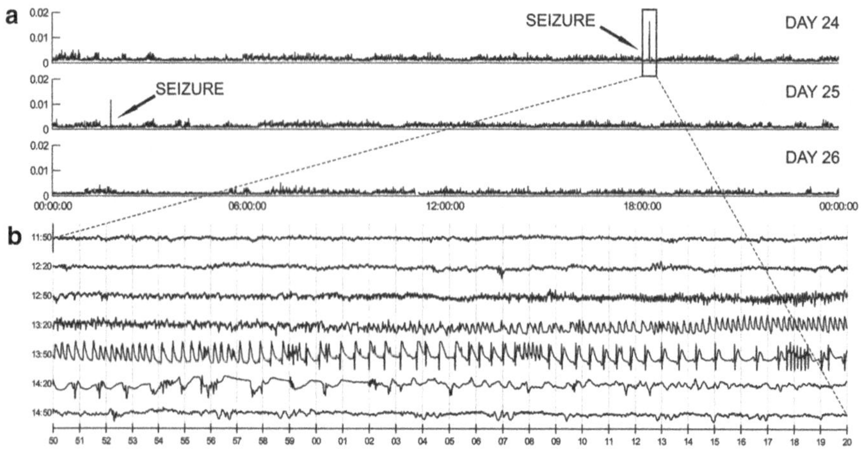

Fig. 31.4 MSO precipitates recurrent seizures. (**a**) Continuous 3-day-record (days 24–26 after surgery) of Teager energy (a weighted measure of signal energy such that high-frequency signals contribute greater energy than low-frequency signals ($E \propto w^2A^2$, where E is the energy, w is the frequency and A is the amplitude of the signal); Energy estimates were obtained at a 1 s resolution) of a single ic (intracranial) electroencephalography (EEG) time-series from a representative animal infused continuously with intrahippocampal MSO (0.625 μg/h). Energy estimates were obtained at 1 s resolution and averaged over a 5 s running window (x-axis). A 24-h-period (midnight to midnight) is displayed in each trace. Two seizures were recorded during the 72-h period. As in human epilepsy, seizures in the MSO model are readily identified by the difference in energy (y-axis) from background icEEG activity. (**b**) Continuous 3.5 min icEEG (from day 24: 18: 11: 50 to 18: 15: 20) displaying the first seizure identified in (**a**) (Adapted from [44] and reproduced with permission from Brain\Oxford University Press)

in hippocampal GS activity by 82–97 % vs. saline group [44] (Fig. 31.4). Some of the MSO-treated animals displayed neuropathological characteristics that were similar to mesial temporal sclerosis, such as hippocampal atrophy and patterned loss of hippocampal neurons.

The low GS activity can trigger the increase in astrocytic and extracellular glutamate, which may account for the hyperexcitibility after MSO administration. On the other side, the deficit of GS also reduces the synthesis of glutamine which can be converted to glutamate after transports into the neurons. Therefore, the outcome of the GS deficiency seems not easy to be speculated. It has been hypothesized that in glutamine-significant depletion situations, the supplement of exogenous glutamine may assume a primary role in the support of excitatory neurotransmission, and inhibition of glutamine synthesis may further compromise the excitatory neurotransmitter synthesis [45]. However, in TLE patients, the loss of GS is spatially restricted to specific areas mostly CA1, CA3 and dentate hilus, which allows the supplement of glutamine from other non-compromised region, therefore the excitatory neurotransmitter synthesis may not be compromised and the accumulation of extracellular glutamate is reasonable [36].

Other evidences highlighting the involvement of GABA deficit in the seizure induction after blocking the GS are also available. In a study of the effect of chronic H1-antihistamine treatment on seizure susceptibility after drug withdrawal, it is found that chronic H1-antihistamines diphenhydramine and pyrilamine treatment produced long-lasting increase in seizure susceptibility together with the reduction of GS activity and glutamine and GABA level [46] (Fig. 31.5). Supplement with glutamine reversed the high susceptibility after diphenhydramine treatment. It suggests that the lack of glutamine can predominantly render the deficiency of GABA release, and subsequently the increase of seizure susceptibility. Moreover, a reduction of evoked inhibitory post-synaptic currents (eIPSC), suggesting the impaired vesicular release of GABA, is found in hippocampal slices after MSO administration [26]. Although these data seem not in accord with the hypothesis in glutamine depletion situations mentioned above, it suggests that the deficiency of GABA synthesis together with the accumulation of glutamate in interstitial space could be the main reasons for the hyperexcitability,

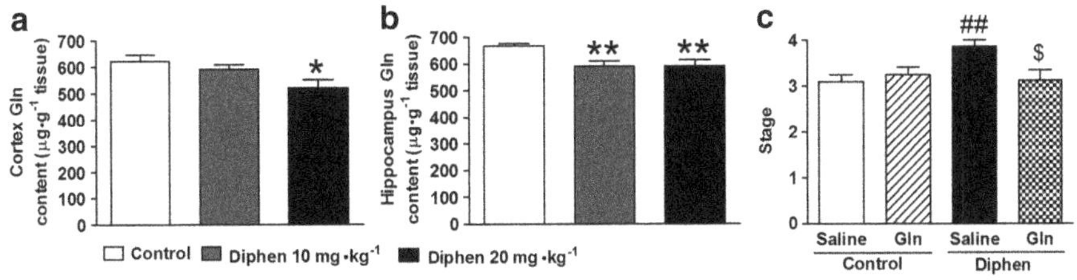

Fig. 31.5 Effect of chronic diphenhydramine treatment on glutamine after withdrawal in rats. Ten days after withdrawal from a 2-week diphenhydramine (diphen) treatment, the total glutamine (Gln) content in the cortex (**a**) and hippocampus (**b**) was determined by high-performance liquid chromatography. The pentylenetetrazol-induced seizure behavioral stage was determined after supplementation with 2 g/kg Gln at 10 days after drug withdrawal from a 2-week 20 mg/kg diphen treatment (**c**). Values are expressed as mean ± SEM. $n = 7$–9 (**a**, **b**); $n = 7$–11 (**c**). $^{*}P < 0.05$, $^{**}P < 0.01$ Compared with control; $^{\#\#}P < 0.01$ compared with saline-treated rats in control group; $\$P < 0.05$ compared with saline-treated rats in diphen group (Adapted from [46] and reproduced with permission from CNS Neurosci Ther\Blackwell Publishing Ltd)

after the inhibition of GS. Further studies are required to elucidate the detailed association between the aberrant glutamine–glutamate–GABA cycle and seizure or epilepsy development.

Other components of glutamine–glutamate–GABA cycle may also be implicated in the development of epilepsy. For instance, GDH activity was decreased in the temporal cortex and hippocampus in MTLE patients, which was negatively correlated with the duration since the first intractable seizure [47]. The expression of GLT-1 and GLAST were also decreased in the epileptogenic hippocampal formation in TLE patients [48]. It suggests that the alteration of any component in the cycle may result in hyperexcitibility and even seizure.

Glutamine is depleted from muscle stores during severe metabolic stress including sepsis and major surgery. Dietary supplementation with nutrients, including glutamine, enhancing immune function is beneficial to patients with surgical and critical illnesses [49]. Glutamine also has been shown to reduce the number of serious neonatal infections in very preterm children. However, the effect of glutamine supplement on the CNS is not well known. Short-term glutamine supplementation after birth increases white matter, hippocampus, and brain stem volumes in very preterm children at school age, however, it may not be a direct effect of glutamine on the brain but associated with the lower incidence of serious neonatal infections [50]. Whereas, from a study in rats it is found that glutamine supplementation during brain development facilitates cortical spreading depression propagation, as judged by the higher cortical spreading depression velocities [51]. Whether glutamine supplementation can be used to treat epilepsy still awaits investigation by abundant experimental or even clinical studies.

Conclusions

Mounting evidence has addressed the critical role of glutamine in the CNS, which orchestrates the communication between astrocytes and neurons by participating in the glutamine–glutamate/GABA cycle. The effective cycling limits the accumulation of toxic glutamate in the extracellular space, and supplies neurotransmitter precursors for reuse in excitatory and inhibitory synapses. Without sufficient conversion from glutamate to glutamine in astrocytes, for example when the GS is downregulated, the increase of glutamine in interstitial space and the insufficiency of GABA synthesis may take place. However, which is the primary reason inducing seizure or the development of epilepsy is still not understood, and further studies are needed to address this issue especially based on human-related evidence. To be noted, new therapeutic strategies targeting glutamine or glutamine–glutamate/GABA cycle may benefit the control of TLE with further investigations.

References

1. Broer S, Brookes N. Transfer of glutamine between astrocytes and neurons. J Neurochem. 2001;77:705–19.
2. Albrecht J, Sonnewald U, Waagepetersen HS, et al. Glutamine in the central nervous system: function and dysfunction. Front Biosci. 2007;12:332–43.
3. Norenberg MD, Jayakumar AR, Rama Rao KV, et al. New concepts in the mechanism of ammonia-induced astrocyte swelling. Metab Brain Dis. 2007;22:219–34.
4. Xu GY, McAdoo DJ, Hughes MG, et al. Considerations in the determination by microdialysis of resting extracellular amino acid concentrations and release upon spinal cord injury. Neuroscience. 1998;86:1011–21.
5. Smith QR. Transport of glutamate and other amino acids at the blood-brain barrier. J Nutr. 2000;130:1016S–22.
6. Norenberg MD. Distribution of glutamine synthetase in the rat central nervous system. J Histochem Cytochem. 1979;27:756–62.
7. Derouiche A, Frotscher M. Astroglial processes around identified glutamatergic synapses contain glutamine synthetase: evidence for transmitter degradation. Brain Res. 1991;552:346–50.
8. Derouiche A, Ohm TG. Glutamine synthetase immunoreactivity in the human hippocampus is lamina-specific. Neurosci Lett. 1994;165:179–82.
9. Chaudhry FA, Reimer RJ, Edwards RH. The glutamine commute: take the N line and transfer to the A. J Cell Biol. 2002;157:349–55.
10. Solbu TT, Bjorkmo M, Berghuis P, et al. SAT1, a glutamine transporter, is preferentially expressed in GABAergic neurons. Front Neuroanat. 2010;4:1.
11. Jenstad M, Quazi AZ, Zilberter M, et al. System A transporter SAT2 mediates replenishment of dendritic glutamate pools controlling retrograde signaling by glutamate. Cereb Cortex. 2009;19:1092–106.
12. Kvamme E, Torgner IA, Roberg B. Kinetics and localization of brain phosphate activated glutaminase. J Neurosci Res. 2001;66:951–8.
13. Bellocchio EE, Hu H, Pohorille A, et al. The localization of the brain-specific inorganic phosphate transporter suggests a specific presynaptic role in glutamatergic transmission. J Neurosci. 1998;18:8648–59.
14. Fremeau Jr RT, Troyer MD, Pahner I, et al. The expression of vesicular glutamate transporters defines two classes of excitatory synapse. Neuron. 2001;31:247–60.
15. Danbolt NC. Glutamate uptake. Prog Neurobiol. 2001;65:1–105.
16. Rothstein JD, Martin L, Levey AI, et al. Localization of neuronal and glial glutamate transporters. Neuron. 1994;13:713–25.
17. Schmitt A, Asan E, Puschel B, et al. Cellular and regional distribution of the glutamate transporter GLAST in the CNS of rats: nonradioactive in situ hybridization and comparative immunocytochemistry. J Neurosci. 1997;17:1–10.
18. Zielke HR, Collins Jr RM, Baab PJ, et al. Compartmentation of [14C]glutamate and [14C]glutamine oxidative metabolism in the rat hippocampus as determined by microdialysis. J Neurochem. 1998;71:1315–20.
19. Hertz L, Zielke HR. Astrocytic control of glutamatergic activity: astrocytes as stars of the show. Trends Neurosci. 2004;27:735–43.
20. Wang XF, Cynader MS. Astrocytes provide cysteine to neurons by releasing glutathione. J Neurochem. 2000; 74:1434–42.
21. Yu AC, Drejer J, Hertz L, et al. Pyruvate carboxylase activity in primary cultures of astrocytes and neurons. J Neurochem. 1983;41:1484–7.
22. Bu DF, Erlander MG, Hitz BC, et al. Two human glutamate decarboxylases, 65-kDa GAD and 67-kDa GAD, are each encoded by a single gene. Proc Natl Acad Sci U S A. 1992;89:2115–9.
23. Jin H, Wu H, Osterhaus G, et al. Demonstration of functional coupling between gamma-aminobutyric acid (GABA) synthesis and vesicular GABA transport into synaptic vesicles. Proc Natl Acad Sci U S A. 2003;100:4293–8.
24. Dennis SC, Lai JC, Clark JB. Comparative studies on glutamate metabolism in synaptic and non-synaptic rat brain mitochondria. Biochem J. 1977;164:727–36.
25. Laake JH, Slyngstad TA, Haug FM, et al. Glutamine from glial cells is essential for the maintenance of the nerve terminal pool of glutamate: immunogold evidence from hippocampal slice cultures. J Neurochem. 1995; 65:871–81.
26. Liang SL, Carlson GC, Coulter DA. Dynamic regulation of synaptic GABA release by the glutamate-glutamine cycle in hippocampal area CA1. J Neurosci. 2006;26:8537–48.
27. Ortinski PI, Dong J, Mungenast A, et al. Selective induction of astrocytic gliosis generates deficits in neuronal inhibition. Nat Neurosci. 2010;13:584–91.
28. Wang L, Maher TJ, Wurtman RJ. Oral L-glutamine increases GABA levels in striatal tissue and extracellular fluid. FASEB J. 2007;21:1227–32.
29. Otis TS, Jahr CE. Anion currents and predicted glutamate flux through a neuronal glutamate transporter. J Neurosci. 1998;18:7099–110.

30. Spencer SS, Spencer DD. Entorhinal-hippocampal interactions in medial temporal lobe epilepsy. Epilepsia. 1994;35:721–7.
31. Riban V, Bouilleret V, Pham-Le BT, et al. Evolution of hippocampal epileptic activity during the development of hippocampal sclerosis in a mouse model of temporal lobe epilepsy. Neuroscience. 2002;112:101–11.
32. Cavus I, Kasoff WS, Cassaday MP, et al. Extracellular metabolites in the cortex and hippocampus of epileptic patients. Ann Neurol. 2005;57:226–35.
33. Cavus I, Pan JW, Hetherington HP, et al. Decreased hippocampal volume on MRI is associated with increased extracellular glutamate in epilepsy patients. Epilepsia. 2008;49:1358–66.
34. During MJ, Spencer DD. Extracellular hippocampal glutamate and spontaneous seizure in the conscious human brain. Lancet. 1993;341:1607–10.
35. Morimoto T, Nagao H, Yoshimatsu M, et al. Pathogenic role of glutamate in hyperthermia-induced seizures. Epilepsia. 1993;34:447–52.
36. Eid T, Behar K, Dhaher R, et al. Roles of glutamine synthetase inhibition in epilepsy. Neurochem Res. 2012;37:2339–50.
37. Petroff OA, Errante LD, Rothman DL, et al. Glutamate-glutamine cycling in the epileptic human hippocampus. Epilepsia. 2002;43:703–10.
38. Eid T, Thomas MJ, Spencer DD, et al. Loss of glutamine synthetase in the human epileptogenic hippocampus: possible mechanism for raised extracellular glutamate in mesial temporal lobe epilepsy. Lancet. 2004;363:28–37.
39. van der Hel WS, Notenboom RG, Bos IW, et al. Reduced glutamine synthetase in hippocampal areas with neuron loss in temporal lobe epilepsy. Neurology. 2005;64:326–33.
40. Laming PR, Cosby SL, O'Neill JK. Seizures in the Mongolian gerbil are related to a deficiency in cerebral glutamine synthetase. Comp Biochem Physiol C. 1989;94:399–404.
41. Letwin NE, Kafkafi N, Benjamini Y, et al. Combined application of behavior genetics and microarray analysis to identify regional expression themes and gene-behavior associations. J Neurosci. 2006;26:5277–87.
42. van Gassen KL, van der Hel WS, Hakvoort TB, et al. Haploinsufficiency of glutamine synthetase increases susceptibility to experimental febrile seizures. Genes Brain Behav. 2009;8:290–5.
43. Szegedy L. Enzyme histochemical studies in the rat hippocampus, cerebellar cortex and brainstem motor nuclei during methionine sulphoximine convulsions. Cell Mol Biol Incl Cyto Enzymol. 1978;23:43–53.
44. Eid T, Ghosh A, Wang Y, et al. Recurrent seizures and brain pathology after inhibition of glutamine synthetase in the hippocampus in rats. Brain. 2008;131:2061–70.
45. Coulter DA, Eid T. Astrocytic regulation of glutamate homeostasis in epilepsy. Glia. 2012;60:1215–26.
46. Hu WW, Fang Q, Xu ZH, et al. Chronic h1-antihistamine treatment increases seizure susceptibility after withdrawal by impairing glutamine synthetase. CNS Neurosci Ther. 2012;18:683–90.
47. Malthankar-Phatak GH, de Lanerolle N, Eid T, et al. Differential glutamate dehydrogenase (GDH) activity profile in patients with temporal lobe epilepsy. Epilepsia. 2006;47:1292–9.
48. Proper EA, Hoogland G, Kappen SM, et al. Distribution of glutamate transporters in the hippocampus of patients with pharmaco-resistant temporal lobe epilepsy. Brain. 2002;125:32–43.
49. Kim H. Glutamine as an immunonutrient. Yonsei Med J. 2011;52:892–7.
50. de Kieviet JF, Oosterlaan J, Vermeulen RJ, et al. Effects of glutamine on brain development in very preterm children at school age. Pediatrics. 2012;130:e1121–7.
51. de Lima DS, Maia LM, Barboza Ede A, et al. L-glutamine supplementation during the lactation period facilitates cortical spreading depression in well-nourished and early-malnourished rats. Life Sci. 2009;85:241–7.

Chapter 32
Glutamine Supplementation in Glutamine Synthetase Deficiency

Johannes Häberle

Key Points

- Inherited glutamine synthetase deficiency is an ultra-rare disorder leading to severe chronic encephalopathy.
- Glutamine supplementation is a rationale approach to treat glutamine deficiency caused by a defect of glutamine synthetase.
- Supplementation of glutamine has as yet been performed in only a single patient affected by glutamine synthetase deficiency and proved to be safe.
- Glutamine supplementation was shown to fully correct the peripheral biochemical phenotype and to improve the central biochemical phenotype.
- Glutamine supplementation should be started as early as possible to avoid the consequences of glutamine deficiency.

Keywords Glutamine synthetase • Glutamine supplementation • Rare metabolic disease • Neonatal onset seizures • Chronic encephalopathy • Chronic hyperammonemia • Therapeutic trial • GABA • Neurotransmitter replenishment

Abbreviations

CSF	Cerebrospinal fluid
EEG	Electroencephalogram
GABA	γ-Aminobutyric acid
GLUL gene	Glutamine ammonia ligase gene
GS	Glutamine synthetase
MRI	Magnetic resonance imaging
MRS	Magnetic resonance spectroscopy
NAA	*N*-acetylaspartate

J. Häberle, M.D. (✉)
Division of Metabolism, University Children's Hospital Zurich, Zürich 8032, Switzerland
e-mail: Johannes.Haeberle@kispi.uzh.ch

R. Rajendram et al. (eds.), *Glutamine in Clinical Nutrition*, Nutrition and Health,
DOI 10.1007/978-1-4939-1932-1_32, © Springer Science+Business Media New York 2015

Introduction

The non-essential amino acid glutamine is a key player for numerous metabolic reactions in all organisms [1]. Amongst other roles, glutamine is pivotal for the temporary storage and transport of nitrogen between different organs [1] and it is the major amino moiety donor for many transamination reactions that are required for the production of other amino acids, glucose precursors, purines and pyrimidines, and adenosine-monophosphate [2]. Besides, glutamine contributes to pH homeostasis in the kidney and to regulation of plasma glucose levels in the pancreas [3, 4], and is in the central nervous system the primary precursor of the most abundant fast excitatory and inhibitory neurotransmitters, namely glutamate and γ-aminobutyric acid (GABA), respectively [5–7].

Given the many pivotal roles of glutamine, it is surprising that there is only one known reaction for endogenous glutamine production in mammals provided by the enzyme glutamine synthetase (GS; Glutamate-ammonia ligase; EC 6.3.1.2) (Fig. 32.1).

GS is ubiquitously expressed, active in the cytosol and can be considered as key enzyme of nitrogen metabolism [1, 8, 9]. The synthesis of glutamine from glutamate and ammonia is ATP-dependent and requires as well the presence of magnesium and manganese as cofactors. The GS reaction is the source for the entire body glutamine pool since there is no intestinal net absorption of glutamine in healthy individuals [10, 11]. In addition to the many roles of glutamine, the GS reaction is vital for many organs, e.g. by balancing the nitrogen pool between different compartments, by detoxifying ammonia and glutamate in astrocytes [12–14] and by supporting osmotic cell homeostasis [13, 15, 16].

Glutamine plays a critical role in humans already during pregnancy, since there is a need for glutamine for normal ontogeny and brain development [17, 18]. Accordingly, GS is expressed in utero in early human fetuses [19] and its function is necessary for early development in mice and drosophila [20, 21]. Moreover, this is supported by the known GS-dependency of de novo glutamine synthesis in the placenta [22]. However, the supply of glutamine from the placenta to the fetus is ceased immediately after birth, while the demand for glutamine continues to increase in infancy and early childhood due to synaptogenesis and establishment of functional neuronal networks [23, 24].

On the basis of the described importance of the function of GS as well as of the availability of its product, glutamine, for the human organism, an inherited defect of GS in humans must be expected to result in a severe phenotype if this is not already early embryonic or fetal lethal. The severity of a GS defect has already been suggested by the clinical course in patients affected by secondary GS impairment [25, 26] and was in addition recently confirmed in the very few patients with an inborn error of endogenous glutamine synthesis [27, 28] caused by mutations in the *glutamine ammonia ligase* (*GLUL*) gene encoding for GS; the *GLUL* gene, located on chromosome 1q25.3 (OMIM *138290) is one of the oldest existing genes [8]. The defect in these patients is named GS deficiency (OMIM #610015) and is inherited in an autosomal recessive mode [27]. All patients with GS deficiency

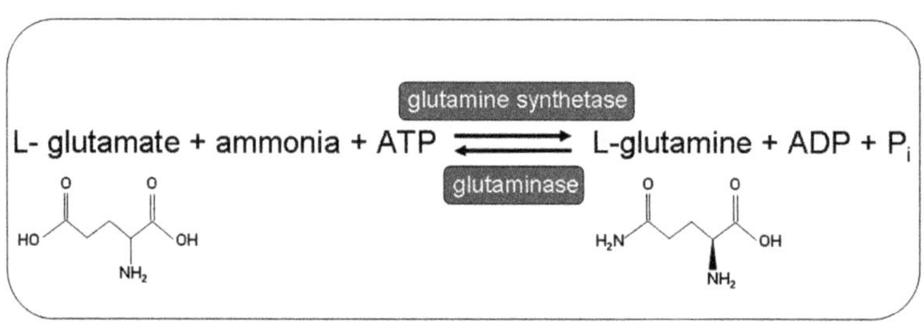

Fig. 32.1 Glutamine synthetase reaction. Reaction of glutamine synthetase as well as the reverse reaction provided by the enzyme glutaminase. Below, structures of glutamate and glutamine are shown illustrating the transamination reaction. *ADP* adenosine diphosphate, *ATP* adenosine triphosphate, P_i inorganic phosphate

suffered from neonatal onset severe epileptic encephalopathy [27, 28] and either died from neonatal multiorgan failure [27, 29] or survived into early childhood [28]. As described in other amino acid synthesis defects [30–32], supplementation of the missing amino acid could in theory have the potential to alleviate the consequences of GS deficiency. This has been recently evaluated also for GS deficiency when in a therapeutic trial performed in a single patient the safety of glutamine supplementation and its potential to influence the course of the disease could be established [24].

This chapter briefly reviews the inherited defect of GS but focuses on our current knowledge and experience of glutamine supplementation in human GS deficiency.

Background to Inherited Glutamine Synthetase Deficiency

An inherited defect of GS has been described in only three patients so far [27, 28]. All three patients presented immediately after birth [27] or early in the neonatal period [28]. The patients were of Turkish or of Sudanese origin and all had a consanguineous background. Interestingly, the mutations identified in the patients all affect the same domain of the *GLUL* gene. Two of the patients carry similar nucleotide exchanges (c.970C>T and c.970C>A, respectively) resulting in missense mutations (p.Arg324Cys and p.Arg324Ser, respectively) affecting the same residue. Another patient carries a missense mutation (c.1021C>T, p.Arg341Cys) in close vicinity. The residues affected are either conserved in all species (Arg324) or conserved in eukaryotes (Arg341) and both are part of active sites: Arg324 is involved in ATP binding and Arg341 is adjacent to the glutamate binding site according to the recently identified GS crystal structure [33] (Fig. 32.2).

It remains unclear whether GS deficiency indeed is an ultra-rare or a sometimes undiagnosed albeit still rare disorder. The only few patients identified so far would support the assumption of an ultra-rare disorder. This would certainly be in line with the outstanding role of GS for the mammalian organism

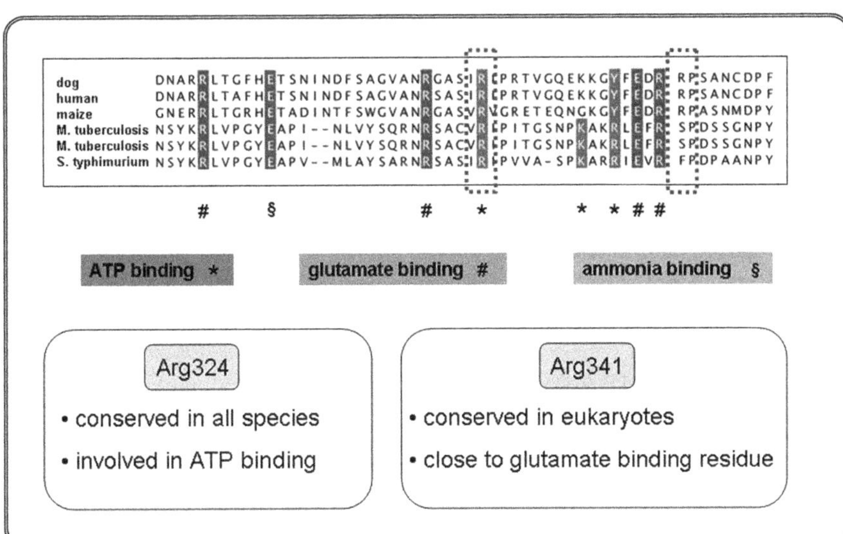

Fig. 32.2 Mutated residues in GS deficiency. Alignment of amino acids 295–349 of the human GS protein with the corresponding sequences from dog, maize, two different M. tuberculosis species as well as from S. typhimurium. Residues involved in ATP, glutamate or ammonia binding, respectively, are indicated by *asterisk*, *hash* or *paragraph signs*, respectively. Residues Arg324 and Arg341 are depicted by *grey dashed frames*. Figure adapted from [33]

during all stages of development. Since already early embryonic stages require the function of GS [19, 21, 34], an inherited defect of this enzyme may indeed lead to early loss of an affected embryo or fetus. On the other hand, all patients with GS deficiency have until now been identified by the same lab suggesting at least to some extent underdiagnosis of this disorder. It is important to note that diagnosis of GS deficiency depends on the cognition of *decreased* levels of an amino acid in plasma, urine or cerebrospinal fluid (CSF) while most metabolic disorders present with *elevated* levels of amino acids.

The Clinical Phenotype in Inherited Glutamine Synthetase Deficiency

The clinical course in the first two patients was already described in detail [27, 29]. In brief, both patients were of Turkish origin and manifested directly after birth with severe epileptic encephalopathy and multiorgan failure. One patient died on day 2 of life while the other survived 4 weeks before succumbing to her multiple problems including seizures, intractable diarrhea and necrolytic erythema of the entire integument. Since the first report of the disorder, only one additional patient was identified and the natural course of this patient over a period of more than 3 years has been recently described [28]. In brief, this patient was born to first cousin parents from Sudan after an uneventful pregnancy. Soon after birth, he was noted to have generalized muscular hypotonia, lower limb hyperreflexia, cloni and episodes of eye staring lasting for 2–3 min. At 13 days of life, generalized tonic–clonic convulsions started and persisted despite extended anticonvulsant therapy contributing to a severe developmental delay. As it was the case in another patient, also this patient suffered from necrolytic erythema when serum glutamine levels were <10 μmol/L at 38 months [28]. The reason for the longer survival of this patient may be a slightly higher level of GS residual activity in case of the missense mutation p.Arg324Ser of the *GLUL* gene identified in the longer surviving patient if compared to the effect of the mutations p.Arg324Cys and p.Arg341Cys in the case of the neonatally deceased patients, respectively, but this is not yet proven (Table 32.1).

Glutamine Supplementation in Glutamine Synthetase Deficiency

Glutamine has gained much interest as a dietary supplement in the general population. Its use has been tested in many studies in healthy adults and the usual conclusion was that of a safe supplement if some potential hazards are taken into account [35, 36]. In the many glutamine supplementation studies in healthy volunteers, doses up to 750 mg/kg/day have proved to be safe during short-term

Table 32.1 Clinical presentation in GS deficiency

Patients	Ethnic background	Onset	Life time	Main symptoms
1	Turkish	Immediately after birth	28 days	Epileptic encephalopathy Multiorgan failure Skin erythema Diarrhea
2	Turkish	Immediately after birth	2 days	Epileptic encephalopathy Multiorgan failure
3	Sudanese	Day 1	6 years	Epileptic encephalopathy Severe retardation Skin erythema (one episode)

application [10, 35, 37–39]. Based on this safety profile and on the severe glutamine deficiency in GS deficiency, its supplementation was considered also for therapeutic purposes in the patient.

In addition, supplementation of an amino acid has already been successfully applied in some of the few other known amino acid biosynthesis disorders, mainly postnatally in a therapeutic way but also as a prophylactic approach to treat affected fetuses during pregnancy [30–32, 40]. It was therefore logical to consider supplementation of glutamine as treatment for GS deficiency.

In the first two patients with GS deficiency, a therapeutic intervention was not feasible because of the early death of the patients. Glutamine supplementation has until now only been tried in a single patient [24]. This intervention was finally undertaken despite concerns about possible increases of plasma and CSF ammonia and of extracellular glutamate concentrations, potentially leading to neurotoxicity and increased susceptibility to seizures [41, 42]. In the following, the glutamine supplementation trial will be described.

The Clinical Situation During the Therapeutic Trial

For many months, the patient had been in a stuporous state with only a few minutes of apparent alertness during daytime. Then, emotional expressions such as satisfaction, hunger or anger could be identified by the parents. The neurological status of the patient was probably the result of the severe changes in cerebral white matter reflecting the longstanding glutamine deficiency, the lack of the metabolic products of glutamine, and the severe chronic epileptic encephalopathy. The observed neurodegeneration is consistent with experimental findings supporting the role of GS for Schwann cell differentiation [43]. On the basis of the described neurological situation, substantial short-term clinical improvement in the patient's condition could not be expected.

The patient was at that time mainly fed via his gastrostomy tube but was also able to suck small amounts of his diet. Convulsions were present every day, but overall, the patient was in a stable condition and vital parameters were all in normal ranges. In this situation, the patient was hospitalized for 4 weeks ensuring close clinical, laboratory and technical monitoring. The therapeutic trial lasted for the entire 4 weeks during which the patient remained clinically stable. A detailed description of the trial was recently published [24].

Practical Aspects of Glutamine Supplementation

The aim of the therapeutic trial was to provide a safe and effective remedy for GS deficiency but at the same time the intervention must ideally be easy to perform to be continued long term and by the family at their home. Thus, an enteral route was primarily addressed so L-glutamine was provided as a powder (Resource® Glutamin, Nestlé Nutrition, Vevey, Switzerland).

A low starting dose of 17 mg/kg/day given in eight dosages equally distributed during day and night time was chosen because of the above-mentioned concerns about the possible toxicity of raising plasma ammonia and glutamate levels. When initially no effect was observed but the intervention was tolerated without problems, glutamine was increased stepwise each day to a final dose of 1,020 mg/kg on day 21 of the trial. For the first 14 days of the trial, fasting glutamine levels obtained immediately before the next enteral dose of glutamine did not raise. Therefore, the interval between single dosages was shortened from 3 to 2 h leading to raising trough levels of plasma glutamine. To improve the practicability of the intervention, 330 mg/kg glutamine was administered during night hours from 12 p.m. until 8 a.m. as a continuous enteral infusion via the gastrostomy tube after dilution of glutamine in 100 mL tap water. Before this infusion has been used, the stability of the glutamine solution was investigated by measurement of glutamine at 0, 6 and 9 h, which yielded steady concentrations.

To provide in addition information on the parenteral dose of glutamine needed for maintaining normal plasma glutamine levels and to hereby prepare for situations in which no enteral application may be tolerated, L-glutamine was given in a dipeptide preparation containing in addition L-alanine (Dipeptiven®, Fresenius Kabi, Stans, Switzerland) during close monitoring of plasma glutamine as a continuous infusion over 6 h at a rate of 21 mg/kg/h and 31 mg/kg/h, respectively, and over 8 h at a rate of 41 mg/kg/h while enteral glutamine supplementation was paused.

Biochemical Monitoring During Glutamine Supplementation

Measuring levels of plasma glutamine generally requires a fasting state with at least 3–4 h time-lag to the last protein containing meal. To meet this requirement during the glutamine supplementation trial, levels of plasma ammonia, glutamine and glutamate (the latter two as part of a complete amino acid profile) were obtained with the largest possible gap to the preceding glutamine dosage and immediately before the next glutamine administration. This rigorous monitoring yielded stable levels of ammonia and glutamate in blood as well as in CSF. Initial fasting concentrations of plasma glutamine were 74 µmol/L (reference range 457–857) and remained unchanged while glutamine was given every 3 h. However, after changing to a two hourly interval and at a dose of 700 mg/kg/day, plasma glutamine levels increased above the lower limit of normal. When glutamine was given as an infusion, plasma glutamine and ammonia levels remained stable as there was no change of the entire clinical situation. Compatible with the improvement in plasma, levels of CSF glutamine constantly increased from 121 at baseline to 146, 171 and 201 µmol/L (reference range 333–658) after 2, 3, and 4 weeks of treatment, respectively, but remained below the lower limit of normal during the limited trial period [24].

Besides, a number of other investigations were performed at baseline and at the end of the trial. These included concentrations of creatine and guanidinoacetate in CSF, which were normal in this patient although baseline creatine was in the upper normal range and showed a similar decrease to that observed by magnetic resonance spectroscopy (MRS). In addition, neurotransmitter metabolites were measured in CSF revealing slightly decreased but over the time of the trial unchanged concentrations of homovanillic acid (171 at baseline and 188 nmol/L at the end of the trial, reference range 211–871). Levels of CSF folates and pterines were always normal as were concentrations of glutamate and total as well as free GABA; details are published in [24].

Technical Monitoring During Glutamine Supplementation

Since the patient suffered from chronic encephalopathy with occasional epileptic seizures, electroencephalogram (EEG) recording was done. At baseline, EEGs were severely abnormal with frontal high amplitude slow waves (0.5–2/s) and intermittent generalized subdelta (0.5/s) waves. During sleep, the amplitude was intermittently attenuated in irregular intervals and partly suppressed for 1–3 s. During the short awake intervals, multifocal sharp waves were present with higher frequency than during sleep. EEG after 1 week of treatment showed a slightly improved background activity and the intermittent amplitude attenuation during sleep seemed to be less distinct. After 3 weeks of glutamine treatment, the background activity had clearly improved with dominant 3–5/s activity in the awake state. At the end of the 4 weeks trial, intermittent amplitude attenuations completely disappeared during sleep and multifocal sharp waves were less frequent in all recordings (both awake and asleep) [24].

In addition, magnetic resonance imaging (MRI) including MRS was performed. At the baseline of the trial, MRI (performed at age 3 years 9 months) showed changes that were not present in the

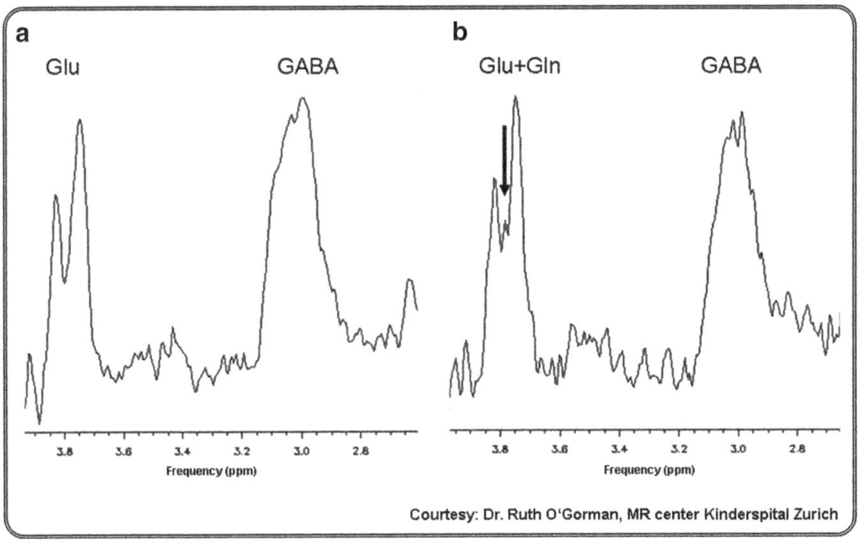

Fig. 32.3 Comparison of MRS spectrum at baseline and at the end of the trial. Brain MRS performed in the patient before the 4 weeks trial (panel **a**) and at the end of the trial (panel **b**). At the beginning of the trial, concentration of glutamate alone (Glu) is given since glutamine was absent. On the *right panel*, concentrations of glutamate and glutamine (Glu + Gln) are shown; the *black vertical arrow* in panel (**b**) indicates the glutamine peak only seen at the end of the trial. GABA concentrations are shown on each *right side* of panel (**a**) and (**b**) (at about 3.0 ppm) demonstrating the decrease in GABA concentrations during the glutamine supplementation trial. Figure adapted from [24]

previous examination at 11 months [28], including increased white matter signal intensity on T2-weighted images, prominent Virchow-Robin-spaces, reduced white matter volume with consequent thinning of the corpus callosum and secondary enlargement of CSF spaces. The basal ganglia were atrophic and no contrast enhancement was present. Two other MRI examinations during the trial did not reveal additional changes.

MRS at baseline demonstrated undetectable glutamine, reduced *N*-acetylaspartate (NAA) and glutamate and elevated creatine, choline, and myo-inositol concentrations, respectively. Monitoring after 2 weeks revealed increased glutamine and glutamate levels and a decrease of creatine and choline with a modest increase in NAA. At the end of the 4 weeks trial, glutamine, glutamate, and NAA levels continued to increase but remained below normal while creatine and choline levels continued to decrease but remained above normal. GABA levels were within the normal range both at baseline and at the end of the trial but there was a trend to lower levels during the trial (Fig. 32.3).

Results of the Therapeutic Trial

The main aim of the trial was to achieve in the patient an improved supply of glutamine mainly to the brain but basically to the entire organism as indicated by increasing concentrations of glutamine in plasma and CSF while avoiding adverse effects. This was considered the prerequisite for an improvement of brain function as indicated by advancement of alertness and the entire clinical status as well as of normalization of the EEG.

Importantly, enteral as well as parenteral L-glutamine was well tolerated during the 4 weeks trial without adverse effects. Of note, enteral glutamine supplementation was entirely sufficient to establish and maintain normal plasma glutamine levels. As an alternative if enteral use is not feasible,

Table 32.2 Summary therapeutic trial

- Improved alertness
- Peripheral glutamine deficiency completely corrected
- Glutamine deficiency in brain partly corrected
- Significant improvement of EEG
- No worsening of hyperammonemia
- No increase of plasma or CSF glutamate

parenteral application of glutamine was also successful in this patient but was considered as second choice for practical reasons and based on the higher invasiveness.

Two weeks after the start of glutamine supplementation, the plasma glutamine concentrations increased with a concomitant improvement in the patient's alertness. This was mainly noted by the parents but could also be confirmed by staff members as there were clearly longer awake intervals during the day. In addition, the intensity of emotional expressions of the patient improved as demonstrated by the "longest ever smile" on the last day of the trial as described by the father. The improvement in alertness of the patient is certainly encouraging with respect to an earlier start of treatment in future patients.

The peripheral biochemical phenotype of GS deficiency, namely the low plasma glutamine level, was normalized under high-dose glutamine supplementation (1,020 mg/kg/day). This is in alignment with earlier reports that, while at normal levels of intake there is no net intestinal absorption of glutamine in healthy individuals, additional supplementation does increase plasma glutamine concentrations [10, 35, 44] and indicates effective absorption of enteral glutamine in GS deficiency. In addition, the central biochemical phenotype was also improved, as indicated by enhanced glutamine availability in CSF and brain tissue.

EEG recordings were much improved both in the awake and sleeping state, suggesting that sufficient amounts of external glutamine can cross the blood–brain barrier and possibly influence neuronal activity. In brain MRS, glutamine concentrations continuously increased from zero to measurable levels, which remained however below those seen in age-matched comparison subjects. While MRS glutamate was also low at baseline, levels increased during the trial but remained low relative to controls. Details to measured levels are documented in [24].

Interestingly, the observed failure of a further build-up of glutamine in brain tissue and in CSF may indicate its increased utilization supported by the advancements in the background EEG activity and by the improved alertness as a sign of amelioration of the encephalopathy. Thus, glutamine supplementation succeeded in increasing the supply of glutamine throughout the body, possibly stimulating cellular metabolism and sustaining normal function [24] (Table 32.2).

Glutamine Supplementation Does Not Aggravate Hyperammonemia

As described above, a main concern of giving glutamine to a patient with GS deficiency was related to the effect of glutamine supplementation on the plasma ammonia levels. This concern was fed by the report of a modest increase (1.6-fold) in cortical ammonia levels in mice affected by a genetic disruption of GS [34]. Also, since the defect GS already resulted in chronic hyperammonemia [28], any additional administration of glutamine was thought to possibly provoke a further increase in plasma and CSF ammonia. However, levels of plasma and CSF ammonia remained stable during the 4 weeks trial even when glutamine supplementation was increased to the final dose of 1,020 mg/kg/day [24].

Conclusions

In summary, there is only a single report of a therapeutic intervention in a patient with an inherited defect of GS [24]. This report demonstrates the feasibility of fully correcting the systemic lack of glutamine and of partly correcting the lack of glutamine in the brain in GS deficiency without worsening preexisting chronic moderate hyperammonemia or provoking toxic CSF ammonia or glutamate levels.

In future patients, glutamine supplementation should begin as early as possible in order to completely avoid the consequences of systemic glutamine deficiency in the milder cases and to alleviate the consequences by replenishing glutamine pools in those patients already affected by severe glutamine deficiency due to insufficient compensation during pregnancy. It remains however to be established whether an earlier intervention can prevent the devastating natural course of chronic encephalopathy in GS deficiency.

Acknowledgements The author acknowledges the family of the patient who underwent the therapeutic trial for their willingness to a close cooperation. Also, colleagues from the State of Qatar (Dr. T. Ben-Omran, Dr. K. Ibrahim and Dr. N. Shahbeck) and from University of Oslo, The Biotechnology Centre and The Centre for Molecular Biology and Neuroscience (Dr. F. Chaudhry) were instrumental for the study on glutamine supplementation. The scientific work on GS deficiency is supported by a grant from Hartmann Müller-Stiftung (grant No. 1492 to JH). Finally, the therapeutic trial as well as further studies into GS deficiency have been supported by a generous grant from Qatar Foundation.

References

1. Häussinger D. Hepatic glutamine transport and metabolism. Adv Enzymol Relat Areas Mol Biol. 1998;72:43–86.
2. Häussinger D, Sies R, editors. Glutamate metabolism in mammalian tissues. Berlin: Springer; 1984. p. 3–15.
3. Solbu TT, Boulland JL, Zahid W, et al. Induction and targeting of the glutamine transporter SN1 to the basolateral membranes of cortical kidney tubule cells during chronic metabolic acidosis suggest a role in pH regulation. J Am Soc Nephrol. 2005;16(4):869–77.
4. Gammelsaeter R, Jenstad M, Bredahl MK, Gundersen V, Chaudhry FA. Complementary expression of SN1 and SAT2 in the islets of Langerhans suggests concerted action of glutamine transport in the regulation of insulin secretion. Biochem Biophys Res Commun. 2009;381(3):378–82.
5. Chaudhry FA, Reimer RJ, Edwards RH. The glutamine commute: take the N line and transfer to the A. J Cell Biol. 2002;157(3):349–55.
6. Chaudhry FA, Boulland JL, Jenstad M, Bredahl MK, Edwards RH. Pharmacology of neurotransmitter transport into secretory vesicles. Handb Exp Pharmacol. 2008;184:77–106.
7. Albrecht J, Sidoryk-Wegrzynowicz M, Zielinska M, Aschner M. Roles of glutamine in neurotransmission. Neuron Glia Biol. 2010;6(4):263–76.
8. Kumada Y, Benson DR, Hillemann D, et al. Evolution of the glutamine synthetase gene, one of the oldest existing and functioning genes. Proc Natl Acad Sci U S A. 1993;90(7):3009–13.
9. Häussinger D, Schliess F. Glutamine metabolism and signaling in the liver. Front Biosci. 2007;12:371–91.
10. Watford M. Glutamine metabolism and function in relation to proline synthesis and the safety of glutamine and proline supplementation. J Nutr. 2008;138(10):2003S–7.
11. Labow BI, Souba WW, Abcouwer SF. Mechanisms governing the expression of the enzymes of glutamine metabolism–glutaminase and glutamine synthetase. J Nutr. 2001;131(9 Suppl):2467S–74. discussion 2486S–2467S.
12. Martinez-Hernandez A, Bell KP, Norenberg MD. Glutamine synthetase: glial localization in brain. Science. 1977;195(4284):1356–8.
13. Suarez I, Bodega G, Fernandez B. Glutamine synthetase in brain: effect of ammonia. Neurochem Int. 2002;41(2–3):123–42.
14. Cooper AJ. The role of glutamine synthetase and glutamate dehydrogenase in cerebral ammonia homeostasis. Neurochem Res. 2012;37(11):2439–55.
15. Häussinger D, Graf D, Weiergraber OH. Glutamine and cell signaling in liver. J Nutr. 2001;131(9 Suppl):2509S–14. discussion 2523S–2504S.
16. Häussinger D. Nitrogen metabolism in liver: structural and functional organization and physiological relevance. Biochem J. 1990;267(2):281–90.

17. Battaglia FC. Glutamine and glutamate exchange between the fetal liver and the placenta. J Nutr. 2000;130(4S Suppl):974S–7.
18. Boulland JL, Rafiki A, Levy LM, Storm-Mathisen J, Chaudhry FA. Highly differential expression of SN1, a bidirectional glutamine transporter, in astroglia and endothelium in the developing rat brain. Glia. 2003;41(3):260–75.
19. Vermeulen T, Görg B, Vogl T, et al. Glutamine synthetase is essential for proliferation of fetal skin fibroblasts. Arch Biochem Biophys. 2008;478(1):96–102.
20. He Y, Hakvoort TB, Vermeulen JL, Lamers WH, Van Roon MA. Glutamine synthetase is essential in early mouse embryogenesis. Dev Dyn. 2007;236(7):1865–75.
21. Caggese C, Caizzi R, Barsanti P, Bozzetti MP. Mutations in the glutamine synthetase I (gsl) gene produce embryo-lethal female sterility in Drosophila melanogaster. Dev Genet. 1992;13(5):359–66.
22. Manso Filho HC, Costa HE, Wu G, McKeever KH, Watford M. Equine placenta expresses glutamine synthetase. Vet Res Commun. 2009;33(2):175–82.
23. Boulland JL, Qureshi T, Seal RP, et al. Expression of the vesicular glutamate transporters during development indicates the widespread corelease of multiple neurotransmitters. J Comp Neurol. 2004;480(3):264–80.
24. Häberle J, Shahbeck N, Ibrahim K, et al. Glutamine supplementation in a child with inherited GS deficiency improves the clinical status and partially corrects the peripheral and central amino acid imbalance. Orphanet J Rare Dis. 2012;7:48.
25. Lichtenstein GR, Yang YX, Nunes FA, et al. Fatal hyperammonemia after orthotopic lung transplantation. Ann Intern Med. 2000;132(4):283–7.
26. Tuchman M, Lichtenstein GR, Rajagopal BS, et al. Hepatic glutamine synthetase deficiency in fatal hyperammonemia after lung transplantation. Ann Intern Med. 1997;127(6):446–9.
27. Häberle J, Görg B, Rutsch F, et al. Congenital glutamine deficiency with glutamine synthetase mutations. N Engl J Med. 2005;353(18):1926–33.
28. Häberle J, Shahbeck N, Ibrahim K, Hoffmann GF, Ben-Omran T. Natural course of glutamine synthetase deficiency in a 3 year old patient. Mol Genet Metab. 2011;103(1):89–91.
29. Häberle J, Görg B, Toutain A, et al. Inborn error of amino acid synthesis: human glutamine synthetase deficiency. J Inherit Metab Dis. 2006;29(2–3):352–8.
30. de Koning TJ. Treatment with amino acids in serine deficiency disorders. J Inherit Metab Dis. 2006;29(2–3): 347–51.
31. de Koning TJ, Klomp LW, van Oppen AC, et al. Prenatal and early postnatal treatment in 3-phosphoglycerate-dehydrogenase deficiency. Lancet. 2004;364(9452):2221–2.
32. Martinelli D, Häberle J, Rubio V, et al. Understanding pyrroline-5-carboxylate synthetase deficiency: clinical, molecular, functional, and expression studies, structure-based analysis, and novel therapy with arginine. J Inherit Metab Dis. 2011;35:761.
33. Krajewski WW, Collins R, Holmberg-Schiavone L, Jones TA, Karlberg T, Mowbray SL. Crystal structures of mammalian glutamine synthetases illustrate substrate-induced conformational changes and provide opportunities for drug and herbicide design. J Mol Biol. 2008;375(1):217–28.
34. He Y, Hakvoort TB, Vermeulen JL, et al. Glutamine synthetase deficiency in murine astrocytes results in neonatal death. Glia. 2010;58(6):741–54.
35. Garlick PJ. Assessment of the safety of glutamine and other amino acids. J Nutr. 2001;131(9 Suppl):2556S–61.
36. Sacks GS. Glutamine supplementation in catabolic patients. Ann Pharmacother. 1999;33(3):348–54.
37. Gleeson M. Dosing and efficacy of glutamine supplementation in human exercise and sport training. J Nutr. 2008;138(10):2045S–9.
38. Ziegler TR, Benfell K, Smith RJ, et al. Safety and metabolic effects of L-glutamine administration in humans. Jpen. 1990;14(4 Suppl):137S–46.
39. Boza JJ, Maire J, Bovetto L, Ballevre O. Plasma glutamine response to enteral administration of glutamine in human volunteers (free glutamine versus protein-bound glutamine). Nutrition. 2000;16(11–12):1037–42.
40. de Koning TJ, Klomp LW. Serine-deficiency syndromes. Curr Opin Neurol. 2004;17(2):197–204.
41. Olney JW, Collins RC, Sloviter RS. Excitotoxic mechanisms of epileptic brain damage. Adv Neurol. 1986;44: 857–77.
42. Albrecht J, Norenberg MD. Glutamine: a Trojan horse in ammonia neurotoxicity. Hepatology. 2006;44(4): 788–94.
43. Saitoh F, Araki T. Proteasomal degradation of glutamine synthetase regulates schwann cell differentiation. J Neurosci. 2010;30(4):1204–12.
44. Lacey JM, Crouch JB, Benfell K, et al. The effects of glutamine-supplemented parenteral nutrition in premature infants. JPEN. 1996;20(1):74–80.

Chapter 33
Plasma Antioxidants and Glutamine Supplementation in HIV

Roberto Carlos Burini, Maria Dorotéia Borges-Santos, Fernando Moreto, and Yong-Ming Yu

Key Points

- HIV+ disease progresses with increased oxidative stress and among the deficient antioxidants is GSH.
- GSH levels can be restored in plasma and intracellularly by oral administration of its amino acids precursors.
- Presently, we restored HIV+ plasma GSH to normal control values by using Gln as dietary supplement.
- The only GSH precursor fully replenished was Gly.
- HIV+ and controls responded similarly to the supplementation by increasing plasma Gln but differently for Glu with much less increase in HIV+.
- The contribution of Gln to higher Gly could be either due to increased protein breakdown or more probably by decreasing Gly catabolism.
- Gly is the major substrate in Ser synthesis in an interconvertible reaction that accounts for almost half of the whole-body Gly flux.
- Moreover, the Gly clearance through GCS accounts for about 25 % of Gly flux leading to both one-carbon (and Hcy synthesis) metabolism and Ser synthesis.
- In both situations the higher Gly catabolism would result in higher formation of Hcy and mainly Ser which were not found here.
- The present findings of GSH restoration by oral GSH supplementation following the increased Gly and reduced Ser levels seem more likely related to a slower breakdown of Gly resulting in lower Ser formation.

Keywords HIV+ • Sulfured-amino acids metabolism • Glutathione antioxidant metabolism • Oral glutamine supplementation • Glycine metabolism

---

R.C. Burini, Ph.D. (✉) • M.D. Borges-Santos • F. Moreto, Ph.D.
Department of Public Health, Centre for Nutritional and Physical Exercise Metabolism, Botucatu Medical School, Sao Paulo State University – UNESP, Distrito de Rubião Junior, s/n, Botucatu, SP, Brazil
e-mail: burini@fmb.unesp.br; doroteia.borges@gmail.com; fer_moreto@yahoo.com

Y.-M. Yu, Ph.D.
Department of Surgery, Shriners Burns Hospital, Massachusetts General Hospital, Harvard Medical School, Boston, MA, USA
e-mail: yyu@partners.org

R. Rajendram et al. (eds.), *Glutamine in Clinical Nutrition*, Nutrition and Health,
DOI 10.1007/978-1-4939-1932-1_33, © Springer Science+Business Media New York 2015

Abbreviations

Arg	Arginine
BMI	Body mass index
Co	Control group
CO_2	Carbon dioxide
Cys	Cysteine
Do	Habitual diet
GCS	Glycine clearance system
Gln	Glutamine
Glu	Glutamate
Gly	Glycine
GSH	Glutathione
GSSG	Oxidized glutathione
HAART	Highly active antiretroviral therapy
Hcy	Homocysteine
HIV+	Group of patients seropositive for human immunodeficiency virus
HPLC	High-performance liquid chromatography
Met	Methionine
NAC	*N*-acetylcysteine
Orn	Ornitine
Pro	Proline
Ser	Serine
SHMT	Serine hydroxymethyltransferase
Tau	Taurine
TCA	Tricarboxylic acid

Introduction

The Role of GSH on Antioxidant Actions

HIV+ patients present higher plasma levels of pro-oxidant and lower antioxidant markers irrespective of their nutritional status and the presence of HAART [1]. The presence of HAART showed some beneficial effects on β-carotene plasma levels but not on the other antioxidant markers [2]. Among those were glutathione (GSH) and its precursors [3]. GSH (L-y-glutamyl-L-cysteinyl-glycine) is the major intracellular hydro-soluble antioxidant agent representing important functions in biochemical processes and cell control, specially the antioxidant and immune defenses [4]. Plasma GSH can also be used as forms of cysteine storage and transport, with consequences for the regulation of signal transduction pathways and gene transcription [5].

GSH is synthesized from the precursor amino acids in two steps catalyzed by the enzymes glutamate cysteine ligase (also known as γ-glutamylcysteine synthetase) and γ-L-glutamyl-L-cysteine:glycine ligase (also known as glutathione synthetase). Plasma GSH arises largely from the liver. The content of GSH in mammalian cells is dynamically maintained by the gamma-glutamyl cycle, using GSH as a substrate for transpeptidases located on their membranes. Tissues that present low transpeptidase

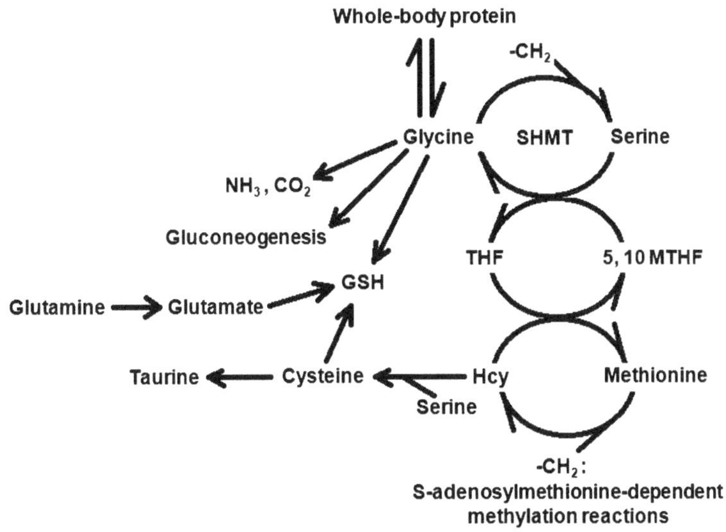

Fig. 33.1 Glutamine, glycine, glutathione metabolism interplay. *SHMT* serine methyltransferase, *THF* tetrahydrofolate, *5, 10 MTHF* 5, 10 methylene tetrahydrofolate, *GSH* glutathione, $-CH_2$ methyl radical

activity (e.g. liver, pancreas, and muscle) export GSH through the blood to cells that have high transpeptidase activity such as kidney [6, 7].

The major contributor to GSH deficiency and associated oxidative stress in humans is a diminished rate of glutathione synthesis, which in turn is due to low availability of its precursor amino acids [8]. GSH is a tripeptide of glutamate, cysteine, and glycine (Fig. 33.1). Cysteine is known to be the rate-limiting substrate for GSH synthesis [9].

The flux of nonessential amino acids (e.g. glutamate, cysteine, and glycine) consists of its release from protein breakdown and from de novo synthesis [8]. Moreover in vivo studies have shown that when healthy adults are fed diets, either deficient in sulfur amino acids [10] or containing reduced amounts of total protein [11], GSH turnover is suppressed. Collectively, these data indicate that GSH deficiency is due in large part to decreased synthesis secondary to a decreased supply of the precursor amino acids that might lead to a decreased de novo synthesis (Fig. 33.1).

The Impact of Dietary Glutamine Supplementation

Improving cysteine availability is the most extensively studied approach for enhancing the cell GSH pool [12]. Among the agents tested are *N*-acetylcysteine (NAC), lipoic acid, cysteamine, and 2-oxothiazolidine 4-carboxylate [13]. However, oral L-glutamine increases its level in plasma of healthy subjects [14] and has also been shown to improve plasma glutathione levels in HIV infection [3, 13]. Glutamine is the preferential substrate of rapidly dividing cells such as enterocytes and immune cells and therefore its supplementation is associated with less-infectious complications in critically ill patients [15]. This study aimed to investigate the responses of the GSH pathway to dietary supplements of Gln in HIV+ drug-treated patients.

Table 33.1 Subjects' demographic, anthropometric, and biochemical data at baseline

Variables	Controls	HIV+ patients	*p* values
Age (years)	24 (23–28)[a]	27 (25–36)	0.070
BMI (kg/m^2)	25 (3.1)[b]	25 (3.0)	0.960
Glucose (MG/dL)	87 (83.5–91)	103 (93.5–117)	0.001
Albumin (g/dL)	4.1 (0.3)	3.9 (0.4)	0.112
Folate (ng/mL)	7.5 (6.3–9.0)	1.9 (1.4–6.6)	0.017
Vitamin B_{12} (pg/mL)	288 (130)	367 (139)	0.115

BMI body mass index
[a]Median (P25-P75)
[b]Mean (SD)

Methodological Considerations

In a randomized controlled supplementation study involving the HIV+ patients under highly active antiretroviral treatment (HAART) for at least 1 year in absence of any renal or liver failure and the ingestion of either vitamins B or GSH precursors and the healthy control group consisting of 20 adults HIV negative and clinically healthy, a dietary supplements containing L-glutamine (Gln 20 g/day) given during consecutive 7-day periods preceded and followed by fasting-blood sampling [3].

The HIV+ patients matched with healthy controls by age, BMI and plasma concentrations of albumin and vitamin B12. Whereas their plasma levels of folate, all but Hcy amino acids and GSH were lower than controls (Tables 33.1 and 33.2).

After 1 week of Gln supplementation the HIV+ group increased GSH (71.4 %) and its precursor amino acids Gly (27.2 %), Glu (13.7 %) and Cys (10.8 %). However, only Met, Hcy, Gly and GSH reached the levels of the controls (Table 33.2).

The plasma concentration of Glu after Gln supplementation increased 3.4 % in controls and decreased 1.0 % in HIV+ patients (Table 33.2). Ser also decreased (25.1 % more than Co), whereas Gly (21.8 %), Tau (14.4 %) and GSH (47.9 %) increased higher than Co (Table 33.2). Therefore after Gln supplementation, both groups presented similar plasma ratio for Tau/Cys with the HIV+ showing higher ratio for Gly/Glu and lower Ser/Gly and Ser/Cys (Fig. 33.2).

Dissecting Out Mechanisms for Glutamine's Actions

The diminished concentrations of GSH precursors could be a result of slower body protein turnover or decreased de novo synthesis [8]. Hence the increased concentration of GSH found after Gln supplement would be the result of increased source of its precursors either by higher protein catabolism or increased de novo synthesis (Fig. 33.1). In the present study, the higher protein breakdown can be excluded because it has been described that Gln administration promotes increasing in lean body mass even in HIV infection [13]. On the other hand, the increased de novo synthesis could be the case for Gly that increased 21.8 % after Gln supplementation. On the other hand, decreased de novo synthesis would be the case of Glu and Ser. Glu is formed from deamination of Gln (by glutaminase) and further deaminated to α-ketoglutarate (2-oxoglutarate) by glutamate dehydrogenase.

Gln supplementation resulted in higher Gln plasma levels in both controls (18.7 %) and HIV+ (19.6 %) groups. However, this similarity was not seen for the Glu levels found as 60 % for controls and only 13.7 % for the patients. Thus HIV+ group showed a lack of response of plasma Glu to the Gln supplementation.

Besides fueling Krebs cycle (with α-ketoglutarate) Glu also participate in biosynthetic processes of other amino acids such as Orn (and Arg), Pro, Gln and Ser. Ser is the main precursor of Gly, another GSH component. Actually, among the GSH precursors Gly was the only amino acid achieving the control values after the Gln supplementation.

Table 33.2 Plasma amino acid and glutathione concentrations in different dietary conditions

Amino acid and group	Usual diet	Glutamine suppl
Methionine (μmol/L)		
Co	30.8 ± 8.8^{aA}	30.3 ± 9.6^{aA}
HIV	20 ± 6.6^{aB}	25.5 ± 11^{aA}
Homocysteine (μmol/L)		
Co	13.9 ± 5.5^{aA}	11.3 ± 2.7^{aA}
HIV	9.8 ± 1.6^{aA}	10.2 ± 1.3^{aA}
Serine (μmol/L)		
Co	108 ± 7.8^{aA}	112 ± 14^{aA}
HIV	86.9 ± 20^{aB}	60.6 ± 17^{bB}
Cysteine (μmol/L)		
Co	413 ± 175^{aA}	420 ± 177^{aA}
HIV	158 ± 10^{aB}	175 ± 26^{aB}
Taurine (μmol/L)		
Co	63.2 ± 3.9^{aA}	63.2 ± 3.9^{aA}
HIV	48.1 ± 3.7^{aB}	57.2 ± 5.6^{bB}
Glutamate (μmol/L)		
Co	94 ± 18.5^{aA}	144 ± 29^{bA}
HIV	56.4 ± 11.3^{aB}	64.1 ± 14^{aB}
Glycine (μmol/L)		
Co	485 ± 68.5^{aA}	480 ± 76^{aA}
HIV	371 ± 20.2^{aB}	472 ± 60^{bA}
Glutamine (μmol/L)		
Co	476 ± 84^{aA}	565 ± 85.4^{bA}
HIV	285 ± 59^{aB}	341 ± 57^{bB}
GSH (μmol/L)		
Co	9.2 ± 2.1^{aA}	8.3 ± 0.8^{aA}
HIV	4.9 ± 0.7^{aB}	8.4 ± 0.4^{bA}
GSSG (μmol/L)		
Co	0.77 ± 0.86^{aA}	0.48 ± 0.23^{aA}
HIV	1.44 ± 0.4^{aB}	1.81 ± 0.17^{bB}
GSSG/GSH (μmol/L)		
Co	0.08 ± 0.07^{aA}	0.06 ± 0.03^{aA}
HIV	0.29 ± 0.06^{aB}	0.2 ± 0.02^{bB}

All values are means ± SD. Data were analyzed by using repeated-measures ANOVA. A significant group × treatment interaction was observed for all amino acids except glutamine and GSSG ($p < 0.05$)

Co control group, *HIV* HIV+ group

^{a,b}Significantly different from habitual diet (baseline) ($p < 0.05$)

^{A,B}Significantly different from control at the same diet ($p < 0.05$)

The Role of Glycine-Serine on Glutamine-GSH Pathway

The major contribution to whole-body Gly flux is the whole-body protein breakdown [16]. Pathways utilizing Gly are the formation of serine, glutathione, protein synthesis, and gluconeogenesis [17] (Fig. 33.1).

Gly and Ser are interconvertible through mitochondrial and cytosolic serine hydroxymethyltransferase (SHMT). These reactions account for approximately 41 % of whole-body Gly flux [18]. The mitochondrial glycine clearance system (GCS) accounts for 22 % of the whole-body Gly flux [19]. The GCS cleaves Gly to CO_2, ammonia, and a 1-carbon unit in the methylene state reacting with folate as 5,10-methylenetetrahydrofolate (Fig. 33.1). SHMT reversibly transfers a 1-carbon group from 5,10-methylenetetrahydrofolate to Gly forming tetrahydrofolate and Ser (Fig. 33.1).

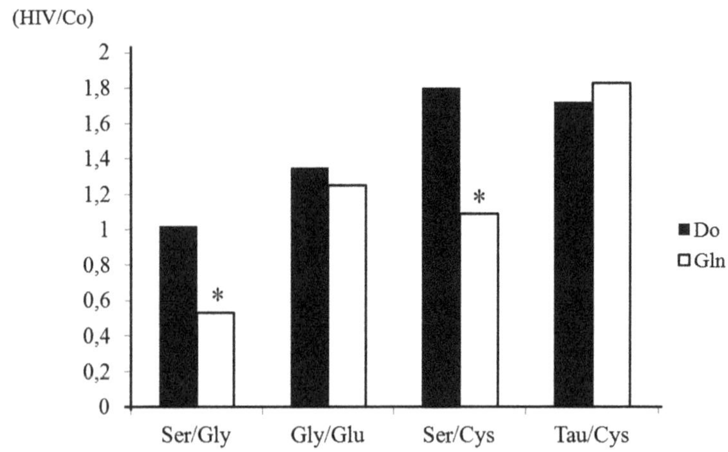

Fig. 33.2 Plasma-derived/precursor amino acid ratio of HIV+ patients in relation to the controls (Co) in both dietary conditions, usual (Do) and Gln supplemented (Gln). $*p<0.05$

The rate of serine synthesis is as high as the rate of Gly cleavage [18]. Hence Gly and Ser are major sources of 1-carbon units released by GCS and SHMT. For each Gly molecule processed, the GCS produces 1 molecule of 5,10-methylenetetrahydrofolate and CO_2. The incorporation of GCS-derived 1-carbon units enter serine synthesis while the other 40 % enter other aspects of 1-carbon metabolism including nucleoside synthesis, homocysteine remethylation, and *S*-adenosyl methionine-dependent methylation reactions [19] (Fig. 33.1). Gly is the major substrate in Ser synthesis and Ser is the major 1-carbon source for homocysteine remethylation [20]. However, it is considered that GCS produces 1-carbon units as 5,10-methylenetetrahydrofolate at a higher rate (approximately 20 times) that needed for Hcy remethylation (to Met) and thus, for methylation demand [17]. Thus nearly all GCS-derived 1-carbon units are consumed in Ser synthesis while a much smaller percentage enters all other reactions of 1-carbon metabolism [21].

In the present chapter the plasma concentrations of Met and Hcy were similar in both groups under both diets, what means preserved transmethylation/remethylation reactions. Interestingly the remethylation reaction of Hcy to Met is folate-dependent [20] whose plasma level was found lower in HIV+ group than the controls.

Besides remethylation reaction (folate/B12 vitamin-dependent) to Met, Hcy can be metabolized to cystathionine by trans-sulfuration reactions (vitamin B6-dependent) consuming Ser and resulting in Cys as end-product (Fig. 33.1). In the present study, differently from Gly and Ser, Cys levels were minimally affected by the Gln supplementation of HIV+ patients. Increased Gly concentration has been described during low vitamin B6 status and slower trans-sulfuration reactions in a tentative to maintain Ser synthesis [19]. This probably would not be the present case once Gln supplementation did not affect significantly Hcy and Cys levels neither maintained Ser levels.

Besides its consumption in trans-sulfuration and remethylation pathways, Ser can be used in the CO_2 formation. Serine dehydratase transforms serine to pyruvate that enters the tricarboxylic acid (TCA) cycle either as oxaloacetate or acetyl-CoA. The carbons of Ser, following conversion to pyruvate, can be converted to CO_2 via the pyruvate dehydrogenase reaction and metabolism of the resulting acetyl-CoA through the TCA cycle. Alternatively, Ser carbons (via pyruvate) also can be converted to CO_2 after the formation of oxaloacetate by pyruvate carboxylase, followed by metabolism in the TCA cycle. Additionally to its oxidation to CO_2, mitochondrial Ser production in humans has been shown to support gluconeogenesis [19]. However, in our data plasma glucose concentrations were similar in both groups [3].

Conclusions

The plasma GSH normalization in HIV+ patients by Gln supplementation with increased Gly and reduced Ser levels in association with mild increase of other GSH precursors (Glu and Cys) seems more related to slower breakdown of Gly (and lower Ser formation) without major consequences on transmethylation/remethylation/trans-sulfuration pathways.

Acknowledgements The authors thank the Brazilian institutions FAPESP and CNPq for the research funding and fellowships.

References

1. Borges-Santos MD, Pereira PCM, Burini RC. Antioxidant deficiency in HIV+patients: a global or specific deficiency of nutrients? Rev Bras Nutr Clin. 2004;19(4):6.
2. Borges-Santos MD, Pardini MI, Burini RC. Effect of the severity of the illness and the antiretroviral medication presence on oxidative stress of HIV+patients. Rev Bras Nutr Clin. 2005;20(3):6.
3. Borges-Santos MD, Moreto F, Pereira PC, Ming-Yu Y, Burini RC. Plasma glutathione of HIV(+) patients responded positively and differently to dietary supplementation with cysteine or glutamine. Nutrition. 2012;28(7–8):753–6.
4. Meister A. Glutathione metabolism and its selective modification. J Biol Chem. 1988;263(33):17205–8.
5. Griffith OW. Biologic and pharmacologic regulation of mammalian glutathione synthesis. Free Radic Biol Med. 1999;27(9–10):922–35.
6. Droge W, Kinscherf R, Mihm S, et al. Thiols and the immune system: effect of N-acetylcysteine on T cell system in human subjects. Methods Enzymol. 1995;251:255–70.
7. Meister A, Anderson ME, Hwang O. Intracellular cysteine and glutathione delivery systems. J Am Coll Nutr. 1986;5(2):137–51.
8. Sekhar RV, Patel SG, Guthikonda AP, et al. Deficient synthesis of glutathione underlies oxidative stress in aging and can be corrected by dietary cysteine and glycine supplementation. Am J Clin Nutr. 2011;94(3):847–53.
9. Fukagawa NK, Ajami AM, Young VR. Plasma methionine and cysteine kinetics in response to an intravenous glutathione infusion in adult humans. Am J Physiol. 1996;270(2 Pt 1):E209–14.
10. Lyons J, Rauh-Pfeiffer A, Yu YM, et al. Blood glutathione synthesis rates in healthy adults receiving a sulfur amino acid-free diet. Proc Natl Acad Sci U S A. 2000;97(10):5071–6.
11. Jackson AA, Gibson NR, Lu Y, Jahoor F. Synthesis of erythrocyte glutathione in healthy adults consuming the safe amount of dietary protein. Am J Clin Nutr. 2004;80(1):101–7.
12. Borges-Santos MD, Burini RC. Metabolic basis of supplemental cysteine. Rev Bras Nutr Clin. 2005;20(4):6.
13. Patrick L. Nutrients and HIV: part three - N-acetylcysteine, alpha-lipoic acid, L-glutamine, and L-carnitine. Altern Med Rev. 2000;5(4):290–305.
14. Valencia E, Marin A, Hardy G. Impact of oral L-glutamine on glutathione, glutamine, and glutamate blood levels in volunteers. Nutrition. 2002;18(5):367–70.
15. Dechelotte P, Hasselmann M, Cynober L, et al. L-alanyl-L-glutamine dipeptide-supplemented total parenteral nutrition reduces infectious complications and glucose intolerance in critically ill patients: the French controlled, randomized, double-blind, multicenter study. Crit Care Med. 2006;34(3):598–604.
16. Gibson NR, Jahoor F, Ware L, Jackson AA. Endogenous glycine and tyrosine production is maintained in adults consuming a marginal-protein diet. Am J Clin Nutr. 2002;75(3):511–8.
17. Lamers Y, Williamson J, Theriaque DW, et al. Production of 1-carbon units from glycine is extensive in healthy men and women. J Nutr. 2009;139(4):666–71.
18. Lamers Y, Williamson J, Gilbert LR, Stacpoole PW, Gregory 3rd JF. Glycine turnover and decarboxylation rate quantified in healthy men and women using primed, constant infusions of [1,2-(13)C2]glycine and [(2)H3]leucine. J Nutr. 2007;137(12):2647–52.
19. Lamers Y, Williamson J, Ralat M, et al. Moderate dietary vitamin B-6 restriction raises plasma glycine and cystathionine concentrations while minimally affecting the rates of glycine turnover and glycine cleavage in healthy men and women. J Nutr. 2009;139(3):452–60.
20. Bailey LB, Gregory 3rd JF. Folate metabolism and requirements. J Nutr. 1999;129(4):779–82.
21. Robinson K, Arheart K, Refsum H, et al. Low circulating folate and vitamin B6 concentrations: risk factors for stroke, peripheral vascular disease, and coronary artery disease. European COMAC Group. Circulation. 1998;97(5):437–43.

Chapter 34
Glutamine, Total Antioxidant Systems and Damage in Renal Ischemia–Reperfusion Injury

Valter Torezan Gouvêa Junior, Cervantes Caporossi, and Carlos Augusto Fernandes Molina

Key Points

- Renal ischemia occurring during the transplant is one of the issues responsible for acute kidney injury.
- The reduction of harmful effects of renal ischemia/reperfusion (I/R) must be considered throughout the whole treatment process, and its minimization can and should be started early on, before the surgery, as a preoperative preparation procedure.
- Ischemia and reperfusion leads to the production of reactive oxygen species (ROS), which initiate lipid peroxidation and protein oxidation of the cell membrane leading to cell death.
- Glutamine (GLN) is the most abundant amino acid found in the blood, one of its most important characteristics is its function as a precursor to glutathione (GSH), which is defined as a potent antioxidant agent.
- Studies have demonstrated that glutamine administration favors the antioxidant system with better preservation of the total antioxidant capacity and renal function.

Keywords Glutamine • Glutamine supplementation • Ischemia–reperfusion • Ischemia–reperfusion kidney • Renal artery occlusion • Kidney transplant • Free radicals antioxidants

Abbreviations

ATP	Adenosine-5′-triphosphate
CATA	Catalase
Cl^-	Chloride ion

V.T.G. Junior, Ph.D. (✉) • C. Caporossi, Ph.D.
Clinical Surgery Department of Julio Muller Hospital, UFMT Brazil (Federal University of Mato Grosso), Rua das Orquídeas 289, Condomínio Residencial Florais Cuiabá, CEP: 78049-420 Cuiabá-MT, Avenida Miguel Sutil 8000, Jardim Mariana sala 1003, Cuiaba-MT, Cuiabá, Mato Grosso 78049-420, Brazil
e-mail: gouvea1910@gmail.com; caporosi@terra.com.br

C.A.F. Molina, Ph.D.
Department of Surgery and Anatomy of São Paulo University, USP, São Paulo, Brazil
e-mail: cafmolina@gmail.com; cirurgia@rca.fmrp.usp.br

R. Rajendram et al. (eds.), *Glutamine in Clinical Nutrition*, Nutrition and Health,
DOI 10.1007/978-1-4939-1932-1_34, © Springer Science+Business Media New York 2015

FNT	Tumor necrosis factor
FR	Free radicals
GLN	Glutamine
GSH	Glutathione
GSH-px	Glutathione peroxidase
GSH-rd	Glutathione reductase
GSSH	Oxidized glutathione
H_2O_2	Hydrogen peroxide
HO_2^-	Hydroperoxide
$HOCl^-$	Hypochlorite radical
I/R	Ischemia–reperfusion
IL-1	Interleukin-1
IL-6	Interleukin-6
L*	Lipid radical
LO*	Alcoxila radical
LTB_4	Leukotriene B_4
LTB_4	Leukotriene B_4
NADPH	Nicotinamide adenine dinucleotide phosphate
NO_2	Nitrogen dioxide
O	Oxygen
O_2	Molecular oxygen
O_2^-	Superoxide
$ONOO^-$	Peroxynitrite
PAF	Platelet-activating factor
pmpca	Per million of the population of a compatible age
PUFA	Polyunsaturated fatty acids
RNS	Reactive nitrogen species
ROS	Reactive oxygen species
SOD	Superoxide dismutase
TAC	Total antioxidant capacity
TROS	Toxic reactive oxygen species
TXA_2	Thromboxane A_2

Introduction

End-stage renal disease is a very relevant problem in public health and there is evidence of increasing occurrence and prevalence of this condition [1]. Data vary a lot, with numbers between 2.5 cases per million of the population of a compatible age (pmpca) in Nigeria, up to 1,403 cases pmpca in the United States [1]. An expressive percentage of these patients require maintenance dialysis treatment or organ transplant [1].

Kidney transplant is recognized as an advance in modern Medicine which can provide years of high quality life to patients with irreversible kidney failure. What was a risky limited experimental treatment option 50 years ago is currently a routine clinical practice in over 80 countries [1].

Renal ischemia occurring during the transplant is one of the issues responsible for acute kidney injury, and with the advent of laparoscopic nephrectomy for live kidney donors there has been an increase in time of this warm ischemia [2]. Ischemia and also kidney reperfusion commonly occur during the operation of several kidney diseases such as renal artery revascularization, treatment of suprarenal aortic aneurysms and partial nephrectomies (especially in laparoscopies) [3].

Reperfusion is essential for the survival of ischemic tissue; however, such a quantity of substrates causes additional injury to cells triggered by a complex series of events which affects the structure and function of all organelles, causing cell death [4]. Free radicals intervene in this cell injury, they are produced when the supply of oxygen is restored through reperfusion [4]. Within these processes what is notable is the generation of reactive oxygen species (ROS), depletion of adenosine-5′-triphosphate (ATP), infiltration of neutrophils, activation of phospholipases and changes in the lipid membrane and the accumulation of intracellular calcium [4].

The reduction of harmful effects of renal ischemia/reperfusion (I/R) must be considered throughout the whole treatment process, and its minimization can and should be started early on, before the surgery, as a preoperative preparation procedure [4].

The intake of pharmaco nutrients may modulate the organism's inflammatory response, thus reducing the harmful power of the physiological cascade of this event [5]. It has been demonstrated that the administration of neutral amino acids such as glycine and alanine protect the renal tubular cells of the lesion caused by ischemia or hypoxemia [4]. Glutamine (GLN) is the most abundant amino acid found in the blood, one of its most important characteristics is its function as a precursor to glutathione (GSH), which is defined as a potent antioxidant agent [6]. It is known that when the kidneys are under oxidant stress, GLN is the limiting factor in the synthesis of GSH just like the beneficial effect of glutamine in the protection of the liver against effects of a lesion by I/R [6]. There is report that the GLN administered in the pretreatment of rats submitted to kidney transplant resulted in the attenuation of tubular cellular apoptosis [7]. Another author observed partial protection from nephrotoxicity induced by cisplatin in rats treated with GLN [8].

Surgery, Ischemia, and Reperfusion

The first kidney transplant was carried out in 1954 in Boston, Massachusetts between twin brothers, and the organ remained in cold ischemia for 82 min until revascularization was complete [9].

Studies on dogs show that recovery after warm ischemia is directly dependent on its duration period [10]. Hence, there is complete rapid recovery if the warm ischemia lasts no longer than 10 min; however, when it is longer than 20 min, renal function recovers only after several hours [10]. With greater periods of 30 min of warm kidney ischemia, recovery comes after 3–9 days, with 60 min, only after weeks, after 120 min this function will be partially reestablished (30–50 %) [10].

Hypoxia is defined as any state in which there is a reduction of available oxygen for cells, and can be caused by the reduction of quantity or saturation of hemoglobin [11]. Ischemia occurs due to a reduction in the blood flow, generally as a consequence of an obstruction in the arterial system or as a result of poor perfusion which occurs as a physiological response to the state of shock [11]. This way, in the ischemic tissues, the anaerobic generation of energy is interrupted after glycolytic substrates are depleted, or the glycolytic function is inhibited by the accumulation of metabolites which should have been removed by the blood flow [26]. Thus the ischemic lesion presents a tendency to damage tissues faster than hypoxia [11].

The consequences of ischemia are quite variable and, in general, depend upon the level of the blood occlusion, collateral circulation and the degree of demand for oxygen in the tissues [12].

In diverse situations in clinical practice ischemia represents a fundamental role in the triggering of physiopathological events that, if they are not reverted in time, can result in irreversible cell damage [12].

At the same time there would be an intense inflammatory reaction in the post-ischemic tissues, leading to a series of biochemical, inflammatory and cellular changes mediated mainly by the formation of free radicals of oxygen or reactive oxygen species (ROS), which, during reperfusion, are freed into circulation, causing damage to other organs in the organism [13]. These effects of the I/R are most frequently observed in the lungs and cardiovascular system, and may result in the possible development of systemic inflammatory response syndrome and multiple organ dysfunction syndrome [13].

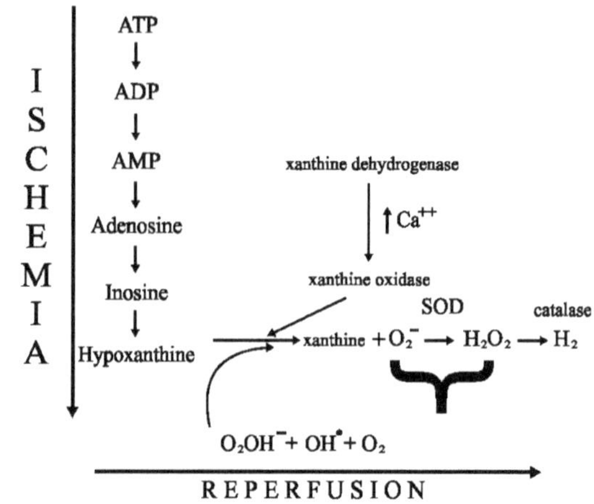

Fig. 34.1 Metabolic pathway for the production of free radicals of O_2 during reperfusion of ischemic tissues by conversion of xanthine dehydrogenase into xanthine oxidase. During the ischemia period, ATP is catabolized into hypoxanthine, which accumulates in the tissues. Hypoxanthine is the first substrate for oxidation by xanthine oxidase, which occurs when the second substrate, oxygen, is supplied during reperfusion, forming reactive oxygen species. *SOD* superoxide dismutase, *ATP* adenosine-5′-triphosphate, *ATP* adenosine-5′-diphosphate

To reverse the ischemic state, one should need to restore blood flow. However, restoring normal blood supply paradoxically may be responsible for injuries even more serious than those of ischemia per se [12].

The origin of free radicals occurs during the ischemia period, ATP is catabolized into hypoxanthine, which accumulates in the tissues [11–14]. As a result of the low energy state, there is cellular homeostasis failure characterized by the loss of ionic gradient across the cell membrane, allowing an influx of Ca^{2+} into the cells, this activates the protease to convert xanthine dehydrogenase into xanthine oxidase [11–14]. Hypoxanthine is the first substrate for oxidation by xanthine oxidase, which occurs when the second substrate, oxygen, is supplied during reperfusion, forming reactive oxygen species from the metabolism of oxygen [11–14] (see Fig. 34.1).

Another source of free radicals would be the production of superoxide radicals by the already mentioned breakdown of electrons in the electron transport system for mitochondria or by the cyclooxygenase pathway for the metabolism of arachidonic acid [14]. For the latter mechanism there would be activation of nonspecific proteases and phospholipases induced by the accumulation of intracellular calcium during the reperfusion period, leading to the synthesis of pro-inflammatory mediators: platelet activating factor (PAF) and eicosanoid compounds (leukotrienes, thromboxanes, and prostaglandins) [11].

Lesions produced like this serve as a stimulus giving rise to an inflammatory reaction [14]. Humoral mediators lead to the chemotaxis of neutrophils at the site of the lesion [12]. The latter interact with the local vascular endothelium, through the action of leukocyte integrins (especially proteins from class CD11/CD18) modulated by leukotriene B_4 (LTB_4), complement component (C5a) and by the platelet activating factor (PAF), as well as endothelial adhesion proteins, most notable are the immunoglobulins from class ICAM-1 and VCAM-1, and selectins, these in turn are modulated by the tumor necrosis factor (TNF) [12, 13]. The endothelial–neutrophil interaction produces an increase in the production of ROS [12, 13]. Proteolytic enzymes such as collagenase, elastase, and myeloperoxidase are then released by the neutrophil [12]. The latter plays an important role, catalyzing the reaction between hydrogen peroxide (H_2O_2) and chloride ion (Cl^-) forming a hypochlorite radical ($HOCl^-$), a potent oxidizing agent [13, 14] (see Figs. 34.2 and 34.3).

The activated neutrophil stimulates the production of pro-inflammatory cytokines [15, 16, 18]. Most notable are the interleukin-1 (IL-1), interleukin-6 (IL-6), arachidonic acid metabolites (leukotriene B_4 and thromboxane A_2), and the FNT [13–15].

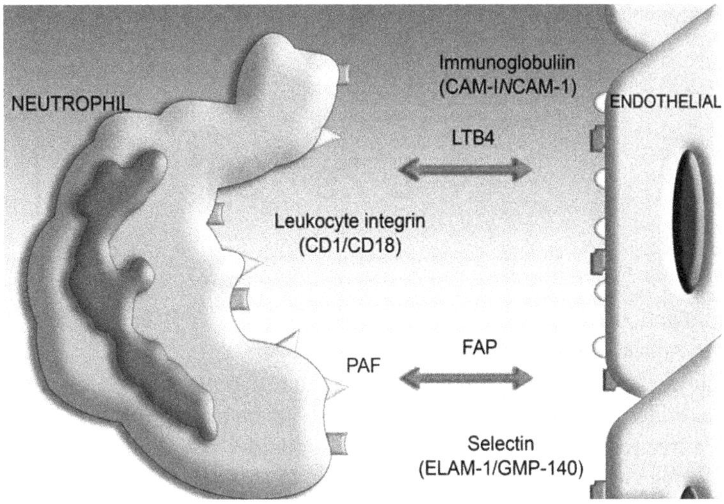

Fig. 34.2 Neutrophil–endothelial interaction and the production of reactive oxygen species. The latter interact with the local vascular endothelium through the action of leukocyte integrins (CD11/CD18) modulated by leukotriene B_4 (LTB_4), complement component (C5a) and by the platelet activating factor (PAF), as well as endothelia's adhesion proteins (ICAM-1 and VCAM-1), the selectins (ELAM-1/GMP-140), these in turn are modulated by the tumor necrosis factor (TNF)

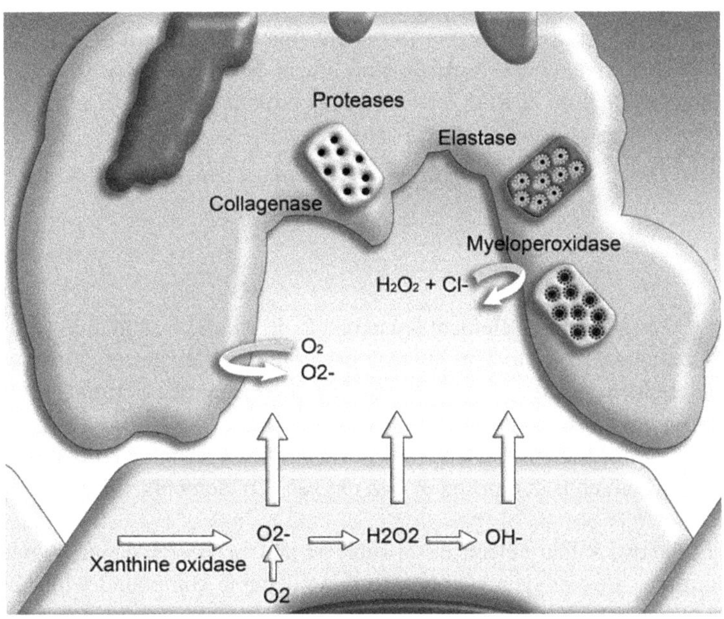

Fig. 34.3 Neutrophil–endothelial interaction and the production of reactive oxygen species. Proteolytic enzymes such as collagenase, elastase and myeloperoxidase are then released by the neutrophil. The latter plays an important role, catalyzing the reaction between hydrogen peroxide (H_2O_2) and chloride ion (Cl^-) forming a hypochlorite radical ($HOCl^-$), a potent oxidizing agent

Fig. 34.4 Electrons layers of molecular oxygen. Distribution of electrons in the electron shell of the element oxygen

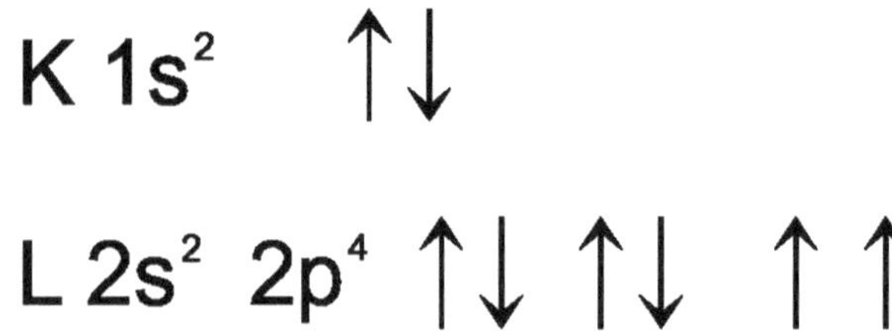

With the amplification of the inflammatory response, other cell lineages come to be recruited, among these are the mastocytes [13–15].

Its decomposition and release of granules give rise to different amines with vasoactive properties such as histamine, proteoglycans, prostacyclins, kinins, leukotrienes, proteases, and nitric oxide [11]. The nitric oxide, a free radical gas, has interesting vasodilatory properties, apart from functioning as an anti-platelet aggregation and being toxic to bacteria [11]. Such functions, particularly beneficial during an inflammatory injury, become harmful due to the interaction of nitric oxide with other radicals, especially superoxide (O_2^-), leading to the production of peroxynitrite ($ONOO^-$) and nitrogen dioxide (NO_2), compounds capable of promoting severe cell damage [12].

Concomitantly with this, capillary flow obstruction with no possibility of perfusion restoration develops in the microcirculation by a mechanism of cell stacking, worsening the ischemic trauma, a phenomenon known as *no-reflow* [13].

Thromboxane A_2 (TXA_2) and leukotriene B_4 (LTB_4) are, respectively, by-products of the cyclooxygenase and lipoxygenase action on arachidonic acid [13]. LTB_4 is a potent leukocyte chemotaxis that promotes neutrophil–endothelial cell interaction with release of free radicals and proteolytic enzymes and TXA_2, as well as inducing neutrophils to release free radicals, is a potent vasoconstrictor and platelet aggregator which reduces the capillary flow after reperfusion [11–15].

Finally, this large production of ROS leads to lipid peroxidation and protein oxidation of the cell membrane leading ultimately to cell death [11–15].

Free Radical

The electronic layers of a chemical element are called K, L, M and N, and their sublevels, s, p, d and f [15]. The term free radical refers to a highly reactive atom or molecule containing an odd number of electrons in its outer electron layer [11–16]. It is this non-pairing of electrons in the outer layer that confers high reactivity to these atoms and molecules [11–16].

We can illustrate the formation of a free radical citing the superoxide radical ($O_2^{-\cdot}$), derived from molecular oxygen (O_2) which is composed of two oxygen (O) elements, the atomic number of which is 8 (see Fig. 34.4).

To form the O_2, the two solitary electrons of sublevel p of an oxygen element interchange with the two electrons from the other oxygen element, forming a stable compound with 12 electrons in the outer layer (L) [16] (see Fig. 34.5).

Remember that reduction reactions imply a gain in electrons and oxidation reactions, a loss. However, when normal metabolism occurs in a reduction of molecular oxygen (O_2), this will gain an electron, forming a superoxide radical (O_2^-), considered unstable as it has an odd number (13) of electrons in the last layer L [16] (see Fig. 34.6).

Thus, free radicals are formed in a scenario of oxidation–reduction reactions, or give up the lone electron, oxidizing, or they receive another, reducing [16, 17].

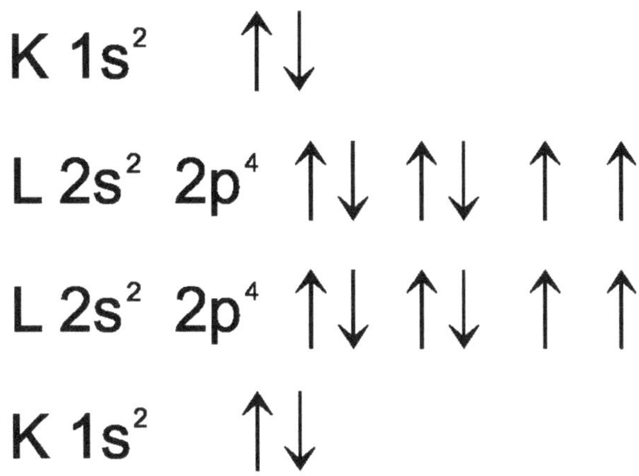

Fig. 34.5 Electrons layers of O_2. To form the O_2, the two solitary electrons of sublevel p of an oxygen element interchange with the two electrons from the other oxygen element, forming a stable compound with 12 electrons in the outer layer (L)

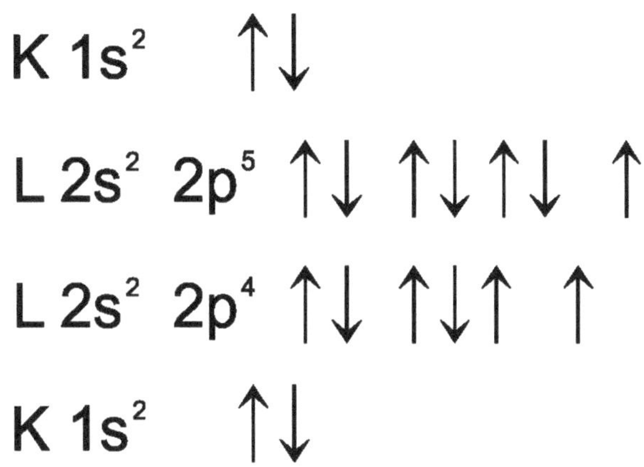

Fig. 34.6 Electrons layers of superoxide radicals (O_2). When normal metabolism occurs in a reduction of molecular oxygen (O_2), this will gain an electron, forming a superoxide radical (O_2), considered unstable as it has an odd number (13) of electrons in the last layer L

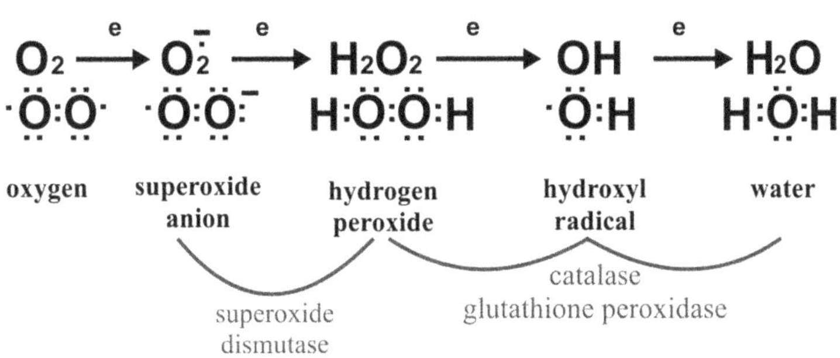

Fig. 34.7 Tetravalent reduction of molecular oxygen (O_2) in the mitochondria until water (H_2O) is formed. Several reactive O_2 species are formed in the process. Normally, the complete reduction of O_2 takes place in the mitochondria, and the reactivity of the ROS is neutralized by the entrance of four electrons. Some antioxidant enzymes are represented

Free radical is not the ideal term to describe reactive pathogenic agents because some of them do not have unpaired electrons in their outer layer [15]. As they are mostly derived from the metabolism of O_2, the term "reactive oxygen species" (ROS) or "toxic reactive oxygen species" (TROS) is used [15–17].

Under physiological conditions of aerobic cellular metabolism, the O_2 undergoes tetravalent reduction with the acceptance of four electrons resulting in the formation of H_2O (see Fig. 34.7) [15–17]. During this process reactive intermediates are formed such as superoxide radicals (O_2^-), hydroperoxide (HO_2), hydroxyl (OH), and hydrogen peroxide (H_2O_2) [15–17].

LH+ OH * (or LO*)------→	L* + H_2O (or LOH)	Iniciation
L*+ O_2 ------→	LOO*	Propagation
LH+ LOO* -------→	L* + LOOH	Propagation
LOO* + L ------→	LOOL	Termination
LOO* + LOO* -------→	LOOL + O_2	Termination

Fig. 34.8 Phases of lipid peroxidation. Lipid peroxidation is a chain reaction, represented by phases of initiation, propagation, and termination. *L* lipid

Normally, the complete reduction of O_2 takes place in the mitochondria, and the reactivity of the ROS is neutralized by the entrance of four electrons [15–17].

These ROS are associated with various diseases, including cancer, liver diseases, atherosclerosis and aging, this is due to the properties of free radicals of provoking cellular injury by attacking membranes, serving as initiators of the process of lipid peroxidation or lipoperoxidation [11–17].

The formation of hydroxyl radicals in biological systems occurs non-enzymatically through the Haber–Weiss reaction and requires the presence of iron (Fe^{3+}) or transition metals [11–17].

Superoxide and hydrogen peroxide free radicals, despite direct action being limited on cellular constituents, are considered aggressive mainly because in the Haber–Weiss reaction they react to produce hydroxyl radicals, those truly responsible for cellular damage [11–17].

Lipoperoxidation

Toxic effects of oxygen on biological components were already known in the late nineteenth century, and have become the subject of intense scientific research in recent years [17]. These effects come from the oxidation of cellular components such as thiols, enzyme cofactors, proteins, nucleotides and lipids, especially polyunsaturated fatty acids (PUFA), mediated by ROS and reactive nitrogen species (RNS), generally known as free radicals (FR) [17].

All cellular components are susceptible to the action of ROS, but the membrane is one of the hardest hit as a result of lipid peroxidation, which leads to changes in the structure and permeability of cell membranes [15]. Consequently, there is a loss of selectivity in the ion exchange and release of the contents of organelles such as lysosomal hydrolytic enzymes, and the formation of cytotoxic products, culminating in cell death [11–17].

Lipid peroxidation is a chain reaction, represented by phases of initiation, propagation, and termination. These phases are shown in the following reactions, where L represents the lipid (see Fig. 34.8) [15].

The above reaction begins with the capturing of hydrogen from polyunsaturated fatty acid (LH) of the cell membrane [15–17]. This capture can be accomplished by OH* or by LO* (alcoxila radical), with the consequent formation of L* (lipid radical) [15–17]. In the first equation of propagation, L* reacts rapidly with O_2 resulting in LOO* (peroxyl radical) which, in turn, captures new hydrogen

$$2\,O_2 + 2H^{+} \xrightarrow{SOD} H_2O_2 + O_2$$

$$2\,H_2O_2 \xrightarrow{CATA} 2\,H_2O_2 + O_2$$

$$2GSH + H_2O_2 \xrightarrow{GSHpx} 2\,H_2O + GSSG$$

Fig. 34.9 Antioxidant enzymatic action. The antioxidant blood system is classified into enzymatic and non-enzymatic, the first being represented mainly by antioxidant enzymes: superoxide dismutase (SOD) that acts on the superoxide radical turning it into hydrogen peroxide, catalase (CATA) and glutathione peroxidase (GSHpx), which act on the hydrogen peroxide transforming it into water. *GSH* Reduced Glutathione, *GSSH* Oxidized glutathione

from polyunsaturated fatty acid, forming L* again in the second propagating equation [15–17]. The termination of lipoperoxidation occurs when the radicals (L* and LOO*) produced in the previous steps propagate to destroy themselves [15–17].

The hydroxyl radical (OH*) is often recognized as the initiator species and the most important in lipoperoxidation associated with iron [15, 17].

Antioxidant Systems

In oxidative stress there is an exaggerated stimulus, with overproduction and consequent imbalance between the pro- and antioxidant system, with a predominance of oxidants and consequent damage [15].

On a physiological level, we can defend ourselves from injury mediated by free radicals using cellular antioxidant reserves [11–17]. The antioxidant blood system is classified into enzymatic and non-enzymatic, the first being represented mainly by antioxidant enzymes: superoxide dismutase (SOD) that acts on the superoxide radical turning it into hydrogen peroxide, catalase (CATA) and glutathione peroxidase (GSHpx), which act on the hydrogen peroxide transforming it into water (see Fig. 34.9) [15–17].

The non-enzymatic antioxidant system consists of many substances, especially GSH, the main intracellular antioxidant compound, tocopherols, ascorbic acid, uric acid and β-carotene, which act on the hydroxyl radical, the true cause of oxidative stress in addition to the transport proteins of transition, such as transferrin, lactoferrin, albumin, metalloproteins and ceruloplasmin, which bind to transition metals preventing them from catalyzing the Haber–Weiss reaction [11–17]. The enzymatic antioxidant system and GSH are present predominantly in the intracellular environment, while the non-enzymatic system is located preferentially in the extracellular environment [7, 8].

Glutathione Antioxidant System

The glutathione antioxidant system is the main non-protein thiol involved in cellular antioxidant defense [18]. It consists of the tripeptide glutathione (g-L-glutamyl-L-cysteinyl-glycine), which is formed by cysteine, glutamic acid and glycine and synthesized primarily by the liver [18]. Its concentration is greater in the intracellular environment, however, it can be found both in plasma and in urine [18].

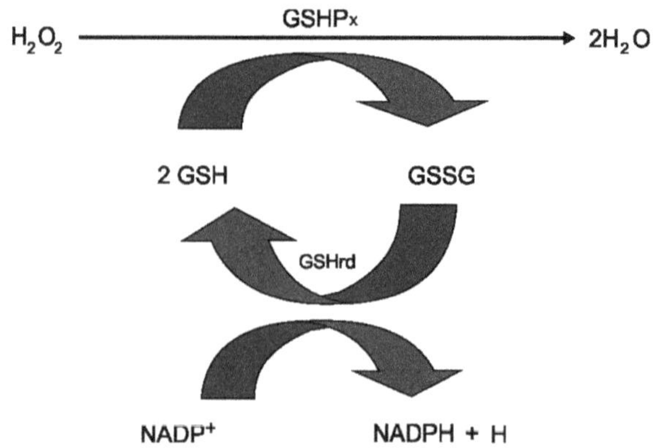

Fig. 34.10 Interconversion of glutathione in its reduced form and oxidized by the action of glutathione peroxidase (GSH-px) and glutathione reductase (GSH-rd) enzymes. GSH-rd does not act directly on the removal of radical species, but it is responsible for the regeneration of glutathione to its reduced form (GSH) in the presence of nicotinamide adenine dinucleotide phosphate (NADPH), aiming to prevent the stoppage of the glutathione metabolic cycle

It exists in the body in its reduced form (GSH) and oxidized (GSSG), acting directly or indirectly in many important biological processes, including the synthesis of proteins, metabolism and cellular protection [19].

This system also consists of the enzymes glutathione peroxidase (GSH-px) and glutathione reductase (GSH-rd) [18, 19]. Both catalyze the action of glutathione [18, 19]. Glutathione peroxidase catalyses the conversion of H_2O_2, produced by superoxide dismutase (SOD), with the dismutation of the superoxide anion (O_2^-), into H_2O [18, 19]. Glutathione reductase contains flavin adenine dinucleotide and uses the reduction of NADPH to reconvert GSSG to 2GSH [18, 19].

Up to now five structural and functional forms of GSH-px are known in mammals and they are all dependent on selenium [20]. Two forms have been identified in blood [20]. GSH-px is 1 of the 25 classes of known selenium proteins; GSH-px acts as an antioxidant by reducing peroxide, such as H_2O_2 [21]. The peptide glutathione (GSH) is a cofactor required in the reduction of peroxides, and acts as a reducing substrate, however it does not display the capacity of the activity of GSH-px [21]. Another enzyme that acts along with the glutathione peroxidase is GSH-rd [19]. This enzyme does not act directly on the removal of radical species, but it is responsible for the regeneration of glutathione to its reduced form (GSH) in the presence of nicotinamide adenine dinucleotide phosphate (NADPH), aiming to prevent the stoppage of the glutathione metabolic cycle [21] (see Fig. 34.10).

Thus, some studies have been developed to determine these enzymes both in cell tissues and in blood plasma [19].

Glutathione and the enzymes, which form part of the catalytic cycle of this peptide, present associations with changes in antioxidants states and with increased oxidative stress [19–21]. Quantification of glutathione may indicate a possible correlation between reduction in the activities of antioxidant enzymes such as glutathione peroxidase, and increase in base levels of DNA harmed due to oxidative damage [19].

Total Antioxidant Capacity

With regard to antioxidants some authors defend the study of total antioxidant capacity (TAC) instead of the analysis of isolated antioxidants, mainly due to the interaction between them in plasma and serum [22]. The analysis of TAC takes into account the cumulative action of all the antioxidants present, an integrated parameter is obtained, capable of revealing nuances about the delicate redox balance existing in vivo [22]. In biological systems, the synergistic activity between antioxidants is very common, as is seen with the actual glutathione [23]. The latter acts by regenerating ascorbate and this regenerates α-tocopherol restoring its properties of suppression of ROS [23]. Therefore, the measure of total antioxidant capacity of a sample can give information more biologically relevant than that obtained by measuring the individual concentration of antioxidants [22].

Renal Ischemia/Reperfusion and Glutamine

Since the publication of the first operations using renal pedicle clamping for vascular control, whether for kidney transplants, partial nephrectomy or correction of aortic aneurysms, this surgical maneuver has been widely used. As the complexity of surgical procedures on the kidney, and in particular, videolaparoscopy as a urological surgical practice, has also increased the time of use of the procedure of renal ischemia and in particular of warm ischemia [2–5].

Consequently, there is a growing interest in the study of injuries resulting from this state of ischemia, adding to this, the injuries related to post-reperfusion syndrome. In understanding this process, numerous experimental models have emerged enabling the study of physiopathological principles governing the lesions now triggered, and possible ways of minimizing them.

Rhoden evaluated the effects of L-arginine in renal I/R [24]. Supplementation with this amino acid led to greater renal damage measured by the malondialdehyde although, paradoxically, there was an improvement of renal function due to the dosage of creatinine [24]. This benefit was observed mainly in the first 96 h of reperfusion [24]. Guz [25], using a similar model in rats subjected to renal ischemia/reperfusion, also demonstrated the beneficial effect of taurine in the preservation of renal function [25]. Several other nutrients were studied in similar studies aiming at providing greater preservation of renal function after I/R [26]. This list of substances includes even synthetic molecules such as mesna (2-mercaptoethane sulfonate) described by Kabasakal [26] preventing renal injury by I/R [26].

One of the most important characteristics of GLN is its relationship with the biosynthesis of glutathione [27]. Glutamine provides glutamate to the glutathione system, which is one of the main sources of antioxidant defense at the cellular level [27]. Glutamate is rarely transported across membranes; glutamine, since it is easily transported, serves as a source of intracellular glutamate [28].

The dose of GLN used is a factor of fundamental relevance.

Johnson [29] demonstrated, in models of animals with breast cancer, that glutamine supplementation at a dose of 1 g/kg/day for 2 weeks almost doubles glutathione levels in breast tissues [29]. Engel [30] also demonstrated that administration of glutamine at a dose of 0.5 g/kg/day in patients undergoing cardiac surgery maintains glutathione levels after surgery [30]. A meta-analysis by Novak [31] demonstrated that a minimum dose of 0.2 g/kg/day is required to obtain a beneficial effect to the critical patient, where the parenteral route in this study showed better results [31]. Another more recent review in which doses from 0.13 to 0.86 g/kg/day were used questions the real benefit of this supplementation in critically ill patients [25]. Gouvêa Junior [32] demonstrated, in an experimental study in rats, that 0.5 g/kg administered by gavage favors the antioxidant system in a model of renal ischemia and reperfusion. We should note that studies show that high doses of GLN in the elderly increase the levels of urea and creatinine, justified by the difficulty of the kidneys in these patients to excrete these substances although there is no clinical significance [33].

The pathway for glutamine administration also deserves special consideration. Luo [34] showed there is no difference in the use of parenteral or enteral GLN regarding the antioxidant capacity and reduction of oxidative stress [34].

The mechanisms related to the preservation of the glutathione system in situations involving I/R injury have been the subject of several studies.

Under normal conditions the binding of glutamate to cysteine is what limits the synthesis of glutathione, but it has been demonstrated that glutamine depletion leads to a decrease in the rate of intracellular glutathione [28]. The level of glutathione is known to gradually decrease during ischemia with subsequent return to baseline levels during reperfusion [28]. Harward [28] showed that GLN supplementation prior to intestinal I/R partly preserves the glutathione in intestinal cells, and reduces lipid peroxidation, suggesting a protective effect in the intestine under this condition [28]. Jia [35], on investigating in an animal model the protective effect of alanyl-glutamine dipeptide against liver damage due to ischemia and reperfusion, concluded there was greater tolerance of liver to warm I/R and high levels of glutathione in these animals [35].

It must be warned that recent studies suggest ischemic preconditioning in organs that are going to be submitted to the stress of I/R [36]. Such preconditioning means a brief induction period of ischemia followed by a brief period of reperfusion before a longer period of ischemia [36]. The role of ischemic preconditioning in the increase of tolerance to ischemia has been described in several organs such as the heart, brain, spinal cord, skeletal muscle, retina, kidneys, intestine, as well as the liver [36]. However, despite studies about why the protective effect of ischemic preconditioning works the real underlying reason for this is still not clearly established [36].

Effect of Glutamine on the Antioxidant System in the I/R Kidney

Glutathione Peroxidase (GSH-px)

Gouvêa Junior [32] demonstrated the preservation of glutathione peroxidase levels in animals subjected to ischemia and reperfusion when there had been administered glutamine supplementation beforehand [32].

This study seems to confirm the beneficial effect of glutamine as a protective cellular agent in ischemia/reperfusion [32]. This same effect was observed by Ezhilan [37] in myocardial cells subjected to oxidative injury [37]. This author noted an increase in total glutathione and glutathione peroxidase in animals previously treated with glutamine [37].

Glutathione peroxidase enzyme activity is essential for the proper functioning of glutathione. Abilés [38], by supplementing glutathione in critically ill patients, showed an increase in glutathione peroxidase proportional to the elevation of glutathione, and inversely with the levels of this enzyme with lipid peroxidation in these patients [38]. Similar results were presented by Kul [39] in animal models using enteral glutamine with an increase in glutathione peroxidase and decrease in lipid peroxidation in the intestine [39].

These findings corroborate with those shown in other experimental models (particularly renal and intestinal I/R) where glutamine supplementation preserved the levels of total glutathione [28, 30]. Contrary to such findings, Gonzáles [40] showed that the administration of 300 mg/kg/day of glutamine by gavage in rats does not increase the activity of the enzymes glutathione reductase, catalase and superoxide dismutase, despite containing decreased glutathione and lipid peroxidation in rats subjected to oxidative stress [40]. This disagreement regarding the findings of the Gouvêa Junior's study [32] may be related to the length of time of use of glutamine [32]. In Gonzáles' study the glutamine was administered by gavage for only 1 day [40], while in the other study, glutamine was administered for 7 days. Furthermore, the dose employed (500 mg/kg/day) is superior to that employed by Gonzalez [32, 40].

Total Antioxidant Capacity (TAC)

The TAC is intended to show the organism's response to the aggressor agent studied, i.e. to the free radicals. It is known that this capacity has a limit [22]. When the production of free radicals surpasses the capacity of antioxidant defense, an "oxidative stress" phenomenon starts resulting in a morphological functional disturbance of the damaged cell [22]. Neto [22] showed that the TAC in the skeletal muscle of rats decreases markedly after lower limb ischemia [22]. Cymrot [41] observed no change in the serum sample of rats submitted to ischemic skin flaps, however they were seen in the tissues within a few days after surgery [41]. According to the authors, this finding is probably due to the fact that the antioxidant changes occurring in the flap are not sufficient to be detected in the systemic circulation, or these changes could have taken place earlier and were not possible to visualize in this experimental model [41].

Gouvêa Junior [32] demonstrated that glutamine supplementation preserves the total antioxidant capacity of plasma in animals subjected to renal ischemia and reperfusion [32]. This effect has previously been observed by Szijártó [42] in an animal model of liver I/R [42]. This may be related to an increase in antioxidant components present in plasma, notably glutathione, or an inhibition in the production of ROS reducing the organic demand for antioxidants.

Effect of Glutamine on Urea, Creatinine and Renal Histology in the I/R Kidney

Renal ischemia of more than 45 min provokes the increase of urea and creatinine with higher levels after 48 h of reperfusion which normalize after the tenth day [43]. Paller [44], in a classic study conducting renal ischemia in rats for 1 h and reperfusion for 15 min after previously administering SOD enzyme, showed lower creatinine levels in the animals treated [44]. These differences were more intense in samples collected after 24 h of ischemia [44].

Tucci [45] observed protection against renal ischemia for 1 h using chlorpromazine beforehand; however the levels of urea and creatinine increased after 24 h of reperfusion [45].

Gouvêa Junior [32] observed no differences in the results of urea and creatinine between animals subjected to renal ischemia and reperfusion using glutamine beforehand [32]. This may be related to the shorter reperfusion period, in this case, only for 1 h [32]. Added to this is the issue, already well established in the literature, of compensatory renal hypertrophy because, in the model used in this study, the animals spent 2 weeks with only one kidney [46].

According to Cologna [47] the first changes in the levels of urea and creatinine occur when renal function is compromised by over 50 % [47]. Maybe if the period of ischemia were higher in this study there would be a difference in the levels of creatinine and urea. Further studies in this line may answer this question using more sensitive methods of measurement of glomerular filtration and consequent diagnosis of earlier renal change.

It is a well known fact that morphological changes consistent with ischemic necrosis of renal tubular cells are confirmed after at least 30 min of ischemia and over 1 h of reperfusion [15]. It is known that very often the cells attacked still manage to survive presenting only sublethal changes which consist of hydropic or vacuolar degeneration with discrete metabolic changes, but still compatible with cell survival [11].

Fuller [7], in their study, registered benefit from the administration of glutamine to kidneys of rats before being subjected to a transplant [7]. In this case there was a protective histological effect primarily in the reduction of renal cell apoptosis, with consequent reduction in tubular necrosis [7].

A beneficial effect of L-alanyl-glutamine was also verified by Stangl [48] in a histological study of liver tissue subjected to I/R [48]. In this case the study took place after 24 h of renal reperfusion [48].

Gouvêa Junior [32] observed no protective effect in animals receiving glutamine prior to kidney I/R [32]. This is justified by the fact that reperfusion having been given for a short time and which was not long enough to lead to changes in cell histology [32]. Starting from the results of this study presented here, it is proposed that longer reperfusion be used in a future study and afterwards investigate whether there is histological evidence to verify benefit found in systemic antioxidant activity resulting from this amino acid.

Finally, attention should be paid to the possible harmful effect of glutamine on the kidneys at high doses (1 g/kg), proven in diabetic animals [49].

Conclusions

In short, the proposal to use glutamine in patients who will be submitted to surgical procedures where renal I/R is necessary, as well as those who will undergo kidney transplant and even in live kidney donors constitutes an innovative procedure.

Based on this, the use of glutamine together with ischemic preconditioning is suggested in subsequent studies in order to maximize its beneficial effects and minimize the damage arising from renal I/R.

References

1. Nogueira PCKo, et al. Estimated prevalence of childhood end-stage renal disease in the state of São Paulo. Rev Assoc Med Bras. [online]. 2011; 57(4): 443–9 [cited 2013-02-11]. ISSN 0104-4230. Available from: http://www.scielo.br/scielo.php?script=sci_arttext&pid=S0104-42302011000400020&lng=en&nrm=iso. http://dx.doi.org/10.1590/S0104-42302011000400020. Accessed on March 2, 2013.
2. Giessing M. Laparoscopic living-donornephrectomy. Nephrol Dial Transplant. 2004;19(4):36–9.
3. Desai MM, Gill IS, Ramani AP, Spaliviero M, Rybicki L, Kaouk JH. The impact of warm ischaemia on renal function after laparoscopic partial nephrectomy. BJU Int. 2005;95:377–83.
4. Kosieradzki M, Rowinski W. Ischemia/reperfusion injury in kidney transplantation: mechanisms and prevention. Transplant Proc. 2008;40(10):3279–88.
5. Singer P, Cohen J, Cynober L. Effect of nutritional state of brain-dead organ donor on transplantation. Nutrition. 2001;17(11–12):948–52.
6. Schuster H, Blanc MC, Bonnefont-Rousselot D, Nakib S, Le Tourneau A, Furst P, et al. Protective effects of glutamine dipeptide and α-tocopherol against ischemia–reperfusion injury in the isolated rat liver. Clin Nutr. 2009;28(3):331–7.
7. Fuller TF, Rose F, Singleton KD, Linde Y, Hoff U, Freise CE, et al. Glutamine donor pretreatment in rat kidney transplants with severe preservation reperfusion injury. J Surg Res. 2007;140(1):77–83.
8. Mora Lde O, Antunes LM, Francescato HD, Bianchi ML. The effects of oral glutamine on cisplatin-induced nefrotoxicity in rats. Pharmacol Res. 2003;47(6):517–22.
9. Merril JP, Murray JE, Harrison JH, Guild WR. Successful homotransplantation of the human kidney between identical twins. JAMA. 1956;160:277–82.
10. Novick AC. Renal hypothermia in vivo and ex-vivo. Urol Clin North Am. 1983;10(4):637–44.
11. Kumar V, Abbas AK, Fausto N. Adaptation, damage and cell death. In: Kumar V, Abbas AK, Fausto N, editors. Robbins and Cotran pathologic basis of disease. 7th ed. Rio de Janeiro: Elsevier; 2007.
12. Silveira M, Yoshida WB. Ischemia and reperfusion in skeletal muscle: injury mechanisms and treatment perspectives. J Vasc Br. 2004;3(4):367–78.
13. Évora PRB, Pearson PJ, Seccombe JF, Schaff HV. Ischemia-reperfusion injury. Pathophysiological and the importance of endothelial function. Arq Bras Cardiol. 1996;66(4):239–45.
14. Granger DN, Hollwarth ME, Parks DA. Ischemia reperfusion injury: role of oxygen-derived free radicals. Acta Physiol Scand. 1986;548 suppl 1:47–63.
15. Ferreira ALA, Matsubara LS. Free radicals: concepts, diseases, defense system and oxidative stress. Rev Assoc Med Bras. 1997;43(1):61–8.
16. Brieger K, Schiavone S, Miller FJ Jr, Krause KH. Reactive oxygen species: from health to disease. *Swiss Med Wkly.* 2012; 142: w13659. DOI: 10.4414/smw.2012.13659. Available at http/www.smw.ch. Accessed on January 4, 2013.
17. Lima SE, Abdalla DSP. Lipid peroxidation: mechanisms and assessment in biological samples. Braz J Pharm Sci. 2001;37(3):293–303.
18. Pastore A, Federicia G, Bertini E, Piemonte F. Analysis of glutathione: implication in redox and detoxification. Clin Chim Acta. 2003;333:19–39.
19. Rover LJ, Höehr NF, Vellasco AP, Kubota LT. Antioxidant system involving the glutathione metabolic cycle associated to electroanalytical methods in the oxidative stress evaluation. *Quim Nova.* 2001; 24(1):112–9. ISSN 0100-4042. Available from: http://www.scielo.br/scielo.php?script=sci_arttext&pid=S0100-40422001000100019&lng=en&nrm=iso. Accessed in January 19, 2013.
20. Zachara BA, Gromadzinska J, Zbrog Z, Swietch R, Wasowicz W, Twardowska E, et al. Selenium supplementation to chronic kidney disease patients on hemodialysis does not induce the synthesis of plasma glutathione peroxidase. Acta Biochim Pol. 2009;56(1):183–7.
21. Battin EE, Brumaghim JL. Antioxidant activity of sulfur and selenium: a review of reactive oxygen species scavenging, glutathione peroxidase, and metal-binding antioxidant mechanisms. Cell Biochem Biophys. 2009;55(1):1–23.

22. Neto AF, Silva JCB, Fagundes DJ, Percário S, Ferreira N, Juliano Y, Neto AAM. Oxidatives alterations, total antioxidant status and nitric oxide study in rats submitted to ischemia and reperfusion of hind limbs. Acta Cir Bras. 2005;20(2): 134–9.
23. May JM, Qu ZC, Whitesell RR. Ascorbic acid recycling enhances the antioxidant reserve of human erythrocytes. Biochemistry. 1995;34(39):12721–8.
24. Rhoden EL, Lucas ML, Pereira-lima L, Rhoden CR, Souto CAV. Effects of I-arginine on the kidney level of malondialdehyde in rats submitted to renal ischaemia-reperfusion. BJU Int. 2001;88(3):273–7.
25. Guz G, Oz E, Lortlar N, Ulusu NN, Nurlu N, Demirogullari B, et al. The effect of taurine on renal ischemia/reperfusion injury. Amino Acids. 2007;32(3):405–11.
26. Kabasakal L, Sehirli AO, Çetinel S, Cilkler E, Gedik N, Sener G. Mesna (2-mercaptoethane sulfonate) prevents ischemia/reperfusion induced renal oxidative damage in rats. Life Sci. 2004;75(19):2329–40.
27. Bollhalder L, Pfeil AM, Tomonaga Y, Schwenkglenks M. A systematic literature review and meta-analysis of randomized clinical trials of parenteral glutamine supplementation. Clin Nutr. 2012;32(2):213–23.
28. Harward TRS, Coe D, Souba WW, Klingman N, Seerger JM. Glutamine preserves gut glutathione levels during intestinal ischemia/reperfusion. J Surg Res. 1994;56(4):351–5.
29. Johnson AT, Kaufmann YC, Luo S, Todorova V, Klimberg VS. Effect of glutamine on glutathione, igf-l, and tgf-β_1. J Surg Res. 2003;111(2):222–8.
30. Engel JM, Muhling J, Kwapisz M, Heidt M. Glutamine administration in patients undergoing cardiac surgery and the influence on blood glutathione levels. Acta Anaesthesiol Scand. 2009;53(10):1317–23.
31. Novak F, Heyland DK, Avenell A, Drover JW, Su X. Glutamine supplementation in serious illness: a systematic review of the evidence. Crit Care Med. 2002;30(9):2022–9.
32. Gouvêa Junior VT, Caporossi C, Salomão AB, Côrtes E, Munhoz MF, Nascimento JE. Effect of glutamine on the total antioxidant system of rats subjected to renal ischemia and reperfusion. Acta Cir Bras. 2011;26(6):445–50.
33. Galera SC, Fechine FV, Teixeira MJ, Coelho ZCB, Vasconcelos RC, Leitão de Vasconcelos PC. The safety of oral use of L-glutamine in middle-aged and elderly individuals. Nutrition. 2010;26:375–81.
34. Luo M, Bazargan N, Griffith DP, Fernández-Estivariz C, Leader LM, Easley KA, et al. Metabolic effects of enteral versus parenteral alanyl-glutamine dipeptide administration in critically ill patients receiving enteral feeding: a pilot study. Clin Nutr. 2008;27(2):297–306.
35. Jia CJ, Daí CL, Zhang X, Cui K, Xu F, Xu YQ. Alanyl-glutamine dipeptide inhibits hepatic ischemia-reperfusion injury in rats. Word J Gastroenterol. 2006;12(9):1373–8.
36. Silva Jr OC, Centurion S, Pacheco EG, Brisoti JL, Oliveira AF, Sasso KD. Basics aspects of the ischemia reperfusion injury and of the ischemic reconditioning. Acta Cir Bras. 2002;17(3):96–100.
37. Ezhilan RA, Rajesh R, Rajaprabhu D, Meena B, Ganesan B, Anandan R. Antioxidant defense of glutamine on myocardial antioxidant status in adriamycin-induced cardiomyopathy in rats. J Cell Anima Biol. 2008;2(5):107–11.
38. Abilés J, Moreno-Torres R, Moratalla G, Castano J, Abúd P, Mudarra A, et al. Efects de la suplementación com glutamina sobre el sistema antioxidante y la peroxidacón lipídica empacientes críticos com nutrición pareteral. Nutri Hosp. 2008;23(4):332–9.
39. Kul M, Vurucu S, Demirkaya E, Tunc T, Aydinoz S, Meral C, et al. Enteral glutamine and/or arginine supplementation have favorable effects on oxidative stress parameters in neonatal rat intestine. J Pediatr Gastroenterol Nutr. 2009;49(1):85–9.
40. Gonzáles S, Polizio AH, Erário MA, Tomaro ML. Glutamine is highly effective in preventing in vivo cobalt-induced oxidative stress in rat liver. Word J Gastroenterol. 2005;11(23):3533–8.
41. Cymrot M, Percário S, Ferreira LM. Comportamento do estresse oxidativo e da capacidade antioxidante total em ratos submetidos a retalhos cutâneos isquêmicos. Acta Cir Bras. 2004;19(1):18–26.
42. Szijarto A, Hahn O, Batmunkh E, Stangl R, Kiss A, Lotz G, et al. Short-term alanyl-glutamine dipeptide pretreatment in liver ischemia–reperfusion model: effects on microcirculation and antioxidant status in rats. Clin Nutr. 2007;26(5):640–8.
43. Eschwège P, Paradis V, Conti M, Holstege A, Richet F, Detève J, Ménager P, Legrand A, Jardin A, Bedossa P, Benoit G. In situ detection of lipid peroxidation by-products as markers of renal ischemia injuries in rat kidneys. J Urol. 1999;162(2):553–7.
44. Paller SM, Hoidal JR, Ferris TF. Oxygen free radicals in ischemic acute renal failure. J Clin Invest. 1984; 74(4): 1156–64.
45. Tucci SJ, Carvalho RN, Celini FM, Cologna AJ, Suaid HJ, Tirapelli LF, Martins ACP. Renal ischemia and reperfusion injury: influence of chlorpromazine on renal function and lipid peroxidation. Acta Cir Bras. 2008;23(1):42–6.
46. Tucci SJ, Carvalho RN, Celini FM, Cologna AJ, Suaid HJ, Tirapelli LF, Martins ACP. Compensatory renal growth and mitochondrial function: the influence of warm ischemia and reperfusion. Acta Cir Bras. 2008;23(1):31–5.
47. Cologna AJ, Lima LVS, Tucci SJ, Suaid HJ, Reis RB, Tirapelli LF, et al. Cyclosporine action on kidneys of rats submitted to normothermic ischaemia and reperfusion. Acta Cir Bras. 2008;23(1):36–41.
48. Stangl R, Szijártó A, Onody P, Tamás J, Tátrai M, Hegedűs V, et al. Reduction of liver ischemia-reperfusion injury via glutamine pretreatment. J Surg Res. 2009;22:1118–25.
49. Alba-Loureiro TC, Ribeiro RF, Zorn TMT, Lagranha CJ. Effects of glutamine supplementation on kidney of diabetic rat. Amino Acids. 2010;38:1021–30.

Chapter 35
Protection by Glutamine After Ischemia/Reperfusion Injury

Kechen Ban and Rosemary A. Kozar

Key Points

- Ischemia/reperfusion (I/R) occurs in a wide range of clinical scenarios and is associated with considerable morbidity and mortality.
- Glutamine has been demonstrated to protect against I/R-induced injury in a number of different organs including the intestine, liver, heart, kidney and brain.
- Glutamine's protective effects include suppression of hyperinflammation, protection against cell apoptosis, and enhancement of cell proliferation.
- Studies in animal models have shown that the protective effect of glutamine on I/R injury are mediated by activation of anti-inflammatory mechanism including peroxisome proliferator-activated receptor gamma and heme oxygenase-1 and suppression of pro-inflammatory mediators including nuclear factor-kappaB, activating protein-1, and inducible nitric oxide synthase.
- To achieve maximum beneficial effect of glutamine, the delivery route, dose and timing have to be optimized.

Keywords Ischemia/reperfusion • Ischemia/reperfusion injury • Glutamine • Glutamine supplementation • Inflammation • Organ

Abbreviations

AP-1	Activating protein-1
HO	Heme oxygenase
IL	Interleukin
HSP	Heat shock protein
iNOS	Inducible nitric oxide synthase

K. Ban, Ph.D. (✉) • R.A. Kozar, M.D., Ph.D.
Department of Surgery, University of Texas Medical School at Houston,
6431 Fannin Street, Houston, TX 77030, USA
e-mail: Kechen.Ban@uth.tmc.edu; Rosemary.A.Kozar@uth.tmc.edu

R. Rajendram et al. (eds.), *Glutamine in Clinical Nutrition*, Nutrition and Health,
DOI 10.1007/978-1-4939-1932-1_35, © Springer Science+Business Media New York 2015

I/R	Ischemia/reperfusion
NF-κB	Nuclear factor-kappaB
PPARγ	Peroxisome proliferator-activated receptor gamma
PPRE	Peroxisome proliferator-activated receptor responsive element
RXR	Retinoid X receptor
TLR	Toll-like receptor
TNF-α	Tumor necrosis factor-α

Introduction

Ischemia/reperfusion (I/R) occurs in a wide range of clinical scenarios including trauma, shock, transplantation, stroke, myocardial infarction, coronary angioplasty, thrombolytic therapy, coronary revascularization, and autoimmune diseases. Ischemia can cause tissue and organ damage due to an insufficient oxygen and glucose, which are necessary for cellular metabolism, which subsequently results in tissue or organ dysfunction. Although reperfusion is necessary to attenuate injury of ischemic tissues, it can trigger a cascade of events leading to additional tissue injury and even remote organ injury. Therefore, I/R injury contributes to the pathophysiology of a wide range of clinical diseases and is associated with considerable morbidity and mortality.

Despite extensive studies, the precise cellular and molecular mechanisms of I/R injury is yet to be fully elucidated. Attempts to develop effective therapies for I/R injury are particularly difficult due to the lack of the fundamental knowledge. However, clinical observations and laboratory studies have demonstrated that an acute inflammatory response triggered by I/R is a crucial event which includes recruitment and activation of neutrophils and platelet and complement activation. In the early stages of I/R, activated neutrophils mediate a hyperinflammatory response through secretion of many inflammatory mediators, including cytokines and chemokines, and reactive oxygen species which are central to innate and adaptive immune processes.

The Role of Glutamine Supplementation in I/R Injury in Different Organs

Glutamine is considered a "conditionally essential" amino acid during stress and critical illness and has been used clinically to improve outcomes. The positive effect of glutamine administration has been well-documented in I/R injury. Although key physiological roles are shared, it is important to understand the different effects of glutamine in each organ I/R injury in order to achieve more efficient therapeutic modalities. Here, we summarize the effect of glutamine administration in different organ I/R injury in preclinical animal models. The role of glutamine supplementation in patients with major surgery or with sepsis, which often accompany I/R injury, will be discussed in Part 4 in this book.

The Role of Glutamine Supplementation in Intestinal I/R Injury

Intestinal I/R injury occurs in a variety of clinical settings, including major trauma, hemorrhage, small bowel transplantation, superior mesenteric artery and vein thrombosis, acute pancreatitis, sepsis, cardiopulmonary bypass, and burn injuries. Intestinal I/R leads to generation of inflammatory factors, release of cytotoxic substances, activation of pathologic enzymes and immune cells in the intestine. These changes can result in intestinal mucosal injury, enhanced intestinal permeability, and hyperinflammation, leading to gut dysfunction or even multiple organ dysfunction syndrome.

Gut-specific therapies to mitigate I/R-induced gut dysfunction are few. Glutamine, however, may represent one such therapy. Glutamine supplementation has been shown to facilitate the maintenance of gut mucosal integrity and to attenuate infectious complications and mortality in adult surgical and critically ill patients [1]. Glutamine is not only the major fuel for enterocytes and colonocytes but also has a key influence in supporting gut functions and integrity [2]. For this reason, research focusing on the use of glutamine as a pharmaconutrient to prevent and treat the physiopathological conditions generated by intestinal I/R has garnered considerable attention.

Previous studies have focused on the effect of glutamine pretreatment. In one study, rats were pretreated with glutamine via orogastric route in a dose of 1 g/kg daily for 4, 7, and 15 days or a dose of 2 g/kg daily for 7 days, followed by 1 h of intestinal ischemia/1 h reperfusion [3]. Interestingly, only pretreatment with glutamine in 1 g/kg for 4 days significantly attenuated I/R-induced elevated plasma endotoxin levels. The longer periods of pretreatment or the higher dose (2 g/kg) did not suppress the elevation of plasma endotoxin levels. The protective effect on histological damage in the intestine was observed only when glutamine pretreatment was given at a dose of 1 or 2 g/kg for 7 days. This study suggests that the dose and timing of administration of glutamine are critical to achieve beneficial effects on I/R intestinal injury. In another study by the same group using the 1 g/kg dose of glutamine for 4 days, glutamine pretreatment significantly attenuated intestinal permeability caused by intestinal I/R but did not prevent histopathological changes in the intestine or decrease plasma endotoxin levels [4].

The protective effect of glutamine pretreatment on intestinal I/R injury was also found by Mederios et al. In their study, rats received 1.5 mg/kg/day of 5 % glutamine daily for 5 days before surgery via gavage followed by 1 h intestinal ischemia/2 h reperfusion [5]. Glutamine significantly suppressed bacterial translocation to mesenteric lymph nodes, liver, and lung, and reduced systemic levels of tumor necrosis factor (TNF)-α and interleukin (IL)-6, indicating that glutamine protects the intestinal barrier integrity and reduces the inflammatory cytokine response during intestinal I/R. Bacterial translocation is the passage of viable indigenous bacteria from the gastrointestinal tract to normally sterile extraintestinal sites, such as the mesenteric lymph nodes, livers, lungs, blood and other tissues [6] and is associated with intestinal mucosal barrier function.

We have shown in a rat model of intestinal ischemia of 60 min and reperfusion of 30 min that 10 mM glutamine administered into an intestinal sac at the onset of ischemia was protective [7]. Glutamine maintained intestinal barrier function through preservation of cytoskeleton integrity, increased incorporation of G-actin into F-actin, and inhibition of intestinal permeability. Recently, in a mouse model of intestinal ischemia of 1 h and reperfusion of 6 h, we found that administration of 60 mM glutamine given enterally at the onset of ischemia also significantly decreased intestinal permeability and inflammation (Fig. 35.1) as well as injury (Fig. 35.2) [8]. Interestingly, alanine failed to demonstrate the beneficial effects of glutamine. This may be due to the ability of glutamine, but not alanine, to increase intestinal ATP [9]. Glutamine, but not alanine, is metabolized by intestinal epithelial cells. These data suggest that the individual amino acid may have differential effects on intestinal barrier function.

To investigate the molecular mechanisms of glutamine's protection, 60 mM glutamine (approximates the concentration of glutamine found in commercially available immune-enhancing enteral diets) was administered and intestinal inflammatory mediators assessed [10]. Glutamine not only inhibited the increased expression of the pro-inflammatory mediator inducible nitric oxide synthase (iNOS) but also enhanced activity of the anti-inflammatory mediator, peroxisome proliferator-activated receptor gamma (PPARγ). Importantly, the PPARγ inhibitor, GW9662, further increased intestinal injury and inflammation and abolished the protective effects of glutamine. Treatment with the iNOS inhibitor, *N*-[3(aminomethyl)benzyl]acetamidine (1,400 W), had synergistic protective effects with glutamine during intestinal I/R. These data suggest that the protective role of glutamine in intestinal I/R is mediated by PPARγ and iNOS. In another experiment using the same model, glutamine suppressed pro-inflammatory activating protein-1 (AP-1) activity and decreased c-jun expression [11].

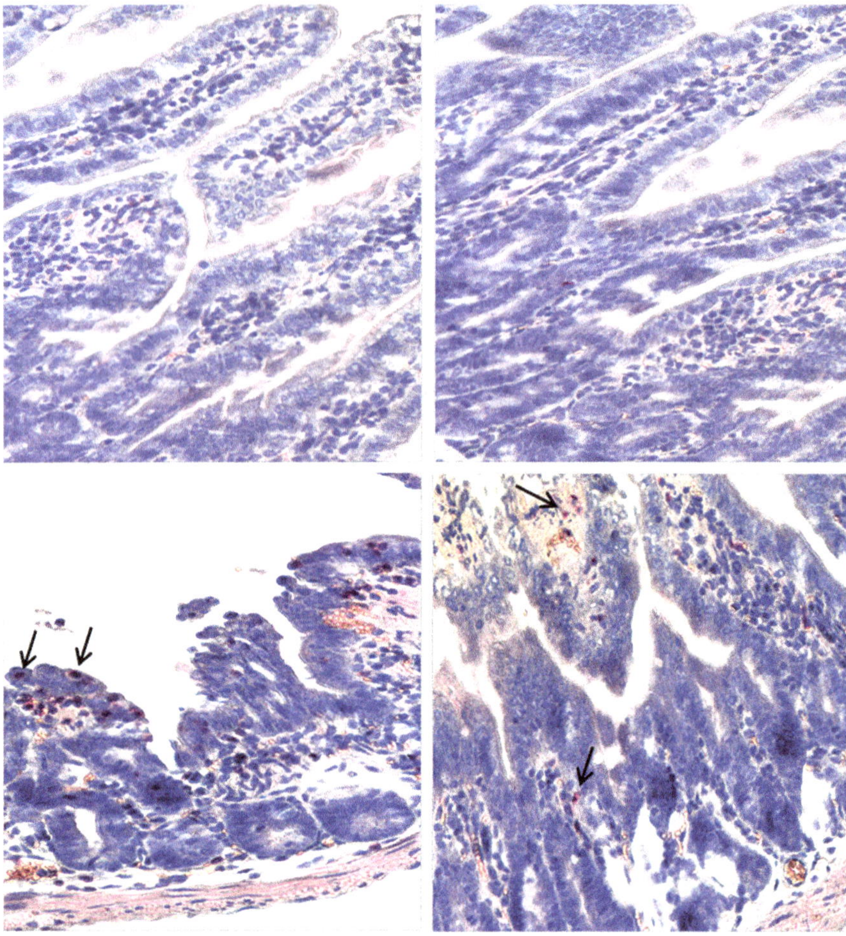

Fig. 35.1 Glutamine given at the onset of reperfusion inhibited intestinal neutrophil infiltration after I/R. Glutamine given at the onset of reperfusion inhibited neutrophil infiltration after intestinal ischemia/reperfusion (I/R). Enteral glutamine was given at the onset of reperfusion in a mouse model of intestinal I/R [8]. Sham groups underwent an identical surgical procedure without I/R. Intestinal sections were stained using a Naphthol AS-D Chloroacetate Esterase Cytochemical Staining kit (Sigma), which identifies specific leukocyte esterases. Representative images were shown. The black arrow indicates a neutrophil which was stained with *red* color. 8 mice/group (unpublished data)

The studies discussed thus far all investigated enteral glutamine. Using a similar rodent model of gut I/R, glutamine-supplemented parenteral nutrition was utilized for 48 h [12]. The results showed that glutamine added to standard parenteral nutrition protected against intestinal injury and permeability, prevented bacterial translocation, and decreased plasma endotoxin levels, compared to standard parenteral nutrition. In another study, 3 % glutamine was infused for 24 h and then rodents were subjected to either 30 or 60 min of intestinal ischemia/60 min of reperfusion [13]. Glutamine supplementation decreased cell membrane lipid peroxidation and maintained intestinal gut glutathione levels during intestinal I/R.

The beneficial effect of parenteral glutamine improved survival in a mouse model of intestinal I/R. Mice that were pretreated with 2 % glutamine-supplemented total parenteral nutrition for 5 days had a significantly higher survival (62 %) than mice fed total parenteral nutrition alone (15 %) [14].

Though most studies show clear benefit from glutamine, there are a number of studies that showed conflicting results. In one study, 2 % glutamine was injected into the duodenum at the onset of 75 min

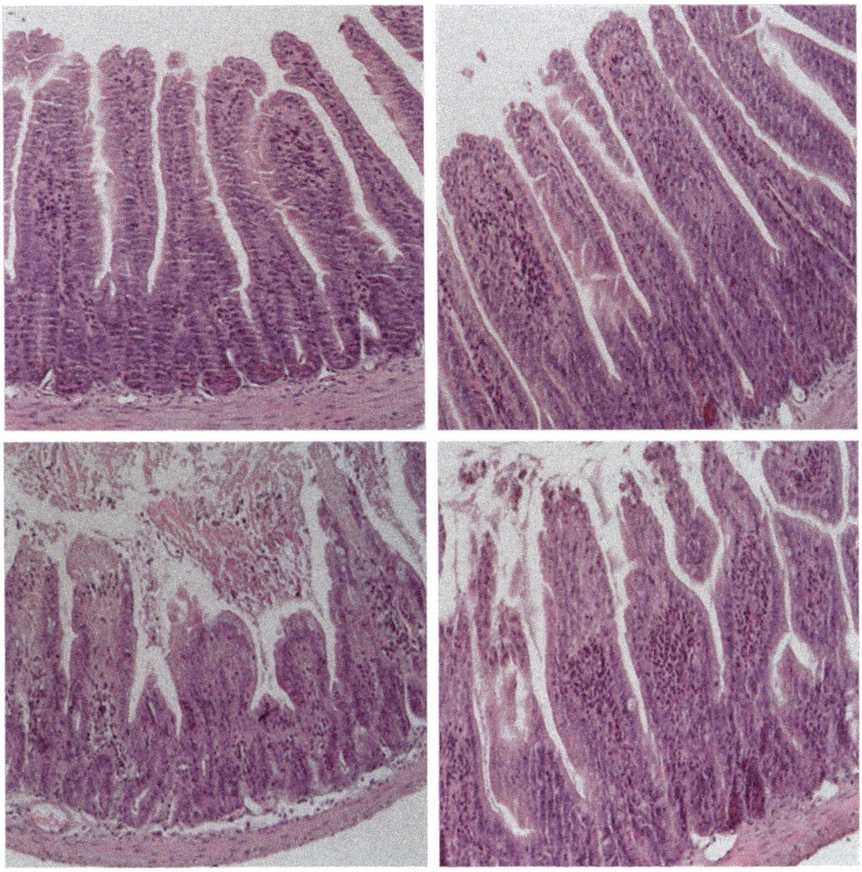

Fig. 35.2 Glutamine given at the onset of reperfusion protected against intestinal injury after I/R. Glutamine given at the onset of reperfusion protected against intestinal injury after ischemia/reperfusion (I/R). Enteral glutamine was given at the onset of reperfusion in a mouse model of intestinal I/R [8]. Sham groups underwent an identical surgical procedure without I/R. Intestinal tissues were stained with hematoxylin and eosin. Representative images were showed. 8 mice/group (unpublished data)

of ischemia [15]. Animals pre-treated with glutamine had lower survival. In a similar experiment, 2 % glutamine was administered after 50 min of ischemia, at the onset of reperfusion. Adhesion molecule CD11b expression and reactive oxygen intermediate production by circulating myeloid cells were significantly increased in glutamine treatment group, suggesting that glutamine enhanced leukocyte activity. Therefore, the authors concluded that intraluminal glutamine during severe intestinal ischemia has detrimental effects on survival associated with promotion of circulating myeloid cell priming and activation. In another study, mice were subjected to 90 min of ischemia and 3 % glutamine was given parenterally [16]. Glutamine treatment was detrimental, showing that the survival rates were 92 % versus 42 % at 12 h and 38 % versus 0 % at 48 h in the control and glutamine-treated groups, respectively. In another set of experiments, mice were subjected to 60 min ischemia followed by 2 or 4 h reperfusion and glutamine was given with same dose and route. Glutamine treatment increased systemic reactive oxygen intermediate production after phorbol myristate acetate stimulation and increased CD11b expression.

In summary, most studies have demonstrated a protective role of glutamine after intestinal I/R injury. The beneficial effects of glutamine include a reduction in intestinal permeability, mucosal

Table 35.1 The effect of glutamine supplementation with different doses, routes, and timing of administration in intestinal I/R models

Specie	Dose	Route	Timing	Effect observed	Reference
Rat	1–2 g/kg	Orally	4 and 7 days before I/R	Attenuated plasma endotoxin levels and protected against intestinal histological damage	[3]
	1 g/kg	Orally	4 days before I/R	Attenuated the intestinal permeability	[4]
	1.5 mg/kg	Gavage	5 days before I/R	Suppressed bacterial translocation and inflammatory cytokine levels	[5]
	60 mM	Enterally	At the onset of ischemia	Attenuated intestinal injury and inflammation	[10]
	10 mM	Enterally	At the onset of ischemia	Maintained intestinal barrier function	[9]
	10 mM	Enterally	At the onset of ischemia	Attenuated intestinal injury	[7]
	2.4 % (164 mM)	Parenterally	After ischemia	Protected against intestinal injury and permeability, prevented bacterial translocation and inhibition of plasma endotoxin levels	[12]
	3 % (205 mM)	Parenterally	24 h before ischemia	Decreased cell membrane lipid peroxidation	[13]
Mouse	60 mM	Enterally	At the onset of ischemia	Attenuated intestinal permeability, inflammation and injury	[17]
	2 % (138 mM)	Parenterally	5 days before I/R	Increased survival	[14]
	2 % (138 mM)	Enterally	At the onset of ischemia	Decreased survival and enhanced leukocyte activity	[15]
	3 % (205 mM)	Parenterally	During ischemia	Increased reactive oxygen intermediate production and vascular permeability	[16]

injury, inflammation, bacterial translocation, production of inflammatory mediators and plasma endotoxin as well as improved survival. The dose of glutamine proven to be efficacious ranged from 10 to 60 mM when delivered intraluminally, 1–2 g/kg when given orally, and 138–205 mM when administrated parenterally. The timing of administration has ranged from as long as 7 days prior to ischemia to the onset of reperfusion. Table 35.1 summarizes the dose, route and timing used and the effect observed in glutamine supplementation in animal models of intestinal I/R injury.

Remote organ injury is also a major consequence of intestinal I/R. Thus far, most glutamine studies focused on gut protection. We have recently demonstrated that enteral glutamine given at the onset of reperfusion not only protects the gut but also has similar protective effects on the lung [8].

The Role of Glutamine Supplementation in Hepatic I/R Injury

Hepatic I/R injury is considered as a key factor that contributes to significant morbidity and mortality associated with liver transplantation, liver resection for cancer, trauma, and hemorrhagic shock. Reperfusion is associated with an accumulation of inflammatory cells, release of inflammatory mediators, production of reactive oxygen species and reactive nitrogen species, leading to hepatic injury due to inflammation, apoptosis, and necrosis [17, 18]. Therefore, an emerging interest has focused on the prevention of liver injury and enhancement of liver recovery, repair, and regeneration after hepatic I/R. Although ischemic preconditioning has been shown to achieve better outcomes [19], this procedure can only be applied as a preventive measure in elective settings. Attempts to develop pharmacologic treatments to mitigate hepatic I/R injury have proven extremely difficult.

There are not many studies examining the effect of glutamine on hepatic I/R injury. In a study by Araugo et al, male Wistar rats were treated with L-alanyl-glutamine (0.75 mg/kg), a stabilized form dipeptide from L-glutamine, intraperitoneally 2 h before laparotomy and then subjected to total hepatic ischemia for 30 min induced by clamping of portal triad [20]. They found that L-alanyl-glutamine preconditioning significantly reduced alanine aminotransferase and lactate dehydrogenase levels in serum and caspase-3 expression in the liver tissue after hepatic I/R, suggesting that glutamine has the protective effect on hepatic I/R injury. Another rat hepatic I/R experiment also showed that pretreatment with glutamine reduced hepatocyte necrosis and apoptosis and improved blood flow in the liver and attenuated inflammatory cytokine monocyte chemotactic protein-1 in serum after hepatic I/R [21]. In an isolated liver I/R experiment, livers isolated from rodents were submitted to no-flow ischemia for 45 min and reperfusion for 45 min in the presence of 2 mM L-alanyl-glutamine [22]. L-ALANYL-GLUTAMINE inhibited an inflammatory response by attenuating NO and TNF-α production, indicating that glutamine has protective effects in I/R-induced hepatic injury. However, glutamine does not always show benefit. In one study, lean Zucker rats were pretreated with intraperitoneal glutamine (0.75 g/kg) 24 and 6 h prior to warm ischemia and then submitted to 75 min of warm ischemia followed by 24 h of liver reperfusion [23]. Glutamine did not affect serum transaminase, hepatic neutrophil accumulation, hepatocyte necrosis or heat shock protein 70 expression in the liver tissue, indicating that glutamine pretreatment did not protect against hepatic warm I/R injury in rats. Therefore, further studies are needed to determine the effect of glutamine after liver I/R.

The Role of Glutamine Supplementation in Myocardial I/R Injury

Myocardial I/R injury is a major cause of cellular damage in various pathophysiological conditions including myocardial infarction, heart transplantation, and cardiovascular bypass surgery. Ischemic heart disease and consequent heart failure are the major cause of morbidity and mortality worldwide [24]. Myocardial ischemia causes a decrease of cellular oxygen tension and an increase of carbon dioxide tension, as well deprivation of nutrients such as glucose, leading to cell death. The initial treatment for patients with myocardial infarction is restoration of myocardial perfusion. Although advances in thrombolysis and percutaneous coronary interventions result in restoration of coronary flow, reperfusion of coronary flow paradoxically triggers the morphological injury of the tissue, referred to as myocardial I/R injury. Thus, I/R injury remains the leading cause of heart failure. It has been well-established that the inflammatory response after reperfusion is the key cause of myocardial I/R injury. Despite many interventions derived from animal models of myocardial I/R and clinically tested in patients, none have shown definitive advantages due to the absence of specific causal-therapeutic treatments [25]. Therefore, new therapeutic interventions to alleviate myocardial I/R injury and improve the prognosis of patients are highly anticipated.

Thus far, only several studies have attempted to identify the role of glutamine in myocardial I/R. In one study, rats were pretreated with alanine–glutamine dipeptide (0.52 g/kg, intraperitoneal) for 18 h and then hearts were isolated and exposed to global ischemia for 15 min followed by reperfusion for 30 min [26]. Analysis revealed that pretreatment of glutamine preserved cardiac output and maintained myocardial tissue glutamate, ATP content, accumulation of myocardial lactate, and glutathione content. These results indicate that pretreatment with glutamine improves post-I/R cardiac function. In an ex vivo study, hearts isolated from rats were given 2.5 mM of glutamine 30 min before the start of ischemia and then subjected to global ischemia followed by reperfusion for 60 min [27]. The results showed that pretreatment with glutamine significantly improved functional recovery and decreased cardiac troponin I release through increases in levels of protein O-linked *N*-acetylglucosamine and ATP. In an in vitro study mimicking to I/R in vivo, cardiomyocytes were exposed to hypoxia/ischemia for various periods followed by reperfusion in the presence of 10 mM glutamine [28]. Glutamine supplementation protected against cardiomyocyte death and promoted recovery of contractile function after I/R. Glutamine protection against cardiac I/R injury awaits clinical evaluation.

The Role of Glutamine Supplementation in Cerebral I/R Injury

Cerebral stroke is a major contributor of morbidity and mortality worldwide. Like other tissues/organs, restoration of blood flow can lead to exacerbation of injury in the brain including neuronal, endothelial and glial cells. Despite much effort, effective therapies for stroke are still largely lacking. One study showed administration of L-alanyl-glutamine (0.75 g/kg) prior to cerebral I/R decreased nucleus degeneration and cell death [29].

The Role of Glutamine Supplementation in Renal I/R Injury

The effect of glutamine administration during renal I/R has also been investigated, and the summary can be found in the pertinent chapter in this book.

In summary, preclinical animal experiments have clearly demonstrated that glutamine supplementation reduced I/R-induced injury, particularly, in the intestine. Further investigations into its clinical efficacy and better understanding of the mechanism of glutamine supplementation are needed. Table 35.2 summarizes the effect of glutamine supplementation on animal I/R models in different organs.

Table 35.2 The effect of glutamine supplementation on animal I/R models in different organs

Organ	Effect observed	Reference
Intestine	Some studies showed a decrease in intestinal injury, permeability, inflammation, bacterial translocation, plasma endotoxin level, cell membrane lipid peroxidation and animal mortality. However, other studies have showed an increase in survival and leukocyte activity, reactive oxygen intermediate production and vascular permeability	[3–5, 7, 9, 10, 12–16]
Liver	Some studies showed a decrease in alanine aminotransferase and lactate dehydrogenase levels in serum, hepatocyte necrosis and apoptosis, inflammation as well as improved blood flow in the liver. But one study showed no changes in serum transaminase, hepatic neutrophil accumulation and hepatocyte necrosis	[20–23]
Heart	Preserved cardiac output and maintained myocardial tissue glutamate, ATP content, accumulation of myocardial lactate and glutathione content, and improved functional recovery and decreased cardiac troponin I release	[26, 27]
Brain	Decreases of nucleus degeneration and cell death	[29]

Mechanisms of Glutamine in Protection Against I/R-Induced Injury

Glutamine regulates a variety of genes involved in major cellular processes, such as, inflammatory response, proliferation, apoptosis and intermediary metabolism. For example, glutamine protected against intestinal epithelial cell death/apoptosis through induction of activity of the extracellular signal-regulated kinase signaling pathway [30] or reduction of specificity protein 3 expression [31]. However, most studies on glutamine's protection in a variety of stress conditions, such as, hypoxia and reactive oxygen species, have focused on the capacity of glutamine in inhibition of inflammation.

Glutamine exerts anti-inflammatory effects during I/R via a variety of pathways including inhibition (NF-κB, AP-1 and signal transducer and activator of transcription) and activation (PPARγ and heat-shock transcription factor 1) of specific transcription factors. For example, glutamine may regulate PPARγ activity via toll-like receptor (TLR) 4 signaling pathway. PPARγ regulates inflammatory pathways through interference with transcription factors including NF-κB, AP-1, signal transducer and activator of transcription and nuclear factor-activated T cell [32]. PPARγ regulates NF-κB by forming a complex with the NF-κB subunit p65 [33]. TLR4 is considered as one of the major contributors to inflammation after I/R and glutamine can specifically inhibit TLR4 receptor expression [34]. The suppression of TLR4 may be one of the mechanisms of glutamine's protection against I/R injury. The protective effects of glutamine on inflammatory injury can also be through upregulation of heat shock proteins (HSPs) [35].

Although multiple factors are involved in I/R injury and preclinical animal studies revealed that glutamine has protective property in intestinal or microvascular permeability, bacterial translocation, inflammation and pro-inflammatory cytokines production, thus far, the mechanisms of glutamine protection in I/R are not well studied and have mainly focused on its anti-inflammatory properties.

PPARγ

The PPAR family of nuclear receptors is composed of PPARα, PPARβ/δ, and PPARγ. The PPARs form permissive heterodimers with the retinoid X receptor (RXR). The PPAR/RXR heterodimers bind to PPAR-responsive elements (PPREs) in the regulatory region of their target gene to regulate gene expression. Relatively high levels of PPARα are found in brown adipose tissue, intestine, liver, heart and kidney, while abundant PPARβ/δ is expressed in the intestine, muscle, skin, gut, placenta, adipose tissue and brain. Although PPARγ is expressed in different organs and cell types, such as, pancreas, liver, kidney and immune cells including lymphocytes, monocytes, macrophages and dendritic cells, the relative abundance of expression is found in the adipose tissue and gut. Except for the control of lipid and glucose metabolism, PPARs play a crucial role in the regulation of the inflammatory response.

A number of animal studies have demonstrated upregulation of PPARγ after I/R. More importantly, preclinical animal studies have shown the therapeutic effect of PPARγ agonists on improving functional outcome after I/R [36, 37].

In a rodent model of transient cerebral ischemia, PPARγ expression levels were markedly elevated in ischemic neurons and administration of a PPARγ agonist mitigated the effects of cerebral ischemia by demonstrating a reduction of infarction size and improvement of neurologic function [36, 37].

In an intestinal epithelial cell line (IEC-6), there was a dose-dependent effect between glutamine and PPARγ DNA binding and transcriptional activities measured by electrophoretic mobility shift and luciferase reporter gene assays, respectively, but the increases of DNA binding and transcriptional activities did not result from the increase of PPARγ protein. Additionally, glutamine itself was not a ligand of PPARγ, confirmed by ligand binding assay [38]. Further investigation using tandem mass spectroscopy demonstrated that glutamine treatment increased 15-S-hydroxyeicosatetraenoic acid and dehydrogenated 13-hydroxyoctaolecadienoic acid, two identified endogenous PPARγ ligands. However, in human epithelial colorectal adenocarcinoma cells (caco-2), treatment of glutamine did not increase but rather decreased PPARγ protein expression and DNA binding activity [39]. This discrepancy may due to the different genetic backgrounds of cells since IEC-6 cells were derived from normal intestinal epithelium and caco-2 cells from a human epithelial colorectal adenocarcinoma.

In a rodent model of intestinal I/R injury, luminal glutamine enhanced PPARγ DNA binding activity [10]. We have recently shown in an intestinal specific conditional PPARγ null mouse that glutamine loses its protective effect (unpublished data).

NF-κB

NF-κB is expressed in almost all cell types and plays a central role in directing the immune response through regulation of the transcription of inflammatory factors such as cytokines, chemokines, and adhesion molecules. The critical role of NF-κB in I/R injury has been well-documented [40–44]. A recent study demonstrated that glutamine significantly reduced NF-κB in the kidney in a rat renal I/R model [45]. When glutamine was administered intraperitoneally prior to reperfusion, the NF-κB p65 subunit was increased in the nuclear fractions isolated from the kidney after 6 h of reperfusion [45].

AP-1

AP-1 dimeric transcription factor is a family of jun and fos proteins that form jun–jun and jun–fos homo- and heterodimers. The major AP-1 proteins include Jun (c-Jun, JunB, JunD) and Fos (c-Fos, FosB) as well as Fra-1 and Fra-2. The various combinations of AP-1 proteins allow AP-1 to regulate most inflammatory mediators because AP-1 contains transcriptional regulator binding sites provided by broad combinatorial possibilities. We have previously found that enteral glutamine supplementation inhibited AP-1 activity determined by electrophoretic mobility shift assay in a rat intestinal I/R model and that supershift analysis confirmed the increased activity of AP-1 was associated with increased levels of c-Jun expression [11].

iNOS

The pro-inflammatory mediator, iNOS, is a nitric oxide synthase which is expressed in various cells and tissues. However, iNOS has low basal expression until activated by an immune response, such as cytokines or oxidative stress. Production of nitric oxide by iNOS is detrimental during I/R and protective effects of iNOS inhibition in renal dysfunction and injury after renal I/R have been reported [46]. Nitric oxide itself can form peroxynitrite with the superoxide radical and then damages the tissue. Glutamine significantly reduced iNOS level in the kidney in a rat renal I/R model [45] and a rat intestinal I/R model [10].

HO-1

Heme oxygenase (HO), the rate-limiting enzyme in heme catabolism, includes three distinct isoforms HO-1, HO-2 and HO-3. Glutamine can enhance HO-1 expression. In rat hepatic I/R, pretreatment with glutamine increased HO-1 expression in the liver [21]. Oxidant stress and inflammation are major factors which contributed to organ injury during I/R. HO-1 is induced by stress including oxidative stress, hypoxia, and cytokines. HO-1 is anti-inflammatory and anti-apoptotic [47]. HO-1 protects against oxidative stress. Protection of HO-1 has been demonstrated in various stress conditions including I/R, hemorrhagic shock, hypoxia, and reactive oxygen species [48]. HO-1 ameliorates hepatic I/R injury [49].

Syndecan-1

Syndecans are a major family of cell surface heparan sulfate proteoglycans, including syndecan-1 to 4. Syndecan-1 is mainly expressed in epithelial cells and plasma cells. Syndecan-1 is not only an integral membrane protein but also involved in many biological activities, such as cell proliferation, apoptosis and migration. Syndecan-1 also shows the capacity to modulate inflammation. The anti-inflammatory properties of syndecan-1 have been documented in inflammatory diseases, cancer, and infection [50]. Although the expression of syndecan-1 in the intestinal tissue during I/R has not been investigated, in an in vitro I/R model, glutamine preserved syndecan-1 expression on the intestinal cell surface and mitigated syndecan-1 shedding [8]. More importantly, in vivo, glutamine reduced intestinal hyperpermeability, inflammation, and injury after intestinal I/R, effects lost in syndecan-1 null mice [8]. Table 35.3 summarizes the regulated genes by glutamine in animal I/R models.

The precise molecular mechanism by which glutamine regulates these genes after I/R injury is still not well understood. However, it is well-documented that PPARγ can negatively regulate NF-κB through either a co-activator competition model that NF-κB and PPARγ use same co-activators, or a direct interaction model that one or both NF-κB and PPARγ is inhibited because of direct interactions between these two nuclear receptors and negatively regulated transcription factors, or a co-repressor-dependent model that NF-κB is transrepressed by PPARγ ligands via inhibition of the signal-dependent clearance of co-repressor complexes [51]. PPARγ can also suppress AP-1 in a ligand-dependent manner [51]. Moreover, PPARγ can dampen the macrophage inflammatory response through inhibition of pro-inflammatory molecules, such as TNF-α, IL-6, and iNOS [52]. PPARγ ligands inhibited the expression of iNOS in part by antagonizing activities of the transcription factors activation protein 1, signal transducer and activator of transcription, and NF-κB [53]. Previous studies also found that NF-κB [54] and AP-1 [55] promoted iNOS activity, while iNOS was inhibited by HO-1 [56]. The mechanism of suppression of inflammation by glutamine is summarized in Fig. 35.3.

Table 35.3 Influence of glutamine supplementation on gene expression/activity in experimental animal I/R models

Organ	Gene regulated	Reference
Liver	Increased HO-1 expression	[21]
Kidney	Reduced iNOS and NF-κB expression	[45]
Intestine	Enhanced PPARγ DNA binding activity	[10]
Intestine	Reduced AP-1 expression	[11]

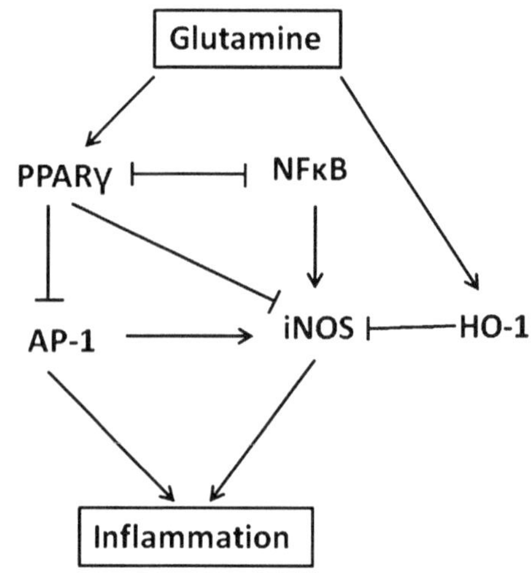

Fig. 35.3 Proposed mechanism of suppression of inflammation by glutamine under I/R-induced stress. Under stress induced by I/R, glutamine activates the activity of PPARγ. Subsequently, PPARγ inhibits the activity of NF-κB and AP-1 and the expression of iNOS. iNOS is also suppressed by HO-1 but is enhanced by AP-1. AP-1 and iNOS then mediate the inflammation

Conclusions

Cumulative evidence has demonstrated the protective effect of glutamine administration in tissue I/R injury of different organs including the intestine, liver, heart, kidney, and brain in preclinical animal models. Although in most studies, the beneficial effects of glutamine were observed with pretreatment with glutamine prior to I/R, promising results were also found when glutamine was administered at the onset of reperfusion, suggesting that glutamine administration can be used not only as a preventive measure but also a therapeutic measure. Glutamine's protective effect is mediated by a variety of physiological aspects including suppression of hyperinflammation, protection against cell apoptosis, and enhancement of cell proliferation. Particularly, in intestinal I/R, glutamine administration preserved gut function including maintenance of absorption, protection against mucosal injury, abrogation of inflammation, enhancement of mucosal blood flow and maintenance of gut barrier function [57]. Studies in preclinical animal models have shown that PPARγ, NF-κB, AP-1, iNOS, and HO-1 mediates the protective effect of glutamine on I/R injury. To achieve maximum beneficial effect of glutamine, the delivery route, dose, and timing need to be optimized. More importantly, further investigation into the precise molecular mechanism underlying glutamine's protective role in I/R injury is warranted.

References

1. Estívariz CF, Griffith DP, Luo M, et al. Efficacy of parenteral nutrition supplemented with glutamine dipeptide to decrease hospital infections in critically ill surgical patients. J Parenter Enteral Nutr. 2008;32:389–402.
2. Kim M, Wischmeyer PE. Glutamine. World Rev Nutr Diet. 2013;105:90–6.
3. Demirkan A, Savaş B, Melli M. Endotoxin level in ischemia-reperfusion injury in rats: effect of glutamine pretreatment on endotoxin levels and gut morphology. Nutrition. 2010;26:106–1011.
4. Demirkan A, Orazakunov E, Savaş B, et al. Enteral glutamine pretreatment does not decrease plasma endotoxin level induced by ischemia-reperfusion injury in rats. World J Gastroenterol. 2008;14:463–8.
5. Medeiros AC, Chacon DA, Sales VS, et al. Glucan and glutamine reduce bacterial translocation in rats subjected to intestinal ischemia-reperfusion. J Invest Surg. 2006;19:39–46.
6. Berg RD, Garlington AW. Translocation of certain indigenous bacteria from the gastrointestinal tract to the mesenteric lymph nodes and other organs in a gnotobiotic mouse model. Infect Immun. 1979;23:403–4011.

7. Kozar RA, Schultz SG, Hassoun HT, et al. The type of sodium-coupled solute modulates small bowel mucosal injury, transport function, and ATP after ischemia/reperfusion injury in rats. Gastroenterology. 2002;123:810–6.
8. Peng Z, Ban K, Sen A, et al. Syndecan 1 plays a novel role in enteral glutamine's gut-protective effects of the post-ischemic gut. Shock. 2012;38:57–62.
9. Kozar RA, Schultz SG, Bick RJ, et al. Enteral glutamine but not alanine maintains small bowel barrier function after ischemia/reperfusion injury in rats. Shock. 2004;21:433–7.
10. Sato N, Moore FA, Kone BC, et al. Differential induction of PPAR-gamma by luminal glutamine and iNOS by luminal arginine in the rodent postischemic small bowel. Am J Physiol Gastrointest Liver Physiol. 2006;290(4):G616–23.
11. Sato N, Moore FA, Smith MA, et al. Immune-enhancing enteral nutrients differentially modulate the early proinflammatory transcription factors mediating gut ischemia/reperfusion. J Trauma. 2005;58:455–4561.
12. Wu GH, Wang H, Zhang YW, et al. Glutamine supplemented parenteral nutrition prevents intestinal ischemia-reperfusion injury in rats. World J Gastroenterol. 2004;10:2592–4.
13. Harward TR, Coe D, Souba WW, et al. Glutamine preserves gut glutathione levels during intestinal ischemia/reperfusion. J Surg Res. 1994;56:351–5.
14. Ikeda S, Zarzaur BL, Johnson CD, et al. Total parenteral nutrition supplementation with glutamine improves survival after gut ischemia/reperfusion. J Parenter Enteral Nutr. 2002;26:169–73.
15. Omata J, Fukatsu K, Ueno C, et al. Intraluminal glutamine administration during ischemia worsens survival after gut ischemia-reperfusion. J Surg Res. 2007;143:260–4.
16. Fukatsu K, Ueno C, Hashiguchi Y, et al. Glutamine infusion during ischemia is detrimental in a murine gut ischemia/reperfusion model. J Parenter Enteral Nutr. 2003;27:187–92.
17. Mendes-Braz M, Elias-Miró M, Jiménez-Castro MB, et al. The current state of knowledge of hepatic ischemia-reperfusion injury based on its study in experimental models. J Biomed Biotechnol. 2012;2012:298657.
18. Montalvo-Jave EE, Escalante-Tattersfield T, Ortega-Salgado JA, et al. Factors in the pathophysiology of the liver ischemia-reperfusion injury. J Surg Res. 2008;147:153–9.
19. Clavien PA, Selzner M, Rüdiger HA, et al. A prospective randomized study in 100 consecutive patients undergoing major liver resection with versus without ischemic preconditioning. Ann Surg. 2003;238:843–50.
20. Araújo Júnior RJ, Silva Júnior RG, et al. Preconditioning with L-alanyl-glutamine reduces hepatic ischemia-reperfusion injury in rats. Acta Cir Bras. 2011;26 Suppl 1:8–13.
21. Zhang SC, Shi Q, Feng YN, et al. Tissue-protective effect of glutamine on hepatic ischemia-reperfusion injury via induction of heme oxygenase-1. Pharmacology. 2013;91:59–68.
22. Schuster H, Blanc MC, Bonnefont-Rousselot D, et al. Protective effects of glutamine dipeptide and alpha-tocopherol against ischemia-reperfusion injury in the isolated rat liver. Clin Nutr. 2009;28:331–7.
23. Noh J, Behrends M, Choi S, et al. Glutamine does not protect against hepatic warm ischemia/reperfusion injury in rats. J Gastrointest Surg. 2006;10:234–9.
24. Rosamond W, Flegal K, Furie K, et al. Heart disease and stroke statistics-2008 update: a report from the American Heart Association Statistics Committee and Stroke Statistics Subcommittee. Circulation. 2008;117:e25–146.
25. Hausenloy DJ, Yellon DM. Myocardial ischemia-reperfusion injury: a neglected therapeutic target. J Clin Invest. 2013;123:92–100.
26. Wischmeyer PE, Jayakar D, Williams U, et al. Single dose of glutamine enhances myocardial tissue metabolism, glutathione content, and improves myocardial function after ischemia-reperfusion injury. J Parenter Enteral Nutr. 2003;27:396–403.
27. Liu J, Marchase RB, Chatham JC. Glutamine-induced protection of isolated rat heart from ischemia/reperfusion injury is mediated via the hexosamine biosynthesis pathway and increased protein O-GlcNAc levels. J Mol Cell Cardiol. 2007;42:177–85.
28. Wischmeyer PE, Vanden Hoek TL, Li C, et al. Glutamine preserves cardiomyocyte viability and enhances recovery of contractile function after ischemia-reperfusion injury. J Parenter Enteral Nutr. 2003;27:116–22.
29. Pires VL, Souza JR, Guimarães SB, et al. Preconditioning with L-alanyl-L-glutamine in a Mongolian gerbil model of acute cerebral ischemia/reperfusion injury. Acta Cir Bras. 2011;26 Suppl 1:14–20.
30. Larson SD, Li J, Chung DH, et al. Molecular mechanisms contributing to glutamine-mediated intestinal cell survival. Am J Physiol Gastrointest Liver Physiol. 2007;293:G1262–71.
31. Ban K, Kozar RA. Glutamine protects against apoptosis via downregulation of Sp3 in intestinal epithelial cells. Am J Physiol Gastrointest Liver Physiol. 2010;299:G1344–53.
32. Santora R, Kozar RA. Molecular mechanisms of pharmaconutrients. J Surg Res. 2010;161:288–94.
33. Kelly D, Campbell JI, King TP, et al. Commensal anaerobic gut bacteria attenuate inflammation by regulating nuclear-cytoplasmic shuttling of PPAR-gamma and RelA. Nat Immunol. 2004;5:104–12.
34. Mbodji K, Torre S, Haas V, et al. Alanyl-glutamine restores maternal deprivation-induced TLR4 levels in a rat neonatal model. Clin Nutr. 2011;30:672–7.
35. Wischmeyer PE, Kahana M, Wolfson R, et al. Glutamine induces heat shock protein and protects against endotoxin shock in the rat. J Appl Physiol. 2001;90:2403–10.

36. Zhao Y, Patzer A, Gohlke P, et al. The intracerebral application of the PPARgamma-ligand pioglitazone confers neuroprotection against focal ischaemia in the rat brain. Eur J Neurosci. 2005;22:278–82.
37. Sundararajan S, Gamboa JL, Victor NA, et al. Peroxisome proliferator-activated receptor-gamma ligands reduce inflammation and infarction size in transient focal ischemia. Neuroscience. 2005;130:685–96.
38. Ban K, Sprunt JM, Martin S, et al. Glutamine activates peroxisome proliferator-activated receptor-γ in intestinal epithelial cells via 15-S-HETE and 13-OXO-ODE: a novel mechanism. Am J Physiol Gastrointest Liver Physiol. 2011;301:G547–54.
39. Fiatte C, Huin C, Collet P, et al. Expression of PPARgamma is reduced by medium supplementation with L-glutamine in human colorectal Caco-2 cells. Int J Mol Med. 2008;22:825–32.
40. Hassoun HT, Zou L, Moore FA, et al. Alpha-melanocyte-stimulating hormone protects against mesenteric ischemia-reperfusion injury. Am J Physiol Gastrointest Liver Physiol. 2002;282:G1059–68.
41. Hassoun HT, Kozar RA, Kone BC, et al. Aischemic hypothermia differentially modulates oxidative stress proteins during mesenteric ischemia/reperfusion. Surgery. 2002;132:369–76.
42. Yeh KY, Yeh M, Glass J, et al. Rapid activation of NF-kappaB and AP-1 and target gene expression in postischemic rat intestine. Gastroenterology. 2000;118:525–34.
43. Zou L, Attuwaybi B, Kone BC. Effects of NF-kappa B inhibition on mesenteric ischemia-reperfusion injury. Am J Physiol Gastrointest Liver Physiol. 2003;284:G713–21.
44. Esposito E, Mondello S, Di Paola R, et al. Glutamine contributes to ameliorate inflammation after renal ischemia/reperfusion injury in rats. Naunyn Schmiedebergs Arch Pharmacol. 2011;383:493–508.
45. Rao J, Qian X, Wang P, et al. All-trans retinoic acid preconditioning protects against liver ischemia/reperfusion injury by inhibiting the nuclear factor kappa B signaling pathway. J Surg Res. 2013;180:e99–106.
46. Chatterjee PK, Patel NS, Kvale EO, et al. Inhibition of inducible nitric oxide synthase reduces renal ischemia/reperfusion injury. Kidney Int. 2002;61:862–71.
47. Otterbein LE, Soares MP, Yamashita K, et al. Heme oxygenase-1: unleashing the protective properties of heme. Trends Immunol. 2003;24:449–55.
48. Zhu X, Fan WG, Li DP, et al. Heme oxygenase-1 system and gastrointestinal inflammation: a short review. World J Gastroenterol. 2011;17:4283–8.
49. Tsuchihashi S, Zhai Y, Bo Q, et al. Heme oxygenase-1 mediated cytoprotection against liver ischemia and reperfusion injury: inhibition of type-1 interferon signaling. Transplantation. 2007;83:1628–34.
50. Teng YH, Aquino RS, Park PW. Molecular functions of syndecan-1 in disease. Matrix Biol. 2012;31:3–16.
51. Ricote M, Glass CK. PPARs and molecular mechanisms of transrepression. Biochim Biophys Acta. 2007;1771:926–35.
52. Welch JS, Ricote M, Akiyama TE, et al. PPARgamma and PPARdelta negatively regulate specific subsets of lipopolysaccharide and IFN-gamma target genes in macrophages. Proc Natl Acad Sci U S A. 2003;100:6712–9717.
53. Ricote M, Li AC, Willson TM, et al. The peroxisome proliferator-activated receptor-gamma is a negative regulator of macrophage activation. Nature. 1998;391:79–82.
54. Pautz A, Art J, Hahn S, et al. Regulation of the expression of inducible nitric oxide synthase. Nitric Oxide. 2010;23:75–93.
55. Cho MK, Suh SH, Kim SG. JunB/AP-1 and NF-kappa B-mediated induction of nitric oxide synthase by bovine type I collagen in serum-stimulated murine macrophages. Nitric Oxide. 2002;6:319–32.
56. Wang WP, Guo X, Koo MW, et al. Protective role of heme oxygenase-1 on trinitrobenzene sulfonic acid-induced colitis in rats. Am J Physiol Gastrointest Liver Physiol. 2001;281:G586–94.
57. Ban K, Kozar RA. Enteral glutamine: a novel mediator of PPARgamma in the postischemic gut. J Leukoc Biol. 2008;84:595–9.

Chapter 36
Glutamine and Cancer Immunosuppression

Ines Hammami and Mario Jolicoeur

Key Points

- Immunosuppression phenomenon is reported in different diseases.
- Glutamine inhibits T-cell priming either by preventing tumor-associated antigens' processing and presentation through major histocompatibility complexes or by down-regulating the expression of co-stimulatory and adhesion molecules.
- High uptake of glutamine by tumor and immunosuppressive cells interferes with glutamine-dependent T-cell immunomodulatory functions.
- Glutamine up-regulated the synthesis of tumor-derived factors which in turn may regulate glutamine metabolism.
- Glutamine metabolism ensures favorable condition for tumor progression.
- Glutamine regulates arginine metabolism by providing cofactors, regulating gene expression and enzyme activities.
- Arginine can be endogenously synthesized from glutamine.
- Glutamine regulates gene levels of key transcription factors implicated in immunosuppression phenomenon.
- Control of glutamine availability and metabolism represents a promising therapeutic strategy to help recovering anti-cancer immune response.

Keywords Glutamine • Cancer • Immunosuppression • Immunesurveillance • Anti-cancer immune response • Myeloid-derived suppressor cells

Abbreviations

APC	Antigen-presenting cells
Arg	Arginine
ARG	Arginase
ASS	Argininosuccinate synthetase

I. Hammami, B.Eng., M.Sc.A., Ph.D. (✉) • M. Jolicoeur, B.Eng., M.Sc.A., Ph.D.
Department of Chemical Engineering, Ecole Polytechnique de Montréal,
2500 Chemin de Polytechnique, Montreal, QC, Canada H3T-1J4
e-mail: ines.hammami@polymtl.ca; mario.jolicoeur@polymtl.ca

R. Rajendram et al. (eds.), *Glutamine in Clinical Nutrition*, Nutrition and Health,
DOI 10.1007/978-1-4939-1932-1_36, © Springer Science+Business Media New York 2015

BM	Bone marrow
CTL	Cytotoxic T lymphocyte
DC	Dendritic cell
G/M-CSF	Granulocyte/macrophage-colony stimulating factor
Gln	Glutamine
HIF	Hypoxia induction factor
IL	Interleukin
ICAM	Intracellular adhesion molecules
IFN	Interferon
iNOS	Inducible nitric oxide synthase
LFA	Lymphocyte function associated antigen
LPS	Lipopolysaccharides
MDSC	Myeloid-derived suppressor cell
MHC	Major histocompatibility complex
mRNA	Messenger ribonucleic acid
MSC-1	Myeloid suppressor cells-1
NF-κB	Nuclear factor κ light chain enhancer of activated B cells
TAA	Tumor-associated antigen
TCA	Tricarboxylic acid
TGF	Tumor growth factor
TNF	Tumor necrosis factor
Treg	T regulatory cell

Introduction

The immunesurveillance process remains one of the most controversial and poorly understood areas of immunity. Cancer and organ transplantation are two clinical situations where the suppression of the immune response has been and is still widely investigated. While the anti-tumor-specific immune function must be enhanced to prevent tumor progression, the situation is the complete opposite in organ transplantation, where the immune response against the grafted organ should be suppressed to ensure transplantation success. Immune suppression has also been reported in several other diseases, the most popular being the human immunodeficiency virus [1], but also in rheumatic diseases [2], neurodegenerative diseases (including Parkinson's disease, Alzheimer's disease, amyotrophic lateral sclerosis, multiple sclerosis, and human immunodeficiency virus-associated neurodegeneration) [3], etc. In the present review, a special focus will be placed on cancer-related immunosuppression.

In fact, a healthy immune system is able to recognize, destroy and prevent the outgrowth of tumors. Briefly, the earliest step for the induction of anti-tumoral immune response, summarized in Fig. 36.1, is the recognition of tumor-associated antigen (TAA) by professional antigen-presenting cells (APCs). TAAs will then be processed and presented on the surface of fully activated and mature APCs through the major histocompatibility complexes (MHCs). Thereafter, $CD4^+$ and $CD8^+$ T-lymphocytes recognize the presented TAAs and differentiate into cytotoxic T lymphocytes (CTLs) that are able to destroy tumor cells [4].

However, the specific anti-tumor immune response is hardly observed in cancer-bearing hosts especially in later stages of cancer. As for immunomodulation, the nutritional status of cancer patients has a profound effect on the tumor escape process. Specifically, glutamine (Gln) has been shown to be crucial for both the immunity and tumor progression (Refer to the Chaps. 4 and 8). These findings have fuelled investigations on the role of Gln in cancer-mediated suppression of immune functions and the aim of this review is to describe and discuss the potential of Gln in the maintenance/eradication of tumor escape phenomenon (Fig. 36.1).

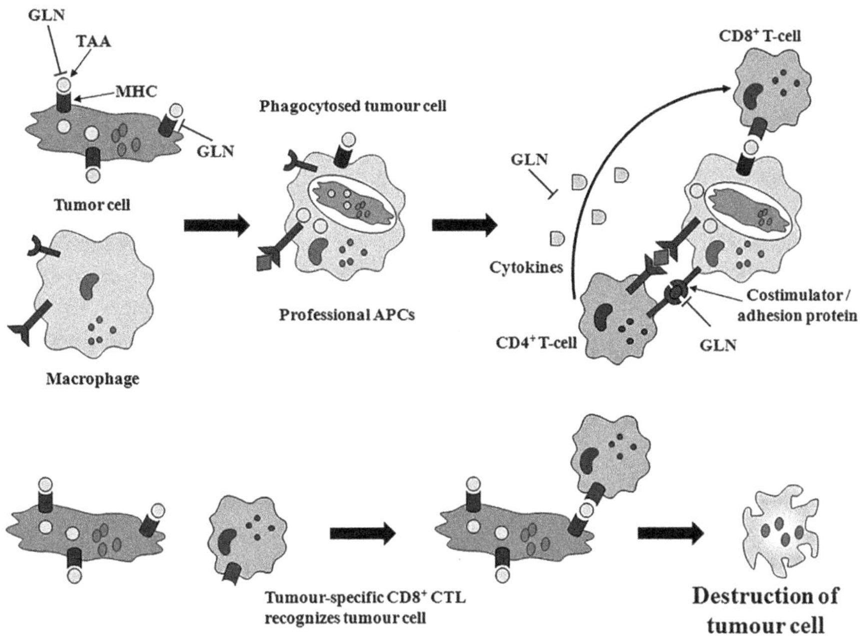

Fig. 36.1 Induction of anti-tumor CTL responses and direct effects of Gln on this process. APCs recognize tumor cells through TAAs they carry on their surfaces. Professional APCs that present TAAs through their MHCs recruit $CD4^+$ helper and $CD8^+$ cytotoxic T cells. Differentiated CTLs are then able to destroy tumor cells without any additional requirements (co-stimulation, $CD4^+$ helper T cells) [4]

Mechanisms of Immunosuppression in Cancer

The concept of tumor immunesurveillance has been first described in 1863 by Rudolph Virchow who observed leukocyte infiltration in tumors [5]. By the time, evidences of the immunological resistance against tumor growth have been accumulated [6]. However, complete tumor regression by the immune system has been rarely reported. In fact, tumors develop several mechanisms to escape the immune-surveillance process.

The first immunosuppressive strategy is related to the primary step of mounting a tumor-specific immune function which is the recognition of TAAs. Tumor cells may not express enough TAAs or simply modify TAAs' peptidic sequence. They can also down-regulate the expression of MHCs, thus preventing the presentation of TAAs, their recognition by effector T cells and further differentiation of APCs [7, 8]. In fact, T-cell priming has, for a long time, been investigated for the development of tumor immune vaccines, since mounting an effective anti-tumor immune response depends on the spatio-temporal release of TAAs and the quality of tumor-associated T-cell priming [6].

The second mechanism of tumor escape relies on the absence of essential co-stimulatory factors (such as the cytotoxic T lymphocyte antigen CTLA-4, the cluster of differentiation CD28) and adhesion molecules (e.g. intracellular adhesion molecules ICAM-1, lymphocyte function-associated antigen-3 LFA-3, mucin-cell-surface-associated 1 MUC-1) [9]. In fact, the binding of CD28, normally presented on T-cell surface, to its ligands B7-1/2, expressed on tumor cell surface, is crucial for the complete activation of T cells [10]. The first two strategies act on the cross-talking between tumor cells and immune effector cells to prevent possible induction of any anti-tumor immune resistance.

Third, tumor cells produce immunosuppressive molecules, called tumor-derived factors (TDFs), such as granulocyte/macrophage-colony stimulating factors (G/M-CSFs), interleukins (ILs), tumor growth factors (TGFs), etc [11]. Namely, TGF-β is a potent inhibitor of T-cell cycle progress. G/M--CSFs and ILs regulate the activities of specific enzymes (as it will be discussed below) and contribute to the maturation and recruitment of immunosuppressive cells [12], which represents the last immunosuppressive strategy.

In fact, tumors recruit T regulatory cells (Tregs), tolerogenic dendritic cells (DCs) and myeloid-derived suppressor cells (MDSCs) in the spleen, blood, lymphoid organ and tumoral microenvironment to control the anti-tumor-specific immune response.

On the one hand, DCs are considered as the most efficient APCs due to their high concentrations in MHCs and co-stimulatory factors as well as their migratory capacity. However, in cancer-bearing hosts, DCs remain immature, so called tolerogenic, allowing immune tolerance [13]. On the other hand, several mechanisms have been proposed to explain Tregs immunosuppressive potential, among these are the secretion of inhibitory cytokines (such as IL-10, IL-35, TGF-β), the down-regulation of co-stimulatory factors' expression, and the induction of APCs death via the perforine/granzyme pathway [14]. Ultimately, MDSCs suppress CTLs' immunomodulatory functions via the L-arginine (L-ARG) metabolism. In fact, MDSCs express two enzymes that metabolize L-Arg: (1) the inducible nitric oxide synthase (iNOS) that, in presence of oxygen and nicotinamide adenine dinucleotide phosphate (NADPH), oxidizes L-Arg to produce nitric oxide (NO) and L-citrulline, and (2) arginase 1 (ARG1) which converts L-Arg into urea and L-ornithine (Fig. 36.2) [11].

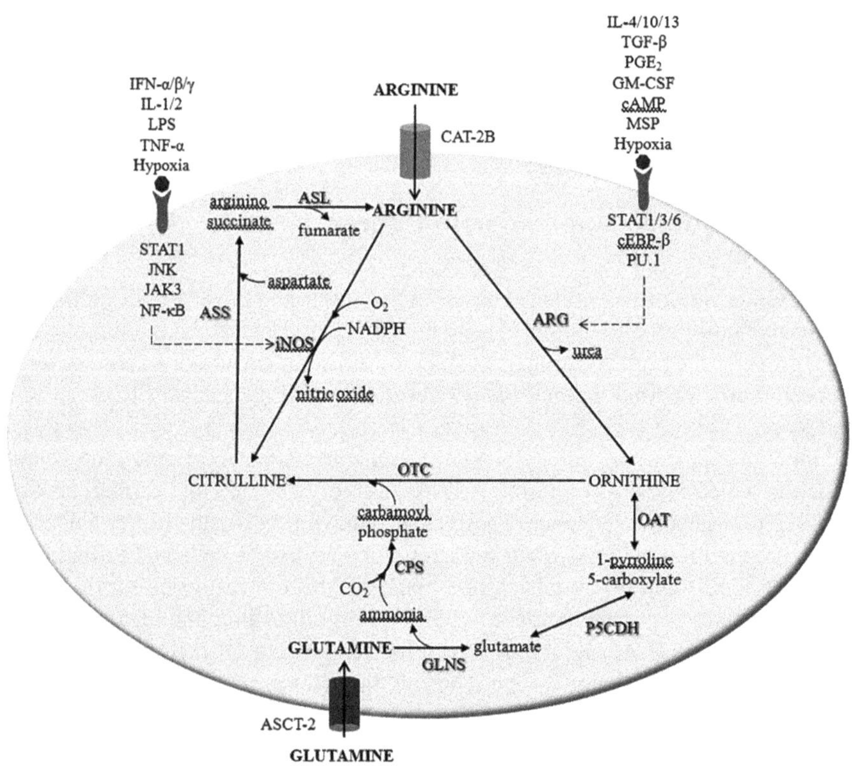

Fig. 36.2 Arg catabolism and Gln-to-Arg pathway in MDSCs [15]. Different stimuli activates iNOS and ARG1 activities (*dashed lines*). iNOS and ARG1 metabolize L-arg which revealed to be endogenously synthesized from L-citrulline and L-glutamine. *OAT* ornithine aminotransferase, *P5CDH* 1-pyrroline-5-carboxylate dehydrogenase, *GLNS* glutaminase, *CPS* carbamoyl phosphate synthetase, *OTC* ornithine transcarbamylase, *JAK* Janus kinase, *JNK* c-Jun N-terminal kinase, *PU.1* Purine rich 1 Box,, *MSP* macrophage stimulating protein, *cAMP* cyclic adenosine monophosphate, *PGE* prostaglandin E, *CAT-2B* cationic amino acid transporter, *ASCT-2* sodium-dependent neutral amino acid transporter

The sparse availability of L-Arg in the blood triggers the loss of the CD3ξ chain of the T-cell receptor and further blocks T-cell proliferation and finally induces their death [16]. Likewise, the metabolism of L-tryptophan and L-phenylalanine by MDSCs results in the arrest of T-cell proliferation [17, 18]. Nitric oxide also reacts with biomolecules both in the generating and target cells to produce reactive nitrogen oxide species. These latter are strong immunosuppressive factors and act at several levels including DNA, proteins, lipids, signaling pathways, cell respiration, etc. to alter T-cell proliferation and induce their death [19]. In addition to L-Arg intake through diet and protein turnover, L-ARG is endogenously produced in MDSCs through enzymatic activities of argininosuccinate synthetase (ASS) and lyase which convert L-citrulline into L-Arg [15]. Moreover, L-citrulline can be synthesized from glutamine, glutamate and proline ensuring MDSCs' autosufficiency in L-Arg [20].

In the following sections, we state and discuss the implication of Gln in each immunosuppressive strategy apart.

Effects of Gln on the Expression of MHC and Adhesion/Co-stimulatory Molecules

The initiation of T-cell responses requires the recruitment of multiple ligands on their specific receptors at the cell surface (Fig. 36.3). Indeed, ICAM-1 triggers the adhesion of APCs to the corresponding receptor LFA-1 expressed by T cells [4]. However, Gln was shown to down-regulate the expression of several components of the immunoglobulin superfamily of cell adhesion molecules. For instance, low Gln reduced the expression of ICAM-1 in arsenic-treated neutrophils, leading to the blockage of neutrophils activation [21]. Likewise, the constitutive expression of ICAM-1 in monocytes was shown to be down-regulated at low Gln concentrations [22]. Supplementation of Gln also lowers LFA-1 and macrophage-associated antigen-1 expression in arsenic-exposed mice [23]. Therefore, Gln has the potential to act at both levels, i.e. APCs and CD4$^+$ T cells, to inhibit their cross-talking and prevent CTLs differentiation.

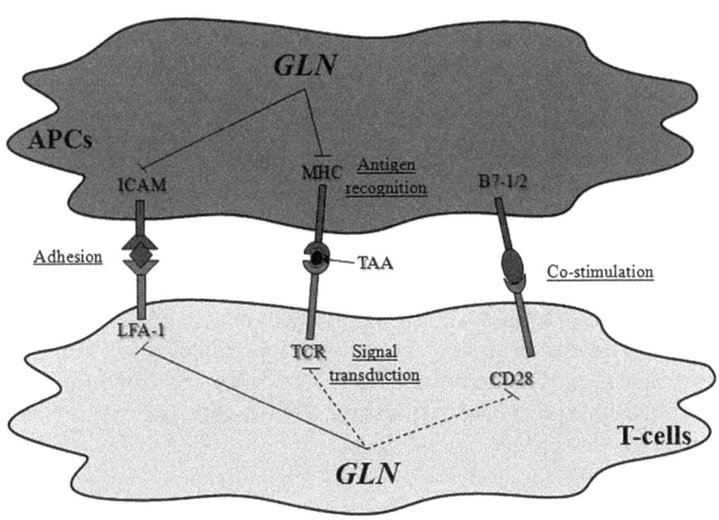

Fig. 36.3 Priming of T-cell response. The initiation of anti-tumor T-cell response requires the recognition of TAA by TCR whose activation launches signaling cascades. This process further requires the presence of adhesion and co-stimulatory molecules to stabilize T cells binding into APCs. The direct and indirect inhibitory effects of Gln on this process are presented in *bold* and *dashed lines* respectively

No direct effect of Gln on the production of co-stimulatory molecules has been reported at the best of our knowledge. However, it has been shown that the expression of glutamine transporter and its activity in lymphocytes is dependent on CD28, a co-stimulatory molecule [24]. Therefore, the tumor-mediated down-regulation of CD28 expression triggers the dysfunction of Gln-dependent physiological functions in T cells, the most important ones being their proliferation and IL-2 receptor signaling pathway (Fig. 36.3).

Likewise, the role of Gln in TAAs expression has not been specifically addressed yet. However, Gln was shown to regulate MHC expression. In fact, Gln supplementation increases the expression level of human leukocyte antigen, a MHC class II, in monocytes of postoperative and trauma patients [25, 26]. So far, evidences of relationships between Gln and immune cell priming were reported in different models of immune effector cells but not in the context of immunosuppression. Nevertheless, it appears to be of extreme importance to investigate whether Gln is implicated in the prevention of anti-tumor-specific immune response initiation. In fact, the complex set of interactions occurring at the tumor edge may have attracted research efforts on the most potent immunosuppressive mechanism which is downstream T-cell priming step.

Metabolism of L-Gln at the Tumor Edge

In addition to preventing APCs differentiation and CTLs activation, the consumption of L-Gln, per se, by tumor cells represents a mechanism of immune tolerance. A similar effect has also been reported in endurance athletes where a decrease of L-Gln concentration is accompanied by transient immunodepression [27]. Namely, the high uptake rate of L-Gln by tumor cells [28] and tumor-infiltrating MDSCs [29] dampens L-Gln availability at the tumor edge and so inhibits the proliferation of immune cells. The in vitro simulation of MDSC maturation showed an increase of L-Gln consumption rate in GM-CSF and IL-6-treated bone marrow (BM) cells [29]. Similarly, L-Gln uptake rate was 5 times higher in lipopolysaccharides (LPS)-treated murine macrophages and human monocytes, which become immunosuppressive via L-Arg metabolism [30]. Furthermore, extensive study of L-Gln metabolism by MDSCs showed that L-Gln significantly contributes to the acidification of the tumor microenvironment [31]. This condition promotes tumor neovascularization, angiogenesis and metastasis [31] and leads to the enforcement of tumor stroma and indirectly to the decrease of L-Gln concentration in the tumor. The in vitro simulation of MDSC maturation process and the inhibition of L-arg metabolizing enzymes (both studies conducted in our laboratory) highlighted the immunosuppression-related metabolic events that are summarized in Fig. 36.4 [29].

L-Gln was also shown to be crucial to the replenishment of tricarboxylic acid (TCA) cycle intermediates in BM-derived MDSCs and MSC-1 cells, an immortalized cell line derived from mouse MDSCs [29, 31]. The high activity of TCA cycle revealed to generate high amounts of NADPH and lactate, and this through the $NADP^+$-dependent malic enzyme that converts malate into pyruvate [29, 31]. In fact, glutaminase and $NADP^+$-dependent malic enzyme activities, as well as glutamine oxidation and lactate secretion, have been shown to be concomitantly up-regulated in LPS/adrenaline/interferon (IFN)-γ-treated macrophages [32]. A similar behavior has been reported in neutrophils, where the high glutamine-derived lactate production rate was related to higher demands in NADPH as compared to lymphocytes or macrophages [33].

The effects of the various tumor-derived factors on glutamine transporter or glutaminolysis enzymes, at the mRNA level, protein expression or enzyme activity in immunosuppressive cells or similar systems (e.g. cytokine-treated macrophages) are not well characterized although the regulation of glutamine uptake and metabolism by cytokines has been reported in other cell types and human or animal models. For instance, IFN-α was shown to up-regulate glutaminase mRNA and protein level in human immunodeficiency virus-associated dementia individuals [34]. A similar effect was reported in TGF-β-treated gluconeogenic porcine kidney cells [35].

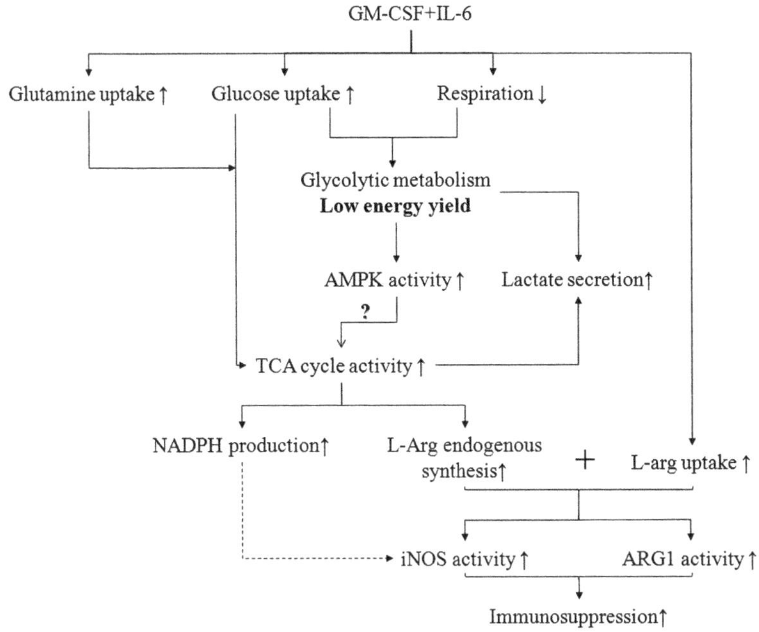

Fig. 36.4 Metabolic events occurring during BM cells maturation into MDSCs. The exposure of BM cells to GM-CSF and IL-6 activates iNOS and ARG1 activities rendering cells immunosuppressive. This was accompanied by an increase in glucose and L-Gln uptake rates. However, cells revealed to exhibit glycolytic metabolism since cells respiration decreases during the maturation process. The AMP-activated protein kinase was activated in response to the energy deficit leading to the increase of TCA cycle activity. Both anaerobic glycolysis and TCA cycle allowed the secretion of high amounts of lactate. Moreover, high TCA cycle activity ensured endogenous synthesis of L-arg and the production of NADPH, one of iNOS cofactor. The chronology of these events is hypothetic due to the lack of understanding of the AMPK regulatory mechanism

However, implication of Gln in the immunosuppressive activity of tolerogenic DCs neither Tregs has been investigated. In fact, in the cancer context, MDSCs are considered as the most potent cells of the tumor immunosuppressive network. They trigger the recruitment of Tregs in the tumor microenvironment and substitute tolerogenic DCs, if suppressed, to ensure tumor escape [36], and so most of the research focusing on Gln in cancer-related immunosuppression have been performed on MDSCs.

Cross-regulation of Gln and Arg Metabolisms

Gln and iNOS Regulation

iNOS enzyme is a bi-domain protein; the C-terminal moiety acts as a reductase domain that contains the bindings site for NADPH, flavin adenine dinucleotide and mononucleotide and calmodulin, and the N-terminal moiety acts as an oxygenase domain that contains the binding domains for L-Arg, heme and tetrahydrobiopterin [37]. As previously discussed, Gln ensures the availability of an iNOS cofactor, i.e. NADPH, by maintaining high TCA cycle activity and sustained flux through the NADP$^+$-dependent malic enzyme [31]. In fact, NO production rate was reduced in the presence of glutaminase inhibitor (6-diazo 5-oxo norleucine) in activated murine macrophages and human monocytes [30]. Likewise, the same study conducted by Murphy et al. showed that culturing these cells in the absence of iNOS substrate, i.e. L-Arg, up-regulated Gln uptake to ensure NO synthesis, suggesting the presence of Gln-to-Arg pathway [30]. Similarly, culturing MSC-1 cells in the absence of Gln attenuated the production of NO derivatives, while ARG1 activity was not affected

[31]. In fact, several studies focused on the potential regulation of iNOS gene and protein expression by Gln. Namely, L-Gln was shown to attenuate iNOS mRNA and protein level in IL-1β-activated hepatocytes preventing NO-induced mitochondria dysfunction [38]. Furthermore, alanine-glutamine dipeptide, a source of Gln, decreases iNOS mRNA level in hemorrhagic shock patients' liver samples [39]. Conversely, Gln did not affect iNOS mRNA level in cytokine-treated or not treated colorectal cancer cell lines [40]. So far, the relationship between Gln and iNOS gene and protein expression has not been yet specifically investigated in immunosuppressive iNOS-expressing cells despite the aforementioned strong evidences of iNOS activity regulation by Gln. Indeed, it has been reported that exposing macrophages to hypoxia and cytokines increases iNOS mRNA level and that iNOS promoter depends on hypoxia-inducible factor 1 (HIF-1) and nuclear factor κ light chain enhancer of activated B cells (NF-κB) [41]. Corzo et al. have showed that MDSCs express HIF-1α to adapt to quasi-hypoxic conditions in tumors [42]. Hammami et al. also reported a decrease of cell respiration by at least 60 % during BM-derived MDSC maturation process [29]. Studies focusing on Gln deprivation effects on human carcinoma cells showed a reduced expression of HIF-1/2α [43]. Furthermore, stable HIF is dependent on the accumulation of TCA cycle intermediates, specifically by fumarate, which inhibits HIF hydroxylases [44]. Gln-dependent high TCA cycle activity and accumulation of fumarate, a by-product of L-Arg endogenous synthesis pathway, has been reported in MDSCs and MSC-1 cells [29, 31]. Gln metabolism may then indirectly favor glycolytic metabolism which is known to be exhibited by both MDSCs [29, 31] and tumor cells [28]. Moreover, Gln was shown to regulate the activation of NF-κB signaling pathway in LPS-treated peritoneal macrophages [45, 46]. Therefore, Gln plays a central role in the iNOS-mediated immune suppression and the control of its metabolism may represent a promising approach to treat several NO-induced pathologies.

Gln and the Endogenous Synthesis of Arg

One of the primary strategies that have been explored to overcome tumor escape was based on Arg deprivation. This strategy was rapidly abandoned since Arg showed to be endogenously synthesized, from citrulline, in several cell types (e.g. kidney cells, aortic endothelial cells, macrophages, etc.) [33]. Moreover, Gln can be converted into citrulline through the enzymatic activities of glutaminase, pyrroline-5-carboxylate synthase, ornithine aminotransferase, ornithine carbamoyltransferase and carbamoyl phosphate synthetase [33]. The activities of these enzymes were up-regulated in bacillus Calmette-Guérin-stimulated macrophages and in the absence of L-Arg to ensure continuous NO biosynthesis [33]. In addition to its role as a carbon and nitrogen source for Arg synthesis, Gln regulates the enzymatic activity and the gene expression level of ASS, the rate-limiting enzyme of the Arg synthesis pathway, through the cytosolic *O*-glycosylation of the transcription factor Sp1 [47]. That is, ASS gene expression also depends on the activation of NF-κB signaling pathway which is, in turn, Gln-dependent [48]. In fact, Gln regulates gene expression of several transcription factors implicated in signaling pathways which, in turn, regulate cell metabolism, inflammatory response and cell proliferation, survival and death [43]. Among these, Gln activates the CCAAT/enhanced binding protein β [43] that has been recently reported as a regulator of MDSC maturation in growing tumors [49].

Gln and Cytokine Production

The last mechanism of Gln-mediated immunosuppression consists in the modulation of cytokine production by Gln itself or its metabolic byproducts. Indeed, all cells present at the tumor edge, including immune, tumor and immunosuppressive cells, produce numerous cytokines that can be used for signaling between different cell compartments or secreted to ensure inter-cellular cross-talk. While Th1 or pro-inflammatory cytokines (e.g. TNF-β, IL-2, IL-6, IL-12 INF-α and γ, etc.) stimulate the immune system, Th2 or anti-inflammatory cytokines (such as TGF-β, IL-4, IL-5 and IL-10, etc.) suppress the immune system. These cytokines regulate L-Arg metabolism; specifically, Th1 and Th2 cytokines induce the activities of iNOS and ARG1, respectively [11]. As in all the aforementioned regulation mechanisms by Gln, the Gln-mediated synthesis of cytokines is cell type-dependent and requires a prior stimulation [50].

First, Gln enhances IL-2 production in challenged immune cells and so the decreased concentration of Gln in the tumor microenvironment reduces IL-2 synthesis and the initiation of the IL-2-dependent signaling pathways, which regulates T-cell immunomodulatory functions [50]. Moreover, the production of TNF-α from macrophages and IL-8 from monocytes are dependent on Gln concentration and high secretion rates of cytokines' secretion can be attenuated in the presence of a glutaminolysis inhibitor or in the absence of Gln [51]. Similarly, the Gln-mediated production of IL-6 and IL-1β was addressed in LPS-treated rat peritoneal macrophages; Yassad et al. suggested that Gln acts at the translational level, since unlike mRNA level, cytokine concentration was affected by Gln supplementation or deprivation [52, 53]. Moreover, the enhancement of IL-4 and IL-6 secretion in phytohemagglutinin-stimulated lymphocytes was shown to be Gln-dependent, as for IFN-γ synthesis by bacillus Calmette-Guérin-treated mononuclear cells [50].

The modulation mechanisms of cytokine synthesis by Gln in stimulated immune effector cells are not completely understood, but the control of gene expression, especially those of transcription factors, by Gln is likely responsible for this regulatory effect. In fact, Gln regulates the LPS-induced IL-8 secretion through the signal transducers and activators of transcription-4 pathway, and Gln deprivation in breast cancer cells increases IL-8 gene expression through NF-κB activation [43]. Further investigation is then required to elucidate the regulatory role played by Gln on cytokine secretion in the immunosuppression context.

Conclusion

A complex set of interactions between growing tumors and the immune system triggers the dysfunction of the adaptive immune ability to recognize tumors and prevent their outgrowth. The most concentrated amino acid in blood, i.e. Gln, plays a central role in the tumor escape process. Gln-mediated immunosuppressive mechanisms have not been only reported in tumor cells but also in immune effector cells and in immunosuppressive cell populations derived from immature immune cells. Gln effects can be divided to direct effects, where Gln affects gene and protein expression levels or enzyme activities, and indirect effects where Gln affects signaling pathways and the distribution of carbon intermediates and energy-rich nucleotides required for multiple physiological functions (Table 36.1).

Indirect effects can also be associated with the role of Gln as a carbon and/or nitrogen source for other amino acids that may also have immunosuppressive potential; this aspect was not reviewed in this chapter due to the high number of potential amino acids. Furthermore, Gln can as well be an essential amino acid for the folding of crucial proteins, and its absence may conduct to the loss of their bioactivity. So far, strong evidences demonstrate that Gln is not only a vital fuel for tumor cells and immune cells, but rather works as an immunosuppressive nutrient. Regulatory mechanisms by which Gln do control several cellular aspects leading to defective immunosurveillance phenomenon are still misunderstood and require further investigation, both in vivo and in vitro, to be able to define efficient therapeutic strategies against Gln-mediated immunosuppression. Box 36.1 states some concerns about the clinic application of Gln-based strategies.

Table 36.1 Summary of Gln possible implication on cancer-related immunosuppression

Cell type	How Gln promotes immunosuppression?
Tumor cells	– High Gln uptake by tumor cells decrease Gln availability and down-regulate Gln-dependent T-cell functions – Gln up-regulates the synthesis of specific cytokines that induce the maturation and recruitment of immunosuppressive cells – Tumor-derived factors may up-regulate glutaminase mRNA and so Gln metabolism – Gln contributes in the acidification of the tumor microenvironment – Potential down-regulatory effect of Gln on MHC expression
Immune cells	– Gln down-regulates the expression of adhesion molecules required for the priming of immune response both in CTLs and T helper cells – Possible regulation of the synthesis of co-stimulatory molecules by Gln – The decreased availability of Gln reduced IL-2 production and prevent the initiation of IL-2 receptor signaling cascade
Immunosuppressive cells	– High Gln uptake by BM-derived MDSCs decrease Gln availability and down-regulate Gln-dependent T-cell functions – Gln ensures high activity of malic enzyme to produce lactate and NADPH, an iNOS cofactor – Gln up-regulates iNOS mRNA level via HIF stabilization and NF-κB activation – Gln may be endogenously converted into Arg whose metabolism represent a very potent immunosuppressive mechanism – Gln up-regulates enzymatic activity and gene expression of ASS through the NF-κB signaling pathway – Gln enhances the expression of Th1/2 cytokines which in turn regulates iNOS and ARG1 activities, respectively

Box 36.1: Lab Work Versus Clinical Applications of Gln-Based Therapeutic Strategies

Despite the considerable progress in the understanding of Gln role in cancer-related immunosuppression, overcoming this role at the clinical point of view is not feasible so far.

Gln revealed to be highly implicated in the promotion of cancer-related immunosuppression. One may suggest to use Gln-depleted diet or to inhibit Gln transporter or enzymes of the glutaminolysis pathway. These strategies may have several beneficial effects both on tumor regression and the correction of anti-tumor-specific immune response.

But, *is it clinically feasible?*

As seen in this book, Gln is crucial for different physiological conditions and is required for the functioning of vital organs including liver, kidney, intestine, central nervous system, etc. Then, depleting Gln from the diet of cancer-bearing hosts should be conducted under strict supervision of overall patients' health. Likewise, the use of chemical compounds to inhibit Gln transport or metabolism should be targeted to specific cells in precise locations. For instance, tumor-infiltrating lymphocytes should be able to consume Gln to ensure its proliferation and immunomodulatory functions. However, drug targeting remains an obstacle for the clinic use of multiple therapeutic strategies that showed to be promising in vitro.

To avoid problems associated with Gln depletion or the inhibition of its uptake or metabolism, researchers and clinicians should act on downstream effects of Gln, such as enzymes activities or signaling pathways, etc. with a special concern for targeting.

References

1. Epeldegui M, Vendrame E, Martinez-Maza O. HIV-associated immune dysfunction and viral infection: role in the pathogenesis of AIDS-related lymphoma. Immunol Res. 2010;48(1–3):72–83.
2. Byng-Maddick R, Ehrenstein M. Infections in biological agents used in rheumatic disease. Br J Hosp Med (Lond). 2012;73(9):517–20.
3. He F, Balling R. The role of regulatory T cells in neurodegenerative diseases. Wiley Interdiscip Rev Syst Biol Med. 2013; 5(2):153–80.
4. Abbas AK, Lichtman AH. Basic immunology: functions and disorders of the immune system. 2006.
5. David H. Rudolf Virchow and modern aspects of tumor pathology. Pathol Res Pract. 1988;183(3):356–64.
6. Zou W. Immunosuppressive networks in the tumor environment and their therapeutic relevance. Cancer. 2005;5:263–74.
7. Restifo NP, Kawakami Y, Marincola F, et al. Molecular mechanisms used by tumors to escape immune recognition: immunogenetherapy and the cell biology of major histocompatibility complex class I. J Immunother Emphasis Tumor Immunol. 1993;14(3):182–90.
8. Seliger B, Harders C, Lohmann S, et al. Down-regulation of the MHC class I antigen-processing machinery after oncogenic transformation of murine fibroblasts. Eur J Immunol. 1998;28(1):122–33.
9. Capece D, Verzella D, Fischietti M, Zazzeroni F, Alesse E. Targeting costimulatory molecules to improve antitumor immunity. J Biomed Biotechnol. 2012;2012:926321.
10. Costello RT, Gastaut JA, Olive D. Tumor escape from immune surveillance. Arch Immunol Ther Exp (Warsz). 1999;47(2):83–8.
11. Serafini P, Borrello I, Bronte V. Myeloid suppressor cells in cancer: recruitment, phenotype, properties, and mechanisms of immune suppression. Semin Cancer Biol. 2006;16(1):53–65.
12. Drake CG, Jaffee E, Pardoll DM. Mechanisms of immune evasion by tumors. Adv Immunol. 2006;90:51–81.
13. Gabrilovich D. Mechanisms and functional significance of tumour-induced dendritic-cell defects. Nat Rev Immunol. 2004;4(12):941–52.
14. Cao X. Regulatory T, cells and immune tolerance to tumors. Immunol Res. 2010;46(1–3):79–93.
15. Morris Jr SM. Enzymes of arginine metabolism. J Nutr. 2004;134 Suppl 10:2743S–7S. discussion 2765S–2767S.
16. Munder M, Schneider H, Luckner C, et al. Suppression of T-cell functions by human granulocyte arginase. Blood. 2006;108(5):1627–34.
17. Boulland ML, Marquet J, Molinier-Frenkel V, et al. Human IL4I1 is a secreted L-phenylalanine oxidase expressed by mature dendritic cells that inhibits T-lymphocyte proliferation. Blood. 2007;110(1):220–7.
18. Fallarino F, Grohmann U, You S, et al. The combined effects of tryptophan starvation and tryptophan catabolites down-regulate T cell receptor zeta-chain and induce a regulatory phenotype in naive T cells. J Immunol. 2006;176(11):6752–61.
19. Mocellin S, Bronte V, Nitti D. Nitric oxide, a double edged sword in cancer biology: searching for therapeutic opportunities. Med Res Rev. 2007;27(3):317–52.
20. Wu G, Bazer FW, Davis TA, et al. Arginine metabolism and nutrition in growth, health and disease. Amino Acids. 2009;37(1):153–68.
21. Hou YC, Hsu CS, Yeh CL, Chiu WC, Pai MH, Yeh SL. Effects of glutamine on adhesion molecule expression and leukocyte transmigration in endothelial cells exposed to arsenic. J Nutr Biochem. 2005;16(11):700–4.
22. Spittler A, Winkler S, Gotzinger P, et al. Influence of glutamine on the phenotype and function of human monocytes. Blood. 1995;86(4):1564–9.
23. Pai MH, Chien YW, Tsai YH, Hu YM, Yeh SL. Glutamine reduces the expression of leukocyte integrins leukocyte function-associated antigen-1 and macrophage antigen-1 in mice exposed to arsenic. Nutr Res. 2008;28(8):544–9.
24. Carr EL, Kelman A, Wu GS, et al. Glutamine uptake and metabolism are coordinately regulated by ERK/MAPK during T lymphocyte activation. J Immunol. 2010;185(2):1037–44.
25. Boelens PG, Houdijk AP, Fonk JC, et al. Glutamine-enriched enteral nutrition increases HLA-DR expression on monocytes of trauma patients. J Nutr. 2002;132(9):2580–6.
26. Spittler A, Sautner T, Gornikiewicz A, et al. Postoperative glycyl-glutamine infusion reduces immunosuppression: partial prevention of the surgery induced decrease in HLA-DR expression on monocytes. Clin Nutr. 2001;20(1):37–42.
27. Castell L. Glutamine supplementation in vitro and in vivo, in exercise and in immunodepression. Sports Med. 2003;33(5):323–45.
28. Wise DR, Thompson CB. Glutamine addiction: a new therapeutic target in cancer. Trends Biochem Sci. 2010;35(8):427–33.

29. Hammami I, Chen J, Murschel F, Bronte V, De Crescenzo G, Jolicoeur M. Immunosuppressive activity enhances central carbon metabolism and bioenergetics in myeloid-derived suppressor cells in vitro models. BMC Cell Biol. 2012;13:18.
30. Murphy C, Newsholme P. Importance of glutamine metabolism in murine macrophages and human monocytes to L-arginine biosynthesis and rates of nitrite or urea production. Clin Sci (Lond). 1998;95(4):397–407.
31. Hammami I, Chen J, Bronte V, DeCrescenzo G, Jolicoeur M. L-glutamine is a key parameter in the immunosuppression phenomenon. Biochem Biophys Res Commun. 2012;425(4):724–9.
32. Costa Rosa LF, Curi R, Murphy C, Newsholme P. Effect of adrenaline and phorbol myristate acetate or bacterial lipopolysaccharide on stimulation of pathways of macrophage glucose, glutamine and O_2 metabolism. Evidence for cyclic AMP-dependent protein kinase mediated inhibition of glucose-6-phosphate dehydrogenase and activation of NADP+-dependent "malic" enzyme. Biochem J. 1995;310(Pt 2):709–14.
33. Newsholme P, Costa Rosa LF, Newsholme EA, Curi R. The importance of fuel metabolism to macrophage function. Cell Biochem Funct. 1996;14(1):1–10.
34. Zhao L, Huang Y, Tian C, et al. Interferon-alpha regulates glutaminase 1 promoter through STAT1 phosphorylation: relevance to HIV-1 associated neurocognitive disorders. PLoS One. 2012;7(3):e32995.
35. Andratsch M, Feifel E, Taylor L, et al. TGF-beta signaling and its effect on glutaminase expression in LLC-PK1-FBPase+cells. Am J Physiol Renal Physiol. 2007;293(3):F846–853.
36. Umansky V. New strategies for melanoma immunotherapy: how to overcome immunosuppression in the tumor microenvironment. Oncoimmunology. 2012;1(5):765–7.
37. Aktan F. iNOS-mediated nitric oxide production and its regulation. Life Sci. 2004;75(6):639–53.
38. Lu J, Wang XY, Tang WH. Glutamine attenuates nitric oxide synthase expression and mitochondria membrane potential decrease in interleukin-1beta-activated rat hepatocytes. Eur J Nutr. 2009;48(6):333–9.
39. Yang R, Tan X, Thomas AM, et al. Alanine-glutamine dipeptide (AGD) inhibits expression of inflammation-related genes in hemorrhagic shock. J Parenter Enteral Nutr. 2007;31(1):32–6.
40. Marion R, Coeffier M, Leplingard A, Favennec L, Ducrotte P, Dechelotte P. Cytokine-stimulated nitric oxide production and inducible NO-synthase mRNA level in human intestinal cells: lack of modulation by glutamine. Clin Nutr. 2003;22(6):523–8.
41. Robinson MA, Baumgardner JE, Otto CM. Oxygen-dependent regulation of nitric oxide production by inducible nitric oxide synthase. Free Radic Biol Med. 2011;51(11):1952–65.
42. Corzo CA, Condamine T, Lu L, et al. HIF-1alpha regulates function and differentiation of myeloid-derived suppressor cells in the tumor microenvironment. J Exp Med. 2010;207(11):2439–53.
43. Brasse-Lagnel C, Lavoinne A, Husson A. Control of mammalian gene expression by amino acids, especially glutamine. FEBS J. 2009;276(7):1826–44.
44. Koivunen P, Hirsila M, Remes AM, Hassinen IE, Kivirikko KI, Myllyharju J. Inhibition of hypoxia-inducible factor (HIF) hydroxylases by citric acid cycle intermediates: possible links between cell metabolism and stabilization of HIF. J Biol Chem. 2007;282(7):4524–32.
45. da Silva Lima F, Rogero MM, Ramos MC, Borelli P, Fock RA. Modulation of the nuclear factor-kappa B (NF-kappaB) signalling pathway by glutamine in peritoneal macrophages of a murine model of protein malnutrition. Eur J Nutr 2012 Eur J Nutr. 2013;52(4):1343–51.
46. Rogero MM, Borelli P, Fock RA, et al. Effects of glutamine on the nuclear factor-kappaB signaling pathway of murine peritoneal macrophages. Amino Acids. 2010;39(2):435–41.
47. Brasse-Lagnel C, Fairand A, Lavoinne A, Husson A. Glutamine stimulates argininosuccinate synthetase gene expression through cytosolic O-glycosylation of Sp1 in Caco-2 cells. J Biol Chem. 2003;278(52):52504–10.
48. Brasse-Lagnel C, Lavoinne A, Loeber D, et al. Glutamine and interleukin-1beta interact at the level of Sp1 and nuclear factor-kappaB to regulate argininosuccinate synthetase gene expression. FEBS J. 2007;274(20):5250–62.
49. Marigo I, Bosio E, Solito S, et al. Tumor-induced tolerance and immune suppression depend on the C/EBPbeta transcription factor. Immunity. 2010;32(6):790–802.
50. Chang WK, Yang KD, Shaio MF. Effect of glutamine on Th1 and Th2 cytokine responses of human peripheral blood mononuclear cells. Clin Immunol. 1999;93(3):294–301.
51. Murphy C, Newsholme P. Macrophage-mediated lysis of a beta-cell line, tumour necrosis factor-alpha release from bacillus Calmette-Guerin (BCG)-activated murine macrophages and interleukin-8 release from human monocytes are dependent on extracellular glutamine concentration and glutamine metabolism. Clin Sci (Lond). 1999;96(1):89–97.
52. Yassad A, Lavoinne A, Bion A, Daveau M, Husson A. Glutamine accelerates interleukin-6 production by rat peritoneal macrophages in culture. FEBS Lett. 1997;413(1):81–4.
53. Yassad A, Husson A, Bion A, Lavoinne A. Synthesis of interleukin 1beta and interleukin 6 by stimulated rat peritoneal macrophages: modulation by glutamine. Cytokine. 2000;12(8):1288–91.

Chapter 37
Combining Exercise with Glutamine Supplementation in Cancer-Cachexia Metabolism

Maria Cristina Cintra Gomes-Marcondes and Emilianne Miguel Salomão

Key Points

- Cancer causes severe changes to carbohydrate, lipid and protein metabolism.
- Exercise ensures good muscle strength and protein turnover, guaranteeing a good quality of life.
- Glutamine is an amino acid that can ensure the activity of cells by providing energy, carbon and nitrogen for several processes.
- Nutritional supplementation with glutamine in combination with exercise can help the cancer-cachectic state in most patients.

Keywords Exercise • Nutritional supplementation • Glutamine • Protein metabolism • Body composition • Cancer • Cachexia

Abbreviations

AMPK	AMP-activated protein kinase
BCAAs	Branched chain amino acids—leucine valine, isoleucine
CaMK	Calmodulin kinase
CP	Creatine phosphate
CPT-1	Carnitine palmitoyltransferase-1
Erk	Extracellular signal-regulated kinase
HSL	Hormone-sensitive lipase
IFN-γ	Interferon-gamma
IGF	Insulin-like growth factor
IL-6	Interleukin-6
IκB	Inhibitor of NFκB
JNK	c-Jun N-terminal kinase
LMF	Lipid-mobilising factor

M.C.C. Gomes-Marcondes, Ph.D. (✉) • E.M. Salomão, Ph.D.
Department of Structural and Functional Biology, Biology Institute, State University of Campinas – UNICAMP, Rua Monteiro Lobato, 255, Campinas, São Paulo 13083-862, Brazil
e-mail: cintgoma@unicamp.br; emisalomao@hotmail.com

R. Rajendram et al. (eds.), *Glutamine in Clinical Nutrition*, Nutrition and Health,
DOI 10.1007/978-1-4939-1932-1_37, © Springer Science+Business Media New York 2015

MAPKs	Mitogen-activated protein kinase
MGF	Mechano-growth factor
mTOR	Mammalian target of rapamycin
NFκB	Nuclear factor-kappa B
PGC-1	Peroxisome-proliferator-activated receptor gamma coactivator-1
PIF	Proteolysis-inducing factor
PKC	Calcium-dependent protein kinase
S6K1	Ribosomal protein S6 kinase
TNF-α	Tumour necrosis factor alpha

Introduction

Physical activity contributes to several beneficial processes including the management, treatment and prevention of various diseases, particularly cardiovascular and metabolic diseases. These well-being and health benefits include the improvement of the circulatory, respiratory and immune systems, reducing the diseases risks. Furthermore, in several studies, cancer prevention has been shown to be related to physical activity [1–3].

Among the methods aimed at increasing physical performance, athletes, coaches and scientists use different nutritional (ergogenic) compounds that can improve an athlete's performance. This chapter presents updated information on the physiological functions of glutamine, especially during exercise, and the use of this amino acid as a nutritional supplement for physical activity. In addition, researchers are interested in the relation between the physiopathological changes in cancer and physical activity as adjuvant therapy [1–3]. Exercise promotes biochemical and physiological adaptations resulting in increased energy reserves, which improves the metabolic profile of various tissues in cancer patients. There are several studies showing the role of physical activity in preventing cancer and reducing cancer incidence. These studies reveal that individuals that have sedentary jobs or do not perform any physical activity have a higher risk of cancer than those who engage in regular physical activity [1–3]. However, this relationship has not been observed for all cancers. For example, there is evidence that physical activity, when practiced regularly, contributes to a reduction of the risk of certain cancers, especially those of the colon and gynaecologic system. Although exercise does not directly reduce the risk of cancer recurrence or delay tumour growth, it is the key component for controlling triggering factors, such as obesity, overweight, and hormonal, immunological, and other metabolic changes [1, 2]. Several possible exercise mechanisms have been postulated: it may act on the immune system (stimulation of natural killer cells by interleukins), via hormonal changes (primarily on oestrogens) and changes in adiposity, via changes in dietary and nutritional habits, and via other secondary actions [1–3]. Cancer causes profound mental and physical changes in patients, and despite increasingly efficient and modern cancer treatments, these changes still compromise quality of life and an individual's ability to cope with treatment. Thus, exercise can be an adjuvant therapeutic modality for improving patient responses.

Physiological Adaptations from Exercise

Human beings have different capacities for physical exercise adaptation according to their anatomical, physiological and behavioural characteristics [4]. Typical aerobic exercise, known as endurance exercise, is continuous and prolonged, and is related to human evolutionary characteristics, as oxygen is necessary for muscle function [4]. Endurance training works many muscle groups in rhythm; walking, running, swimming and cycling are classic examples of aerobic exercise. The stimulation induced by endurance exercise generates individual responses during each exercise session that result in a chronic adaptive response. Among these responses are an increase in muscle glycogen and lipid content, higher intracellular mitochondrial density, and increased protein turnover dedicated to the synthesis of proteins, including metabolic enzymes, antioxidants, chaperones, and myofilament proteins and mitochondrial carrier proteins [5]. This category of exercise brings many benefits to the body; for example, it reduces the cardiovascular disease risk, as moderate physical activity decreases the synthesis of C-reactive protein and tumour necrosis factor (TNF-α). Moreover, moderate training improves quality of life and life expectancy, as it induces slight increases in serum creatine kinase and lactate, which induces fat mobilisation. In addition to local skeletal muscle responses, endurance training also induces systemic adaptations relevant to the treatment and prevention of pathological conditions, such as diabetes, cardiovascular disease, dyslipidaemia and cancer, and this is the main focus of this chapter [1, 2, 6].

During aerobic exercises, muscle cells consume more oxygen to produce energy. Thus, the cells consume large amounts of energy produced during aerobic exercise. Under these conditions, glucose is converted into pyruvic acid, which enters into the mitochondrial compartment after being converted to acetyl-CoA, and this conversion produces 36 ATPs under aerobic conditions (18-fold more than anaerobic exercise). Anaerobic exercise includes any intense physical activity that works different muscle groups continuously and rhythmically under high intensity for a short time; examples of anaerobic activities are bodybuilding, sprinting, jumping, or any other type of exercise involving quick high-intensity movements. Anaerobic exercise is usually practiced by athletes to develop strength and muscle mass. The muscle tissue develops better performance under anaerobic conditions because creatine phosphate is the main source of energy and anaerobic glycolysis, in which glucose is used in the absence of oxygen, provides only 2 ATPs (unlike aerobic exercise). Lactic acid, a by-product, is efficiently removed by adapted, trained muscles.

In endurance exercise, the body adapts to preserve glucose because glucose preservation is essential for the functioning of other tissues such as the brain and blood cells. Thus, energy from glucose is replaced by energy provided by beta-oxidation of fatty acids, which are derived mainly from adipose tissue and muscle [7]. Thus, this skeletal muscle response consists of a three- to eightfold increase in body metabolic rate that remains for hours after exercise, even in moderate exercise. This residual effect of physical activity is largely responsible for its high energy expenditure, and there is an additional adaptation to gain muscle protein mass, causing an increase in lean mass and a reduction in fat mass. During the course of physical training, the muscles adapt to oxidise a higher proportion of fatty acids because the enzymes involved in the mechanism of beta-oxidation increase in proportion to physical activity. Several studies show that endurance exercise results in divergent responses in signalling pathways, even in pre- and post-training conditions. Exercise is a potent stimulus for several kinases, including mitogen-activated protein kinase (MAPKs, such as extracellular signal-regulated kinase (ERK1/2)) and the stress-activated kinases p38 MAPK and c-Jun N-terminal kinase (JNK). The local and systemic metabolism factors induced by exercise lead to phosphorylation of MAPK signalling pathway proteins and the transcriptional regulation of important genes. Protein kinase B/Akt is a serine/threonine kinase with two isoforms (Akt1 and Akt2) that are implicated as important targets of insulin action. Akt activation leads to glycogen synthesis, GLUT4 translocation and glucose transport, and the regulatory responses of these genes in skeletal muscle [8]. Moreover, during exercise, an increase in the sarcoplasmic Ca^{2+} level stimulates the generation of ATP, participates in actin/myosin coupling that causes contraction, and activates transcriptional responses through calcium-dependent signalling pathways via calmodulin kinase (CaMK), calcium-dependent protein kinase (PKC) and the Ca^{2+}/calmodulin-dependent phosphatase calcineurin [9]. AMP-activated protein kinase (AMPK) appears to be the condition sensor in muscle energy. Intense and sub-maximal exercises increase the activity of AMPK α1 and α2, respectively, but this increase is moderated by the availability of glycogen in the muscle [9–11]. On the other hand, individual participation in exhaustive exercise results in acute and chronic effects of peroxisome-proliferator-activated receptor γ coactivator-1α (PGC-1α) on mitochondrial biogenesis [9, 12, 13]. As mentioned above, skeletal muscles require a large amount of calories for their activity during aerobic activity, and energy from the β-oxidation of fatty acids supplies much of this energy. During activity, there is an intense and rapid activation of MAPK, especially the ERK1/2 isoforms, which leads to the activation of hormone-sensitive lipase (HSL) [14, 15]. HSL is also regulated by PKC and consequently mobilises intramuscular triglyceride [7]. Moreover, AMPK stimulates muscle fatty acid oxidation by inhibiting acetyl-CoA carboxylase and activating malonyl-CoA; this removes the inhibition of mitochondrial fatty acyl-CoA translocation by carnitine palmitoyltransferase-1 (CPT-1) [9]. Physical training allows muscle tissue to adapt to higher energy consumption, thus increasing muscle mass. Thus, mechanical contraction and hormonal stimulation, either individually or in combination, activate muscle cell signalling, ensuring protein synthesis [16, 17]. The actions of insulin on protein metabolism are particularly important in muscle; in addition to the action of insulin, the insulin-like growth factors (IGFs) are able to stimulate cell growth and protein synthesis, thus increasing mRNA transcription [16, 18]. After exercise, cell signalling modulates muscle hypertrophy by specific pathways that increase the diameter and fibre length (an increase in the number of fibres in a cross-sectional area) [19, 20]. Endurance exercise results in less hypertrophy than rapid short-term exercise, such as bodybuilding [20]. Insulin also mediates the anabolic effects of exercise by inhibiting proteolysis, thus suppressing amino acid release and oxidation. Mammalian target of rapamycin (mTOR) is activated by various stimuli including insulin, growth factors and amino acids. This kinase is crucial for the protein synthesis because it activates ribosomal protein S6 kinase 1 (S6K1) in response to mechanical stimuli [17, 21]. The contractile activity of a muscle appears to be critical for increasing muscle mass and precedes the endocrine signals to deplete muscle proteins. The mechanotransduction stimulus promotes muscle synthesis of mechano-growth factor (MGF, an IGF isoform) [21, 22]. MGF exerts a potent hypertrophic effect in response to strength training. The increased muscle work promotes several biochemical reactions associated with increased amino acid uptake by skeletal muscle [20, 23, 24]. Studies with isolated muscles show that the rate of amino acid transport is directly linked to contractile activity. Few studies have evaluated the effects of physical training on muscle protein turnover and glucose metabolism in cancer-cachexia states.

Cancer-Cachexia Metabolic Changes

Cancer modifies the harmony of metabolic processes through extensive pathophysiological changes in the body. These changes are related to anorexia, the consumption of specific substrates by neoplastic cells, stimulation of catabolic pathways, and quantitative and qualitative transformation of the internal medium. These changes lead to a condition called cachexia, which is associated with the increased release of substances synthesised by cancer or host cells [25, 26]. Cachexia is characterised by involuntary body weight loss due to deep lean body mass loss and decreased fat stores, and accounts for over 20 % of all cancer deaths. The metabolic changes that occur in cachexia and anorexia include deviations from the homeostatic metabolism of carbohydrates, lipids, and especially proteins.

Involuntary body weight loss that occurs during cancer-cachexia may be related to lower nutrient intake and increased basal energy expenditure, which occurs through the mobilisation of glycogen and fat stores and muscle protein mass. To expand, the healthy subject (adult male, ~70 kg) adapts to a chronic food intake reduction that maintains glycaemia following these phases. In the first phase, blood glucose is maintained within normal limits (4–5.5 mmol/L) due to exogenous glucose. In the second phase (considered acute fasting), blood glucose is supplied by the hepatic glycogen reserves, and depleted in less than 24 h. In the third phase (transition from acute to prolonged fasting), blood glucose is obtained mainly via gluconeogenesis from the oxidation of amino acids from muscle catabolism; at this stage, there is a daily protein loss of approximately 75 g. In the fourth phase (adaptation to prolonged fasting), the body protein mass is preserved, reducing the gluconeogenesis process, and some cells (for example, those in the central nervous system) obtain energy from fat metabolism, thus saving lean body mass and obtaining energy from body fat sources. This adaptation allows only a 2 % total muscle mass loss in 20 days.

In the presence of cancer, the patient loses the ability to adapt his or her metabolism. Thus, gluconeogenesis remains high, and the hypercatabolic state with higher nitrogen excretion due to intense protein catabolism persists, reducing lean body mass. Tumour cells, particularly those from pancreatic, colon and stomach cancers, primarily use glucose as an energy source, altering glucose homeostasis. The glucose demand by tumour cells is increased because of the use of glucose-6-phosphate and fructose 6-phosphate for the synthesis of purines, pyrimidines, DNA and RNA and because tumour cells are unable to maintain an adequate level of intracellular ATP for more than 4 h in the absence of glucose (normal cells can maintain an adequate level for approximately 24 h). Thus, this anaerobic metabolism of glucose in tumour cells results in greater lactate production. This lactate is converted into glucose by the liver via the Cori cycle, increasing the inefficiency of cellular energy generation. The activity of the Cori cycle accounts for 50 % of glucose turnover in cachectic patients, against to 20 % in healthy individuals. New glucose synthesis is also increased by the gluconeogenic substrates alanine, glutamine, and glycerol, which corresponds to an increase of hepatic glucose production in weight loss patients of approximately 40 % (Fig. 37.1). In this case, the Cori cycle is partly responsible for the higher negative energy balance in patients, especially those with lung or pancreatic cancer [25, 27]. These changes in carbohydrate metabolism can be the most important factor exacerbating the cancer-cachexia state.

The fat body, which represents the largest energy stock, is used to fill the increased metabolic demand caused by tumour growth in the host. The mobilisation of fatty acids can occur even before the loss of body weight. In this case, lipid-mobilising factor (LMF) [25, 26] acts directly on adipose tissue, promoting the release of fatty acids and glycerol by elevating intracellular cAMP (cyclic adenosine monophosphate) levels. Furthermore, LMF and other cytokines, such as TNF-α, inhibit lipoprotein lipase, preventing the removal of fatty acid from plasma lipoproteins, and resulting in increased circulating lipids in these patients.

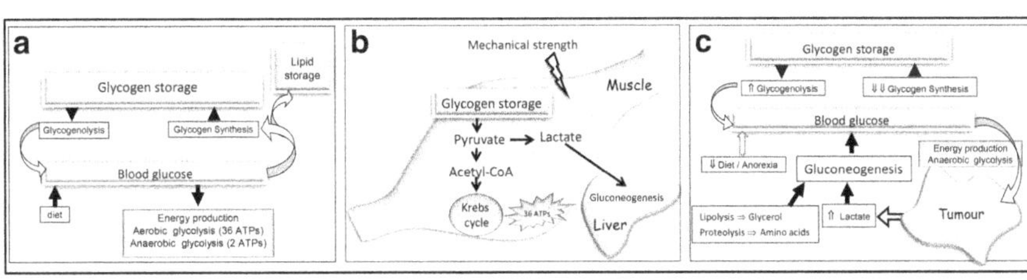

Fig. 37.1 Carbohydrate metabolism. Scheme (**a**) represents a healthy subject: the supply of glucose/carbohydrate diet provides the substrate for the glycogen storage glycogenesis process and also supplies the lipid deposit, and the maintenance of blood glucose (~5 mmol/L in fasting state) is guaranteed by the mobilisation of glycogen through glycogenolysis. Scheme (**b**) represents carbohydrate metabolism during endurance exercise. In Scheme (**c**), the catabolic state represents the cancer patient; glycogen stores are depleted because glycogenolysis mobilises the glycogen store to provide blood glucose, which is decreased due to reduced dietary intake or anorexia. Blood glucose provides energy to tumour cells, and the high glucose demand is ensured by gluconeogenesis from lactate produced by the tumour cells (through anaerobic glycolysis) and by tissue catabolism (adipocyte storage, which provides glycerol, and muscle tissue, which provides amino acids)

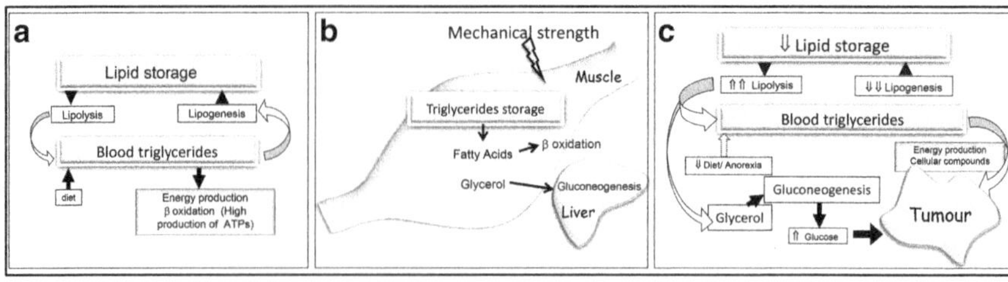

Fig. 37.2 Lipid metabolism. Scheme (**a**) represents a healthy subject, in which the triacylglycerol supply is provided by the diet, and most of the energy supply is obtained through the fatty acid β-oxidation process, thus ensuring high ATP production. In addition, the high levels of triacylglycerol ensure the lipid stock process (adipose tissue through lipogenesis). Scheme (**b**) represents energy distribution during endurance exercise. Scheme (**c**) represents the cachexia-cancer state, in which the high glucose demand by neoplastic cells causes an increase in glucose production from the gluconeogenesis process; due to this deposit, the lipid is mobilised (lipolysis), thus ensuring the provision of triacylglycerol, free fatty acids and glycerol to supply power to the host cells. These substrates are also used (to a lesser extent) by neoplastic cells for components for cellular synthesis and energy

The adipocytes of cancer patients respond 2–3 times better to the lipolytic effects of catecholamines and natriuretic peptides than those of healthy people. These adipocytes have a 50 % higher mRNA expression of hormone-sensitive lipase, which can be stimulated by LMF [25, 26]. Interleukin-6 (IL-6) levels increase in cancer-cachectic patients, indicating an inflammatory state mainly in adipocyte tissue. Many authors consider cancer-cachexia a chronic inflammatory disease (Fig. 37.2).

The loss of lean body mass is the major factor contributing to the reduction of survival time in cancer patients. The increased catabolism associated with reduced protein synthesis is present in the skeletal muscles of patients and experimental animals with cancer. Protein synthesis during cachexia is approximately 8 % of that in healthy individuals, who have approximately 53 % total body protein synthesis. Moreover, certain tissues or organs may have increased protein synthesis, such as the liver, which secretes acute phase proteins. The most significant metabolic effect in cancer is the loss of body protein, reflected by an increase in urinary nitrogen excretion and the presence of a negative nitrogen balance. Protein spoliation during cancer is mainly related to three different proteolytic pathways responsible for the catabolism of skeletal muscle [25, 26, 28]. The lysosomal proteolytic pathway involves the degradation of proteins, including mainly extracellular and surface membrane proteins. A second cytosolic calcium-dependent system operates in trauma situations, tissue necrosis and autolysis by protein breakdown. The third and most important proteolysis process is known as the ATP-dependent ubiquitin-proteasome proteolytic pathway, which also occurs during fasting, and extreme conditions, such as sepsis, denervation atrophy and metabolic acidosis, and is responsible for the accelerated proteolysis in cancer-cachexia [28, 29]. This ubiquitin-ATP-dependent proteolytic pathway also contributes to the high energy expenditure observed in cancer-cachexia patients [26, 30]. Muscle catabolism and weight loss in patients and experimental animals with cancer is also associated with cytokines (TNF-α, IL-6 and interferon-γ (IFN-γ)) [26, 28, 29, 31–33] and proteolysis-inducing factor (PIF) [25, 26, 33, 34]. PIF acts by directly stimulating the ubiquitin-proteasome in muscle cells, the key element for protein catabolism in cancer-cachexia. Thus, protein catabolism provides amino acids, which can stimulate the gluconeogenesis process, increasing the energy needs of the host and neoplastic cells. Some amino acids are preferentially used by neoplastic cells because they cannot be synthesised; this results in increased amino acid demand by the patient. Glutamine, for example, is not synthesised by various types of cancer cells, but is a protein and nucleotide precursor in neoplastic cells. In cancer cells, protein synthesis is accelerated due to the increase of enzymes responsible for the biosynthesis of DNA, purines and pyrimidines. A consequence of this high demand and activity in neoplastic cells is that the host's protein intake is insufficient to provide nitrogen balance. Furthermore, healthy subjects adapt to low nutrient intake, increasing fatty acid mobilisation (Fig. 37.2) and

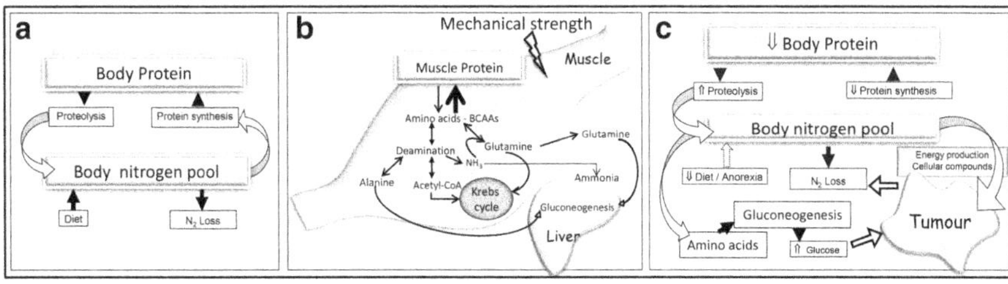

Fig. 37.3 Protein metabolism. Scheme (**a**): in healthy subjects, the supply of body amino acids/nitrogen is provided by the diet, which directs the substrates to protein synthesis and reuse from the catabolic process, ensuring the equilibrium of protein turnover and nitrogen balance. Scheme (**b**) represents protein metabolism during endurance exercise. In Scheme (**c**), the cancer patient is unable to adapt to the chronic lack of substrates imposed by anorexia. In this case, there is an increase in the proteolysis and a decrease in synthesis because the amino acids mobilised from body protein will be consumed by tumour growth. Furthermore, the amino acids are used for the synthesis of glucose via gluconeogenesis to fulfil the high energy demand of tumour cells

reducing protein catabolism, a condition which would produce less glucose from amino acids. The lack of nutrients and anorexia caused by the evolution of the cancer promote the non-adaptation of the cancer patient's protein metabolism, resulting in the severe loss of lean body mass (Fig. 37.3).

Physical Activity, Glutamine and Cancer

Physical exercise promotes primary and secondary preventive effects against the development of various types of cancer, but little is known about the use of physical exercise during treatment. During cancer development and treatment, many patients experience physical side effects, including asthenia, anaemia, nausea, vomiting, sarcopenia, osteopenia, neutropenia, changes in body composition, reductions in vascular and cardiopulmonary function, pain and fatigue. Other psychological factors, such as anxiety, mood changes, reduced self-esteem, and depression, are also present during cancer evolution. These effects can persist for months or years after treatment [35, 36]. Fatigue and loss of physical performance characterise the reduced quality of life in cancer patients before, during and after treatment [35–39] and can affect more than 75 % of patients in the first cycle of chemotherapy [35]. On the other hand, studies show that aerobic exercise, when properly monitored, improves physical performance in cancer patients, reducing fatigue and muscle loss and consequently, enhancing host responses and quality of life [40]. Nutritional intervention and exercise can help to reduce the rates of tumour growth and metastasis in mice, thus decreasing neoplastic symptoms [37, 38, 41, 42]. Studies show that supplementation with amino acids, particularly leucine, decreases protein degradation and stimulates skeletal muscle protein synthesis due to an anabolic effect on muscle protein metabolism [43–46]. Glutamine may also be involved in the increased protein synthesis of skeletal muscle and also decreases catabolism [29, 41]. A diet supplemented with glutamine in combination with exercise improved immune function and reduced tumour growth in an experimental cachexia model [24, 47–50].

Glutamine is synthesised by various tissues and is the most abundant amino acid in the body, where approximately 80 % is found in skeletal muscle; muscle glutamine concentrations (15–20 mmol/L) are 30 times higher than those in plasma (0.6 mmol/L) [44, 47]. In a hypercatabolic state, such as infection and cancer, where a negative nitrogen balance and increased muscle breakdown occur, glutamine demand increases, resulting in a significant reduction in plasma levels. In contrast, low- and medium-intensity exercises have beneficial effects on the immune system when compared to sedentary states. The plasma glutamine concentration decreases immediately after exhaustive exercise and during an exercise recovery period, suggesting that there could be an immunosuppression mechanism that acts on lymphocyte proliferation and macrophage phagocytosis [48]. Glutamine is a major cellular substrate; additionally, it is an energy source for cell proliferation and an important vehicle for nitrogen and carbon transport from various tissues as well as a substrate for the synthesis of other substances, such as nucleic acids. Glutamine is synthesised and released into the blood compartment through muscle tissue; in particular, exercise may differentially affect the production of glutamine by muscle cells and its plasma availability [47]. During rest, different types of muscle fibres have different concentrations of glutamine, depending on physical training and nutrition. The muscle fibres of type I (oxidative fibres) and type I/II (mixed fibres) have high amounts of glutamine, which can ensure greater availability of ATP for cellular activity. The intramuscular concentration of ATP is small enough for short periods of muscle contraction. During intense exercise, the increased ATP demand is met by re-synthesis of ATP from creatine phosphate (CP). Subsequently, ATP is supplied by anaerobic glycolysis, forming lactic acid, which occurs during intense exercise. However, during moderately intense exercise, the large supply of ATP by oxidative phosphorylation occurs under aerobic conditions. In oxidative phosphorylation, the amino acids also provide a supply of ATP. In moderate intensity endurance exercise, the main substrate used for ATP supply is glycogen; muscle glycogen stores are depleted, increasing the metabolism of branched chain amino acids (BCAAs) and fatty acids. In this case, the concentration of glutamine in the muscle increases during the first moments of exercise activity, and returns to normal after glutamine is released into the circulation. Glutamine is used for gluconeogenesis primarily in the liver and kidneys. Glutamine and alanine act as transporters of the ammonia resulting from deamination of BCAAs. This process avoids the accumulation of toxic ammonia in the muscle. In addition, as glycogen storage is related to the cell volume, glutamine promotes glycogen deposition in the muscles and liver, because this amino acid is co-transported with sodium, which increases the volume of intracellular water. Thus, the uptake of glutamine by muscle causes an increase in water uptake and glycogen re-synthesis after exercise. The increase in cell volume also modulates the activity of glycogen synthase, most likely resulting in stimulation of glycogen synthase phosphatase [48]. Glutamine also provides the carbon-chain for glycogen re-synthesis. In the Krebs cycle, glutamine is converted to α-ketoglutarate, which under the action of malic enzyme, forms malate, which is subsequently converted into phosphoenolpyruvate. The other reactions that lead to gluconeogenesis characterise glucose-6-phosphate synthesis; specifically, it is not possible to transform glutamine into free glucose in muscle cell due to the absence of glucose-6-phosphatase. Thus, the increased availability of glucose-6-phosphate stimulates the activity of the enzyme glycogen synthase. Another possible role of glutamine is to increase the intramuscular content of other Krebs cycle intermediates during the first minute of the exercise, which then increases the energy generated via oxidative phosphorylation, thereby affecting athletes' performance. This hypothesis is confirmed experimentally by glutamine supplementation (0.125 g/kg body weight) 1 h prior to an ergometric cycle of 70 % of VO_2 max exercise. This supplementation increases the pool of Krebs cycle intermediates after 10 min of exercise, most likely due to α-ketoglutarate [51]. However, no change in endurance capacity is observed because the depleted phosphocreatine content and accumulation of lactate do not restrict flow to the Krebs cycle. Among supplements, glutamine can act on physical performance because it can regulate the acid–base balance by increasing the buffering capacity of the blood and tissues in situations of acidosis resulting from high-intensity exercise, as shown by the increased lactate concentration associated with H^+ ion content. Supplementation with 2 g of glutamine results in increased plasma bicarbonate ions (HCO_3), altering the acid–base balance in healthy subjects after an absorptive period of 90 min. Moreover, in experimental cachexia, lactate production is decreased in Walker tumour-bearing rats subjected to 4 % glutamine-rich diets and exercise (Fig. 37.4) [50]. In the case of exercise, the progressive increase in intensity during 6 weeks of exercise significantly enhances the plasma glutamine content at rest. This physiological adaptation is necessary to protect the body from glutamine depletion. In intense catabolism, such as that which occurs in cancer, muscle tissue increases the rate of glutamine synthesis and release into the

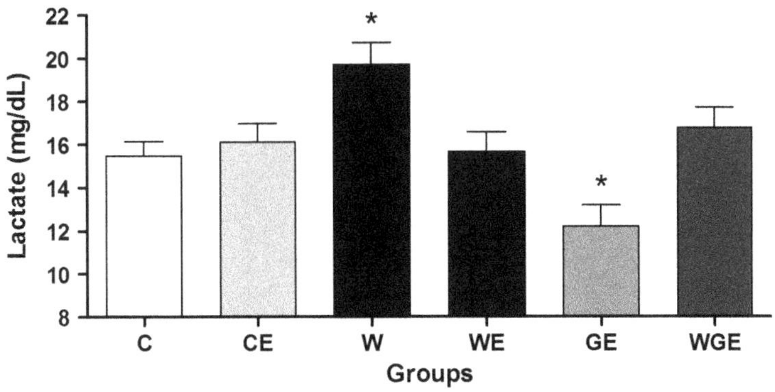

Fig. 37.4 Serum lactate content in young tumour-bearing rats subjected to a glutamine-rich diet (4 %) and aerobic exercise (swimming). C, control rats; CE, exercised rats; W, Walker 256 tumour-bearing rats; WE, exercised tumour-bearing rats; GE, exercised rats fed a glutamine-rich diet; WGE, exercised tumour-bearing rats fed a glutamine-rich diet

bloodstream in response to the increased glutamine demand from other organs and tissues, especially tumour cells. Glucocorticoids rise during these catabolic states, leading to physiological changes, such as increased flow of glutamine from muscle due to the enhanced activity of glutamine synthetase and decreased muscle glutamine store [52]. All of these changes seem to be insufficient to maintain plasma glutamine levels because the glutamine use exceeds the rate of synthesis and release from muscle tissue, decreasing the plasma concentration. Deficiency of glutamine metabolism under conditions of intense catabolism, which occurs in cancer, can lead to progressive intestinal atrophy and may result in septic syndrome and multiple organ failure. Some clinical studies have shown that glutamine supplementation can lead to shorter hospitalisations by reducing the catabolism of BCAAs in skeletal muscle of cachectic patient, decreasing the muscle release of glutamine and alanine. As mentioned above, in the cancer catabolic state, glutamine metabolism is highly diverted to the gluconeogenic process, energy production and cellular activity. Glutamine can produce an increase in cell differentiation because glutamine also participates in the proliferation of neoplastic cells, as this cell machinery prioritises the use of glutamine for synthesis and energy processes. However, tumour cells contain a lower amount of intracellular glutathione, a sub-product of glutamine metabolism, leading to increased toxicity from chemotherapy and radiotherapy in these cells [53]. This lack of glutathione occurs in neoplastic cells because of the imbalance of intracellular reduced and oxidised glutathione; glutathione redox balance would modulate the redox-sensitive protein kinases protecting against oxidative injury, as part of natural antioxidant system in normal cell. Furthermore, glutathione directly influences the phosphorylation of IkB, activating nuclear factor-kappa B (NFkB), which initiates the inflammatory process and, in muscle, activates the proteolytic process. The immune cells use large amounts of glutamine and its demand is high in skeletal muscle and other organs during intense exercise. Moreover, glutamine supplementation in combination with exercise can divert the supply of nutrients for tumour growth, increasing the proliferation of immune cells and resulting in an improvement of the cachectic state in tumour-bearing animals [50]. Glutamine supplementation and exercise can increase protein synthesis, improve nitrogen balance, and enhance glutathione concentration in the liver after exercise. Increased liver glutamine concentration increases the process of detoxification and antioxidant defence, reflecting the body's ability to combat reactive oxygen species and decrease oxidative stress. Glutamine influences cell function and signalling pathways. In experimental models of cachexia, glutamine supplementation can minimise the loss of myosin, the major muscle protein, and improve protein balance in trained animals (Fig. 37.5) [50]. Thus, glutamine can reduce the rate of infection, delaying the inflammatory response and activation of T cells in the cancer host. Moreover, glutamine can reduce the toxic effects that occur due to radiotherapy and chemotherapy, thus

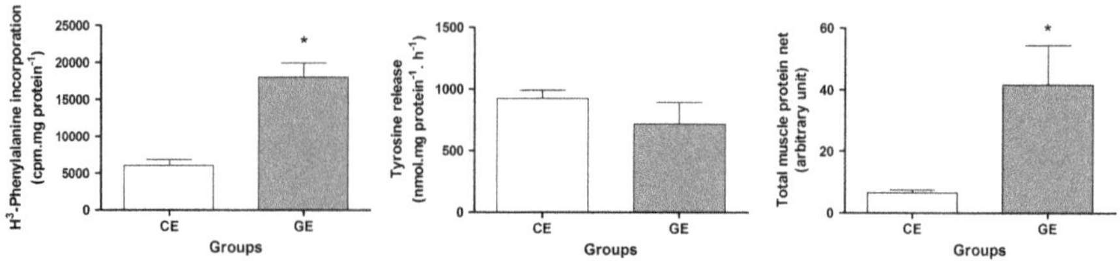

Fig. 37.5 Effects of a glutamine-rich diet and aerobic exercise on protein synthesis (**a**), degradation (**b**) and total muscle protein (**c**) in tumour-bearing animals. The right gastrocnemius muscles from all experimental groups were incubated with [3H]phenylalanine for 2 h, as protein synthesis is based on this radio-labelled amino acid (nmol/mg/h). The contralateral gastrocnemius muscle was similarly incubated for 2 h with cycloheximide to measure protein breakdown based on released tyrosine (nmol/μg/h). CE, exercised control rats; GE exercised group fed a glutamine-rich diet (4 % glutamine). The columns represent the means ± standard error. The number of animals per group is eight. $*P<0.05$ against CE group

improving the quality of life for cancer patients. Currently, there is great interest in understanding the role of glutamine as a link between the metabolism of muscles and immune cells during and after exercise. In acute and chronic exercise, there is greater glutamine uptake and utilisation by certain tissues, cells and organs, while skeletal muscle glutamine release is increased during catabolic states, such as cancer. Therefore, there is interest in the use of nutritional supplements, especially amino acids, which may help to maintain glutamine concentrations and improve the cancer-cachectic patient.

Conclusions

Amino acid supplementation and exercise increase the protein synthesis, improve nitrogen balance, and increase glutamine and glutathione synthesis; these changes improve the oxidative stress and immune responses. Glutamine enhances muscle energy and increases muscle mass and strength when associated with endurance exercise. In the cancer catabolic state, glutamine nutritional supplementation and exercise as adjuvant therapy can improve patient response, quality of life and survival.

References

1. Irwin ML, Mayne ST. Impact of nutrition and exercise on cancer survival. Cancer J. 2008;14(6):435–41.
2. Kushi LH, Doyle C, McCullough M, Rock CL, Demark-Wahnefried W, Bandera EV, et al. American Cancer Society Guidelines on nutrition and physical activity for cancer prevention: reducing the risk of cancer with healthy food choices and physical activity. CA Cancer J Clin. 2012;62(1):30–67.
3. Rock CL, Doyle C, Demark-Wahnefried W, Meyerhardt J, Courneya KS, Schwartz AL, et al. Nutrition and physical activity guidelines for cancer survivors. CA Cancer J Clin. 2012;62(4):243–74.
4. Lieberman DE. What we can learn about running from barefoot running: an evolutionary medical perspective. Exerc Sport Sci Rev. 2012;40(2):63–72.
5. Baar K, Nader G, Bodine S. Resistance exercise, muscle loading/unloading and the control of muscle mass. Essays Biochem. 2006;42:61–74.
6. Doyle C, Kushi LH, Byers T, Courneya KS, Demark-Wahnefried W, Grant B, et al. Nutrition and physical activity during and after cancer treatment: an American Cancer Society guide for informed choices. CA Cancer J Clin. 2006;56(6):323–53.
7. Bacurau RF, Bassit RA, Sawada L, Navarro F, Martins Jr E, Costa Rosa LF. Carbohydrate supplementation during intense exercise and the immune response of cyclists. Clin Nutr. 2002;21(5):423–9.
8. Hawley JA, Burke LM, Phillips SM, Spriet LL. Nutritional modulation of training-induced skeletal muscle adaptations. J Appl Physiol. 2011;110(3):834–45.

9. Hawley JA, Hargreaves M, Zierath JR. Signalling mechanisms in skeletal muscle: role in substrate selection and muscle adaptation. Essays Biochem. 2006;42:1–12.
10. Camera DM, West DW, Burd NA, Phillips SM, Garnham AP, Hawley JA, et al. Low muscle glycogen concentration does not suppress the anabolic response to resistance exercise. J Appl Physiol. 2012;113(2):206–14.
11. Coffey VG, Hawley JA. The molecular bases of training adaptation. Sports Med. 2007;37(9):737–63.
12. Benziane B, Widegren U, Pirkmajer S, Henriksson J, Stepto NK, Chibalin AV. Effect of exercise and training on phospholemman phosphorylation in human skeletal muscle. Am J Physiol Endocrinol Metab. 2011;301(3):E456–66.
13. Stepto NK, Benziane B, Wadley GD, Chibalin AV, Canny BJ, Eynon N, et al. Short-term intensified cycle training alters acute and chronic responses of PGC1alpha and Cytochrome C oxidase IV to exercise in human skeletal muscle. PloS One. 2012;7(12):e53080.
14. Alsted TJ, Nybo L, Schweiger M, Fledelius C, Jacobsen P, Zimmermann R, et al. Adipose triglyceride lipase in human skeletal muscle is upregulated by exercise training. Am J Physiol Endocrinol Metab. 2009;296(3): E445–53.
15. Steinberg GR. Role of the AMP-activated protein kinase in regulating fatty acid metabolism during exercise. Appl Physiol Nutr Metab. 2009;34(3):315–22.
16. Seene T, Kaasik P, Alev K. Muscle protein turnover in endurance training: a review. Int J Sports Med. 2011; 32(12):905–11.
17. Yamada AK, Verlengia R, Bueno Junior CR. Mechanotransduction pathways in skeletal muscle hypertrophy. J Recept Signal Transduct Res. 2012;32(1):42–4.
18. Kimball SR, Jefferson LS. Signaling pathways and molecular mechanisms through which branched-chain amino acids mediate translational control of protein synthesis. J Nutr. 2006;136 Suppl 1:227S–31.
19. Shavlakadze T, Chai J, Maley K, Cozens G, Grounds G, Winn N, et al. A growth stimulus is needed for IGF-1 to induce skeletal muscle hypertrophy in vivo. J Cell Sci. 2010;123(Pt 6):960–71.
20. Phillips SM. The science of muscle hypertrophy: making dietary protein count. Proc Nutr Soc. 2011;70(1):100–3.
21. Hornberger TA. Mechanotransduction and the regulation of mTORC1 signaling in skeletal muscle. Int J Biochem Cell Biol. 2011;43(9):1267–76.
22. Riddoch-Contreras J, Yang SY, Dick JR, Goldspink G, Orrell RW, Greensmith L. Mechano-growth factor, an IGF-I splice variant, rescues motoneurons and improves muscle function in SOD1(G93A) mice. Exp Neurol. 2009;215(2):281–9.
23. Glover EI, Phillips SM. Resistance exercise and appropriate nutrition to counteract muscle wasting and promote muscle hypertrophy. Curr Opin Clin Nutr Metab Care. 2010;13(6):630–4.
24. Phillips GC. Glutamine: the nonessential amino acid for performance enhancement. Curr Sports Med Rep. 2007;6(4):265–8.
25. Tisdale MJ. Cancer cachexia. Curr Opin Gastroenterol. 2010;26(2):146–51.
26. Tisdale MJ. Mechanisms of cancer cachexia. Physiol Rev. 2009;89(2):381–410.
27. Laviano A, Meguid MM, Inui A, Muscaritoli M, Rossi-Fanelli F. Therapy insight: cancer anorexia-cachexia syndrome–when all you can eat is yourself. Nat Clin Pract Oncol. 2005;2(3):158–65.
28. Costelli P, Baccino FM. Mechanisms of skeletal muscle depletion in wasting syndromes: role of ATP-ubiquitin-dependent proteolysis. Curr Opin Clin Nutr Metab Care. 2003;6(4):407–12.
29. Costelli P, Muscaritoli M, Bonetto A, Penna F, Reffo P, Bossola M, et al. Muscle myostatin signalling is enhanced in experimental cancer cachexia. Eur J Clin Invest. 2008;38(7):531–8.
30. Tisdale MJ. Cancer anorexia and cachexia. Nutrition. 2001;17(5):438–42.
31. Gomes-Marcondes MC, Smith HJ, Cooper JC, Tisdale MJ. Development of an in-vitro model system to investigate the mechanism of muscle protein catabolism induced by proteolysis-inducing factor. Br J Cancer. 2002;86(10): 1628–33.
32. Gomes-Marcondes MC, Tisdale MJ. Induction of protein catabolism and the ubiquitin-proteasome pathway by mild oxidative stress. Cancer Lett. 2002;180(1):69–74.
33. Tisdale MJ. Catabolic mediators of cancer cachexia. Curr Opin Support Palliat Care. 2008;2(4):256–61.
34. Yano CL, Ventrucci G, Field WN, Tisdale MJ, Gomes-Marcondes MC. Metabolic and morphological alterations induced by proteolysis-inducing factor from Walker tumour-bearing rats in C2C12 myotubes. BMC Cancer. 2008;8:24.
35. Escalante CP, Kallen MA, Valdres RU, Morrow PK, Manzullo EF. Outcomes of a cancer-related fatigue clinic in a comprehensive cancer center. J Pain Symptom Manage. 2010;39(4):691–701.
36. Ingram C, Wessel J, Courneya KS. Evaluating the benefits of exercise for women receiving adjuvant therapy for breast cancer: research challenges. Can Oncol Nurs J. 2010;20(2):96–8.
37. Argiles JM, Busquets S, Lopez-Soriano FJ, Costelli P, Penna F. Are there any benefits of exercise training in cancer cachexia? J Cachexia Sarcopenia Muscle. 2012;3(2):73–6.
38. Penna F, Busquets S, Pin F, Toledo M, Baccino FM, Lopez-Soriano FJ, et al. Combined approach to counteract experimental cancer cachexia: eicosapentaenoic acid and training exercise. J Cachexia Sarcopenia Muscle. 2011;2(2):95–104.

39. Dimeo F. Exercise for cancer patients: a new challenge in sports medicine. West J Med. 2000;173(4):272–3.
40. Adamsen L, Quist M, Midtgaard J, Andersen C, Moller T, Knutsen L, et al. The effect of a multidimensional exercise intervention on physical capacity, well-being and quality of life in cancer patients undergoing chemotherapy. Support Care Cancer. 2006;14(2):116–27.
41. Toledo M, Busquets S, Sirisi S, Serpe R, Orpi M, Coutinho J, et al. Cancer cachexia: physical activity and muscle force in tumour-bearing rats. Oncol Rep. 2011;25(1):189–93.
42. Bacurau RF, Belmonte MA, Seelaender MC, Costa Rosa LF. Effect of a moderate intensity exercise training protocol on the metabolism of macrophages and lymphocytes of tumour-bearing rats. Cell Biochem Funct. 2000;18(4):249–58.
43. Holecek M. Glutamine and branched-chain amino acids – practical importance of their metabolic relations. Cas Lek Cesk. 2005;144 Suppl 3:9–12.
44. Holecek M. Relation between glutamine, branched-chain amino acids, and protein metabolism. Nutrition. 2002;18(2):130–3.
45. Barbosa AW, Benevides GP, Alferes LM, Salomao EM, Gomes-Marcondes MC, Gomes L. A leucine-rich diet and exercise affect the biomechanical characteristics of the digital flexor tendon in rats after nutritional recovery. Amino Acids. 2012;42(1):329–36.
46. Ventrucci G, Mello MA, Gomes-Marcondes MC. Proteasome activity is altered in skeletal muscle tissue of tumour-bearing rats a leucine-rich diet. Endocr Relat Cancer. 2004;11(4):887–95.
47. Agostini F, Biolo G. Effect of physical activity on glutamine metabolism. Curr Opin Clin Nutr Metab Care. 2010;13(1):58–64.
48. Cruzat VF, Rogero MM, Tirapegui J. Effects of supplementation with free glutamine and the dipeptide alanyl-glutamine on parameters of muscle damage and inflammation in rats submitted to prolonged exercise. Cell Biochem Funct. 2010;28(1):24–30.
49. dos Santos RV, Caperuto EC, de Mello MT, Batista Jr ML, Rosa LF. Effect of exercise on glutamine synthesis and transport in skeletal muscle from rats. Clin Exp Pharmacol Physiol. 2009;36(8):770–5.
50. Salomao EM, Gomes-Marcondes MC. Light aerobic physical exercise in combination with leucine and/or glutamine-rich diet can improve the body composition and muscle protein metabolism in young tumor-bearing rats. J Physiol Biochem. 2012;68(4):493–501.
51. Bruce M, Constantin-Teodosiu D, Greenhaff PL, Boobis LH, Williams C, Bowtell JL. Glutamine supplementation promotes anaplerosis but not oxidative energy delivery in human skeletal muscle. Am J Physiol Endocrinol Metab. 2001;280(4):E669–75.
52. Rowbottom DG, Keast D, Morton AR. The emerging role of glutamine as an indicator of exercise stress and overtraining. Sports Med. 1996;21(2):80–97.
53. Paccagnella A, Morassutti I, Rosti G. Nutritional intervention for improving treatment tolerance in cancer patients. Curr Opin Oncol. 2011;23(4):322–30.

Chapter 38
Glutamine and Skeletal Muscle

Julio Tirapegui and Vinicius Fernandes Cruzat

Key Points

- Conditional essential amino acids are a group of amino acids naturally produced in the body, although during catabolism processes the consumption and utilization of these amino acids exceed the synthesis capacity, given exogenous supply.
- Glutamine is one of the most important amino acids of the intermediate metabolism during the catabolism process, especially to muscle cells.
- Oxidative damage leads to the activation of the inflammatory process contributing to the catabolism of muscle mass by oxidative stress, activating heat shock proteins (HSPs) and lowering glutamine–glutathione (GSH) axis.
- Free amino acids or dipeptides supply, like exogenous L-glutamine or L-alanyl–L-glutamine, are important nutritional solutions to attenuate the lower availability of glutamine in the body.
- The differences of the effects in skeletal muscle of free and dipeptides forms of L-glutamine still remain to be clarified.

Keywords Amino acids • Glutathione • Glutamate • Heat shock proteins • Supplementation

Abbreviations

BCAA	Branched chain amino acids
CNS	Central nervous system
GLS	Glutaminase
GLUD	Glutamate dehydrogenase
GS	Glutamine synthetase
GSH	Glutathione
GSRd	Glutathione disulphide reductase
HSP	Heat shock proteins
HSPs	Heat shock proteins

J. Tirapegui, Ph.D. (✉) • V.F. Cruzat
Department of Food Science and Experimental Nutrition, Faculty of Pharmaceutical Sciences, University of São Paulo, Av. Professor Lineu Prestes, 580, Bloco 14, São Paulo, SP 05508-900, Brazil
e-mail: tirapegu@usp.br; vinifc@usp.br

R. Rajendram et al. (eds.), *Glutamine in Clinical Nutrition*, Nutrition and Health,
DOI 10.1007/978-1-4939-1932-1_38, © Springer Science+Business Media New York 2015

JNK	Janus kinase
MAPK	p38 Mitogen-activated protein kinase
NFkB	Nuclear factor kappa-B
NH_3	Ammonia
NH_4^+	Ammonium ion
NO	Nitric oxide
PgE_2	Prostaglandin E_2
PKC	Protein kinase C
TNF-α	Tumor necrosis factor alpha

Introduction

Of the group of 20 amino acids which covalently bonded in linear sequences to form all proteins from the oldest bacteria to the most complex forms of life, glutamine deserves special attention. For many mammals, including human beings, glutamine, especially intermediate metabolism of amino acids of muscle cells, is the most abundant free amino acid in the body and is important in many cell types, playing an important role in a number of essential functions. In high catabolism conditions, such as diseases and exhausting exercise, the synthesis of glutamine does not supply the needs demanded by the organism. In this process, one of the most important sites of glutamine synthesis is the skeletal muscle, not for its synthesis capacity per se, but because it represents at least 40 % of total bodily mass. Furthermore, studies demonstrate, by means of molecular biology, that glutamine can also influence a number of cell signaling pathways, specially the heat shock proteins (HSPs) expression response and the antioxidant system, mainly mediated by glutathione (GSH). As it is a conditionally essential amino acid, science has been searching for exogenous forms for its replacement, mainly focusing on attenuating the reduction of muscle stores of glutamine in areas ranging from the clinic to sports. The present chapter shows and discusses aspects of glutamine metabolism in the skeletal muscle tissue as well as its supplementation and possible benefits in catabolic situations in healthy patients and recovery from disease.

Glutamine Metabolism and Functions in Skeletal Muscle

The first scientific reports to consider glutamine as molecule with biologically important properties date back to the eighteenth century. Hlaziwetz and Habermann, Schulze and Bosshard, and Damodaran and his collaborators significantly contributed to the description and understanding of glutamine metabolism. However, only after the work of Sir Hans Krebs, who in 1935 showed the cell capacity for synthesizing or degrading glutamine, did a number of researchers show greater interest in this part of metabolism.

After World War II, studies by Eagle showed that glutamine is important for cell growth and maintenance. In culture, cells utilize glutamine in quantities greater than any other amino acid [1]. This fact had been already verified by Eagle et al. who observed the structural degeneration of isolated fibroblasts of mice cultivated in conditions deprived of glutamine, followed by cell death. Other works with diverse types of cells, such as lymphocytes, macrophages, enterocytes and HeLa cells showed that cell development can be increased and cell structures and functions can be maintained in cultures containing glutamine. In every cell, glutamine can donate nitrogen atoms to the synthesis of purines, pyrimidines and amino sugars [2]. Such results show the importance of glutamine for a large number of metabolic pathways and these mechanisms, depending on glutamine, have been called glutaminolithic pathways.

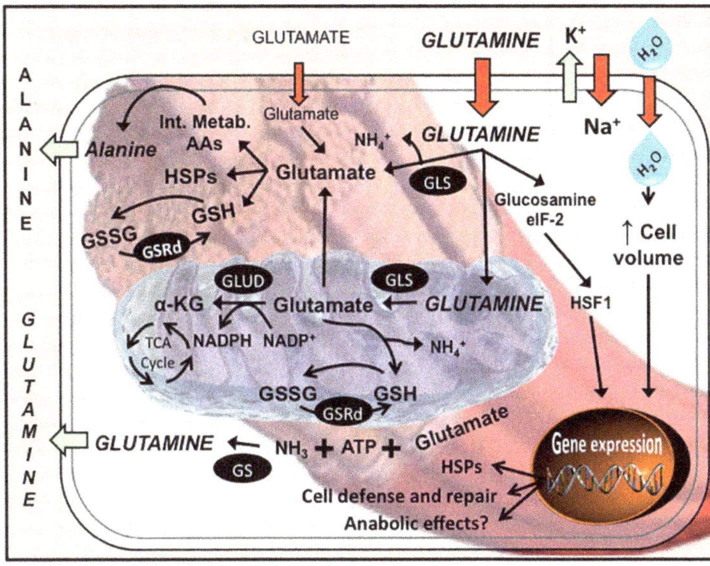

Fig. 38.1 Glutamine metabolism in skeletal muscle cells. From glutamine, glutamate is produced through glutaminase activity (GLS), releasing ammonium ion (NH_4^+). Inside mitochondria or in the cytosol, glutamate is an important precursor for the synthesis of the intermediate metabolism of amino acids, such as alanine, antioxidant defenses, such as glutathione (GSH) and cell repair, such as heat shock proteins (HSP). Cells, especially muscle cells, can synthesize glutamine through glutamine synthetase (GS), using glutamate, ATP and ammonia (NH_3). Glutamine is transported inside the cell through active transport with sodium (Na^+) potassium (K^+) ATPase, which increases the absorption of water, altering the volume of the cell, stimulating the resistance to damage, and can also serve as anabolic stimuli

Individuals considered healthy, weighing about 70 kg show an amount of 70–80 g of glutamine, distributed in a number of body tissues. In blood, glutamine concentration is about 500–700 µmol/L. Whether it is in tissue or in blood, glutamine concentration can suffer influence in accordance with the activity of enzymes involved in the glutamine metabolism, namely, glutaminase (GLS, EC 3.5.1.2) and glutamine synthetase (GS, EC 6.3.1.2). There are a number of enzymes that are found in the glutamine metabolism; however, starting from the availability of glutamate and ATP, glutamine synthetase promotes glutamine synthesis, as it is an endergonic reaction of $\Delta G<0$. It is important to note that glutamate is synthesized from alpha-ketoglutarate and ammonia (NH_3). Glutamine hydrolysis occurs by means of the glutaminase enzyme, releasing the ammonium ion (NH_4) [3] (Fig. 38.1).

Some types of cells, such as the immune system cells, the kidneys and the intestine, show a higher use of glutamine, by means of glutaminase enzyme, and are therefore considered predominantly glutamine consuming tissues. Glutaminase is seen in a number of metabolic processes and can be found in bacteria, plants and animals. In mammalians, glutaminase can be found in two isoforms: one (less frequent) in the liver and the other in all other tissues, such as the kidneys, the brain, leucocytes and the intestinal tract [4]. However, its more active form mainly appears in the mitochondria [3]. On the other hand, the skeletal muscles, the lungs, the liver, the brain and fat tissues have a higher capacity for glutamine synthesizing by means of the glutamine synthetase enzyme, and therefore are predominantly considered glutamine synthesizing tissues (Fig. 38.2a). As the organism can synthesize glutamine, it is nutritionally classified as a non-essential or dispensable amino acid. This classification, however, depends on body homeostasis and if we consider the glutamine compounds family, in catabolic situations such as sepsis, infections [5], surgeries, trauma [6], and intense and prolonged physical exercise [7], the glutamine synthesis does not supply the needs required by the organism (Fig. 38.2b).

The liver is the tissue that exhibits the highest capacity for glutamine synthesis. However, quantitatively, the main tissue for glutamine synthesis, storage and release is the skeletal muscle. Actually, this is not due to a high glutamine synthetase activity per se, but to the capacity of metabolizing amino

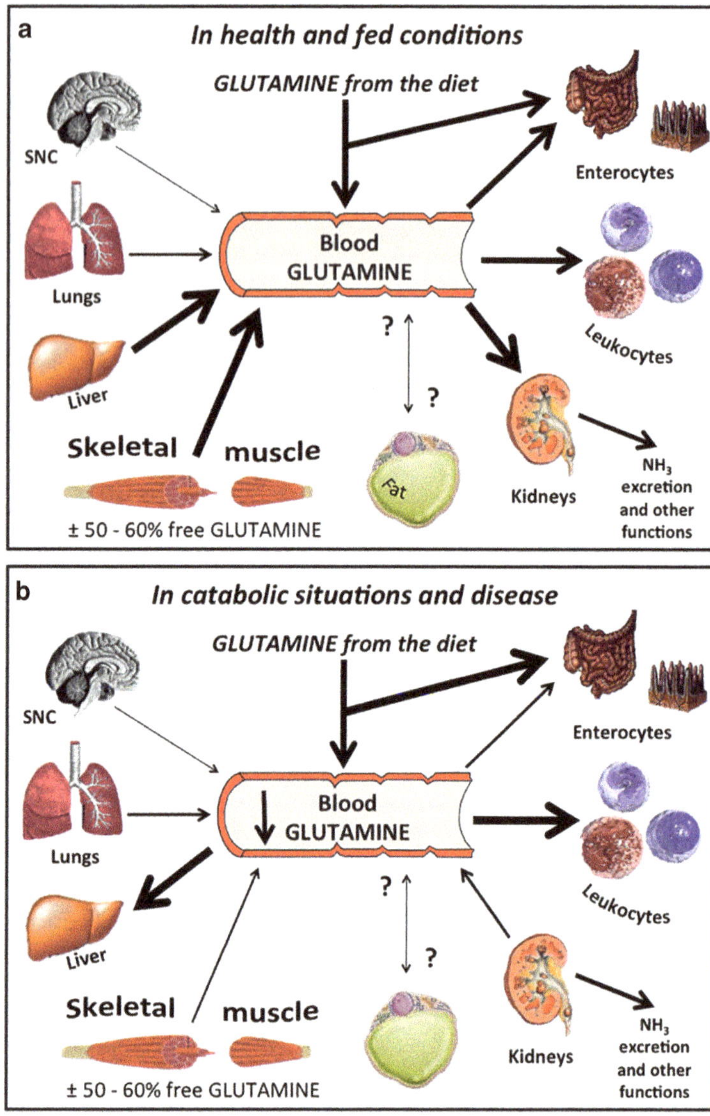

Fig. 38.2 Predominance (*thick arrows*) in the synthesis and degradation of glutamine in various tissues and organs in a healthy or fed state (**a**), and catabolic situations or disease (**b**). *CNS* central nervous system, NH_3 ammonia, *GLN* glutamine. Adapted from [11]

acids of the branched chain amino acids, which contributes to the glutamine metabolism [8], and because this tissue represents an average of 40 % of the total bodily mass [3]. The BCAA are predominantly metabolized on the skeletal muscle tissue, which means that they are outside the liver metabolism, quickly increasing their plasma concentration after ingestion. In the intermediary metabolism of amino acids, the BCAA play an important role through transamination as an energy source or for the synthesis of other amino acids. This is the case of the glutamine synthesis, which can be synthesized in the skeletal muscle from the BCAA by branched chain amino acids aminotransferase. Studies demonstrate that BCAA can be transaminated, releasing α-ketoglutarate and glutamate, which can supply its amino group to pyruvate, generating alanine or incorporate free ammonia, for de novo synthesis of glutamine (Fig. 38.3).

The glutamine synthesis ratio in the skeletal muscle is approximately 50 mmol/h, higher than any other amino acid [2]. During the catabolism process, a number of organs and tissues such as the immune system cells and liver show a high demand for glutamine, and the skeletal muscle tissue

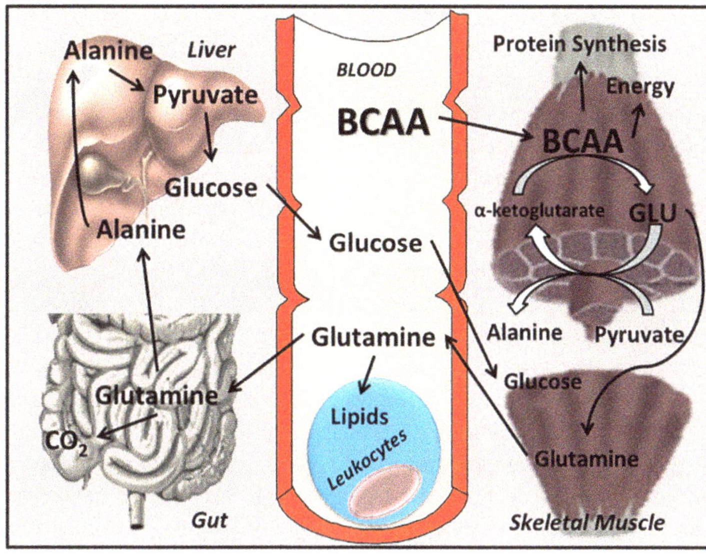

Fig. 38.3 The glutamine metabolism in skeletal muscles, and its relationship with intermediate metabolism of amino acids. *BCAA* branched chain amino acids, *GLU* glutamate

Table 38.1 Concentration of alanine, glutamine and glutamate, and the type of fibers predominant in skeletal muscles at rest

	Skeletal muscle tissues		
Amino acids	Vastus lateralis (human)	Gastrocnemius (mouse)	Soleus (mouse)
Alanine (μmol/g fresh tissue)	1.7–3.2	0.8–2.7	1.1–2.3
Glutamine (μmol/g fresh tissue)	12.8–18.2	2.6–5.2	7.8–17.3
Glutamate (μmol/g fresh tissue)	2.3–4.8	0.8–2.1	3.6–11.0

Adapted from [13]

becomes an important site for the synthesis and release of this amino acid. Additionally, in catabolic situations [6], an intense muscle proteolysis is observed, and a number of tissues begin to depend on the ability of the skeletal muscle to supply the organism glutamine needs through the plasma [3]. This effect can contribute to the disequilibrium of the intermediary metabolism, with the loss of homeostasis in the kidneys, intestine and lymphoid organs as the glutamine synthesis and degradation capacity represent an important form of metabolic interaction [9]. Additionally, glutamine serves as an important energetic and metabolic substrate, acting as a major respiratory fuel, gluconeogenic precursor, and carrier of nitrogen [4].

While in plasma the glutamine concentration is about 20 % of the total free amino acids, in skeletal muscle this percentage is about 40–60 %. The predominance of the muscle fiber type can influence the glutamine synthesis [10]. According to Table 38.1, type 1 fibers have about three times more glutamine storage that type 2 fibers [10, 11]. This fact is attributed to a higher activity of glutamine synthetase and to the higher availability of ATP for glutamine synthesis. Depending on the muscle under study, when the de novo synthesis of glutamine is inhibited, the intramuscular storages can be depleted in about 7 h. The synthesis of glutamine in the skeletal muscle, during the post-absorptive state, can occur through the availability and uptake of glutamate from the blood circulation. Glutamate is responsible for 40 % of the glutamine synthesis, and, compared to other amino acids, is the most abundant intracellular amino acid (reported concentrations vary between 2 and 20 mM), and glutamine is the most abundant extracellular amino acid in vivo (0.7 mM compared to an approximate L-glutamate concentration of 20 μM) [9, 12]. L-glutamate cannot readily cross the cell wall of skeletal muscles because it has an overall charge of −1 at pH 7.4, and the amino acid transporter is able to transport glutamate into the cell, present at low density in the plasma membrane [9]. Hence, in order to increase glutamine concentration in skeletal muscles and the availability of glutamate in these tissues, glutamate cannot be replaced by glutamic acid, but rather must be in the form of glutamine supplementation. It is important to note that in the skeletal muscles of mammalian species the quantities of amino acids other than glutamine and glutamate, such as alanine and glycine, are high [12] (Table 38.1).

Hormones like insulin and insulin growth factors (IGFs) stimulate glutamine transport to the intracellular medium, whereas glucocorticoids stimulate the release of glutamine to the extracellular medium [12]. The transmembrane gradient for glutamine through the skeletal muscle is high, while its diffusion through the cell membrane is restricted. In this way, glutamine needs to be transported in an active form to inside the cells, through a sodium-dependent channel system (Fig. 38.1), whose outcome is a consumption of ATP. Additionally, it is important to remark that the transport of glutamine through the cell membrane is faster than all the other 20 amino acids [14].

When transported inside the cell, glutamine simultaneously promotes the absorption of water and the release of potassium (K^+), which increases the cell hydration state and influences its volume (Fig. 38.1) [15]. The increase in cell volume can stimulate the protein synthesis, which is considered an anabolic signal or resistance to injury [11, 15]. During intense exercise, for example, the skeletal muscle fibers volume changes rapidly, and must return to its normal value during recovery. It is likely that membrane depolarization contributes to cell swelling during exercise, and the acidification accompanying intracellular lactate production acts to preserve cell volume and resistance to damage [15].

The lower glutamine availability in the organism impairs the intracellular supply of glutamate to the synthesis of the most important and more concentrated non-enzymatic antioxidant in the cell, the γ-L-glutamyl–L-cysteinylglycine (GSH). Made up of cysteine residues, glutamic acid and glycine, GSH is found in high concentrations in cells and can directly react with reactive oxygen species (ROS) in non-enzymatic reactions, as well as acting as an electron donor in the peroxide reduction, catalyzed by glutathione peroxidase enzyme (GPx) [6, 7].

During catabolic states, which include diseases such as sepsis and exhausting physical exercises, an elevated oxidative stress can be observed as the intracellular redox state is raised. This shift can be obtained from the ratio between the intracellular concentration of glutathione disulfide (GSSG) and GSH, which is the ratio [GSSG]/[GSH], resulting in a reduction of GSH and an increase in the amounts of GSSG [16]. The redox state of the cells is consequently related to GSH concentrations, which are also influenced by the availability of amino acids. A higher glutamine/glutamate ratio reinforces the substrates availability for GSH. This mechanism can be seen by observing the GSH metabolism in red blood cells and, hepatic and muscle cells. The effects or consequences of oxidative stress are shown in Fig. 38.4.

According to the cell type and the mechanism involved, GSH has high concentration, protecting the cell's membrane, maintaining the concentration of a number of proteins and its sulfhydryl group (–SH) in the reduced form, which are necessary for the antioxidant synthesis. In this way, deficiencies in the GSH synthesis in animal cells have very serious consequences, such as, for instance, the lyse of erythrocytes [17].

Quantitatively, the liver is the main organ for the de novo synthesis of GSH, being responsible for nearly 90 % of the circulating GSH in physiological conditions. The elevated concentration of hepatic GSH is mainly due to the high activity of glutathione reductase in this tissue. In the liver, the presence of compounds that are transformed into mercapturic acids, such as paracetamol, diminishes the GSH concentration, and consequently, the liver's ability to eliminate peroxides by the action of GPx is also reduced. In this way, the generation of large quantities of hydrogen peroxide by the cells can promote high amounts of oxidized glutathione (GSSG). The GSH self-oxidation can also be catalyzed by iron and copper ions, leading to the formation of the tiil radical as an intermediary and further generation of GSSG, the superoxide radical ($O_2^{\cdot -}$), hydroxyl radical ($OH^{\cdot}$) and hydrogen peroxide (H_2O_2). Other important oxygen and nitrogen reactive species are shown in Table 38.2.

In catabolic situations, the liver, under hormonal influence, exports GSH to the plasma, especially through glucagon, vasopressin and catecholamines. The muscle tissue is responsible for the increased

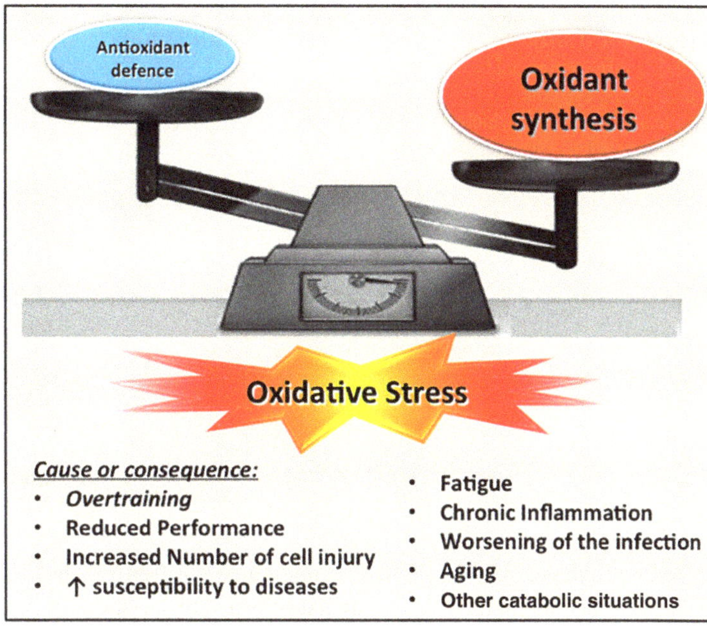

Fig. 38.4 In some cases, excess of oxidative stress affects health and many other parameters in athletes

Table 38.2 Important oxygen and nitrogen reactive species

	Name	Symbol
Free radicals	Superoxide anion	$O_2^{\cdot -}$
	Hydroxyl radical	$OH^{\cdot}$
	Alkoxyl	$RO^{\cdot}/LO^{\cdot}$
	Peroxyl	$ROO^{\cdot}/LOO^{\cdot}$
	Hydroperoxyl radical	$HO_2^{\cdot}$
	Nitric oxide	$NO^{\cdot}$
	Nitric dioxide	$NO_2^{\cdot}$
Not radical compounds	Hydrogen peroxide	H_2O_2
	Hypochlorous acid	HOCL
	Ozone	O_3
	Singlet oxygen	$^1DO_2$
	Lipid peroxides	LOOH
	Peroxynitrite	ONOOH

capture of GSH from plasma, mainly with the function of the compensation of the increased production of ROS. However, the GSH synthesis depends on the cysteine and glycine concentrations, and mainly on glutamate (Fig. 38.5), which represents the first and probably the most important step in the synthesis of integrating GSH compounds, and is dependent on the availability and transport of glutamine to inside the cell.

Glutathione depletion in skeletal muscle can increase caspase-independent signaling, as well as increasing mitochondrial-associated apoptotic events to subsequent cell death stimuli [18]. It is important to notice that alternatives to increase the GSH concentration through its supplementation or even glutamate, are not effective and can be toxic, sometimes accelerating the cell senescence process [19]. A number of studies demonstrate that glutamine supplementations can represent an effective option when the increase of the availability of GSH in the organism is required [7, 20]. Furthermore, is important to note that gradual stimuli, such physical activity stimulates per se the *hormesis* and adaptation of the organism, stimulating the antioxidant mechanism [19, 21, 22].

On the other hand, the importance of glutamine for the induction of heat shock proteins (HSPs) response, specifically HSP-70, is well-documented [23]. HSPs are a family of polypeptides clustered

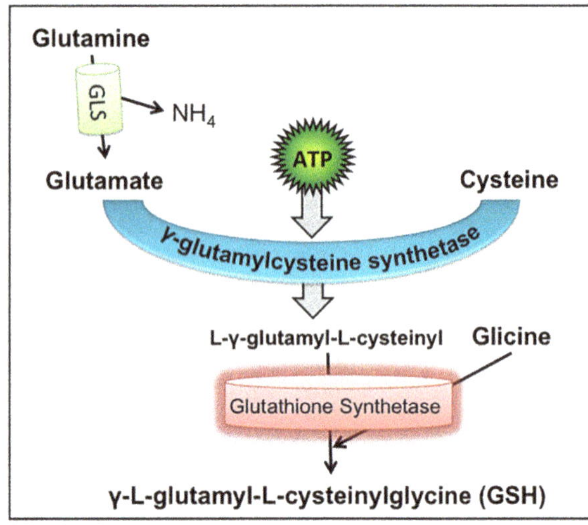

Fig. 38.5 Route of synthesis of glutathione (GSH) involving three amino acids as precursors, cysteine, glycine and glutamate, which can be donated by the hydrolysis of glutamine

according to molecular weight, whose main inductor factor is the occurrence of denatured proteins in the intracellular medium. This mainly happens due to variations in body temperature, the inflammatory process, and oxidative stress. The first report on them was documented in the salivary gland cells of *Drosophila buskii* after a serendipitous heat shock by Ritossa in 1962 [24]. At lower temperatures, genes decrease the strength of these proteins. Thus these proteins, described in 1974, were denominated temperature-sensitive; in other words, thermal or heat shock proteins [24].

Actually, HSPs could also be more properly called stress-sensitive proteins, as further studies by Ritossa showed that a number of agents or metabolic stressing conditions stimulate the HSPs. Being stress-sensitive, various events such as exposition to heavy metals, UV radiation, amino acid analogs, bacterial or viral infections, inflammation, cyclooxygenase inhibitors (including acetylsalicylic acid), oxidative stress, cytostatic drugs (anti-cancer), growth factors, cell development and differentiation can induce the expression of HSPs [24]. All of these factors strongly activate the transcription of the main thermal shock eukaryotic factor (heath shock factor—HSF-1), leading to the expression of HSP-70 [25].

HSF-1 is a transcriptional factor found in its inactive form not bonded to DNA, and its activation occurs as a result of a number of stress stimuli that trigger inactive latent monomers phosphorylation of this transcriptional factor, found in the cytoplasm of the cells. As phosphorylated, these monomers combine and form a homotrimer. The HSF-1 homotrimers, being activated, migrate to the nucleus of the cell and bond to specific sites of the promoting region of the HSP genes, denominated thermal shock elements (HSEs). This mechanism allows specific signs to initiate the process of synthesis, transcription and translation of RNAm of the HSPs. The higher rate of HSPs has been related to a stronger resistance of cells to death under stress challenging situations [26]. Glutamine is an important stimulus for HSP-70, and the reduction of the concentration of glutamine in the body may contribute to cell death. This relation is not dependent and may still be controversial, especially in skeletal muscle cells [27, 28].

Supplementation of Glutamine: Effects on Skeletal Muscle

In vitro studies with various cell types, such as muscle cells, intestinal mucosa, the immune system, and specific neurons of the central nervous system, hepatocytes, β cells, among others, have demonstrated that glutamine, when added to a culture medium, can alter a variety of cell functions [14, 29].

Table 38.3 Common types of glutamine supplements available on sports market or hospital solutions

Name	Form	Most common utilization
L-Glutamine	Free	Oral solution
L-Alanyl–L-glutamine	Dipeptide	Parenteral solution
L-Glycyl–L-glutamine	Dipeptide	Parenteral solution
L-Arginyl–L-glutamine	Dipeptide	Parenteral solution

Whether it is to transport ammonia between tissues, to contribute to the intermediary metabolism or gluconeogenesis, it is difficult to imagine the survival, maintenance and proliferation of cells without the participation of glutamine.

As glutamine is a conditionally essential amino acid, science aims to study the possible effects of exogenous replacement with L-glutamine through supplementation. The exogenous administration of L-glutamine is usually made by utilizing its free form, as an isolated amino acid. Another very common form is the supplementation of L-glutamine together with another amino acid, usually the dipeptide L-alanyl–L-glutamine.

The effects of the utilization of L-glutamine in dipeptide form on glutamine availability has been attributed to the fact that enterocytes have a more efficient transport mechanism for the absorption of dipeptides and tripeptides than for the absorption of free amino acids. The glycopeptide transport protein (PepT-1), which is located in the luminal membrane of the jejunum, followed by the ileum, has a broad substrate specificity and actively transports dipeptides and tripeptides from the diet into the intestines of humans and animals [30, 31]. Research utilizing radioactively labeled glutamine dipeptides has shown that nearly 90 % of the radioactivity accumulates intact in the cytosol. In this manner, glutamine can avoid intracellular hydrolysis and subsequent metabolism by enterocytes, proceeding directly to systemic circulation [32, 33]. On the other hand, rates above 50 % of total free L-glutamine absorbed from the small intestine are subsequently metabolized in this tissue and the liver, weakly contributing to the muscle cells or even the immune system. Parenteral solutions seem to be more effective than oral or enteral solutions when the maintenance of glutamine concentration in the body is desired. The most common glutamine solutions available are cited in Table 38.3.

Research on the transport and utilization of glutamine in the small intestine is very important when the dietitian desires muscle and systemic effects of L-glutamine supplementation. The importance of L-glutamine supplementation is well-documented in diverse post-surgical patients submitted to total parenteral nutrition (TPN), to which L-glutamine was added, either in free form or as a dipeptide form. Certain studies show that the supplementation of L-glutamine in parenteral nutrition enhanced the clinical conditions of individuals with transplanted bone marrow [34], cutting the reduction of GSH [6], diminishing muscular atrophy during the metabolic stress of surgery, reducing the rate of hospital infection [35], and improving the nitrogen balance, thereby lowering the overall hospital costs. Most of these studies with postoperative patients show that a daily i.v. or TPN L-glutamine dosage (20–30 g) or 0.3–0.5 g/kg body weight can reduce the dramatic decrease in glutaminemia and glutamine in tissues such as skeletal muscles [36]. Additionally, in i.v. or TPN, L-glutamine is typically given as a dipeptide, L-alanyl–L-glutamine, which can be found in commercial product in concentration of 200 g/L, with an osmolality <900 mOsm. In this sense, parenteral solutions seem to be more effective than oral or enteral solutions, when the maintenance of glutamine concentration in the body is desired [36]. However, these solutions are very invasive and may expose the patient to increased risk of infections, so that, as far as possible, enteral alternatives should be chosen. Moreover, enteral routes are much more physiological and provide the physiological generation of other amino acid derivatives (e.g. citrulline and arginine), which can only be accounted for if L-glutamine is given enterally [37]. Thus L-glutamine has become an effective supplement in clinical nutrition, especially parenteral nutrition.

However, the same utilization as a nutritional supplement for sports or enteral nutrition has raised many doubts and controversies [32].

The muscle glutamine metabolism can be altered in a number of catabolic conditions, including cancer, sepsis, diabetes, prolonged or exhausting physical exercise [38]. Serious muscle damage and catabolism lead to the activation of local and acute inflammatory response [33]. These processes increase the cell consumption of glutamine, promoting the imbalance of the synthesis and degradation of this amino acid [14]. The lower concentration of ATP and glutamate in skeletal muscles under catabolic stimuli can also inhibit the action of the key enzyme for glutamine synthesis, glutamine synthetase. This avoids the removal of ammonia in the form of glutamine. Ammonia can be toxic to the cells promoting cell apoptosis and hyperammonemia [39]. The reduction of the glutamine concentration and the higher inflammatory response increase the protein breakdown, which can reduce the cell antioxidant concentration and promote immunosuppression [38].

Interestingly, in other catabolic situations, such as diabetes, a disease essentially related to the concentrations of glucose and lipids, little is known about the alterations in the concentration of amino acids, the metabolism and the eventual effects of in vivo supplementation [40]. In a recent study, the concentration of glutamine in patients diagnosed for type 2 diabetes showed a significant reduction (20 %), when compared to healthy individuals [41]. Besides glutamine, arginine amino acid also showed low plasma concentration in type 2 diabetic individuals [41].

As glutamine can be transaminated and converted into arginine, its reduction in the organism has an effect on the intermediary metabolism of the arginine, which is a precursor of nitric oxide (NO), a free radical essential for the signaling in intracellular molecules, which is responsible for the regulation of blood flux, arterial pressure and function of cells in the immune system. In a study with type 2 diabetic subjects, the concentration of nitric oxide metabolites (e.g. nitrite and nitrate) was reduced in the skeletal muscle, which could be related to the worsening of the resistance to insulin [42]. Hyperglycemia and the high concentration of free fatty acids induce the activation of signaling pathways to stress and pro-inflammatory sensitive proteins, which alters the secretion and action of insulin, aggravating diabetes type 2. Among the intracellular signaling pathways involved in this process, the pathways of Nuclear Factor Kappa-B (NFkB), p38 Mitogen-Activated Protein Kinase (MAPK), Janus Kinase (JNK) and Protein Kinase C (PKC) are included. More recently, mechanisms such the expression of HSPs and their relation to intra- and extracellular concentration, can be involved in the pathogenesis development of type 2 diabetes [43].

The supplementation with L-glutamine has been studied with the aim of reducing the catabolic effects associated with the reduction of glutamine concentration in humans and in animal models. However, the efficacy of this oral nutritional intervention is frequently questioned due to the high metabolization of glutamine by the small intestine, and the alternative to break through the intestinal barrier has been the utilization of L-alanyl–L-glutamine.

Studies in animal models with acute oral L-glutamine supplementation, in free form or as a dipeptide, demonstrate an increase in the plasmatic glutamine concentration between 30 and 120 min after supplementation [44]. The concentration and the area under the curve of the dipeptide acutely supplemented group was 26 % superior to the free L-glutamine supplemented group, 30 min after the supplementation [44]. This result can be explained by the higher presence of the peptide transporter 1 (Pept-1), which actively transports dipeptides inside the enterocytes and intracytoplasmatic dipeptidases, which increase the release of glutamine and alanine deriving from acute supplementation with L-alanyl–L-glutamine, and consequently promotes a higher release into the circulation. The same study shows a higher liver and muscle glutamine concentration after the chronic supplementation with L-alanyl–L-glutamine. In another study, animals submitted to exhausting physical exercise and chronic supplementation with L-alanyl–L-glutamine demonstrated that the nutritional intervention may attenuate the reduction of glutamine concentration in soleus and gastrocnemius muscles immediately and 1 h after the exhausting exercise [32].

However, the hypothesis that the dipeptide composition could affect its more efficient absorption and further release into blood was not tested. It was observed that supplementation with the L-alanyl–L-glutamine dipeptide and a solution containing L-glutamine and L-alanine, both in free form, in rats submitted to training and long duration exercises, was able to increase the hepatic and muscular concentration of glutamine and glutamate, which in turn increased the tissue concentration of GSH antioxidant, attenuating the oxidative stress induced by long duration physical exercise [7]. In another study, the same supplementations reduced the release of creatine kinase and pro-inflammatory cytokines, such as tumor necrosis factor alpha (TNF-α) and prostaglandin E_2 (PgE_2), in trained animals submitted to exhausting exercise [33].

Under catabolic stimuli, active muscles release alanine and glutamine into the circulation (60 % of the overall amino acid delivery into the blood). Alanine can be synthesized from pyruvate with nitrogen, and glutamine from ammonia production with glutamate and ATP [45, 46]. These events are important mechanisms for cell defense and survival, trying to maintain homeostasis. Both amino acids are important and can alter the intermediate metabolism during and after the catabolic process in skeletal muscle. Nutritional solutions with glutamine supplementations (dipeptide vs. free amino acids) are important when the effects on skeletal muscle and other tissues than the gut are considered; however, results from pancreatic β cells (which are also tightly dependent on alanine and glutamine metabolism) shed light on another possible mechanism explanation. Accordingly, L-alanine oxidation was required for the synergistic effect on glucose-stimulated insulin secretion and was also accompanied by an increase in intracellular glutamate concentration [2], while glutamine is important for β-cell viability and function [46, 47]. Furthermore, alanine may protect cells from apoptosis induced by pro-inflammatory cytokines (the same observed in endotoxemic states), by enhancing antioxidant defenses [47]. In another study, subjects were supplemented with L-glutamine in the free form and as dipeptide form (L-alanyl–L-glutamine) or free L-glutamine from wheat protein. The results showed a greater increase in glutaminemia with L-alanyl–L-glutamine and free L-glutamine from wheat protein, compared to controls and free L-glutamine alone [48].

Orally taken together, free L-glutamine *plus* L-alanine supplementation seems to have similar metabolic effects when compared to L-alanyl–L-glutamine dipeptide, and either form could be utilized in clinical and sports nutrition, although certain controversies still remain, especially regarding the mechanisms involved in this process.

Conclusions

Glutamine is a conditional essential amino acid which is important for many cells and their functions, especially the recovery of muscle cells and survival of diseases. If there is insufficient glutamine available in the body, the exogenous supply is needed to enhance cell defenses and prevent apoptosis or excess of inflammation, but many questions on the type of supplementation of glutamine when given orally can be discussed. In clinical nutrition, physicians and dietitians may use glutamine in i.v. or TPN solutions, and the efficacy of this nutritional intervention is clearly important for the intermediate metabolism of amino acids and the recovery of the patient. However, in sports nutrition glutamine supplementation should be provided only when really necessary, especially for non-professional athletes. The standard dosage of L-glutamine supplementation is 20–30 g per day or 0.3–0.5 g/kg body weight, although the frequency of this nutritional intervention needs to be observed and controlled. Based on the literature in the area, the total amount of L-glutamine per day may be divided to more than one single dosage, observing the kinetics of glutamine in plasma. The exact frequency and other questions, like the efficacy of administration together with other amino acids, need to be studied. It is important to note that L-glutamine supplementation may not prevent the inflammatory response and muscle damage or enhance performance, but may help the recovery of cells, including skeletal muscle.

References

1. Curi R, Lagranha CJ, Doi SQ, Sellitti DF, Procopio J, Pithon-Curi TC. Glutamine-dependent changes in gene expression and protein activity. Cell Biochem Funct. 2005;23:77–84.
2. Newsholme P, Procopio J, Lima MMR, Pithon-Curi TC, Curi R. Glutamine and glutamate – their central role in cell metabolism and function. Cell Biochem Funct. 2003;21:1–9.
3. Neu J, Shenoy V, Chakrabarti R. Glutamine nutrition and metabolism: where do we go from here? FASEB J. 1996;10:829–37.
4. Labow BI, Souba WW, Abcouwer SF. Mechanisms governing the expression of the enzymes of glutamine metabolism–glutaminase and glutamine synthetase. J Nutr. 2001;131 Suppl 9:2467S–74.
5. Rogero MM, Borelli P, Vinolo MA, Fock RA, Pires ISD, Tirapegui J. Dietary glutamine supplementation affects macrophage function, hematopoiesis and nutritional status in early weaned mice. Clin Nutr. 2008;27:386–97.
6. Flaring UB, Rooyackers OE, Wernerman J, Hammarqvist F. Glutamine attenuates post-traumatic glutathione depletion in human muscle. Clin Sci. 2003;104:275–82.
7. Cruzat VF, Tirapegui J. Effects of oral supplementation with glutamine and alanyl-glutamine on glutamine, glutamate, and glutathione status in trained rats and subjected to long-duration exercise. Nutrition. 2009;25:428–35.
8. Shimomura Y, Murakami T, Nakai N, Nagasaki M, Harris RA. Exercise promotes BCAA catabolism: effects of BCAA supplementation on skeletal muscle during exercise. J Nutr. 2004;134:1583S–7.
9. Newsholme P, Lima MMR, Porcopio J, et al. Glutamine and glutamate as vital metabolites. Braz J Med Biol Res. 2003;36:153–63.
10. Walsh NP, Blannin AK, Clark AM, Cook L, Robson PJ, Gleeson M. The effects of high-intensity intermittent exercise on the plasma concentrations of glutamine and organic acids. Eur J Appl Physiol Occup Physiol. 1998;77:434–8.
11. Rowbottom DG, Keast D, Morton AR. The emerging role of glutamine as an indicator of exercise stress and overtraining. Sports Med. 1996;21:80–97.
12. Manso Filho HC, McKeever KH, Gordon ME, et al. Developmental changes in the concentrations of glutamine and other amino acids in plasma and skeletal muscle of the standard bred foal. J Anim Sci. 2009;87:2528–35.
13. Graham TE, MacLean DA. Ammonia and amino acid metabolism in skeletal muscle: human, rodent and canine models. Med Sci Sports Exerc. 1998;30:34–46.
14. Curi R, Newsholme P, Procopio J, Lagranha C, Gorjao R, Pithon-Curi TC. Glutamine, gene expression, and cell function. Front Biosci. 2007;12:344–57.
15. Usher-Smith JA, Huang CLH, Fraser JA. Control of cell volume in skeletal muscle. Biol Rev. 2009;84:143–59.
16. Galley HF. Oxidative stress and mitochondrial dysfunction in sepsis. Br J Anaesth. 2011;107:57–64.
17. Whillier S, Garcia B, Chapman BE, Kuchel PW, Raftos JE. Glutamine and alpha-ketoglutarate as glutamate sources for glutathione synthesis in human erythrocytes. FEBS J. 2011;278:3152–63.
18. Dam A, Mitchell A, Rush JE, Quadrilatero J. Elevated skeletal muscle apoptotic signaling following glutathione depletion. Apoptosis. 2012;17:48–60.
19. Finkel T, Holbrook NJ. Oxidants, oxidative stress and the biology of ageing. Nature. 2000;408:239–47.
20. Cruzat VF, Rogero MM, Ou AK, Pires ISO, Tirapegui J. Effect of alanyl-glutamine supplementation on muscle damage in rats submitted to exhaustive exercise. Ann Nutr Metab. 2007;51:386–7.
21. Lamb GD, Westerblad H. Acute effects of reactive oxygen and nitrogen species on the contractile function of skeletal muscle. J Physiol. 2011;589:2119–27.
22. Powers SK, Talbert EE, Adhihetty PJ. Reactive oxygen and nitrogen species as intracellular signals in skeletal muscle. J Physiol. 2011;589(Pt 9):2129–38.
23. Kim M, Wischmeyer PE. Glutamine. World Rev Nutr Diet. 2013;105:90–6.
24. Heck TG, Scholer CM, de Bittencourt PI. HSP70 expression: does it a novel fatigue signalling factor from immune system to the brain? Cell Biochem Funct. 2011;29:215–26.
25. Xue H, Slavov D, Wischmeyer PE. Glutamine-mediated dual regulation of heat shock transcription factor-1 activation and expression. J Biol Chem. 2012;287:40400–13.
26. Singleton KD, Wischmeyer PE. Glutamine's protection against sepsis and lung injury is dependent on heat shock protein 70 expression. Am J Physiol Regul Integr Comp Physiol. 2007;292:R1839–45.
27. Meador BM, Huey KA. Glutamine preserves skeletal muscle force during an inflammatory insult. Muscle Nerve. 2009;40:1000–7.
28. Lightfoot A, McArdle A, Griffiths RD. Muscle in defense. Crit Care Med. 2009;37:S384–90.
29. Rogero MM, Borges MC, Fock RA, et al. Glutamine in vitro supplementation decreases glucose utilization by the glycolytic pathway in Lps-activated peritoneal macrophages. Ann Nutr Metab. 2009;55:455.
30. Nässl A-M, Rubio-Aliaga I, Fenselau H, Marth MK, Kottra G, Daniel H. Amino acid absorption and homeostasis in mice lacking the intestinal peptide transporter PEPT1. Am J Physiol Gastrointest Liver Physiol. 2011; 301:G128–37.

31. Ingersoll SA, Ayyadurai S, Charania MA, Laroui H, Yan Y, Merlin D. The role and pathophysiological relevance of membrane transporter PepT1 in intestinal inflammation and inflammatory bowel disease. Am J Physiol Gastrointest Liver Physiol. 2012;302:G484–92.
32. Rogero MM, Tirapegui J, Pedrosa RG, de Castro IA, Pires ISD. Effect of alanyl-glutamine supplementation on plasma and tissue glutamine concentrations in rats submitted to exhaustive exercise. Nutrition. 2006;22:564–71.
33. Cruzat VF, Rogero MM, Tirapegui J. Effects of supplementation with free glutamine and the dipeptide alanyl-glutamine on parameters of muscle damage and inflammation in rats submitted to prolonged exercise. Cell Biochem Funct. 2010;28:24–30.
34. Ziegler TR, Young LS, Benfell K, et al. Clinical and metabolic efficacy of glutamine-supplemented parenteral nutrition after bone marrow transplantation. A randomized, double-blind, controlled study. Ann Intern Med. 1992;116:821–8.
35. Grau T, Bonet A, Minambres E, et al. The effect of L-alanyl-L-glutamine dipeptide supplemented total parenteral nutrition on infectious morbidity and insulin sensitivity in critically ill patients. Crit Care Med. 2011;39:1263–8.
36. Wernerman J. Clinical use of glutamine supplementation. J Nutr. 2008;138:2040S–4.
37. Krause MS, de Bittencourt PIHJ. Type 1 diabetes: can exercise impair the autoimmune event? The L-arginine/glutamine coupling hypothesis. Cell Biochem Funct. 2008;26:406–33.
38. Newsholme P, Krause M, Newsholme EA, Stear SJ, Burke LM, Castell LM. A-Z of nutritional supplements: dietary supplements, sports nutrition foods and ergogenic aids for health and performance Part 18. Br J Sports Med. 2011; 45:230–2.
39. Newsholme P. Why is L-glutamine metabolism important to cells of the immune system in health, postinjury, surgery or infection? J Nutr. 2001;131(9 Suppl):2515S–22.
40. Newsholme P, Abdulkader F, Rebelato E, et al. Amino acids and diabetes: implications for endocrine, metabolic and immune function. Front Biosci. 2011;16:315–39.
41. Menge BA, Schrader H, Ritter PR, et al. Selective amino acid deficiency in patients with impaired glucose tolerance and type 2 diabetes. Regul Pept. 2010;160(1–3):75–80.
42. Krause M, Rodrigues-Krause J, O'Hagan C, et al. Differential nitric oxide levels in the blood and skeletal muscle of type 2 diabetic subjects may be consequence of adiposity: a preliminary study. Metabolism. 2012;61:1528–37.
43. Rodrigues-Krause J, Krause M, O'Hagan C, et al. Divergence of intracellular and extracellular HSP72 in type 2 diabetes: does fat matter? Cell Stress Chaperones. 2012;17:293–302.
44. Rogero MM, Tirapegui J, Pedrosa RG, Pires ISD, de Castro IA. Plasma and tissue glutamine response to acute and chronic supplementation with L-glutamine and L-alanyl-L-glutamine in rats. Nutr Res. 2004;24:261–70.
45. Newsholme P, Bender K, Kiely A, Brennan L. Amino acid metabolism, insulin secretion and diabetes. Biochem Soc Trans. 2007;35(Pt 5):1180–6.
46. Newsholme P, Brennan L, Rubi B, Maechler P. New insights into amino acid metabolism, beta-cell function and diabetes. Clin Sci. 2005;108:185–94.
47. Cunningham GA, McClenaghan NH, Flatt PR, Newsholme P. L-Alanine induces changes in metabolic and signal transduction gene expression in a clonal rat pancreatic beta-cell line and protects from pro-inflammatory cytokine-induced apoptosis. Clin Sci. 2005;109:447–55.
48. Harris RC, Hoffman JR, Allsopp A, Routledge NB. L-glutamine absorption is enhanced after ingestion of L-alanylglutamine compared with the free amino acid or wheat protein. Nutr Res. 2012;32:272–7.

Chapter 39
Glutamine and Myostatin Expression in Muscle Wasting

Fabio Penna, Andrea Bonetto, Francesco M. Baccino, and Paola Costelli

Key Points

- Skeletal muscle mass depends on the balance between protein synthesis and degradation rates.
- Muscle wasting in pathological states is mainly associated with activation of protein breakdown above control levels.
- Myostatin is a negative regulator of skeletal muscle mass, acting on both myogenesis and protein turnover.
- Increased myostatin expression is a frequent finding in diseases characterized by the occurrence of muscle atrophy.
- Glutamine levels are generally decreased in acute and chronic illnesses, and glutamine supplementation to critically ill patients results in improved clinical conditions.
- Myotube atrophy induced by glucocorticoid or proinflammatory cytokine exposure can be reverted by glutamine treatment. Such an effect is associated with normalization of myostatin hyperexpression and signaling.
- Glutamine effectiveness in restoring normal myostatin pathway could depend on the inhibition of proinflammatory cascades as well as on the regulation of microRNA expression.

Keywords Muscle wasting • Protein breakdown • Myostatin • Glutamine • Proinflammatory cytokines • Nutritional strategies

Abbreviations

ActRII	Activin receptor II
ALK	Activin-like kinase
AMPK	Adenosine monophosphate (AMP)-activated kinase

F. Penna, Ph.D. (✉) • F.M. Baccino, Ph.D. • P. Costelli, Ph.D.
Department of Clinical and Biological Sciences, University of Turin, Corso Raffaello 30, Torino 10125, Italy
e-mail: fabio.penna@unito.it; francesco.baccino@unito.it; paola.costelli@unito.it

A. Bonetto, Ph.D.
Indiana University School of Medicine - IUPUI,
980 W. Walnut Street, R3-C540, Indianapolis, IN 46202, USA
e-mail: abonetto@iupui.edu

R. Rajendram et al. (eds.), *Glutamine in Clinical Nutrition*, Nutrition and Health,
DOI 10.1007/978-1-4939-1932-1_39, © Springer Science+Business Media New York 2015

BMP	Bone morphogenetic proteins
ERK	Extracellular signal-regulated kinase
FLRG	Follistatin-related gene
FoxO	Forkhead box O
GASP-1	Growth and differentiation factor-associated protein-1
GLUT-4	Glucose transporter type 4
HSP70	Heat shock protein 70
IGF-1	Insulin-like growth factor 1
IL-6	Interleukin-6
JNK	c-Jun N-terminal kinase
LPS	Lipopolysaccharide
MAPK	Mitogen-activated protein kinases
MuRF1	Muscle ring finger 1
Myd88	Myeloid differentiation primary response gene (88)
NF-κB	Nuclear factor κB
PI-3K	Phosphoinositide 3 kinase
Smad	Small mother against decapentaplegic
TGFβ	Transforming growth factor β
TLR	Toll-like receptor
TNFα	Tumor necrosis factor α
TRAF	TNF receptor-associated factor

Introduction

The skeletal muscle has been considered for a long time just a protein storage tissue, despite the relevance of its contribution to whole body metabolism. Indeed, it contributes to regulate energy balance, heat production, and insulin sensitivity, also producing humoral mediators called myokines.

The skeletal muscle mass mainly reflects protein content, and strictly depends on the balance between protein synthesis and degradation rates, that is regulated by both anabolic and catabolic signals [1]. Alterations in this equilibrium lead to mass accretion (hypertrophy) or depletion (atrophy), depending on the prevailing pathways (anabolic or catabolic).

Muscle hypertrophy has long believed to essentially depend on increased protein synthesis rates, although many years ago also modulations of protein degradation have been proposed to play a role. By contrast, muscle atrophy describes a change occurring as a result of disuse (e.g., immobilization, denervation, muscle unloading), aging, starvation, and a number of disease states (sepsis, diabetes, cancer cachexia). Several molecular triggers and signaling pathways differently contribute to the generation of muscle wasting in the above conditions, leading to a marked increase in protein degradation, associated or not with reduced protein synthesis rates, that results in decreased protein content and myofiber diameter. However, most of the signaling pathways involved in atrophy also play a role in the induction of hypertrophy, and in this regard considering the former just as the converse of the latter could be questionable (see [1]).

Skeletal Muscle Wasting

Several chronic and degenerative pathologies are characterized by significant loss of skeletal muscle mass. Functionally, hypotrophy results in decreased muscle strength, with asthenia and reduced physical performance, and declining efficiency of respiratory muscles with hypoventilation and respiratory

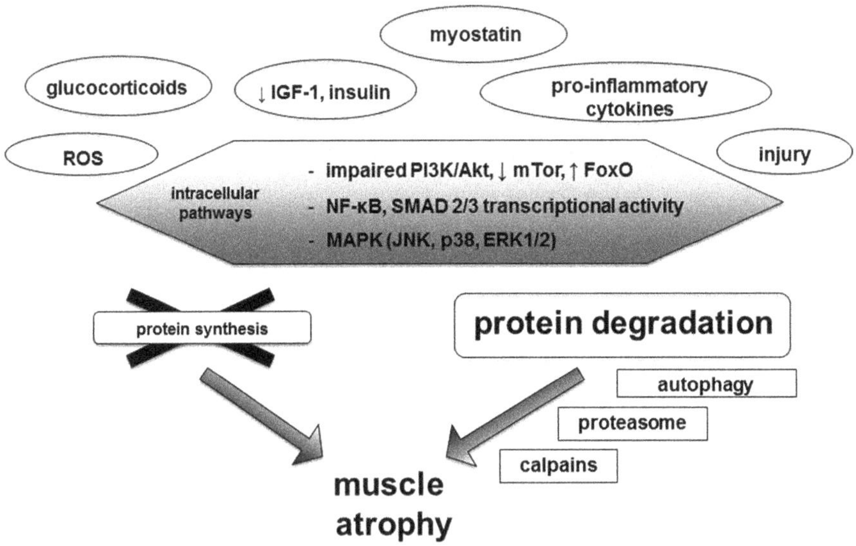

Fig. 39.1 Mechanisms involved in the pathogenesis of skeletal muscle wasting. Several factors, of extracellular and/or intracellular origin, may activate signaling pathways that directly or indirectly converge to modulate protein turnover rates, eventually resulting in skeletal muscle atrophy

failure. In some circumstances, the mobilization of muscle protein may serve the purpose of providing substrates for energy production and gluconeogenesis, synthesis of acute phase reactants or other anabolic processes. In other instances, however, muscle protein depletion in wasting syndromes appears basically purposeless, in part at least, and it is obviously so if the catabolic state persists when excess nutrients are supplied by parenteral feeding. Protein loss may primarily affect the skeletal muscle compartment (primary or neurogenic muscular disorders) or may reflect the role of skeletal muscle as main protein reserve of the organism (wasting syndromes). However, despite this dichotomy, at least some of the mechanisms operating in the wasting syndromes (Fig. 39.1) appear to apply also to muscle atrophy occurring in primary or neurogenic muscular disorders.

As reported above, muscle atrophy mainly depends on enhanced protein breakdown rates. The role played by the different intracellular proteolytic systems in this regard, however, is still controversial, since the Ca^{2+}-dependent, the ATP-ubiquitin-dependent and the autophagic lysosomal pathways have all been involved [1].

Muscle protein hypercatabolism in chronic diseases has been frequently associated with increased levels of proinflammatory cytokines, TNFα in particular, as suggested by studies performed in experimental models as well as in human subjects (see references in [1]). Consistently, activation of NF-κB, one of the main targets of TNFα, has been involved in causing muscle atrophy by downregulating the muscle-specific transcription factor MyoD. This observation has been confirmed by a study reporting that NF-κB activation in mice overexpressing in the skeletal muscle a constitutively active form of IκB kinase β results in severe wasting (reviewed in [1]). TNFα may concur to skeletal muscle wasting also by downregulating anabolic signaling pathways such as those activated by insulin and IGF-1. As an example, inhibition of insulin signaling by TNFα has been demonstrated in different cell types such as adipocytes, hepatocytes, or C2C12 myocytes. Such an effect seems to rely on reduced phosphorylation of both the insulin receptor and the insulin receptor substrates, together with downregulated expression of the glucose transporter GLUT-4 (reviewed in [2]).

IGF-1 is an anabolic growth factor that stimulates muscle protein synthesis as well as proliferation and differentiation of satellite cells, the muscle-specific stem cell population. IGF-1 has been reported to exert anti-apoptotic effects on muscle cells, to suppress proteolysis and to inhibit both the ubiquitin-proteasome system and the autophagic degradation [1]. Catabolic states such as sepsis and cancer have been associated with reduced levels of circulating IGF-1 (reviewed in [2]) as well as with increased concentrations of proinflammatory cytokines, such as TNFα (see references in [1]). The interplay between IGF-1 and TNFα has also been proposed in an experimental model of sepsis, where the autocrine production of muscle IGF-1 is impaired by LPS administration to rats, and similar observations have been reported in C2C12 myocyte cultures exposed to TNFα (reviewed in [2]). Engagement of both the insulin and the IGF-1 receptors results in the activation of different signal transduction pathways. Particularly relevant to the homeostasis of muscle mass seems to be the insulin receptor substrate-1/PI-3K/Akt axis, which has been involved not only in the activation of protein synthesis but also in the downregulation of protein degradation by maintaining transcription factors of the FoxO family in the inactive state [1].

In addition to IGF-1, other signaling pathways have been involved in the pathogenesis of skeletal muscle atrophy. Particularly relevant, in this regard, is the one regulated by myostatin, that, in some circumstances at least, has been shown to be modulated by TNFα [3, 4].

Myostatin

Myostatin ("growth and differentiation factor-8") is a factor belonging to the BMP/TGF-β superfamily (reviewed in [5]). It has been characterized by McPherron in 1997 (see [5]), and very rapidly has emerged as an important regulator of skeletal muscle mass and repair. Indeed, its expression is largely restricted to the skeletal muscle, while small amount of myostatin mRNA have been detected also in the adipose tissue. Muscle myostatin expression is different between genders, being lower in males than in female mice, in face of higher body and muscle mass. An opposite phenotype can be observed in mice genetically deprived of myostatin, females being bigger than males ([5] and references therein).

Inactivating mutations in the myostatin gene have been identified in cattles, sheeps and dogs showing muscle hypertrophy, and also in human beings. Consistently, both targeted deletion of the myostatin gene and myostatin blockade by short hairpin RNA lead to increased muscle mass in experimental animals (reviewed in [5]). Expression of truncated or inactive forms of myostatin results in increased muscle fiber number (hyperplasia) and/or size (hypertrophy). In this regard, satellite cells lacking myostatin show a proliferative advantage compared with cells from wild-type animals [5], suggesting that myostatin exerts its growth-promoting effect by increasing satellite cell/myofiber number. However, according to other reports myostatin would regulate muscle mass just by inducing hypertrophy (discussed in [5]). In this regard, blocking myostatin in the *mdx* mouse, an experimental model of Duchenne muscular dystrophy, results in improved skeletal muscle mass associated with increased fiber cross-sectional area but not with changes in the number of fibers or myonuclei. Similar observations have been reported in healthy animals treated with anti-myostatin antibodies (see [5]).

Consistently with its role as negative regulator of muscle mass, myostatin hyprexpression generally results in muscle atrophy. High myostatin gene expression and circulating levels have been associated with weight loss in patients with AIDS, and muscle myostatin protein levels are increased in the sarcopenia of aging, as well as in atrophy due to denervation or unloading (see [5]). Upregulation of myostatin expression and myostatin-dependent signaling have been reported in experimental cancer cachexia as well as in cancer patients [3, 6]. In addition, pathological states characterized by muscle wasting frequently present with high glucocorticoid circulating levels, associated with myostatin upregulation [7], and increased myostatin expression has been shown in experimental models of Addison's disease or chronic obstructive pulmonary disease. Finally, confirming the existence of a cross-talk between muscle and the adipose tissue, this latter too is affected by increased myostatin levels (see [5]).

The mechanisms by which myostatin hyperexpression induces muscle atrophy are not completely understood. As reported above, myostatin has been proposed to interfere with myogenesis, modulating both satellite cell proliferation and differentiation [5]. On the other side, muscle wasting is well known to be associated with activation above control levels of different intracellular proteolytic pathways. Among these, myostatin has been involved in the activation of the ubiquitin-proteasome system, leading to increased transcription of the muscle-specific ubiquitin ligases atrogin-1 and MuRF1. Indeed, the signaling pathway activated by myostatin has been demonstrated to inhibit the IGF-1/PI-3K/Akt axis, previously shown to play a role in maintaining FoxO transcription factors in the inactive state, thus modulating protein breakdown rates (see [1, 5]).

Expression, Processing, and Binding of Myostatin Protein

Similar to other TGF-β family members, myostatin is produced as a secreted protein, first synthesized as a precursor and then processed by proteolysis. Following removal of the 24 amino acid signal peptide, myostatin is further cleaved into an amino-terminal propeptide and a 110 amino acid biologically active carboxyl terminus. The cleavage occurs at a dibasic cleavage site, but the nature of the enzyme responsible for this event is unknown, although in cell-based systems co-expression of furin proved capable of increasing active myostatin levels. Circulating myostatin is maintained in the inactive conformation by binding to the propeptide itself or to other myostatin-binding proteins [5].

Several experimental evidences suggest that the propeptide may regulate myostatin activity both in vivo and in vitro. Myostatin-producing Chinese hamster ovary cell lines secrete a biologically inactive carboxy-terminal dimer non-covalently bound to the propeptide. This complex can be activated by heat or acid treatment in a way similar to the activation of TGF-β latent complexes. Moreover, propeptide has been shown to bind to the mature carboxy-terminal dimer and to inhibit its activity. Further, increased muscle mass is observed in mice injected with purified propeptide and in transgenic mice overexpressing the propeptide itself. Finally, the propeptide is one of the proteins associated with myostatin in human or mouse serum (see [5]).

Among other myostatin-binding proteins, particularly interesting is follistatin, originally shown to inhibit the secretion of follicle stimulating hormone. Follistatin can bind to and inhibit myostatin activity with high affinity, as proved by simultaneously overexpressing both molecules in adult skeletal muscle, thus preventing myostatin ability to induce muscle loss [5]. Targeted follistatin overexpression in skeletal muscle has been shown to cause a marked increase in tissue weight, resulting from a combination of hyperplasia and hypertrophy. Remarkably, the increase in muscle mass is far greater than that observed following myostatin gene deletion. One possible explanation for these differences is that follistatin is likely to antagonize other molecules in addition to myostatin that may also act as muscle growth inhibitors ([5] and references therein).

In addition to follistatin, also FLRG and GASP-1 can complex with mature myostatin, resulting in its inhibition. The former, in particular, is able to interact also with other members of the TGF-β family [5].

Following activation of the latent complex, the mature myostatin carboxy-terminal dimer binds to receptors and activates a signal transduction cascade similar to that described for TGF-β (Fig. 39.2). Active myostatin binds with high affinity the ActRIIB and, to a lesser extent, the related ActRIIA, leading to recruitment of a low affinity type I receptor, either ALK-4 or ALK-5, to form a heteromeric complex. ActRIIB can thus transphosphorylate ALK-4/5 and activate its serine/threonine kinase domain, leading to phosphorylation of Smads 2 and 3 and to their interaction with co-Smad 4. The resulting complex translocates to the nucleus, where it regulates the transcription of myostatin target genes [5]. In addition to receptor-regulated Smads and co-Smads, there are also inhibitor Smads such as Smad 6 and Smad 7. While the former takes part primarily to the BMP signaling pathway, inhibiting its activity through competition with the receptor-regulated Smads (Smad 1 and 5) for the Smad 4 cofactor, the latter has been implicated as a negative regulator of TGF-β signaling.

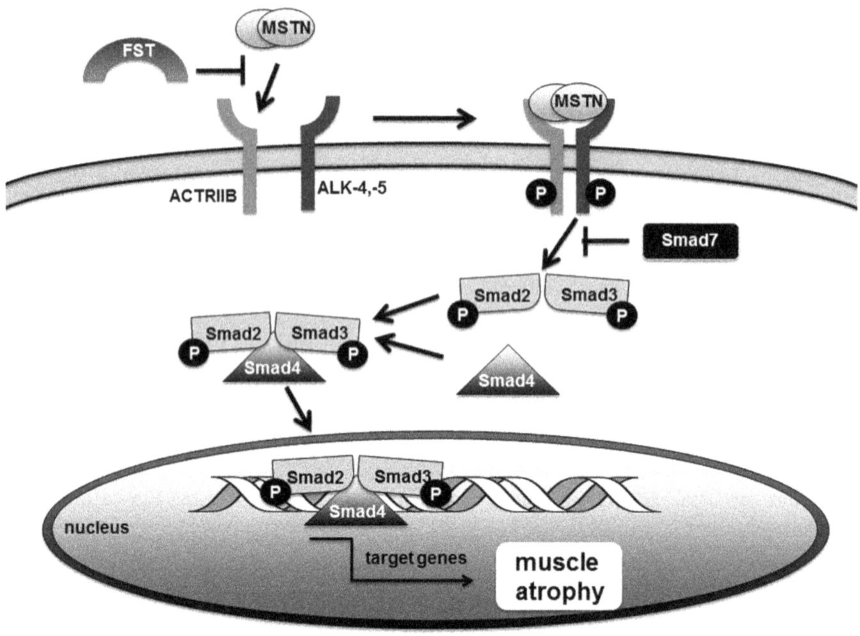

Fig. 39.2 Myostatin-dependent signaling pathway. Engagement of the ActRIIB results in dimerization with ALK-4,5 followed by recruitment and phosphorylation of Smad 2/3, binding to Smad 4 and subsequent nuclear localization and transcriptional activation. Smad 7 can inhibit this signaling pathway by interfering with Smad 2/3 interaction with the active receptor complex

Interestingly, both TGF-β and myostatin signaling induce Smad 7 mRNA, probably activating a negative feedback loop to inhibit TGF-β signaling. Moreover, Smad 7 has been reported to accelerate myogenic differentiation, leading to cellular hypertrophy through a positive feedback loop with MyoD, which, in turn, can activate the Smad 7 promoter. Therefore, Smad 7 may physically associate with MyoD and potentiate its transactivation properties [5].

In addition to the canonical Smad-dependent transduction pathway, myostatin has been reported to signal also by activating the ERK/MAPK [8] or the JNK-dependent [9] pathways.

Experimental Anti-myostatin Approaches

Taking into account the involvement of myostatin as negative regulator of skeletal muscle mass, as well as the occurrence of myostatin increased levels and activity in different conditions associated with muscle atrophy, it is not surprising that several strategies have been developed to inhibit myostatin-dependent signaling (Table 39.1).

Anti-myostatin antibodies such as JA16 or PF-354 have been pioneers in this regard. Their use in preclinical studies have led to the first phase I/II clinical trial using the humanized antibody MYO-029 in patients affected by muscle dystrophy (see references in [5]).

Besides neutralizing antibodies, a number of potential inhibitors of myostatin have been made available that might be used as therapeutic agents. In this regard, myofiber hypertrophy has been reported in mice after myostatin inhibition by plasmid-mediated delivery of mutant myostatin propeptide [10]. Another work shows that SB-505124 inhibits the activity of TGF-β type I receptors

Table 39.1 Molecules and mechanism of action of myostatin inhibitors

Molecule	Mechanism
Myostatin propeptide	Interacts with mature myostatin, blocking the myostatin/receptor interaction
Follistatin	Endogenous inhibitor, blocks myostatin/receptor interaction
FSTL3 (FLRG)	Follistatin-like 3, blocks myostatin/receptor interaction
GASP-1	Interacts with propeptide and mature myostatin, blocks myostatin/receptor interaction
sActRIIB	Soluble activin IIB receptor/Fc fusion protein, blocks myostatin/receptor interaction
Anti-myostatin Ab	Myostatin neutralizing antibody
Anti-myostatin oligo	Small interfering or antisense RNA
SB505124	ALK-4,-5 inhibitor, prevents Smad 2/3 phosphorylation
Valproic acid	Histone deacetylase inhibitor, induces follistatin expression
Trichostatin A	Histone deacetylase inhibitor, induces follistatin expression
Smad7	Competes with Smad4 avoiding the formation of the transcriptional complex Smad2/3/4

See [5, 10–13, 15, 16] and references therein

ALK-4/-5, thus reducing Smad 2/3 phosphorylation [11]. However, further studies are needed to clarify whether SB-505124 could effectively prevent the activation of myostatin signaling both in vitro and in vivo. Also follistatin has been proposed as a successful inhibitor of myostatin, although it may also inhibit other TGF-β family members. Furthermore, follistatin expression has been recently reported to be enhanced in satellite-derived myotubes and embryonic muscles by nitric oxide production. This may foster fusion-induced hypertrophy of myotubes (see references in [5]).

Interesting results have been reported demonstrating the possibility to improve muscle wasting in experimental cancer cachexia by treatment with an ActRIIB-extracellular domain/Fc fusion protein [12]. These observations have been confirmed by another study showing reduced muscle wasting and prolonged survival in tumor-bearing animals administered soluble ActRIIB [13].

Small interfering or antisense RNA approaches have proved effective in reducing muscle myostatin protein expression and increasing muscle mass in murine models (see [5]). Similarly, systemic myostatin inhibition obtained in dystrophic mice through liver-targeted gene transfer of a secretable dominant negative myostatin has been shown to improve muscle phenotype [14].

Finally, histone deacetylase inhibitors have been described as very promising tools in the treatment of muscle wasting diseases, muscle dystrophies in particular [15]. Despite this report, treatment of mice bearing the C26 colon adenocarcinoma with the histone deacetylase inhibitor valproic acid effectively counteracts the increased myostatin levels and activity, without modifying muscle wasting [16].

Modulation of Myostatin Expression/Activity by Nutritional Factors

As described in the Introduction, muscle mass depletion results from protein degradation exceeding protein synthesis rates. Consistently, low dietary protein intake leads to muscle hypotrophy associated with negative nitrogen balance, that until a certain point can be easily counteracted by refeeding. While this is a well accepted concept, little is known about the involvement of myostatin in calorie restriction-induced muscle atrophy, as well as about the regulation of myostatin expression by nutritional factors. In this regard, circulating myostatin remains comparable to control levels in healthy volunteers fasted for 72 h [17]. Also patients affected by type II diabetes do not show changes in circulating myostatin, but its gene expression in the skeletal muscle is significantly increased [18]. Recently, myostatin expression has been shown to be upregulated in experimental animals prone to develop obesity when fed a high fat diet (see [5]), and increased myostatin secretion from the muscle has been reported in obese subjects [19].

Circulating myostatin appears regulated also by physical activity. In this regard, resistance training programs have been shown to decrease the plasma levels of myostatin and to increase those of GASP-1, one of the myostatin-binding proteins (see above). Such an effect is potentiated when volunteers assume creatine during the training period [20]. Creatine is frequently used to increase skeletal muscle mass and performance, effects that have been ascribed to its ergogenic properties. The study by Saremi and coworkers [20] discusses the possibility that creatine effectiveness could result from stimulation of satellite cell activation over that induced by exercise training. This hyperstimulation is suggested to depend on reduced myostatin production, especially in type II glycolytic myofibers.

Finally, supplementation with protein and amino acids is frequently used as a mean to both enhance muscle protein synthesis and reduce degradation. As an example, protein and/or amino acid assumption have been reported to preserve muscle strength after bed rest and to improve disuse-induced muscle wasting and protein hypercatabolism [21]. By contrast, protein and amino acid supplementation does not appear to exert any effect on myostatin hyperexpression in the atrophic muscle of immobilized human volunteers [22]. Another study reports that an essential amino acid supplement provided to volunteers during bed rest and the subsequent active recovery effectively corrects muscle myostatin hyperexpression only when coupled to resistance training exercise [23].

Glutamine and Myostatin

Glutamine is the most abundant amino acid in the body, mainly synthetized in the skeletal muscle from glutamic acid. It is an important nutrient for rapidly dividing cells such as lymphocytes, enterocytes, or tumor cells, and is a precursor for the endogenous antioxidant glutathione. In particular, muscle levels of reduced glutathione and glutamine positively correlate in critically ill patients (reviewed in [24]). Glutamine participates to nitrogen transport in the body, induces the expression of stress proteins and stimulates nucleotide synthesis. Signals involved in the regulation of cell differentiation, such as the ERK MAPK, are activated by glutamine [25]. Reduced muscle glutamine levels are associated with cell shrinkage; this modification has been proposed to act as a sensor that modulates protein catabolism. Consistently, a relation among myotube size, inferred from intracellular water content, nitrogen balance and glutamine content has been shown in catabolic patients (reviewed in [24]).

Glutamine is a “conditional essential amino acid” in catabolic states [24]. Its muscle levels markedly decrease in severe illnesses despite increased muscle production and release. Not only, in addition also chronic pathologies characterized by muscle wasting are associated with reduced glutamine availability. As an example, plasma glutamine levels in tumor-bearing rats are markedly decreased [26], and low circulating glutamine has been associated with worse prognosis in septic patients (see [24]). Reduced glutamine availability could result in activation of the metabolic sensor AMPK. This kinase regulates energy-saving strategies, inhibiting processes that need ATP while potentiating those involved in the maintenance of cell integrity [24].

Glutamine supplementation to critically ill patients results in decreased morbidity and mortality, also reducing the duration of hospital stay. Acute diseases are frequently associated with increased circulating glucocorticoids, and glutamine effectiveness has been proposed to derive from action on these hormones. Indeed, glutamine has been shown to prevent glucocorticoid or sepsis-induced muscle atrophy [7, 27]. Not only, glutamine supplementation attenuates muscle protein waste in cancer patients [28] and glutamine administration to LPS-treated mice has been demonstrated to preserve muscle force without modifying circulating TNFα, suggesting that glutamine target(s) is/are downstream of cytokine production [29]. Finally, glutamine treatment results in improved muscle atrophy by modulating protein turnover in diabetic rats [30].

Some years ago the possibility that glutamine improvement of muscle wasting could be associated with effects exerted on myostatin has been taken into consideration, starting from the observation that

Table 39.2 Diseases and conditions characterized by muscle wasting and general inflammatory state, and associated with reduced glutamine levels, and increased myostatin signaling

Disease state	Reduced glutamine levels	Increased myostatin signaling
HIV/AIDS	✓	✓
Sepsis	✓	✓
Cancer	✓	✓
Burn injury	✓	✓
Sarcopenia	✓	✓
COPD	✓	✓
Heart failure	✓	✓
Kidney failure	✓	✓
Ulcerative colitis	✓	Unknown
Chronic fatigue syndrome	✓	Unknown
Overtraining syndrome	✓	Unknown

See [24, 44] and references therein

pathological states associated with low circulating glutamine also present with increased myostatin signaling (Table 39.2). Just few studies explored such possibility, however. Salheian and coworkers [27] have investigated if glutamine effectiveness on glucocorticoid-induced muscle atrophy reflects modulations of myostatin expression. Muscle wasting induced in rats by dexamethasone treatment is associated with activation of proteasome-dependent proteolysis and with increased myostatin expression at both gene and protein levels. The action of glucocorticoids on myostatin transcription may depend on the presence, on the myostatin promoter, of several glucocorticoid responsive elements ([7] and references therein). Consistently, dexamethasone-induced myostatin hyperexpression can be abrogated by treatment with the glucocorticoid receptor antagonist RU486 [7]. Recent observations propose that the mechanism by which glucocorticoid induce muscle atrophy also involves a myostatin-dependent inhibition of satellite cell activation and self-renewal [31]. Glucocorticoid administration also results in depletion of both muscle and circulating glutamine. When this amino acid is provided to glucocorticoid-treated animals at doses markedly higher than those normally introduced with the diet, significant improvement of muscle atrophy and partial normalization of myostatin expression can be observed [27]. These observations have also been confirmed in C2C12 myocytes exposed to dexamethasone in the presence or in the absence of glutamine. In particular, glutamine addition to C2C12 myoblast culture medium results in about 50 % inhibition of myostatin promoter transcription [27], that increases from two- to threefold after dexamethasone exposure [7]. The authors suggest that also the reduced myostatin expression attained by glutamine administration in the whole animal could derive from direct or indirect inhibition of glucocorticoid interaction with the glucocorticoid responsive elements on the myostatin promoter.

Myostatin expression and protein hypercatabolism can be modulated in C2C12 myocytes as well as in tumor-bearing rats by the proinflammatory cytokine TNFα [3, 16]. Starting from these observations, Bonetto and coworkers [4] have investigated if glutamine supplementation can restore normal levels of myostatin expression and activity as well as of Ca^{2+}-dependent proteolysis in C2C12 myotube cultures exposed to TNFα.

The procatabolic effect exerted by this proinflammatory cytokine on muscle cells is well known: in myotubes exposed to TNFα the levels of myosin heavy chain (MyHC) are markedly reduced, while those of the muscle-specific ubiquitin ligase atrogin 1 are increased ([4] and references therein). Also the Ca^{2+}-dependent proteolysis [4] and the proteasome proteolytic system (Table 39.3A) are hyperactivated by TNFα in C2C12 myotube cultures, while recent observations have shown that the autophagic lysosomal degradative system is perturbed as well [32]. Treatment of C2C12 cells with TNFα results in significant myostatin hyperexpression associated with unchanged follistatin, indicating an activation of the myostatin-dependent signaling pathway above control levels [4]. This is further confirmed by

Table 39.3 Molecular modifications induced by glutamine or valproic acid in C2C12 myotubes exposed to TNFα

A		Atrogin-1	
		TNF	TNF+Gln
mRNA	6 h	$110\pm2^{*}$	$91\pm1^{*,\$\$}$
	24 h	108 ± 2	99 ± 16

B		Follistatin		Myostatin	
		TNF	TNF+VPA	TNF	TNF+VPA
mRNA	24 h	222 ± 72	136 ± 13	$222\pm20^{*}$	$136\pm34^{\$}$
	48 h	131 ± 33	$218\pm16^{**,\$}$	61 ± 20	75 ± 4
Protein	24 h	67 ± 12	$225\pm61^{*,\$}$	$147\pm21^{*}$	$36\pm10^{**,\$\$}$
	48 h	80 ± 8	$157\pm35^{\$}$	72 ± 7	69 ± 20

A: Atrogin-1 mRNA expression in C2C12 exposed to either TNFα or TNFα+Gln for 6 and 24 h. B: Follistatin and myostatin mRNA and protein expression in C2C12 myotubes exposed to either TNFα or TNFα+VPA for 24 and 48 h. Data (means±SD; $n=3$) are expressed as percentage of controls (C). Significance of the differences: $^{*}p<0.05$, $^{**}p<0.01$ versus C; $^{\$}p<0.05$, $^{\$\$}p<0.01$ versus TNFα

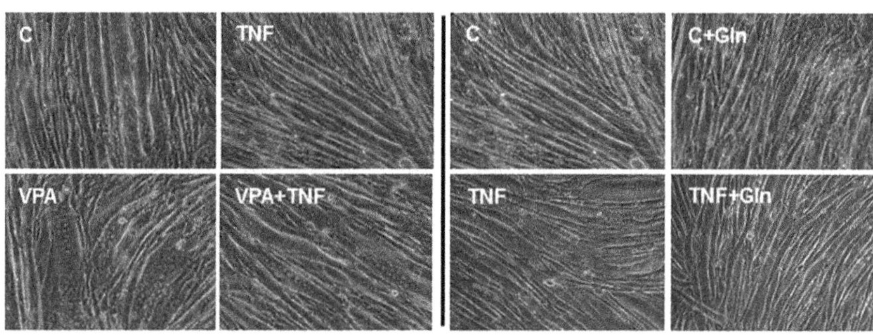

Fig. 39.3 Treatment of C2C12 cells exposed to TNFα with glutamine or valproic acid. Phase contrast images of myotube cultures treated for 24 h with TNFα (100 ng/ml) in the presence or in the absence of glutamine (8 mM) or valproic acid (5 mM)

the increased Smad 2/3 DNA-binding activity [4]. Similar observations have been reported in rats bearing the Yoshida ascites hepatoma AH-130. In these animals, treatment with pentoxifylline, an inhibitor of TNFα synthesis, results in significant protection against muscle wasting and perturbations of myostatin expression and signaling [3].

No information are available about the modulations of myostatin expression pattern in tumor-bearing rats supplemented with glutamine, but Bonetto and coworkers clearly show that when this amino acid is added to C2C12 myotube cultures exposed to TNFα, normal myostatin levels are restored. Interestingly, also the levels of active calpain [4] and atrogin-1 (Table 39.3A) are reduced to values close to those of control cells. Normalization of myostatin expression has also been obtained by treating C2C12 cells exposed to TNFα or mice bearing the C26 tumor with the histone deacetylase inhibitor valproic acid (Fig. 39.3, Table 39.3B) [16]. Deacetylase inhibitors represent a prototype of epigenetic drugs. The therapeutic versatility of these compounds has been demonstrated by treating different pathologies, including cancer, genetic diseases (i.e. muscular dystrophy) and degenerative disorders. The knowledge that histone acetyltransferases promote and deacetylases inhibit skeletal muscle gene expression has suggested the potential effectiveness of deacetylase inhibitors in modulating skeletal myogenesis (see references in [16]). The effects exerted by valproic acid on TNFα-induced myostatin hyperexpression are likely due to the epigenetic modifications. However, recently, glutamine synthetase activity has been shown to be transiently increased in the hippocampus of rats exposed prenatally to valproic acid [33], suggesting that a similar mechanism could operate also in the skeletal muscle, possibly contributing to the effects of valproic acid on myostatin and follistatin expression.

Glutamine supplementation has been reported to improve glucose homeostasis and muscle atrophy in experimental diabetes, but no data are available about its possible effectiveness on myostatin hyperexpression [18]. Myostatin has been proposed to act as a pro-oxidant factor [34], and oxidative stress is a well-known causative factor for muscle atrophy in diabetes [35]. In addition, the hyperproduction of reactive oxygen species also appear to induce myostatin expression itself [34]. In this regard, glutamine effectiveness on muscle wasting in diabetes, and likely on myostatin hyperexpression, could depend on the antioxidant property displayed by this amino acid [36].

Recent observations report that exogenous myostatin induces autophagy in C2C12 myocytes [37]. Autophagy is a physiological process required for the degradation of cellular constituents. Basal levels of autophagy can be increased in stress conditions such as nutrient deprivation, organelle damage, and death-inducing stimuli. The hyperactivation of autophagy has been demonstrated in several experimental models of muscle atrophy, such as fasting, denervation, or cancer [1, 32]; and recently, myostatin hyperexpression has been shown to induce atrophy in trout myotubes activating both autophagy and the proteasome [38]. Amino acids, leucine in particular, have long been known as potent inhibitors of autophagy. As for glutamine, its depletion or supplementation have been demonstrated to result in hyperactivation or inhibition of autophagy, respectively (reviewed by [39]). In this regard, there is the possibility that glutamine effect on autophagy may depend, at least in part, on downregulation of myostatin hyperexpression. This hypothesis, however, remains to be demonstrated.

The mechanisms underlying glutamine effectiveness in reducing myostatin hyperexpression and muscle/myotube atrophy are completely unknown. In this regard, a recent report suggests that the low myostatin expression that accounts for the double-muscle phenotype in Piedmontese cattles is associated with upregulation of microRNA-27b (miR-27b) [40]. The hypertrophy-promoting effect of miR-27b has previously been shown in cardiomyocytes (see references in [40]). Myostatin 3′-untranslated region contains a putative binding site for miR-27a and b, suggesting that modulating the expression of this microRNA could well result in regulation of myostatin levels. Consistently, myostatin hyperexpression induced by glucocorticoid treatment appears to depend on downregulation of miR-27a and b [41] and/or upregulation of miR-1 [42]. No information are actually available about the expression of miR-27b in skeletal muscle atrophy, and no report link glutamine to the regulation of miR-27b. However, essential amino acid administration to human volunteers has been shown to result in upregulation of some miRs (1, 23a, 208b, 499, pri-miR-206), associated with decreased myostatin gene expression and increased follistatin mRNA levels in skeletal muscle biopsies [43]. In this regard, glutamine behaves as an essential amino acid exclusively during disease states (see above). Glucocorticoid-induced miR1 upregulation in muscle has been shown to result in reduced expression of the HSP70. The expression of this constitutively active, cytoprotective protein, is known to increase in stress conditions. Consistently, HSP70 hyprexpression results in protection against sarcopenia of aging or muscle damage, while reduced HSP70 levels have been reported in conditions characterized by skeletal muscle wasting. The protection afforded by HSP70 hyperexpression toward muscle wasting could partially rely on its direct association with the glucocorticoid receptor in the cytoplasm, thereby preventing its nuclear translocation. When miR1 is upregulated, HSP70 levels are reduced, resulting in enhanced activation of the glucocorticoid receptor ([42] and references therein). Keeping in mind the data reported by Ma and coworkers [7], myostatin promoter contains several glucocorticoid responsive elements, thus reduced HSP70 expression could contribute to the increased expression of myostatin in glucocorticoid-treated skeletal muscle. Interestingly, glutamine has been shown to induce both transcription and synthesis of heat shock proteins [44], providing another possible mechanism to explain its effectiveness in inhibiting myostatin hyperexpression in glucocorticoid-treated skeletal muscle.

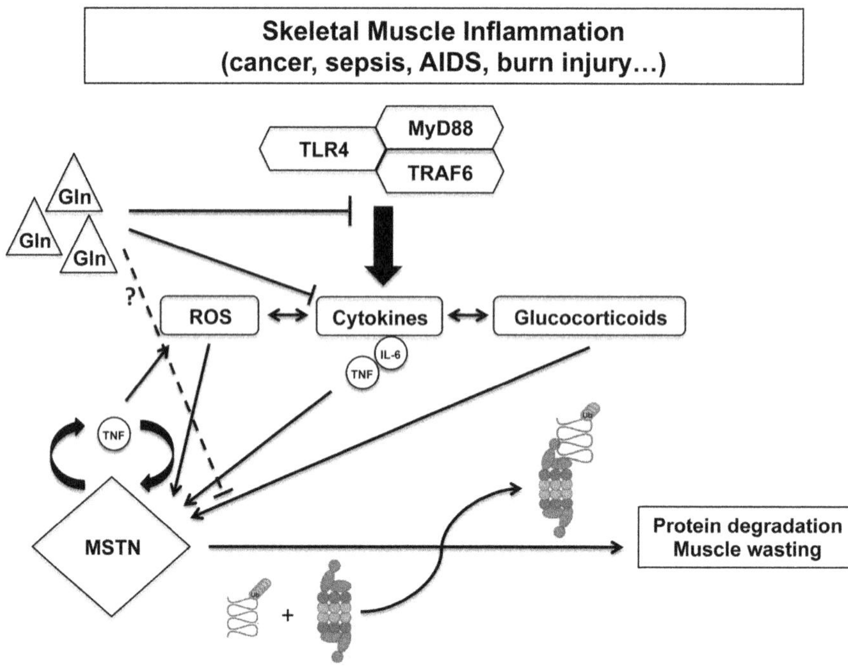

Fig. 39.4 Hypothetical mechanism by which glutamine supplementation could modulate myostatin expression. Local and/or systemic inflammation may result in muscle wasting by activating intracellular pathways that lead to reciprocal interference among cytokines, glucocorticoids and reactive oxygen species. All of these enhance myostatin expression and eventually protein breakdown rates and muscle atrophy. Glutamine may exert a protective effect by inhibiting both the activity of inflammation-driven transcription factors and cytokine production

Finally, glutamine has been proposed as an immunonutrient. The concept of immunonutrition derives from the observation that immune functions are frequently impaired in conditions characterized by malnutrition. The rationale of immunonutrition is to supply supranormal quantities of nutrients in order to achieve pharmacological effects via the enteral or parenteral route [44]. Previous observations have shown that glutamine is able to inhibit proinflammatory cascades such as those activated by lipopolysaccharide involving the TLR4, MyD88, and TRAF6 (reviewed in [44]). More recently, glutamine has been shown to inhibit IL-6 and TNFα in human monocytes stimulated with lipopolysaccharide. Glutamine-induced reduction of proinflammatory cytokines has also been reported in septic patients and in other stress situations such as postoperative period or pancreatitis ([45] and references therein). On this basis, a mechanistic hypothesis trying to explain the overall glutamine effects on the regulation of myostatin expression is proposed in Fig. 39.4.

Conclusions

Glutamine is among the most studied amino acids. Plasma and muscle glutamine pools have been found to decrease in life-threatening conditions associated with muscle wasting such as sepsis, cancer cachexia, burn injury and trauma, while the expression of the muscle negative regulatory factor myostatin is frequently increased (see Table 39.1). Such an apparent inverse correlation between myostatin and muscle wasting on one side and the extent of glutamine pools on the other have suggested that glutamine supplementation may prove effective in correcting both muscle depletion and myostatin hyperexpression. Indeed, improvement in clinical outcome and nitrogen balance has been reported when glutamine and glutamine-containing dipeptides are given to critically ill patients (see above). In addition, glutamine supplementation results in correction of myostatin hyperexpression in glucocorticoid or TNFα-induced muscle/myotube atrophy. The mechanisms underlying such effects are unknown at present, and a couple of hypotheses have been proposed in the present review. Another very interesting point is whether modulations of the myostatin pathway either follow or precede the activation of muscle protein breakdown that leads to tissue wasting. In this regard, treatments known to affect protein breakdown directly (glutamine supplementation; [4, 27]) or cytokine blockade (pentoxifylline) [3], are able to modulate myostatin expression/signaling pathway, suggesting that this factor can causally contribute to the hypercatabolic state.

Therefore, the evaluation of this signaling pathway as a target of nutritional strategies aimed at preventing or delaying the onset of muscle wasting is conceivable.

References

1. Bonaldo P, Sandri M. Cellular and molecular mechanisms of muscle atrophy. Dis Model Mech. 2013;6:25–39.
2. Grounds MD, Radley HG, Gebski BL, et al. Implications of cross-talk between tumour necrosis factor and insulin-like growth factor-1 signalling in skeletal muscle. Clin Exp Pharmacol Physiol. 2008;35:846–51.
3. Costelli P, Muscaritoli M, Bonetto A, et al. Muscle myostatin signaling is enhanced in cancer cachexia. Eur J Clin Invest. 2008;38:531–8.
4. Bonetto A, Penna F, Minero V, et al. Glutamine prevents myostatin hyperexpression and protein hypercatabolism induced in C2C12 myotubes by tumor necrosis factor-α. Amino Acids. 2010;40:585–94.
5. Elliott B, Renshaw D, Getting S, et al. The central role of myostatin in skeletal muscle and whole body homeostasis. Acta Physiol. 2012;205:324–40.
6. Aversa Z, Bonetto A, Penna F, et al. Changes in myostatin signaling in non weight-losing cancer patients. Ann Surg Oncol. 2012;19:1350–6.
7. Ma K, Mallidis C, Bhasin S, et al. Glucocorticoid-induced skeletal muscle atrophy is associated with upregulation of myostatin gene expression. Am J Physiol Endocrinol Metab. 2003;285:E363–71.
8. Yang W, Chen Y, Zhang Y, et al. Extracellular signal-regulated kinase 1/2 mitogen-activated protein kinase pathway is involved in myostatin-regulated differentiation repression. Cancer Res. 2006;66:1320–6.
9. Huang Z, Chen D, Zhang K, et al. Regulation of myostatin signaling by c-Jun N-terminal kinase in C2C12 cells. Cell Signal. 2007;19:2286–95.
10. Hu S, Chen C, Sheng J, et al. Enhanced muscle growth by plasmid-mediated delivery of myostatin propeptide. J Biomed Biotechnol. 2010;2010:862591.
11. DaCosta Byfield S, Major C, et al. SB-505124 is a selective inhibitor of transforming growth factor-beta type I receptors ALK4, ALK5, and ALK7. Mol Pharmacol. 2004;65:744–52.
12. Benny Klimek ME, Aydogdu T, Link MJ, et al. Acute inhibition of myostatin-family proteins preserves skeletal muscle in mouse models of cancer cachexia. Biochem Biophys Res Commun. 2010;391:1548–54.
13. Zhou X, Wang JL, Lu J, et al. Reversal of cancer cachexia and muscle wasting by ActRIIB antagonism leads to prolonged survival. Cell. 2010;142:531–43.
14. Morine KJ, Bish LT, Pendrak K, et al. Systemic myostatin inhibition via liver-targeted gene transfer in normal and dystrophic mice. PLoS One. 2010;5:e9176.
15. Minetti GC, Colussi C, Adami R, et al. Functional and morphological recovery of dystrophic muscles in mice treated with deacetylase inhibitors. Nat Med. 2006;12:1147–50.
16. Bonetto A, Penna F, Minero GV, et al. Deacetylase inhibitors modulate the myostatin/follistatin axis without improving cachexia in tumor-bearing mice. Curr Cancer Drug Targ. 2009;9:608–16.
17. Vamvini MT, Aronis KN, Chamberland JP, et al. Energy deprivation alters in a leptin- and cortisol-independent manner circulating levels of activin A and follistatin but not myostatin in healthy males. J Clin Endocrinol Metab. 2011;96:3416–23.
18. Brandt C, Nielsen AR, Fischer CP, et al. Plasma and muscle myostatin in relation to type 2 diabetes. PLoS One. 2012;7:e37236.
19. Hittel DS, Berggren JR, Shearer J, et al. Increased secretion and expression of myostatin in skeletal muscle from extremely obese women. Diabetes. 2009;58:30–8.
20. Saremi A, Gharakhanloo R, Sharghi S, et al. Effects of oral creatine and resistance training on serum myostatin and GASP-1. Mol Cell Endocrinol. 2010;317:25–30.

21. Paddon-Jones D. Interplay of stress and physical inactivity on muscle loss: nutritional countermeasures. J Nutr. 2006;136:2123–6.
22. Bunn JA, Buford TW, Serra MC, et al. Protein and amino acid supplementation does not alter proteolytic gene expression following immobilization. J Nutr Metab. 2011;2011:539690.
23. Brooks NE, Cadena SM, Vannier E, et al. Effects of resistance exercise combined with essential amino acid supplementation and energy deficit on markers of skeletal muscle atrophy and regeneration during bed rest and active recovery. Muscle Nerve. 2010;42:927–35.
24. Roth E, Oehler R. Hypothesis: muscular glutamine deficiency in sepsis–a necessary step for a hibernation-like state? Nutrition. 2010;26:571–4.
25. Rhoads JM, Argenzio RA, Chen W, et al. L-glutamine stimulates intestinal cell proliferation and activates mitogen-activated protein kinases. Am J Physiol. 1997;272:G943–53.
26. Tessitore L, Costelli P, Bonetti G, et al. Cancer cachexia, malnutrition, and tissue protein turnover in experimental animals. Arch Biochem Biophys. 1993;306:52–8.
27. Salehian B, Mahabadi V, Bilas J, et al. The effect of glutamine on prevention of glucocorticoid-induced skeletal muscle atrophy is associated with myostatin suppression. Metabolism. 2006;55:1239–47.
28. Yoshida S, Kaibara A, Ishibashi N, et al. Glutamine supplementation in cancer patients. Nutrition. 2001;17:766–8.
29. Meador BM, Huey KA. Glutamine preserves skeletal muscle force during an inflammatory insult. Muscle Nerve. 2009;40:1000–7.
30. Lambertucci AC, Lambertucci RH, Hirabara SM, et al. Glutamine supplementation stimulates protein-synthetic and inhibits protein-degradative signaling pathways in skeletal muscle of diabetic rats. PLoS One. 2012;7:e50390.
31. Dong Y, Pan JS, Zhang L. Myostatin suppression of akirin1 mediates glucocorticoid-induced satellite cell dysfunction. PLoS One. 2013;8:e58554.
32. Penna F, Costamagna D, Pin F, et al. Autophagic degradation contributes to muscle wasting in cancer cachexia. Am J Pathol. 2013;182:1367–78.
33. Bristot Silvestrin R, Bambini-Junior V, Galland F, et al. Animal model of autism induced by prenatal exposure to valproate: altered glutamate metabolism in the hippocampus. Brain Res. 2013;1495:52–60.
34. Sriram S, Subramanian S, Sathiakumar D, et al. Modulation of reactive oxygen species in skeletal muscle by myostatin is mediated through NF-κB. Aging Cell. 2011;10:931–48.
35. Mastrocola R, Reffo P, Penna F, et al. Muscle wasting in diabetic and tumor-bearing rats: role of oxidative stress. Free Rad Biol Med. 2008;44:584–93.
36. Tsai PH, Liu JJ, Yeh CL, et al. Effects of glutamine supplementation on oxidative stress-related gene expression and antioxidant properties in rats with streptozotocin-induced type 2 diabetes. Br J Nutr. 2012;107:1112–8.
37. Lee JY, Hopkinson NS, Kemp PR. Myostatin induces autophagy in skeletal muscle in vitro. Biochem Biophys Res Commun. 2011;415:632–6.
38. Seiliez I, Taty Taty GC, Bugeon J, et al. Myostatin induces atrophy of trout myotubes through inhibiting the TORC1 signaling and promoting Ubiquitin-Proteasome and Autophagy-Lysosome degradative pathways. Gen Comp Endocrinol. 2013;186C:9–15.
39. Lin TC, Chen YR, Kensicki E, et al. Autophagy: resetting glutamine-dependent metabolism and oxygen consumption. Autophagy. 2012;8:1477–93.
40. Miretti S, Martignani E, Accornero P, et al. Functional effect of mir-27b on myostatin expression: a relationship in piedmontese cattle with double-muscled phenotype. BMC Genomics. 2013;14:194.
41. Allen DL, Loh AS. Posttranscriptional mechanisms involving microRNA-27a and b contribute to fast-specific and glucocorticoid-mediated myostatin expression in skeletal muscle. Am J Physiol Cell Physiol. 2011;300:C124–37.
42. Kukreti H, Amuthavalli K, Harikumar A, et al. Muscle-specific microRNA1 (miR1) targets heat shock protein 70 (HSP70) during dexamethasone-mediated atrophy. J Biol Chem. 2013;288:6663–78.
43. Drummond MJ, Glynn EL, Fry CS, et al. Essential amino acids increase microRNA-499, -208b, and -23a and downregulate myostatin and myocyte enhancer factor 2C mRNA expression in human skeletal muscle. J Nutr. 2009;139:2279–84.
44. Kim H. Glutamine as an immunonutrient. Yonsei Med J. 2011;52:892–7.
45. Raspé C, Czeslick E, Weimann A, et al. Glutamine and alanine-induced differential expression of intracellular IL-6, IL-8, and TNF-α in LPS-stimulated monocytes in human whole-blood. Cytokine. 2013;62:52–7.

Chapter 40
Web-Based Resources and Suggested Readings

Rajkumar Rajendram, Vinood B. Patel, and Victor R. Preedy

Key Points

- Glutamine has significant clinical value in modern medicine.
- This chapter lists the most up-to-date resources on the regulatory bodies, journals, books, professional bodies and websites that are relevant to an evidence-based approach to the use of glutamine.

Keywords Glutamine • Evidence • Resources • Books • Journals • Regulatory bodies • Professional societies

Introduction

The role of glutamine in metabolism has been recognized for over 40 years. Glutamine is an essential nutrient for all rapidly proliferating cells and growing tissues, including cancer. Glutamine supplementation may be beneficial to patients with longstanding inflammatory activity, who are not producing sufficient quantities of glutamine. The availability of glutamine may be reduced by malnutrition or failure to meet the demands of imposed by critical illnesses [1]. This is supported by observations suggesting that glutamine supplementation may be beneficial in critically ill patients, particularly those who have suffered trauma or burns. Although results are contradictory, some large multicentre studies have shown that glutamine may reduce infectious complications and improve insulin sensitivity [1].

Examples of the applications of glutamine can be found in this book and also via the recommended resources in the tables below.

R. Rajendram, M.R.C.P., F.R.C.A., F.F.I.C.M. (✉)
Royal Free Hospital, Pond Street, Hampstead, London NW3 2QG, UK
e-mail: rajkumarrajendram@doctors.org.uk

V.B. Patel, B.Sc., Ph.D.
Department of Biomedical Sciences, Faculty of Science and Technology,
University of Westminster, 115 New Cavendish Street, London W1W 6UW, UK
e-mail: v.b.patel@westminster.ac.uk

V.R. Preedy, B.Sc., Ph.D., D.Sc.
Nutritional Sciences Division, Department of Nutrition and Dietetics, School of Biomedical and Health Sciences, King's College London, Franklin-Wilkins Building,
150 Stamford Street, London SE1 9NH, UK
e-mail: victor.preedy@kcl.ac.uk

R. Rajendram et al. (eds.), *Glutamine in Clinical Nutrition*, Nutrition and Health,
DOI 10.1007/978-1-4939-1932-1_40, © Springer Science+Business Media New York 2015

Tables 40.1, 40.2, 40.3, 40.4, and 40.5 list the most up-to-date information on the regulatory bodies (Table 40.1), professional bodies (Table 40.2), journals (Table 40.3), books (Table 40.4), and websites (Table 40.5) that are relevant to an evidence-based use of glutamine in health and disease.

Table 40.1 Organizations and regulatory bodies with interests in glutamine

American Association for Cancer Research www.aacr.org/
American Society for Parenteral and Enteral Nutrition (ASPEN) www.nutritioncare.org
British Association for Cancer Research www.bacr.org.uk
Centers for Disease Control and Prevention www.cdc.gov
Department of Health and Human Services www.hhs.gov
European society for clinical nutrition and metabolism (ESPEN) www.espen.org
Food and Drug Administration www.fda.gov
Institute of Cancer Research www.icr.ac.uk
Johns Hopkins School of Public Health www.jhsph.edu
National Cancer Institute www.cancer.gov
National Institutes of Health www.nih.gov
Nutrition www.nutrition.gov
SBNPE www.sbnpe.com.br
US National Library of Medicine and National Institutes of Health www.ncbi.nlm.nih.gov/pubmed
World Health Organization www.who.int/en

This table lists the regulatory bodies and organizations relevant to glutamine

Table 40.2 Professional societies

American Association of Cancer Research www.aacr.org
American Association of Immunologists www.aai.org
American Cancer Society www.cancer.org
American Chemical Society www.acs.org
American Gastroenterological Association (AGA) www.gastro.org
American Physiological Society www.the-aps.org
American Society for Nutrition www.nutrition.org

(continued)

Table 40.2 (continued)

American Society for Neurochemistry
American Society for Parenteral and Enteral Nutrition https://www.nutritioncare.org
AminoAcids.com www.aminoacids.com/index.html
Brazilian Society of Food and Nutrition www.sban.com.br
European Society of Intensive Care Medicine www.esicm.org
European Wound Management Association (EMWA) www.ewma.org/english.html
Federation of American Societies for Experimental Biology (FASEB) www.fasebj.org
International Council on Amino Acids Science www.icaas-org.com
International Society for Hepatic Encephalopathy and Nitrogen Metabolism (ISHEN) www.ishen.org
Italian Society for Human Nutrition www.sinu.it
Italian Society for Artificial Nutrition and Metabolism www.sinpe.org
Nutrition Society www.nutritionsociety.org
Sociedad Española de Nutrición Parenteral y Enteral (SENPE) www.senpe.com
Società Italiana di Nutrizione Artificiale e Metabolismo www.sinpe.org
Society for Inherited Metabolic Disorders www.simd.org
Society for Nutrition Education and Behavior www.sneb.org
Society of Nuclear Medicine www.snm.org
Society on Sarcopenia, Cachexia and Wasting Disorders (SCWD) www.cachexia.org

This table lists the professional societies involved with glutamine

Table 40.3 Journals on glutamine

Acta Cirúrgica Brasileira www.scielo.br/scielo.php?script=sci_serial&pid=0102-8650&lng=en&nrm=iso
American Journal of Clinical Nutrition ajcn.nutrition.org
Am. J. Physiology GI and Liver Physiology ajpgi.physiology.org
Amino Acids www.link.springer.com/journal/726
BMC Cancer www.biomedcentral.com/bmccancer
Cancer Cell www.cell.com/cancer-cell

(continued)

Table 40.3 (continued)

Cancer Immunology, Immunotherapy www.springer.com/medicine/oncology/journal/262
Cancer Research cancerres.aacrjournals.org
Cell Metabolism www.cell.com/cell-metabolism
Clin Dev Immunol www.hindawi.com/journals/cdi/2012/749189
Clinical Hemorheology and Microcirculation www.iospress.nl/journal/clinical-hemorheology-and-microcirculation
Clinical Nutrition www.journals.elsevier.com/clinical-nutrition
Critical Care Medicine journals.lww.com/ccmjournal
European Wound management (EMWA) Journal ewma.org/english/publications/ewma-journal/latest-issues.html
Helicobacter onlinelibrary.wiley.com/journal/10.1111/(ISSN)1523-5378
International Journal of Diabetes & Metabolism ijod.uaeu.ac.ae
J Endocrinol Metab jcem.endojournals.org
Journal of Immunology jimmunol.org
Journal of Infectious Diseases jid.oxfordjournals.org
Journal of Neurochemistry onlinelibrary.wiley.com/journal/10.1111/(ISSN)1471-4159
Journal Nuclear Medicine jnm.snmjournals.org
Journal of Nutrition jn.nutrition.org
Journal of Nutrition and Metabolism www.hindawi.com/journals/jnume/2011/617597
Journal of Nutritional Biochemistry www.jnutbio.com
Journal of Parenteral and Enteral Nutrition pen.sagepub.com
Journal of Physiology and Pharmacology www.jpp.krakow.pl
Mediterr J Nutr Metab www.springer.com/food+science/journal/12349
Metabolic Brain Diseases link.springer.com/journal/11011
Neurotoxicology www.journals.elsevier.com/neurotoxicology/CachedSimilar
Nuclear Medicine and Biology www.sciencedirect.com/science/journal/09698051
Nutrition www.nutritionjrnl.com
Nutricion Hospitalaria www.nutricionhospitalaria.com
Toxicological Sciences www.bioxbio.com/if/html/TOXICOL-SCI.html

This table lists the journals publishing original research and review articles related to glutamine

Table 40.4 Relevant books

Abbas AK, Litchman AHH. Basic Immunology. Elsevier, 2006, USA
Campos ACL. Tratado de Nutrição e Metabolismo em Cirurgia, Editora Rubio, 2013, Brazil
Dink T. Global Perspective on Diabetic Foot Ulcerations. InTech Europe, 2011, Croatia
Hall JE. Guyton and Hall Textbook of Medical Physiology. Saunders, 2011, USA
Katz DL. Nutrition in Clinical Practice, 2nd Edition. Lippincott Williams & Wilkins, 2008, USA
Kindt TJ, Goldsby RA, Osborne BA. Immunology. W.H. freeman and Company, 2007, New York, USA
Mahan LK, Escott-Stump S, Raymond JL. Krause's Food & the Nutrition Care Process. Saunders, 2011, USA
Mora J. Glutamine: Metabolism, Enzymology, and Regulation. Academic Press Inc., 1980, USA
Salway JG. Metabolism at a Glance. Blackwell Publishing Ltd, 2004, USA
Seyfried T. Cancer as a Metabolic Disease: On the Origin, Management, and Prevention of Cancer. John Wiley & Sons, Inc., 2012, USA
Tirapegui J. Nutrição, Metabolismo e Suplementação na Atividade Física (Nutrition, Metabolism and Supplementation on Physical Activity). Atheneu, 2012, Brazil
Tirapegui J. Nutrição - Fundamentos e Aspectos Atuais (Nutrition fundamentals and current aspects). Atheneu, 2006, Brazil
Hassinger DH, Sies H. Glutamine Metabolism in Mammalian Tissue, Springer Verlag, 1984, Germany
Waitzberg DL. Nutrição oral, enteral e parenteral na prática clínica. Editora Atheneu, 2009, Brazil

This table lists books on glutamine

Table 40.5 Relevant internet resources

Bioparadigms
www.bioparadigms.org
BodyBuilding.com, LLC
www.bodybuilding.com/fun/bbinfo.php?page=Glutamine
British Nutrition Foundation
www.nutrition.org.uk
Complementary Medicine
www.umm.edu/altmed/articles/glutamine-000307.htm
COSMIC
cancer.sanger.ac.uk/cancergenome/projects/cosmic
Critical Care Nutrition at the Clinical Evaluation Research Unit, Kingston General Hospital, Canada
www.Criticalcarenutrition.com
DISEASES
diseases.jensenlab.org
GenMANIA
www.genemania.org
HighWire
highwire.stanford.edu
Human Protein Reference Database
www.hprd.org/
KEGG Pathway
www.genome.jp/kegg/pathway.html
Livestrong Glutamine supplement
www.livestrong.com/glutamine/
National Institutes of Health grants:
www.nih.gov
NCI Gastric Cancer home page
https://www.google.com/#q=nci+gastric+cancer
Overview of the major metabolic pathways
www2.ufp.pt/~pedros/bq/integration.htm

(continued)

Table 40.5 (continued)

PESCADOR platform
cbdm.mdc-berlin.de/tools/pescador/
Pubmed
www.ncbi.nlm.nih.gov/pubmed
Purine and Pyrimidine Metabolism
library.med.utah.edu/NetBiochem/pupyr/pp.htm
Scielo
www.scielo.org
ToppGene Suite
toppgene.cchmc.org
Transporter Classification Database
www.tcdb.org/
University of Maryland Medical Center
umm.edu/health/medical/altmed/supplement/glutamine
UpToDate
www.uptodate.com/home
Worthington Enzyme Manual
www.worthington-biochem.com/index/manual.html

This table lists some internet resources on glutamine

Acknowledgements We would like to thank the following authors for contributing to the development of this resource: J. Ampuero, M. Aschner, K. Ban, G. Briassoulis, M.R. Ciriolo, A. Cooper, P. Costelli, J.F. Cunha Filho, K. Frauwirth, L. Gianotti, M.C.C. Gomes-Marcondes, C. Grewer, S. Hagen, I. Hammami, W. Hu, M. Jones, H. Kung, A. Le, C.H. Lehmann, P.R. Leitão de Vasconcelos, G. Mercadal, R.K. Rao, S. Sookoian, G.C. Teodoro, J. Tirapegui.

References

1. Wischmeyer PE. Glutamine: mode of action in critical illness. Crit Care Med. 2007;35(Suppl):S541–4.

Index

R. Rajendram et al. (eds.), *Glutamine in Clinical Nutrition*, Nutrition and Health,
DOI 10.1007/978-1-4939-1932-1, © Springer Science+Business Media New York 2015

T

U

V

W

Y

Z

CPSIA information can be obtained
at www.ICGtesting.com
Printed in the USA
BVHW011301030119
536976BV00003B/3/P

9 781493 919314